Handbook of Genetic Skin Disorders

FRED M. NOVICE, MD
Henry Ford Hospital
Detroit, Michigan

DANIEL W. COLLISON, MD
Assistant Professor of Medicine (Dermatology)
Section of Dermatology
Dartmouth-Hitchcock Medical Center
Lebanon, New Hampshire

WALTER H.C. BURGDORF, MD
Professor and Chairman, Department of Dermatology
University of New Mexico
School of Medicine
Albuquerque, New Mexico

NANCY B. ESTERLY, MD
Professor of Pediatrics and Dermatology
Medical College of Wisconsin
Children's Hospital of Wisconsin
Milwaukee, Wisconsin

W.B. SAUNDERS COMPANY
A Division of Harcourt Brace & Company

Philadelphia
London Toronto Montreal Sydney Tokyo

Handbook of Genetic Skin Disorders

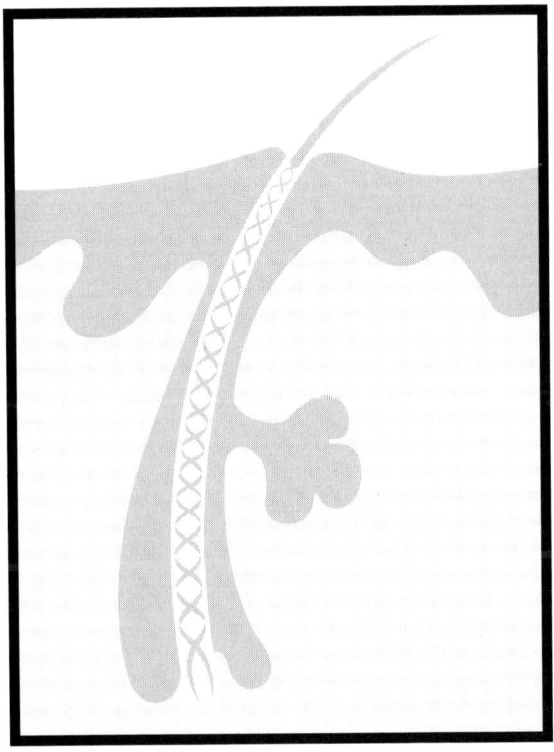

W.B. SAUNDERS COMPANY
A Division of
Harcourt Brace & Company

The Curtis Center
Independence Square West
Philadelphia, Pennsylvania 19106

Library of Congress Cataloging-in-Publication Data

Handbook of genetic skin disorders / Fred M. Novice . . . [et al.].—1st ed.

p. cm.

ISBN 0–7216–3803–1

1. Skin—Diseases—Genetic aspects. I. Novice, Fred M.
[DNLM: 1. Skin Diseases—physiopathology. 2. Skin Diseases—genetics. WR 140 G328 1994]

RL793.G45 1994 616.5′042—dc20

DNLM/DLC 93-25389

Handbook of Genetic Skin Disorders ISBN 0–7216–3803–1

Printed in the United States of America

Last digit is the print number: 9 8 7 6 5 4 3 2 1

This book is lovingly dedicated to

Jo-Anne Novice
Karlee and Taylor Novice

Joan Collison
Charlie Collison

Dorothee Burgdorf

Sarah Devany
Anne, John, and Henry Esterly

whose support and sacrifices have made it possible for
us to research, teach, and write

Preface

This book is a clinical guide to the diagnosis of hereditary diseases of the skin, hair, nails, and mucous membranes. Our goal is to place a conceptual "net" over the often confusing and ever-expanding set of diseases loosely termed *genodermatoses.* The book is not intended to be a textbook of pediatric dermatology or a reference in genetics. Rather, our book should give its user a clinical overview of genodermatoses, with salient details provided for more common, important, or otherwise prominent entities.

Why is such a book needed? The literature dealing with genodermatoses is scattered in many sources. We hope to bridge the gap between texts and journals of pediatrics, dermatology, and medical genetics. The variety and, in some cases, rarity of hereditary skin diseases may also stymie the physician interested in investigating a diagnosis. This book presents key features and references for a wide variety of hereditary skin disorders in a convenient format.

We have mainly limited the scope of the book to mucocutaneous diseases with mendelian inheritance. Diseases that are often sporadic but occasionally familial are listed in an appendix. Acquired entities and malformation syndromes are briefly discussed only when they are of particular differential diagnostic value or when useful for a didactic purpose or point of clarification. For example, epidermolysis bullosa acquisita is briefly discussed along with hereditary forms of epidermolysis bullosa. This is also not a book of dysmorphology, even though such syndromes may have cutaneous findings such as dermatoglyphic changes. We have only rarely included congenital disorders of environmental cause (i.e., teratogenic diseases), again, when useful for didactic purposes.

We have tried to be as inclusive as possible in cataloging the diseases. We have included most of the hereditary skin diseases mentioned in the three outstanding sources of information in this field, namely, the textbooks of Gorlin[1], Rook[2], and McKusick[3]. In addition, we include scores of diseases from the journal literature that have not yet been included in dermatologic textbooks. However, in a book of limited size and scope, there are syndromes and individual case reports of purported genodermatoses that we have missed or intentionally omitted. Although all newly described diseases arise from a single initial observation, it is often impossible early on to predict the accuracy and relevance of such reports. In general, case reports limited to a single patient are not included in this book. On the other hand, the reporting of singular observations is essential for the eventual recognition of a new disease or syndrome. With time, outside input, and new information, we hope that future editions of this book will encompass more entities and delineate those already included more clearly.

In addition to the difficulties of judging the relevance of rare or obscure entities, nomenclature has also been a source of particular difficulty. Some entities have multiple designations (e.g., "hypohidrotic ectodermal dysplasia," "anhidrotic ectodermal dysplasia," and "X-linked ectodermal dysplasia" are synonyms; less obvious examples of synonyms are "tooth and nail syndrome" and "hypodontia and nail dysgenesis"). In other instances, the same designation refers to more than one disorder (e.g, Bazex syndrome referring to both acrodermatitis paraneoplastica and to the syndrome of follicular atrophoderma and basal cell carcinomas).

Although we have made every effort to be accurate and complete, we have surely omitted or overlooked important information. Therefore, we invite notification of all errors of omission and commission. Our manuscript is computerized in a database, allowing us to easily update the manuscript.

REFERENCES

1. Gorlin RJ, Cohen MM Jr, Levin LS. Syndromes of the Head and Neck. 3rd ed. New York, Oxford University Press, 1990
2. Champion RH, Burton JL, Ebling FJG, eds. Rook's Textbook of Dermatology. 5th ed. Oxford, Blackwell Scientific Publications, 1992
3. McKusick VA, ed. Mendelian Inheritance in Man. 10th ed. Baltimore, Johns Hopkins University Press, 1992

Book Organization

Diseases are broadly grouped into chapters according to the major clinical features or etiologies. In the many instances where major clinical findings would permit entries in more than one chapter, the entity is placed arbitrarily in one chapter and occasionally cross-referenced in the other.

Within each chapter, diseases are grouped with other diseases of similar nosology. For example, all the ichthyoses are grouped together in Chapter 1, entitled "Disorders of Cornification." These groups, in turn, are listed in an arbitrary order of importance, often based on frequency of occurrence. Thus, the ichthyoses are listed before the palmoplantar keratodermas. Note, however, that a rare disease may be listed in the chapter before a common one if it makes better sense to keep the rare disease grouped with similar diseases of more frequent occurrence. For example, a rare ichthyosis syndrome may be grouped with the more common ichthyoses.

To save space and to give some sense of priority, rarer or otherwise less important diseases are listed in a more abbreviated style, and smaller print, at the end of the chapter. Again, the format used for each disease was chosen in an arbitrary manner, but with an attempt to reflect the relative incidence of a given disease.

In the final analysis, a book contains whatever information the authors wish. Nevertheless, we would like to explain some of our biases in advance. The main emphasis is on clinical findings, especially those of the skin and its adnexae. Information regarding each disease is presented according to a stereotyped template, which is explained below. The template is not completely fleshed out for every disease. For example, histopathologic findings are listed only when they are essential or very helpful for diagnosis or in excluding other entities, since in most cases exhaustive histopathologic descriptions are available in other textbooks. Similarly, treatment recommendations, which may rapidly become outmoded, are kept to a minimum and are not consistently present. In the case of very rare entities, the disease name and a reference may be the only information presented. If the disease name and article convey inadequate information, then a short clinical description is included.

Proceeding according to the full template of information for a given disease, the first decision was disease nomenclature. In general, we favored the most prevalent **designation**, as long as it was accurate and was not a frank misnomer. Whenever possible, we avoided eponyms, since they are not as informative as descriptive designations. However, certain eponyms are so well established that they prevailed in some instances. We then listed prevalent **synonyms**, although no attempt was made to be exhaustive. Although we are sensitive to giving credit where credit is due, we did not feel qualified to arbitrate among warring disciples or historians in terms of who discovered what first. Rather, we list synonyms so that readers may use these terms when searching the medical literature. Occasionally we point out misnomers or controversies in nomenclature or nosology in the discussion section.

We divided the **clinical manifestations** under the headings of "Skin" and "Non-Skin." The former rubric includes findings involving the skin, mucous membranes, hair, nails, and teeth. The non-skin heading includes all other findings, including partially ectodermally derived manifestations such as craniofacial features and ocular and central nervous system abnormalities. This separation reflects our primary interest in the skin and its adnexae. Occasionally, however, we vary from this schema for the purpose of clarity.

The mode of inheritance is featured in the **genetics** section. Abbreviations used include "AD" for autosomal dominant inheritance, "AR" for autosomal recessive inheritance, "XLR" for X-linked recessive inheritance, and "XLD" for X-linked dominant inheritance. Occasionally we point out the chromosomal location of the gene defect, if known. Since information regarding exact genetic mechanisms is advancing at an extremely rapid pace, including the detection of carriers and prenatal diagnosis, we want to strongly emphasize the importance of consulting knowledgeable geneticists in appropriate cases for genetic counseling. Besides MEDLINE, McKusick's database is an up-to-date resource on genetic markers for specific mendelian disorders.

As noted earlier, our primary goal was to list diseases with mendelian inheritance. For purposes of differential diagnosis or didactics, we have occasionally included sporadically occurring diseases (i.e., those diseases that are neither clearly mendelian nor familial).

We would like to call attention to certain congenital diseases that are commonly mistaken for inherited disorders. For instance, there are some congenital malformation syndromes, such as Sturge-Weber syndrome, that are included only because some readers will expect to find discussion here. We wish to emphasize that these diseases are *not* mendelian and are only rarely familial. This distinction is obviously of great importance when performing genetic counseling of a patient or a patient's relative.

The **pathophysiology** section is used when the biochemical etiology of a disease is known or important information is available. This section appears in a minority of diseases since information on pathophysiology is not available or is unclear for so many of these diseases.

The **laboratory** section includes pertinent diagnostic data obtainable by laboratory examinations. These data include findings from cutaneous histopathology, serology, biochemical studies, radiologic studies, and so forth. This section was frequently omitted, since in many cases information such as cutaneous histopathology was not deemed to be of special diagnostic or didactic value.

As mentioned earlier, information regarding **treatment** is most likely to become out-of-date in a textbook, along with the changing prognosis as therapy affects morbidity and mortality. Therefore, treatment is not a key feature of this book.

We use the **discussion** section to air controversies in the literature, point out difficult areas in diagnosis, and otherwise present information requiring explanation. Disease variants or differential diagnosis may be included in the discussion section; these diseases are identified by a bullet symbol (■). Sporadic or acquired entities are included when deemed appropriate. Alternatively, variants or diseases in the differential diagnosis may follow independently in the text. No attempt was made to be exhaustive in differential diagnosis.

The **reference** section begins with the "McKusick number," a six-digit number used in Victor McKusick's catalog of genetic diseases, *Mendelian Inheritance in Man.* McKusick's book is updated in print about every 2 years. A computerized version, *Online Mendelian Inheritance in Man* (OMIM) is available nearly 24 hours a day for consultation of text and further references. Use of the McKusick number bypasses some of the difficulties of nosology and nomenclature, although we did not agree with McKusick's nosology or information in every instance. Following the McKusick number are salient references from the literature, sometimes including the original article, with particular emphasis placed on dermatologic articles and reviews.

Acknowledgments

Book research was invaluably supported by the facilities of the Department of Dermatology at Henry Ford Hospital, Detroit, Michigan, under the auspices of chairman Edward A. Krull, MD. Search of the medical literature was assisted by superb help at Sladen Library of Henry Ford Hospital. Additional research was supported by the Section of Dermatology at the Dartmouth-Hitchcock Medical Center, Lebanon, New Hampshire, under the chairmanship of Steven K. Spencer, MD.

Several chapters were improved by the unselfish input of reviewers, although we are responsible for any remaining errors in chapter content. We would like to thank the following physicians: Richard M. Haber, MD, of Toronto, Canada, reviewed an early version of Chapter 2 on bullous diseases. Dianne Levisohn, MD, of Bremerton, Washington, reviewed Chapter 10 on nail disorders. At Henry Ford Hospital in Detroit, David Fivenson, MD, reviewed Chapter 15 on Metabolic Disorders, and Dennis R. Ownby, MD, reviewed Chapter 14 on immune disorders.

The cover art is based upon a sketch expertly rendered by Lynette Morgan.

Among the many generous physicians acknowledged in photo legends, Benjamin K. Fisher, MD, of Toronto, and Lester Weiss, MD, of Detroit, were especially helpful in providing access to their superb collections of rare clinical transparencies.

Mechanics of Manuscript Production

For those interested in such details, the use of microcomputers greatly facilitated research and manuscript preparation. Each disease in the book is represented by a HyperCard (Claris Corporation, Cupertino, CA) record in a database on a Macintosh microcomputer (Apple Computer, Cupertino, CA), which had a data field for each section of the disease template (e.g., disease name, synonyms, skin findings). Additional information regarding each disease (such as literature search strategies) is included in each database record. The manuscript is generated by a computer program written in the "Hypertalk" language of HyperCard. Formatting and laser printing of drafts were done using "Microsoft Word" for the Macintosh (Microsoft Corporation, Redmond, WA). Literature searches were automated using "QuicKeys" and "MockWrite" (CE Software, West Des Moines, IA), "McSink" (Dave McWherter and Preferred Publishers, Memphis, TN), and "TermWorks" (James Rhodes and Horizon Software, Lufkin, TX). Literature searches were then imported into "EndNote Plus" (Niles and Associates, Berkeley, CA) bibliography software, which translated the literature searches into the desired format. Additional computerized literature searches were greatly facilitated by the online resources provided by Dartmouth College, including Dartmouth's superb database interface software such as "DCIS Navigator," "Online Library," and "InfoSpeak."

Communication among the coauthors was facilitated by the use of a text field in the Hypercard database called "authors' notes," whereby queries regarding each disease were passed back and forth between the authors. The "authors' notes" were saved as an electronic paper trail, which proved helpful in retracing the lines of thought about difficult points in research. The use of computer modems and telecommunications software (ZTerm, Alverson Software, Mason, OH) to pass the manuscript back and forth over telephone lines was an invaluable timesaver. In the early stages of manuscript preparation, it took 90 minutes to send a 300-page manuscript over the phone lines. Changes in technology over the years shortened the modem transfer time to 20 minutes for an 800-page manuscript. Macintosh computers also evolved from bulky, 20-pound luggables into slim, high-powered notebooks that are easily transported around medical libraries.

Contents

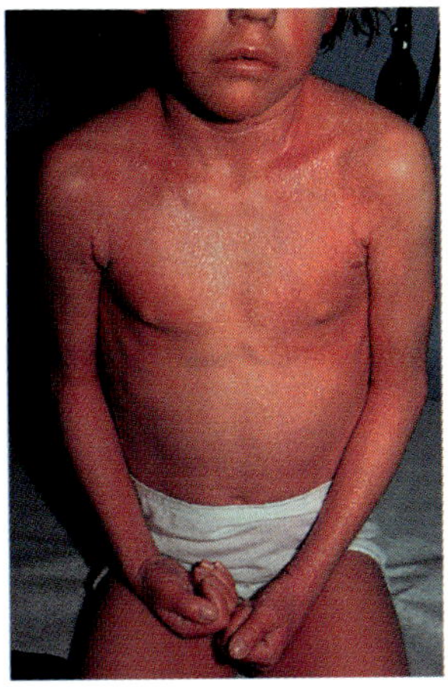

COLOR FIGURE 1–1
Nonbullous congenital ichthyosiform erythroderma. The entire body surface, including the flexural areas, shows fine branny scaling and intense erythema.

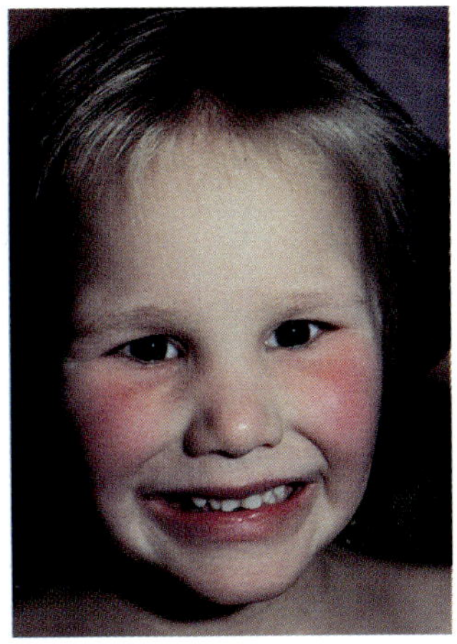

COLOR FIGURE 3–1
Diffuse erythema of both cheeks and sparse brows, lashes, and anterior scalp hair in a young girl with Rothmund-Thomson syndrome.

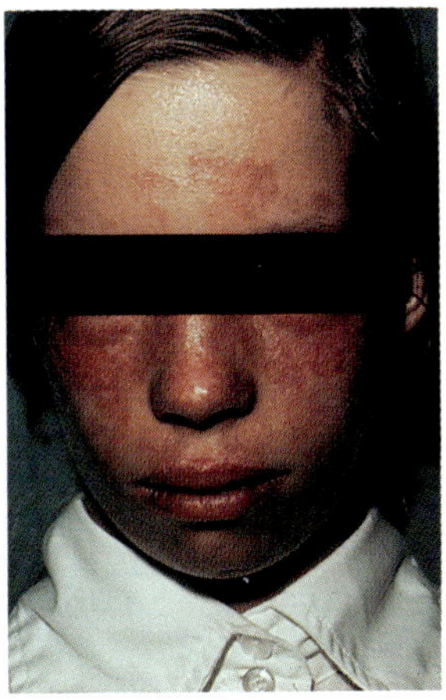

COLOR FIGURE 3–2
Patient with Bloom syndrome showing the characteristic photo-induced erythematous, telangiectatic facial eruption in a butterfly distribution.

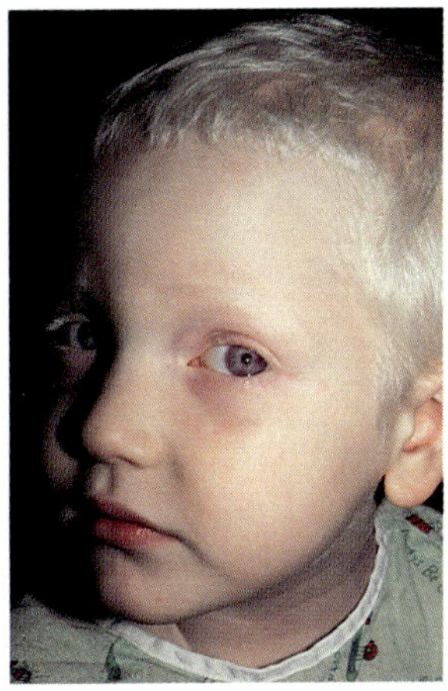

COLOR FIGURE 5–1
Tyrosinase-negative oculocutaneous albinism. The patient has pale white skin and hair and pink irides.

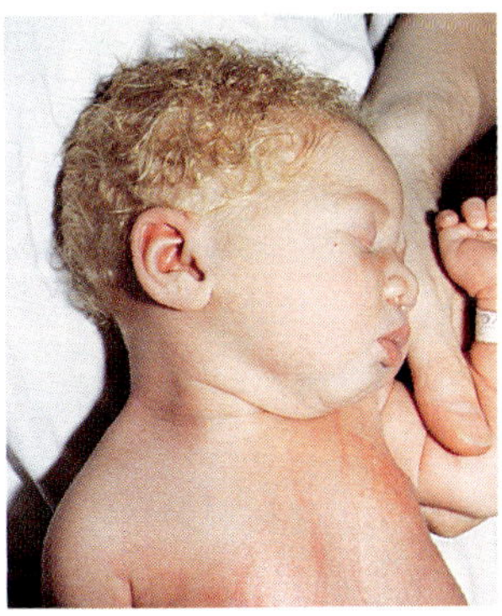

COLOR FIGURE 5–2
Black infant with tyrosinase-positive oculocutaneous albinism. The skin is pink, and the hair is yellow.

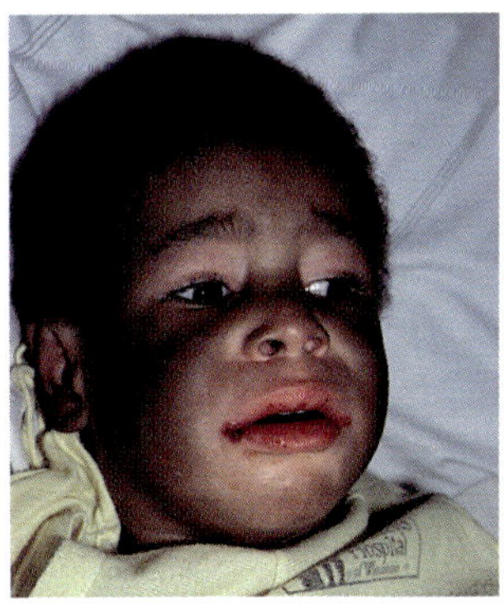

COLOR FIGURE 5–3
Pigmentary dilution, most pronounced over the central face, in a young boy with Chédiak-Higashi syndrome. His hair had a peculiar metallic sheen. There was chronic perlèche.

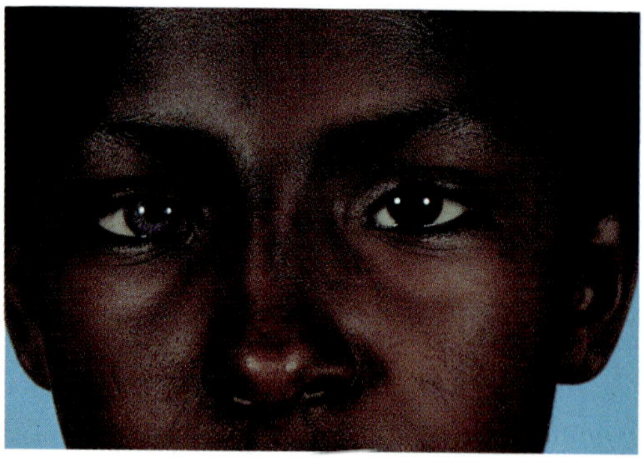

COLOR FIGURE 5–4
Heterochromia iridis in a patient with Waardenburg syndrome. (Courtesy of Lester Weiss, MD, Detroit, Michigan)

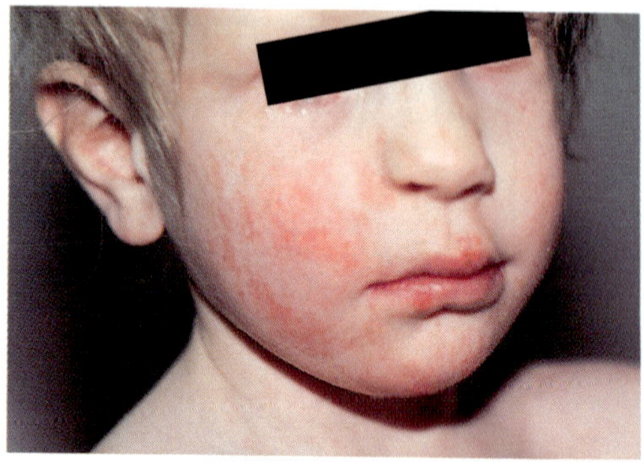

COLOR FIGURE 8–1
Focal dermal hypoplasia. Right eye coloboma and erythematous atrophic patches on the cheek.

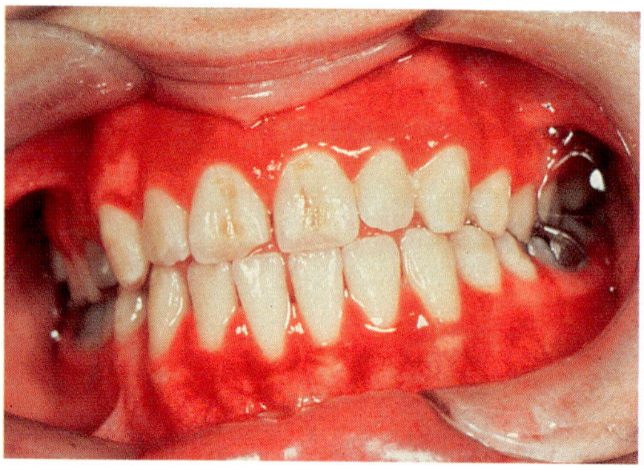

COLOR FIGURE 11–1
Mucoepithelial dysplasia syndrome. The gingivae are typically fiery red. Both the free and attached gingivae are involved. (Courtesy of Robert J. Gorlin, DDS, MS, Minneapolis, Minnesota)

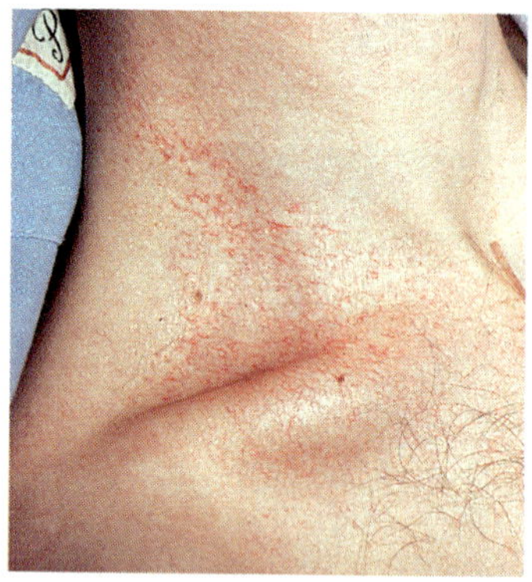

COLOR FIGURE 12–1
Multiple telangiectases on the lateral neck and clavicular area of a patient with ataxia-telangiectasia. (Courtesy of Benjamin K. Fisher, MD, Toronto, Ontario)

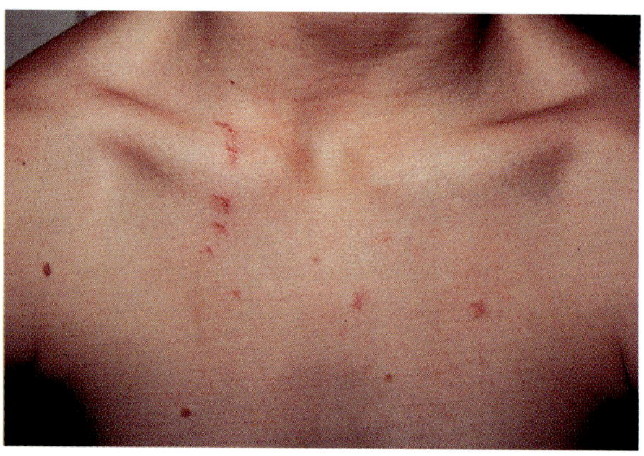

COLOR FIGURE 13–1
Hereditary benign telangiectasia. Multiple telangiectases on the chest of a young boy whose mother had identical lesions.

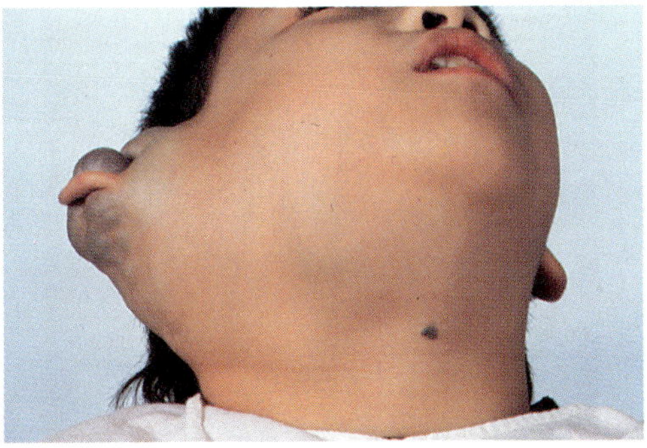

COLOR FIGURE 13–2
This child with blue rubber bleb nevus syndrome has a skin-colored, compressible mass involving the neck, mandible, and periauricular skin as well as a bluish rubbery mass directly involving the pinna. Note the small blue lesion on the neck in midline. (Courtesy of Julie Prendiville, MD, Vancouver, British Columbia)

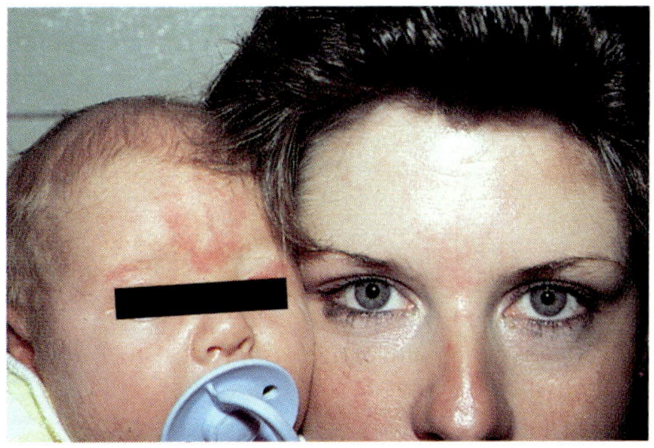

COLOR FIGURE 13–3
Familial nevus flammeus. Glabellar salmon patches in mother and infant.

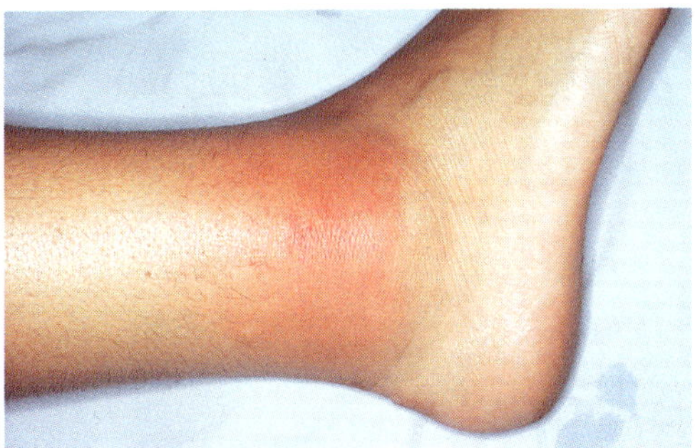

COLOR FIGURE 15–1
Familial Mediterranean fever. Indurated reddened plaque on the lower leg resembling erysipelas. (Courtesy of Benjamin K. Fisher, MD, Toronto, Ontario)

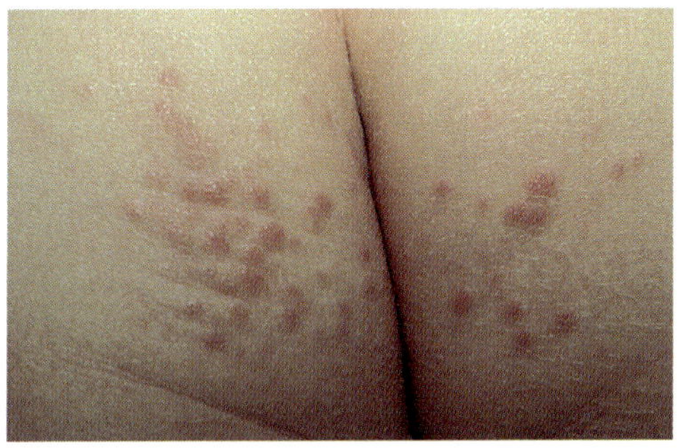

COLOR FIGURE 15–2
Multiple eruptive xanthomas on the buttocks of a patient with hepatic failure.

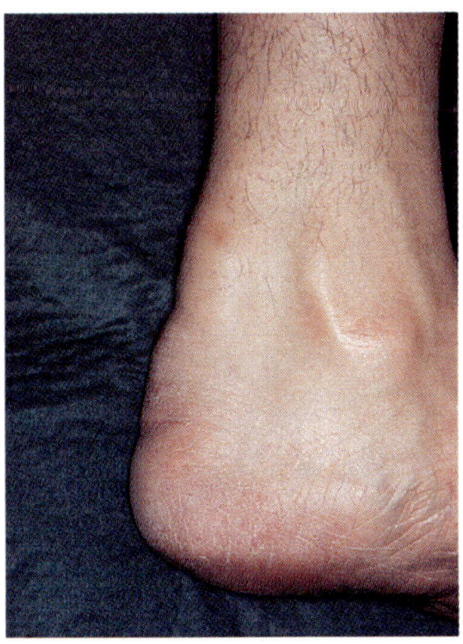

COLOR FIGURE 15–3
Tendinous xanthomas of the Achilles tendon. (Courtesy of Donald Rosenthal, MD, Hamilton, Ontario)

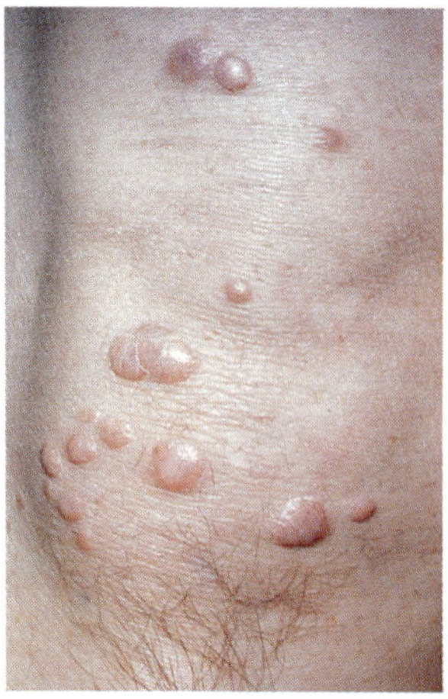

COLOR FIGURE 15–4
Multiple nodular tuberous xanthomas. (Courtesy of Donald Rosenthal, MD, Hamilton, Ontario)

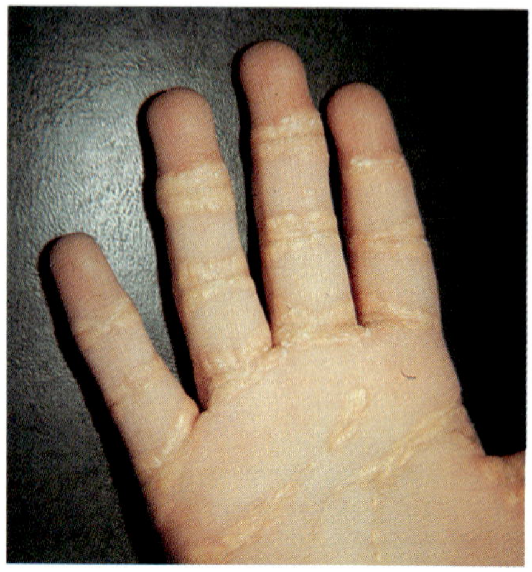

COLOR FIGURE 15–5
Palmar xanthomas in a 5-year-old boy. Note the linear configuration.

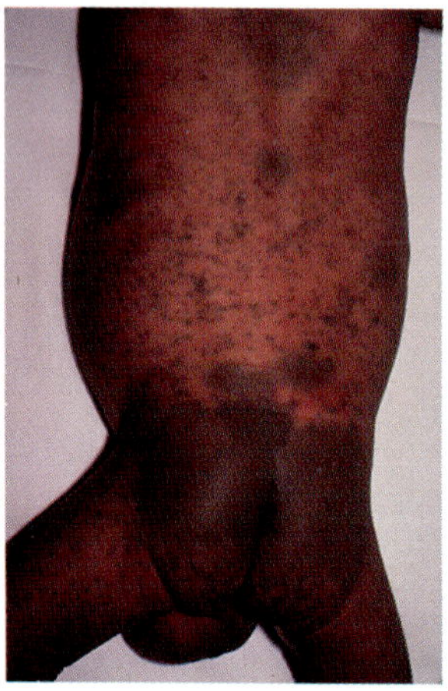

COLOR FIGURE 15–6
Multiple mongolian spots of varying sizes in a 6-month-old infant with GM1 gangliosidosis. These lesions have increased in number since birth. (Courtesy of Mary Spraker, M.D., Atlanta, Georgia)

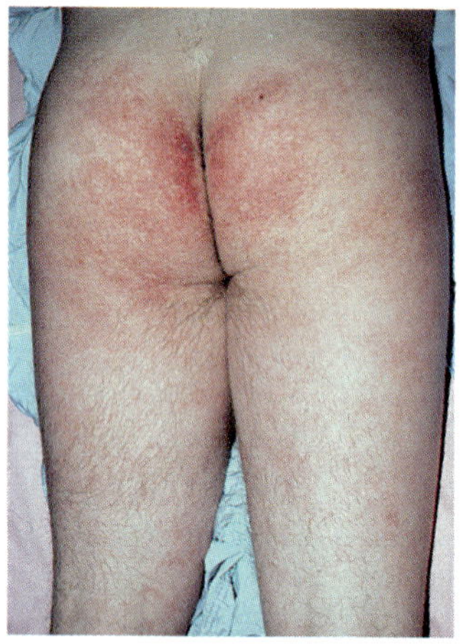

COLOR FIGURE 15–7
Multiple tiny angiokeratomas scattered over the buttocks and thighs of a man with Fabry disease. (Courtesy of Benjamin K. Fisher, MD, Toronto, Ontario)

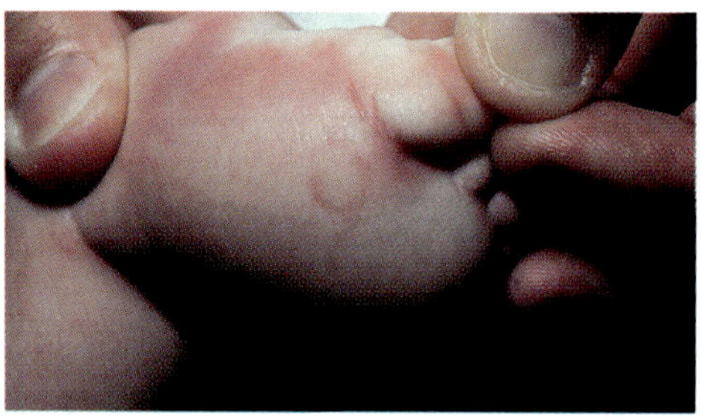

COLOR FIGURE 16–1
Characteristic pedal hemangiomas in a patient with Turner syndrome.

CHAPTER

1

Disorders of Cornification

A large group of disorders characterized by a thickened stratum corneum and excessive scaling are discussed in this chapter. The ichthyoses represent a major subset. Although the etiology and pathogenesis of many of these diseases are poorly understood, it is likely that most are far too complex to be labeled as simply disorders of cornification. Nevertheless, we have included the classification system proposed by Williams and Elias, which designates and numbers all ichthyoses as *disorders of cornification* (DOCs), and have also used this term as the chapter heading, recognizing that, in time, more appropriate terminology may be devised based on a better understanding of the biochemical and structural defects responsible for these conditions.

Ichthyoses

The ichthyoses are a large and varied group of inherited disorders of keratinization or cornification. Van Scott, Frost, and Weinstein published the first scientific classification of this group. Hyperproliferative ichthyoses with increased epidermal turnover were distinguished from the retention ichthyoses with decreased shedding. Histopathologically, hyperproliferative ichthyoses showed variable parakeratosis overlying epidermal hyperplasia; mitotic figures were increased. Retention ichthyoses showed orthohyperkeratosis with minimal to no acanthosis.

Traupe's classification separates the ichthyoses into four categories: (1) isolated vulgar ichthyoses, (2) associated vulgar ichthyoses, (3) isolated congenital ichthyosis, and (4) associated congenital ichthyosis. The disorders are categorized by determining the presence or absence of skin changes at birth as well as abnormalities of other organs. Associated cutaneous and systemic abnormalities, histopathologic findings, and mode of inheritance allow further narrowing of the diagnostic possibilities.

A very useful concept for understanding the effect of epidermal structure

TABLE 1–1
DISORDERS OF CORNIFICATION (THE ICHTHYOSES)

Type (DOC Number)	Inheritance	Skin	Skin Disease Present at Birth	Hair, Teeth, Nails	Non-Skin	Histopathology
Ichthyosis vulgaris (DOC 1)	AD	Presents in first year of life (or later), not at birth; fine white scales, especially extensor, groin; flexures spared; follicular keratosis; increased palmar markings	No		Atopy in 50%	Compact hyperkeratosis with decreased granular layer; distinctive abnormal keratohyaline granules on electron microscopy
X-linked recessive ichthyosis; steroid sulfatase deficiency (DOC 2)	XLR	Brownish to greenish adherent scales in first weeks of life, not at birth; neck is most involved; face spared	No		Corneal opacities; cryptorchidism, testicular cancers; mothers of affected infants have slow, weak labor	Compact hyperkeratosis; normal granular layer; failure to desquamate because of high levels of cholesterol sulfate
Bullous congenital ichthyosiform erythroderma; epidermolytic hyperkeratosis (DOC 3)	AD	Widespread bullous disease at birth, with transition to ridged verrucous hyperkeratosis (spiny ridges)	Yes	Hair casts; nail dystrophy		Epidermolytic hyperkeratosis—vacuolar changes in upper epidermis with clumped keratin; prenatal diagnosis by skin biopsy possible
Classic lamellar ichthyosis, recessive type (nonerythrodermic) (DOC 4)	AR	Collodion baby; large dark scales; severe ectropion; minimal erythroderma; palmoplantar keratoderma	Yes			Papillomatous, psoriasiform appearance; compact hyperkeratosis
Nonbullous congenital ichthyosiform erythroderma (erythrodermic lamellar ichthyosis) (DOC 5)	AR	Collodion baby (most common cause); erythroderma; fine white scales; ectropion	Yes	Alopecia; nail dystrophy		Acanthosis; parakeratosis
Lamellar ichthyosis, dominant type (DOC 6)	AD	Similar to DOC 4 but more keratoderma; may present as collodion baby	Yes			Papillomatosis; alternating orthokeratosis and parakeratosis; thickened granular layer
Harlequin fetus (DOC 7)	AR	Infant encased in massive, grotesque hyperkeratotic plates; survivors have erythroderma and sheets of scale	Yes		Usually die young	Heterogeneous; compact hyperkeratosis and parakeratosis
Ichthyosis hystrix (Curth-Macklin type) (DOC 8)	AD	Wide range of findings from keratoderma to linear to widespread verrucoid hyperpigmented plaques	Yes			Epidermolytic hyperkeratosis; on electron microscopy, binucleate corneocytes and unbroken concentric shells of tonofibrils surround nucleus
Netherton syndrome (including ichthyosis linearis circumflexa [ILC]) (DOC 9)	AR	Generalized erythroderma at or shortly after birth; evolves into ILC or congenital ichthyosiform erythroderma phenotypes	Yes	Trichorrhexis invaginata; other hair shaft defects	Failure to thrive; growth defects; immune defects	If ILC is present, parakeratotic stratum corneum overlying upper stratum malpighii, intracellular edema and spongiosis; otherwise, psoriasiform epidermal acanthosis with overlying eosinophilic material in stratum corneum and subcorneal cleft

Sjögren-Larsson syndrome (DOC 10)	AR	Similar to DOC 4, DOC 5; usually worse flexurally and on lower abdomen; eventually papillomatous; affects predominantly those of northern Swedish heritage	Yes		Mental retardation; neuromuscular spasticity; retinopathy	Papillomatosis; compact hyperkeratosis
Refsum disease (phytanic acid storage disorder) (DOC 11)	AR	Resembles DOC 1; may be limited to palmoplantar keratoderma; dermal nevi often yellow	No		Retinitis pigmentosa; night blindness; peripheral neuropathy; cerebellar ataxia	Compact hyperkeratosis with reduced to absent granular layer; keratinocytes may be vacuolated and contain lipid droplets
Dorfman-Chanarin syndrome (neutral lipid storage disorder) (DOC 12)	AR	Some patients are collodion babies; ichthyotic erythroderma; fine scales; ectropion resembles that in DOC 5	Yes		Myopathy; neurologic problems; cataracts	Papillomatosis; compact hyperkeratosis; lipid vacuoles in keratinocytes (and in peripheral blood granulocytes)
Trichothiodystrophy (Tay syndrome) (IBIDS); variants (BIDS, PIBIDS) (DOC 14)	AR	Some patients are collodion babies; diffuse fine dark scales	Yes	Hair is sparse and brittle; occasional nail ridging and koilonychia	Growth defects; short stature; intellectual impairment; decreased fertility	Compact hyperkeratosis; reduced granular layer
Keratitis-ichthyosis-deafness (KID) syndrome (DOC 15)	AD	Congenital erythroderma, then focal hyperkeratotic plaques	Yes	Hypotrichosis and nail dystrophy	Keratitis; deafness; recurrent infections	Papillomatosis; compact hyperkeratosis
Congenital hemidysplasia-ichthyosis-limb defects (CHILD) syndrome (DOC 16)	XLD	Unilateral psoriasiform rash; striking respect of midline	Yes	Ipsilateral scalp alopecia and nail dystrophy	Congenital hemidysplasia; limb defects; stippled epiphyses; multiple other defects	Psoriasiform epidermal hyperplasia
X-linked dominant chondrodysplasia punctata (DOC 17)	XLD	Ichthyotic erythroderma at birth, evolves into whorled linear hyperkeratotic lesions, follicular atrophoderma	Yes		Chondrodysplasia punctata (one of several variants); cataracts	Compact hyperkeratosis; reduced granular layer
Erythrokeratodermia variabilis (Mendes da Costa syndrome) (DOC 18)	AD	Two components: shifting erythemas and fixed plaques	Yes			Plaques: papillomatosis; compact hyperkeratosis
Peeling skin syndrome (DOC 21)	AR	Two types: (1) symptomatic noninflammatory peeling and (2) congenital erythroderma	Yes			Two patterns: hyperkeratosis with stratum corneum split and psoriasiform hyperkeratosis
Ichthyosis bullosa of Siemens (no DOC number)	AD	Lichenified hyperkeratosis, no erythroderma, localized	Yes			Epidermolytic hyperkeratosis

Reference: Williams ML, Elias PM. Genetically transmitted, generalized disorders of cornification. Dermatol Clin 1987;5:155–178.

and function on ichthyosis is the "bricks and mortar" model of Williams and Elias. The bricks are analogous to the structural proteins of keratin, while mortar is analogous to the epidermal lipids. Most keratin abnormalities are inherited in an autosomal dominant fashion (as is typical for many structural disorders), while most of the lipid problems are autosomal recessive (as for many enzyme disorders). The ichthyoses associated with lipid abnormalities frequently have central nervous system manifestations.

The clinical and histopathologic features of ichthyoses are highly variable and not always helpful in establishing the correct diagnosis. For example, biopsy specimens obtained from patients with ichthyosis vulgaris usually lack a granular layer, but this is an inconstant and, therefore, unreliable finding. The improvements in classification made first by Anton-Lamprecht using ultrastructural evaluation and subsequently by many groups using biochemical and molecular techniques have proved the limitations of clinical descriptions such as "dirty scales" and light microscopic criteria such as a "prominent granular layer." Moreover, although histopathologic findings of epidermolytic hyperkeratosis may be unmistakable, several forms of ichthyosis share this distinctive pattern. Nevertheless, electron microscopy may occasionally be helpful in diagnosis; for example, ichthyosis vulgaris has very characteristic abnormal keratohyaline granules. Ultimately, one often must rely on the combined clinical, genetic, histopathologic, and biochemical information to arrive at a diagnosis.

The salient features of the ichthyoses are shown in Table 1–1. We have used the classification system proposed by Williams and Elias, which designates and numbers all ichthyoses as disorders of cornification.

Frost P, Van Scott EJ. Ichthyosiform dermatoses: classification based on anatomic and biometric observations. Arch Dermatol 1966;94:113–126

Frost P, Weinstein GD, Bothwell JW, Wildnauer R. Ichthyosiform dermatoses: studies of transepidermal water loss. Arch Dermatol 1968;98:230–233

Frost P, Weinstein GD, Van Scott EJ. The ichthyosiform dermatoses: autoradiographic studies of epidermal proliferation. J Invest Dermatol 1966;47:561–567

Traupe H. The Ichthyoses: A Guide to Clinical Diagnosis, Genetic Counseling and Therapy. Berlin, Springer Verlag, 1989

Williams ML, Elias PM. Genetically transmitted, generalized disorders of cornification. Dermatol Clin 1987;5:155–178

ICHTHYOSIS VULGARIS

Synonyms

- ichthyosis simplex
- autosomal dominant ichthyosis
- DOC 1

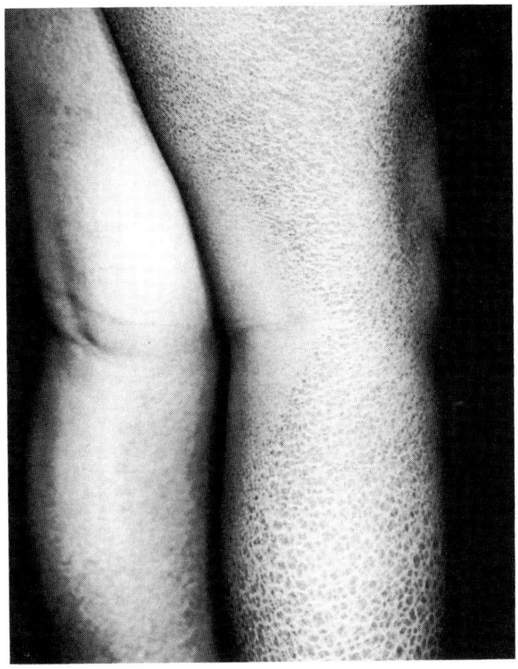

FIGURE 1–1
Sparing of the flexures is an important feature of ichthyosis vulgaris. (Courtesy of Edward A. Krull, MD, Detroit, Michigan)

Skin

small, fine, white to light gray-brown scales, most prominent on the extensor surfaces, especially elbows and knees; flexures are invariably spared, as usually is the face (Fig. 1–1)

onset after birth; 40% of patients are affected by age 3 months and most by age 4 years

may improve in warm weather or after puberty

increased palmoplantar creases

frequent keratosis pilaris

no ectropion, eclabium, or mucosal involvement

areas of ichthyosis have decreased sweat and sebum production

Non-Skin

associated with atopy in about 50%

possibly associated with cryptorchidism (cf. more well-documented association with X-linked ichthyosis)

Genetics

AD

1 in 250 births

Laboratory Data

histopathology: compact hyperkeratosis with decreased or nearly absent granular layer; the leg is the best site for biopsy

retention hyperkeratosis; mitotic activity is normal

electron microscopy: distinctive abnormal keratohyaline granules

decreased profilaggrin and filaggrin

Discussion

milder forms of the disease overlap in appearance with simple asteatosis ("dry skin"), which is especially apparent on the legs of blacks

REFERENCES

McK 146700

Fartasch M, Diepgen TL, Hornstein OP. Are hyperlinear palms and dry skin signs of a concomitant autosomal ichthyosis vulgaris in atopic dermatitis? Acta Derm Venereol Suppl 1989;144:143–145

Kuokkanen K. Ichthyosis vulgaris: a clinical and histopathological study of patients and their close relatives in the autosomal dominant and sex-linked forms of the disease. Acta Derm Venereol Suppl 1969;49(suppl 62):1–72

Mevorah B, Krayenbuhl A, Bovey EH, Van Melle GD. Autosomal dominant ichthyosis and X-linked ichthyosis: comparison of their clinical and histological phenotypes. Acta Derm Venereol 1991;71:431–434

Mevorah B, Marazi A, Frenk E. The prevalence of accentuated palmoplantar markings and keratosis pilaris in atopic dermatitis, autosomal dominant ichthyosis and control dermatological patients. Br J Dermatol 1985;112:679–685

Okano M, Kitano Y, Yoshikawa K, et al. X-linked ichthyosis and ichthyosis vulgaris: comparison of their clinical features based on biochemical analysis. Br J Dermatol 1988;119:777–783

Shwayder T, Ott F. All about ichthyosis. Pediatr Clin North Am 1991;38:835–857

Traupe H. The Ichthyoses: A Guide to Clinical Diagnosis, Genetic Counseling and Therapy. Berlin, Springer Verlag, 1989:49

Wells RS, Kerr CB. Clinical features of autosomal dominant and X-linked recessive ichthyosis in an English population. Br Med J 1966;1:947–950

X-LINKED ICHTHYOSIS

Synonym

- DOC 2

Skin

large, often dark scales in generalized distribution; flexural areas may be involved (Figs. 1–2 and 1–3); palms and soles spared

onset in early infancy; one third have involvement at birth, which may be manifested as a generalized peeling

neck may appear "dirty" and is often the most severely involved area

improves with warm weather

scalp, neck, and face may improve with time, but abdomen and popliteal fossae may worsen

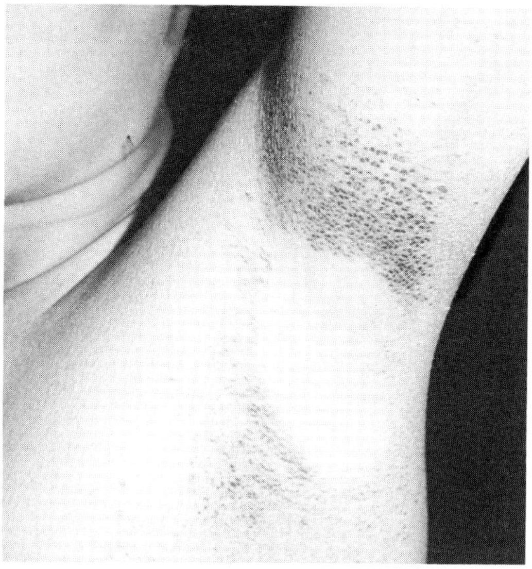

FIGURE 1–2
Sparing of the flexures is noted in this boy with X-linked ichthyosis. Clinically this disorder can be confused with ichthyosis vulgaris.

Non-Skin

corneal opacities involving Descemet's membrane, although traditionally reported to be an important diagnostic feature, have been absent or found only in low percentages of patients in recent studies

posterior embryotoxon, a congenital malformation of the corneoscleral junction, was detected in 7 of 17 patients and 2 of 10 carriers in one study

associations with anosmia and hypogenitalism (Kallmann syndrome), cryptorchidism, and/or testicular malignancies reported

rare oligophrenia

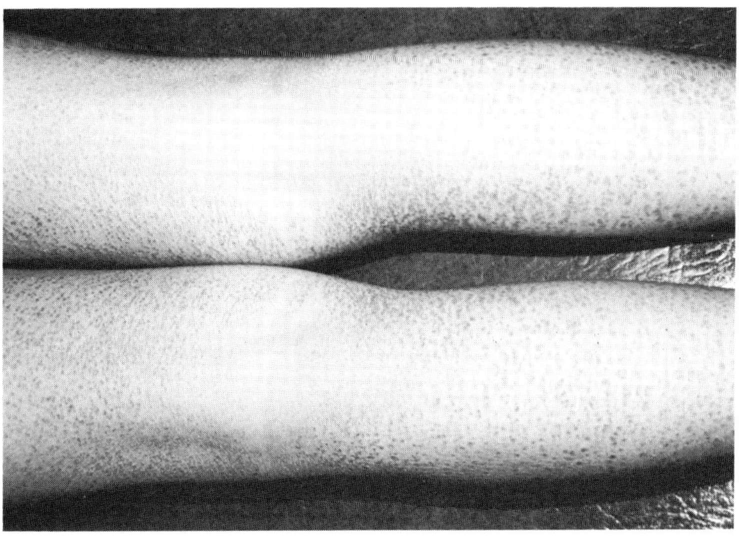

FIGURE 1–3
Variable sparing of the flexures is seen in X-linked ichthyosis.

Genetics

XLR; 1 in 6000 male births

chromosomal abnormalities have been detected in some patients

Laboratory Data

histopathology: hyperkeratosis, usually with a normal or thickened granular layer; however, a decreased granular layer (as in ichthyosis vulgaris) may also be seen

decreased steroid sulfatase and aryl sulfatase C activity; female carriers have half of normal activity

increased cholesterol sulfate located in stratum corneum, red blood cell membranes and serum

increased cholesterol sulfate in low-density lipoproteins results in increased mobility on lipoprotein electrophoresis

steroid sulfatase locus on the distal short arm of the X chromosome

prenatal diagnosis is possible

Discussion

heterozygous females may have mild ichthyosis

although the face is generally reported to be spared, one study noted that 93% of patients had preauricular involvement, compared with 17% in patients with ichthyosis vulgaris

clinical features overlap with those of ichthyosis vulgaris, but palmar involvement and keratosis pilaris are generally absent

mothers of affected children may have slow, weak labor

REFERENCES

McK 308100

de Unamuno P, Martin-Pascual A, Garcia-Perez A. X-linked ichthyosis. Br J Dermatol 1977;97:53–58

Hebert AA, Hood OJ. Diagnosis of X-linked ichthyosis. Pediatr Dermatol 1988;5:211–212

Matsumoto T, Sakura N, Ueda K. Steroid sulfatase activity in nails: screening for X-linked ichthyosis. Pediatr Dermatol 1990;7:266–269

Mevorah B, Krayenbuhl A, Bovey EH, Van Melle GD. Autosomal dominant ichthyosis and X-linked ichthyosis: comparison of their clinical and histological phenotypes. Acta Derm Venereol 1991;71:431–434

Okano M, Kitano Y, Yoshikawa K, et al. X-linked ichthyosis and ichthyosis vulgaris: comparison of their clinical features based on biochemical analysis. Br J Dermatol 1988;119:777–783

Pike MG, Hammerton M, Edge J, et al. A family with X-linked ichthyosis and hypogonadism. Eur J Pediatr 1989;148:442–444

Shackleton C, Williams ML, Epstein EH Jr. Diagnostic tests for recessive X-linked ichthyosis. Pediatr Dermatol 1988;5:211

Shapiro LJ, Cousins L, Fluharty AL, et al. Steroid sulfatase deficiency. Pediatr Res 1977;11:894–897

Shapiro LJ, Weiss R, Buxman MM, et al. Enzymatic basis of typical X-linked ichthyosis. Lancet 1978;2:756–757

Shapiro LJ. X-linked ichthyosis. Int J Dermatol 1981;20:26–31

Sunohara N, Sakuragawa N, Satoyoshi E, et al. A new syndrome of anosmia, ichthyosis,

hypogonadism, and various neurological manifestations with deficiency of steroid sulfatase and arylsulfatase C. Ann Neurol 1986;19:174–181
Voss M, Jüneman R. Ophthalmologic findings in X-linked ichthyosis. Dermatol Monatsschr 1986;172:209–211; abstracted in J Am Acad Dermatol 1986;15:717
Williams ML. A new look at the ichthyoses: disorders of lipid metabolism. [Review]. Pediatr Dermatol 1986;3:476–486

MULTIPLE SULFATASE DEFICIENCY (DOC 13; SULFATIDOSIS)

features of X-linked ichthyosis combined with phenotypic features of the other individual sulfatase deficiencies (e.g., Maroteaux-Lamy syndrome, Hunter syndrome, Morquio syndrome, and Sanfilippo syndrome type A [see entries elsewhere in book]); at least nine sulfatases are known to be deficient

McK 272200
Burch M, Fensom AH, Jackson M, Pitts-Tucker T, Congdon PJ. Multiple sulphatase deficiency presenting at birth. Clin Genet 1986;30:409–415

LAMELLAR ICHTHYOSIS

Synonyms

- classic lamellar ichthyosis
- nonerythrodermic lamellar ichthyosis
- DOC 4

Skin

may be encased in shiny, "collodion"-like membrane at birth (Fig. 1–4), which is shed in first few days, revealing generalized erythema and scaling

scales gradually thicken and darken, becoming large and polygonal ("fish-like"), involving entire body, especially flexural surfaces including the antecubital fossae, axillae, groin, and neck (Fig. 1–5)

unilateral distribution rarely

keratoderma of the palms and soles may be massive, commonly with deep fissures

greasy, varnished appearance of face

hyperhidrosis of palms, soles, face, and flexures may lead to maceration and malodor; hypohidrosis of other areas, primarily due to blockage of sweat pores, may cause heat intolerance

buccal or nasal mucosae rarely thickened

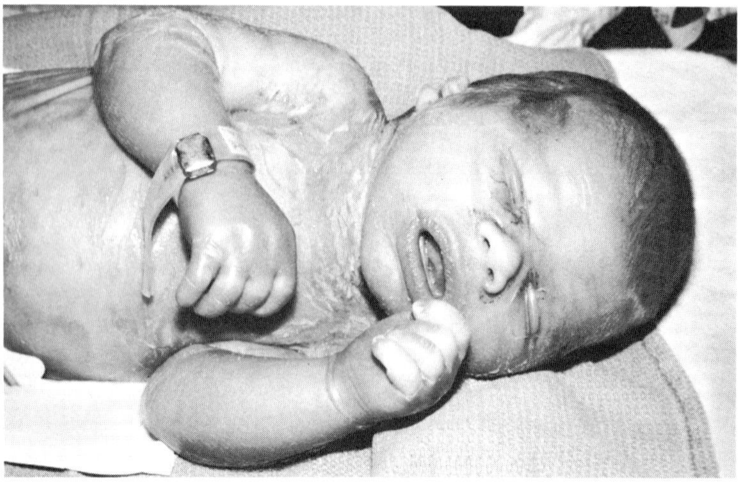

FIGURE 1–4
"Collodion baby" presentation of lamellar ichthyosis. The parchment-like membrane has ruptured in the flexural areas and over the thorax, where there are maceration and secondary infection. Additional characteristic features are ectropion, eclabium, and taut skin over the digits, rendering them inflexible.

hair may be fine and sparse, yet hair and nails may grow at two to three times the normal rate

other nail abnormalities include subungual hyperkeratosis and transverse or longitudinal ridging or stippling

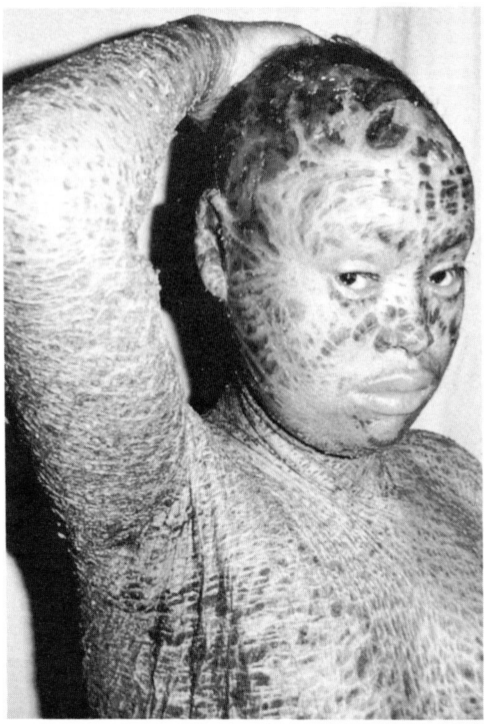

FIGURE 1–5
Lamellar ichthyosis. The entire skin surface including the flexural areas is covered with large, dark, plate-like scales. (Courtesy of Benjamin K. Fisher, MD, Toronto, Ontario)

Non-Skin

bilateral conjunctivitis, lower eyelid ectropion, and eclabium

ears may appear small and deformed

Genetics

AR

1 in 300,000 births

Laboratory Data

histopathology: compact hyperorthokeratosis; normal or thickened granular layer; psoriasiform epidermal acanthosis with papillomatosis

proliferation hyperkeratosis with increased mitoses, decreased epidermal transit time

stratum corneum total lipids and free sterols are increased, but n-alkanes are normal

Prognosis

the disease progresses until adulthood and hyperkeratosis persists; erythema may mostly subside but commonly persists on the face

Discussion

amounts of n-alkanes in stratum corneum are normal, in contrast with the increased levels reported in nonbullous congenital ichthyosiform erythroderma (NCIE); total lipids and free sterols are decreased in NCIE. However, these findings have not been confirmed in all studies and should not be used to make a definitive diagnosis. The n-alkanes being measured may be exogenous and unrelated to the pathogenesis of the disease.

REFERENCES

McK 242100

Bernhardt M, Baden HP. Report of a family with an unusual expression of recessive ichthyosis: review of 42 cases. Arch Dermatol 1986;122:428–433

Hazell M, Marks R. Clinical, histologic, and cell kinetic discriminants between lamellar ichthyosis and nonbullous congenital ichthyosiform erythroderma. Arch Dermatol 1985;121:489–493

Küster W, Melnik B, Plewig G. n-Alkanes in the skin. Arch Dermatol 1991;127:1727–1728

Williams ML, Elias PM. Heterogeneity in autosomal recessive ichthyosis: clinical and biochemical differentiation of lamellar ichthyosis and nonbullous congenital ichthyosiform erythroderma. Arch Dermatol 1985;121:477–488

LAMELLAR ICHTHYOSIS, DOMINANT TYPE (DOC 6)

affected infant may present as collodion baby

palm and sole involvement may be less marked than in recessive lamellar ichthyosis (DOC 4), while pruritus may be more prominent no extracutaneous findings

AD

histopathology: alternating orthokeratosis and parakeratosis and a markedly thickened "transformation layer" between the granular layer and stratum corneum measuring four to six cells thick

McK 146750

Melnik B, Kuster W, Hollmann J, et al. Autosomal dominant lamellar ichthyosis exhibits an abnormal scale lipid pattern. Clin Genet 1989;35:152–156

Toribio J, Fernandez-Redondo V, Peteiro C, et al. Autosomal dominant lamellar ichthyosis. Clin Genet 1986;30:122–126

Traupe H, Kolde G, Happle R. Autosomal dominant lamellar ichthyosis: a new skin disorder. Clin Genet 1984;26:457–461

LAMELLAR ICHTHYOSIS OF THE NEWBORN (SELF-HEALING COLLODION BABY)

a collodion membrane is present at birth, but skin is usually normal after 3 to 10 weeks

AR

the nomenclature should not be confused with lamellar ichthyosis

McK 242300

Frenk E, de Techtermann F. Self-healing collodion baby; evidence for autosomal recessive inheritance. Pediatr Dermatol 1992; 9:95–97

Reed WB, Herwick RP, Harville D, Porter PS, Conant M. Lamellar ichthyosis of the newborn. Arch Dermatol 1972;105:394–399

NONBULLOUS CONGENITAL ICHTHYOSIFORM ERYTHRODERMA

Synonym

- DOC 5

Skin

affected infant may present at birth with collodion membrane

generalized fine white scales and prominent erythroderma; erythroderma may fade later in life (see Color Fig. 1–1)

hyperkeratotic palms and soles

alopecia and nail dystrophy in some

Non-Skin

ectropion

Genetics

AR

Laboratory Data

histopathology: less marked hyperkeratosis and more severe parakeratosis than in lamellar ichthyosis (DOC 4); acanthosis

Discussion

this subtype was formerly not distinguished from lamellar ichthyosis

scales are smaller and finer and ectropion is less marked than in lamellar ichthyosis

increased epidermal turnover rates and epidermal n-alkanes reported (up to 25% of total stratum corneum lipids; normally 5% to 10%); however, findings related to n-alkanes have not been confirmed in all studies and should not be used to make a definitive diagnosis; the n-alkanes being measured may be exogenous and hence be unrelated to the pathogenesis of the disease

REFERENCES

McK 242100

Bergers M, Traupe H, Dunnwald SC, et al. Enzymatic distinction between two subgroups of autosomal recessive lamellar ichthyosis. J Invest Dermatol 1990;94:407–412

Bernhardt M, Baden HP. Report of a family with an unusual expression of recessive ichthyosis. review of 42 cases. Arch Dermatol 1986;122:428–433

Elias PM, Williams ML, Rehfeld SJ. n-Alkanes in the skin: function or fancy? Arch Dermatol 1991;126:868–870

Hazell M, Marks R. Clinical, histologic, and cell kinotic discriminants between lamellar ichthyosis and nonbullous congenital ichthyosiform erythroderma. Arch Dermatol 1985;121:489–493

Küster W, Melnik B, Plewig G. n-Alkanes in the skin. Arch Dermatol 1991;127:1727–1728

Rossmann RI, Anton-Lamprecht I, Swanbeck G. A mother and two children with nonbullous congenital ichthyosiform erythroderma. Arch Dermatol 1986;122:559–564

Williams ML, Elias PM. Elevated n-alkanes in congenital ichthyosiform erythroderma: phenotypic differentiation of two types of autosomal recessive ichthyosis. J Clin Invest 1984;74:296–300

Williams ML, Elias PM. Heterogeneity in autosomal recessive ichthyosis: clinical and biochemical differentiation of lamellar ichthyosis and nonbullous congenital ichthyosiform erythroderma. Arch Dermatol 1985;121:477–488

Williams ML, Elias PM. Ichthyosis: genetic heterogeneity, genodermatoses, and genetic counseling. Arch Dermatol 1986;122:529–531

Williams ML. The ichthyoses—pathogenesis and prenatal diagnosis: a review of recent advances. [Review]. Pediatr Dermatol 1983;1:1–24

BULLOUS CONGENITAL ICHTHYOSIFORM ERYTHRODERMA

Synonyms

- epidermolytic hyperkeratosis
- bullous ichthyotic erythroderma of Brocq
- bullous ichthyosis
- DOC 3

Skin

at birth or shortly thereafter, flaccid blisters may form on erythematous or hyperkeratotic skin; these blisters are induced spontaneously or mechanically and may result in widespread denudation

areas of blisters heal normally, resulting in islands of more normal-appearing skin in the middle of erythematous or hyperkeratotic plaques

later in childhood, patients develop characteristic thick, hyperkeratotic, verrucous brown plaques, most prominent over flexures; plaques are ridged or "spine-like" (Figs. 1–6 and 1–7)

maceration and bacterial colonization of the hyperkeratotic plaques lead to a characteristic malodor

incidence of blisters decreases with age and may even cease, but some patients continue to form blisters, especially in the summer

erythroderma also diminishes with age, but hyperkeratosis remains severe

involvement of palms and soles ranges from none to severe (Fig. 1–8)

occasional nail dystrophy

hair, teeth, and mucous membranes are spared except for the occurrence of hair casts

Non-Skin

eyes are normal; specifically, ectropion is not seen

Genetics

AD

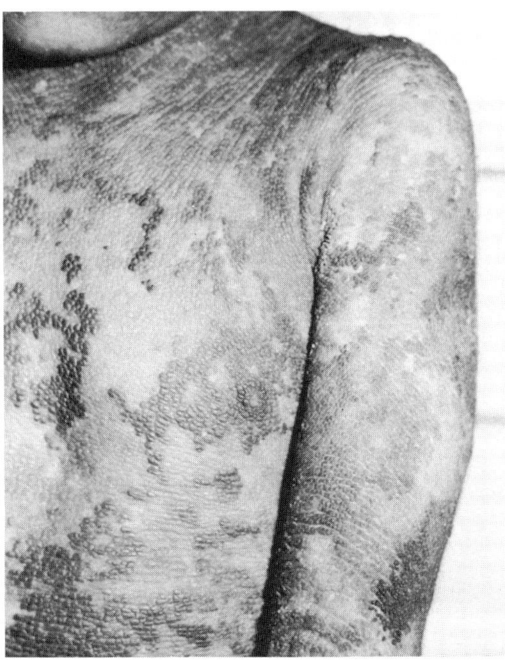

FIGURE 1–6
Bullous congenital ichthyosiform erythroderma. Dark, thick, shotty scales, in some areas showing a characteristic ridge-like pattern. Note the flexural involvement.

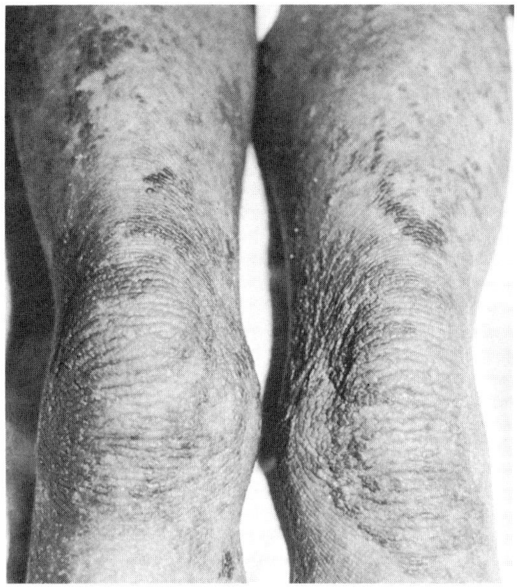

FIGURE 1–7
Thick dark scales over the legs with characteristic ridging over the knees of a patient with bullous congenital ichthyosiform erythroderma.

Pathophysiology

genetic basis for bullous congenital ichthyosiform erythroderma resides in mutations in genes encoding keratins 1 and 10 on chromosomes 12g and 17g, respectively.

Laboratory Data

histopathology: epidermolytic hyperkeratosis (hyperkeratosis and vacuolar changes in upper layers of the stratum malpighii with clumped keratohyaline granules)

proliferation hyperkeratosis (mitotic figures five times normal)

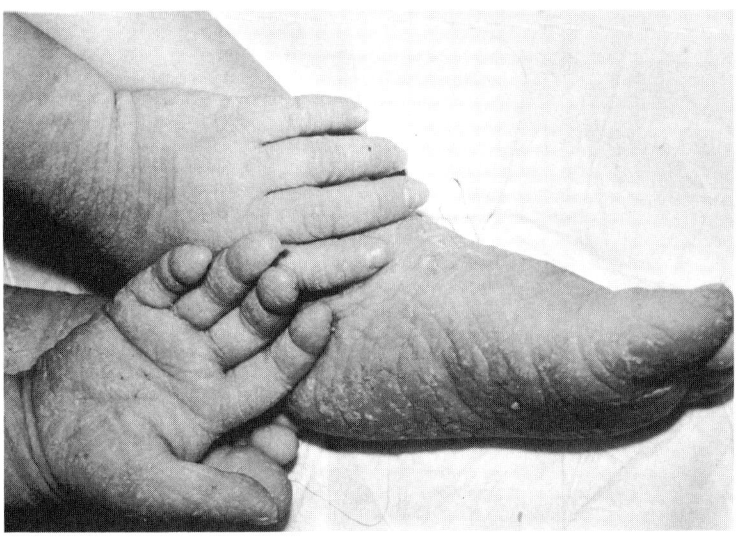

FIGURE 1–8
Hyperkeratosis of the palms and soles in a patient with bullous congenital ichthyosiform erythroderma.

electron microscopy: perinuclear tonofilament shells and irregular clumps of tonofibrils in upper spinous and granular layers

prenatal diagnosis by fetal skin biopsy is possible

Prognosis

increased incidence of eczema vaccinatum and herpeticum; other secondary infections also contribute to mortality and morbidity

Discussion

there have been reports of several families in which a parent with linear epidermal nevi with the histologic features of epidermolytic hyperkeratosis has had a child with bullous congenital ichthyosiform erythroderma; knowledge of this fact is important for genetic counseling

the term *epidermolytic hyperkeratosis* should probably be reserved as a histologic description and not as the name of a particular disease. Epidermolytic hyperkeratosis is present in many diseases, including epidermolytic palmoplantar keratoderma, in single or multiple epidermolytic acanthomas and some epidermal nevi, and as an incidental finding in many other lesions.

REFERENCES

McK 113800

Cheng J, Syder AJ, Yu QC, et al. The genetic basis of epidermolytic hyperkeratosis: a disorder of differentiation-specific epidermal keratin genes. Cell 1992;70:811–819

Epstein EH Jr. The morbid cutaneous anatomy of the human genome. Arch Dermatol 1993;129:1417–1423

McGrath J, Cerio R, Wilson-Jones E. The phenotypic heterogenicity of bullous ichthyosis: a case report of three family members. Clin Exp Dermatol 1991;16:25–27

Mills C, Marks R. Acral epidermolytic hyperkeratosis. Br J Dermatol 1993;128:342–347

Nazzaro V, Ermacora E, Santucci B, et al. Epidermolytic hyperkeratosis: generalized form in children from parents with systematized linear form. Br J Dermatol 1990;122:417–422

Traupe H: The Ichthyoses: A Guide to Clinical Diagnosis, Genetic Counseling and Therapy. Berlin, Springer Verlag, 1989:139–153

ICHTHYOSIS BULLOSA OF SIEMENS

Skin

circumscribed, dark gray, lichenified, hyperkeratotic plaques, predominantly on arms and legs

superficial denuded areas resemble those in epidermolysis bullosa simplex clinically but result from intracorneal blisters; lesions heal without scarring

no erythroderma

Genetics

AD

Laboratory Data

histopathology: epidermolytic hyperkeratosis (hyperkeratosis and vacuolar changes with clumped keratohyaline granules) of superficial spinous and granular layers

electron microscopy: enlarged keratohyaline granules and bulky perinuclear tonofilament clumps are present, but perinuclear tonofilament shells, as seen in bullous congenital ichthyosiform erythroderma, are absent

Discussion

ichthyosis bullosa of Siemens may be a variant of bullous congenital ichthyosiform erythroderma, but they differ ultrastructurally

REFERENCES

Steijlen PM, Perret CM, Schuurmans Stekhoven JH, et al. Ichthyosis bullosa of Siemens: further delineation of the phenotype. Arch Dermatol Res 1990;282:1–5

Traupe H, Kolde G, Hamm H, et al. Ichthyosis bullosa of Siemens: a unique type of epidermolytic hyperkeratosis. J Am Acad Dermatol 1986;14:1000–1005

ICHTHYOSIS HYSTRIX, CURTH-MACKLIN TYPE (DOC 8)

varied clinical findings including widespread verrucoid hyperpigmented plaques

AD

histopathology: epidermolytic hyperkeratosis (hyperkeratosis and vacuolar changes in upper layers of the stratum malpighii with clumped keratohyaline granules) common

electron microscopy: binucleate keratinocytes characteristic; unbroken concentric shells of tonofibrils surround nucleus; no tonofilament clumps; tonofilament attachment to desmosomes not disturbed

McK 146590

Curth HO, Macklin MT. The genetic basis of various types of ichthyosis in a family group. Am J Hum Genet 1954;6:371–381

Traupe H: The Ichthyoses: A Guide to Clinical Diagnosis, Genetic Counseling and Therapy. Berlin, Springer Verlag, 1989:139–153

HARLEQUIN ICHTHYOSIS

Synonyms

- harlequin baby
- harlequin fetus
- DOC 7

Skin

a severe form of ichthyosis; infants are born encased in thick armor-like skin split into polygonal plates separated by deep fissures; the pattern resembles the costume of a harlequin clown (Fig. 1–9)

nails and hair may be hypoplastic or absent

erythroderma and sheets of scale in survivors

Non-Skin

infants are usually born prematurely

ectropion, eclabium, deformed or rudimentary ears, and flexion contractures of limbs and digits

respiratory and sucking movements are restricted by the thick skin

Genetics

probably AR; very rare

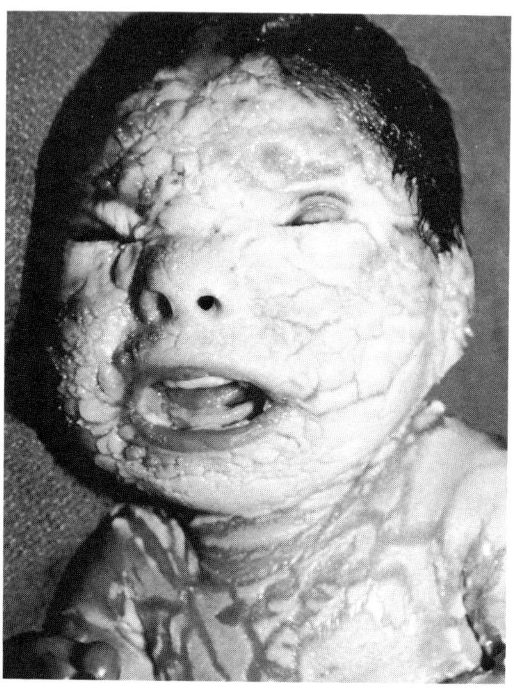

FIGURE 1–9
Harlequin ichthyosis. Markedly thickened horny layer on the head and torso with irregular deep erythematous fissures. Note the extreme ectropion and eclabium. The ears are entirely obscured by the massively thickened epidermis. (Courtesy of Adelaide Hebert, MD, Houston, Texas.)

Laboratory Data

prenatal diagnosis is possible by fetoscopic skin biopsy

Prognosis

secondary infection and septicemia are common

death usual in first weeks of life; rarely, infants survive (e.g., with systemic retinoid therapy)

Discussion

some consider this a unique ichthyosis, while others believe it may be a phenotype representing a heterogeneous group of disorders or that it may be a severe form of autosomal recessive nonbullous congenital ichthyosiform erythroderma or lamellar ichthyosis

various abnormalities in epidermal keratinization including keratin and filaggrin expression and lamellar granule defects suggest genetic heterogeneity

REFERENCES

McK 242500

Dale BA, Holbrook KA, Fleckman P, et al. Heterogeneity in harlequin ichthyosis, an inborn error of epidermal keratinization: variable morphology and structural protein expression and a defect in lamellar granules. J Invest Dermatol 1990;94:6–18

Elias S, Mazur M, Sabbagha R, et al. Prenatal diagnosis of harlequin ichthyosis. Clin Genet 1980;17:275–280

Lawlor F, Peiris S. Progress of a harlequin fetus treated with etretinate. J R Soc Med 1985;11:19–20

Roberts LJ. Long-term survival of a harlequin fetus. J Am Acad Dermatol 1989;21:335–340

Rogers M, Scraf C. Harlequin baby treated with etretinate. Pediatr Dermatol 1989; 6:216–221

Unamuno P, Pierola JM, Fernandez E, et al. Harlequin foetus in four siblings. Br J Dermatol 1987;116:569–572

Ward PS, Jones RD. Successful treatment of a harlequin fetus. Arch Dis Child 1989; 64:1309–1311

CHILD SYNDROME

Synonyms

- DOC 16
- Congenital hemidysplasia, ichthyosiform erythroderma, and limb defects

Skin

unilateral ichthyosiform erythroderma with prominent involvement of body folds at birth or in early infancy (Fig. 1–10); occasional patchy involvement of contralateral side following lines of Blaschko

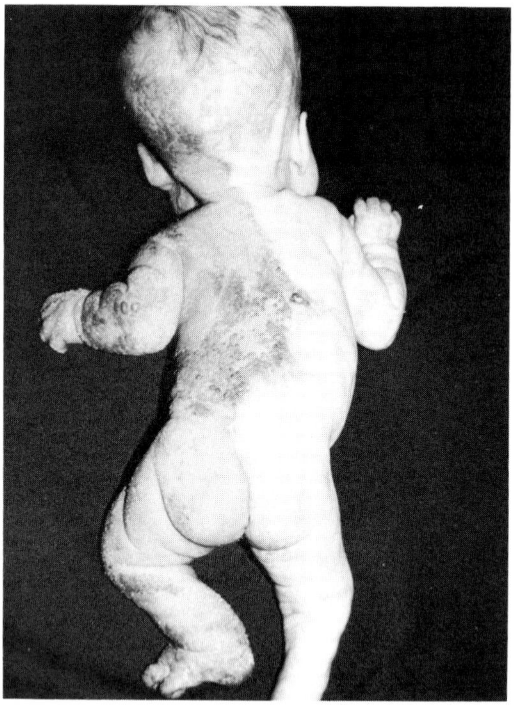

FIGURE 1–10
Posterior view of an infant with CHILD syndrome showing an extensive unilateral dermatosis consisting of erythema and thick yellow-brown hyperkeratosis.

occasional ipsilateral nail abnormalities including onychogryposis and brittleness (Fig. 1–11)

occasional partial alopecia of scalp

Non-Skin

limb defects including skeletal hypoplasia, aplasia, or other anomalies of long bones ipsilateral to the skin eruption

cardiac, especially septal, and renal abnormalities

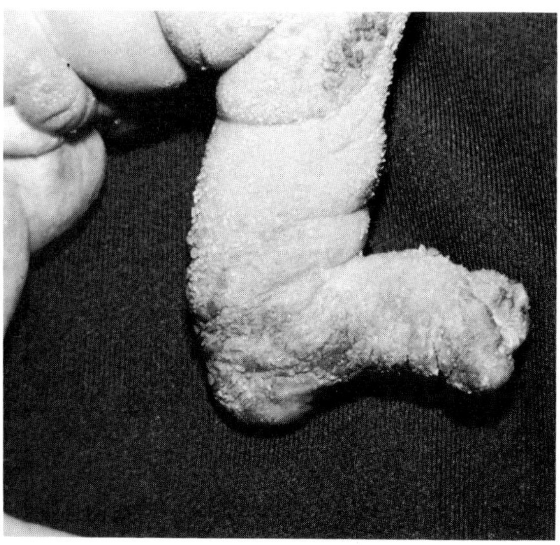

FIGURE 1–11
Same patient as in Figure 1–10. Note extreme hyperkeratosis, nail dystrophy, and absence of the fourth toe.

pulmonary, central nervous system, and endocrinologic abnormalities and ipsilateral hypoplasia of various viscera also reported

Genetics

XLD, though AD and AR also proposed

affected males very rare

Pathophysiology

peroxisomal abnormality reported

Laboratory Data

histopathology: psoriasiform epidermal hyperplasia with pale-staining stratum corneum

keratinization abnormalities, including lamellar granule defects, seen in ultrastructural studies

radiographs may show punctate epiphyseal calcifications, which disappear with time

Prognosis

skin condition may improve with time

REFERENCES

McK 308050

Christiansen JV, Overgaard PH, Sgaard H. The CHILD syndrome—congenital hemidysplasia with ichthyosiform erythroderma and limb defects: a case report. Acta Derm Venereol 1984;64:165–168

Emani S, Rizzo WB, Hanley KP, Taylor JM, Goldyne ME, Williams ML. Peroxisomal abnormality in fibroblasts from involved skin of CHILD syndrome. Arch Dermatol 1992;128:1213–1222

Happle R, Koch H, Lenz W. The CHILD syndrome: congenital hemidysplasia with ichthyosiform erythroderma and limb defects. Eur J Pediatr 1980;134:27–33

Happle R. Psychotropism as a cutaneous feature of the CHILD syndrome. J Am Acad Dermatol 1990;23:763–766

Hebert AA, Esterly NB, Holbrook KA, et al. The CHILD syndrome: histologic and ultrastructural studies. Arch Dermatol 1987; 123:503–509

NETHERTON SYNDROME

Synonyms

- DOC 9
- Comèl-Netherton syndrome

Skin

three principal features of the disease: (1) ichthyosis; (2) hair shaft defects, e.g., trichorrhexis invaginata; and (3) atopic diathesis (Figs. 1–12 and 1–13)

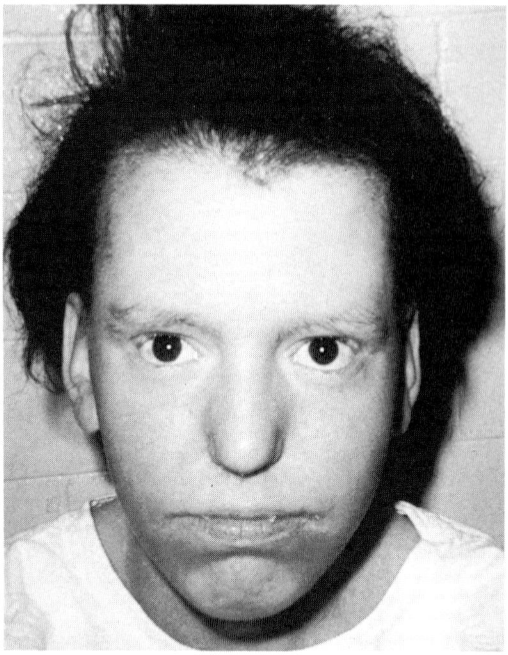

FIGURE 1–12
Sparse lusterless hair, eyebrows, and eyelashes with blepharitis and cheilitis in a patient with Netherton syndrome.

generalized erythroderma is first sign of the disease, occurring at or shortly after birth; evolves into ichthyosis linearis circumflexa (ILC) or congenital ichthyosiform erythroderma (CIE) phenotypes

ILC is manifested as a migratory polycyclic, circinate, and serpiginous eruption with distinctive double-edged scale on trunk and limbs; antecubital/popliteal fossae lichenified and hyperkeratotic; persistent perioral erythema may be present

CIE phenotype has marked generalized erythroderma and scaling; hypotrichosis more pronounced in this variant

hair is brittle and breaks easily

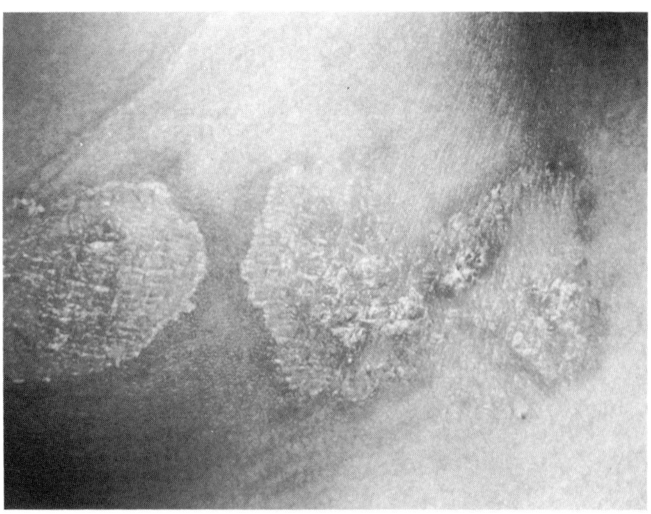

FIGURE 1–13
Hyperkeratotic plaques with figurate borders and doubled-edged scale (ichthyosis linearis circumflexa) on the limb of a patient with Netherton syndrome. (Courtesy of Edward A. Krull, MD, Detroit, Michigan)

trichorrhexis invaginata ("bamboo hair") has a "pencil in cup" appearance microscopically; predominantly involves the scalp; eyebrows, eyelashes, and body hair less commonly involved

trichorrhexis nodosa, pili torti, braid-weave, and other hair shaft abnormalities also noted in some individuals

increased incidence of urticaria and angioedema; concurrence of true atopic dermatitis is controversial

Non-Skin

increased incidence of asthma and recurrent upper respiratory tract infections

failure to thrive and growth defects

occasional mental deficiency and epilepsy

immunodeficiency with recurrent infections (sometimes fatal) and enteropathy with diarrhea, particularly with CIE phenotype

generalized lymphadenopathy in some patients

Genetics

AR

Laboratory Data

histopathology: hyperparakeratosis, strongly eosinophilic material in stratum corneum and subcorneal cleft; psoriasiform epidermal acanthosis; areas of double-edged scale show spongiosis and intracellular edema, occasionally forming vesicles or vesiculopustules

inconstant aminoaciduria (histidine, serine, glycine, and argininosuccinic acid)

rare hypogammaglobulinemia

marked hypernatremic dehydration may be seen in patients with erythroderma due to defective barrier function

markedly increased serum IgE in some

Discussion

- *ichthyosis linearis circumflexa*

  may occur as an isolated entity apart from Netherton syndrome

  may worsen at puberty but postpubertal remissions may occur

  AR; XLR also reported

REFERENCES

McK 256500

Brodin MB, Porter PS. Nertherton's syndrome. Cutis 1980;26:185–188

Caputo R, Vanotti P, Bertani E. Netherton's syndrome in two adult brothers. Arch Dermatol 1984;120:220–222

Greene SL, Muller SA. Netherton's syndrome: report of a case and review of the literature. J Am Acad Dermatol 1985;13:329–337

Hersle K. Netherton's disease and ichthyosis linearis circumflexa: report of a case and review of the literature. Acta Derm Venereol 1972;52:298–302

Kassis V, Nielsen JM, Klem-Thomsen H, et al. Familial Netherton's disease. Cutis 1986; 38:175–178

Krafchik BR. Netherton syndrome. Pediatr Dermatol 1992;9:157–160

Murphy GM, Griffiths WA, Grice K. Netherton's syndrome. J R Soc Med 1989;82:683–684

Nabai H, Mehregan AH. Ichthyosis linearis circumflexa. J Cutan Pathol 1979;6:148–149

Yoshiike T, Manabe M, Negi M, Ogawa H. Ichthyosis linearis circumflexa: morphological and biochemical studies. Br J Dermatol 1985;112:277–283

TAY SYNDROME

Synonyms

- DOC 14
- IBIDS (Ichthyosis, Brittle hair, Impaired intelligence, Decreased fertility, and Short stature)

Skin

diffuse fine scales and erythema (lamellar ichthyosis–like) present at birth; some affected infants born with collodion membrane

palmoplantar keratoderma

hair is sparse and brittle

occasional nail hypoplasia, ridging and koilonychia

Non-Skin

low birth weight

close-set eyes, beaked nose, sunken cheeks, and decreased subcutaneous fat gives a progeric appearance

short stature and mental retardation

hypogonadism

increased susceptibility to bacterial infections in some

Genetics

AR

Laboratory Data

hair has reduced cystine content (trichothiodystrophy); transverse bands seen under polaroscopy

flattening and ribbon-like folding of the hair shaft; trichoschisis is the most common hair shaft abnormality, but atypical trichorrhexis nodosa or other abnormalities may be seen

Discussion

some authors think that PIBIDS syndrome is the combination of Tay syndrome (IBIDS) and xeroderma pigmentosum; see PIBIDS and IBIDS syndromes under Trichothiodystrophy in Chapter 9 on disorders of hair

REFERENCES

McK 242170

Happle R, Traupe H, Grobe H, et al. The Tay syndrome (congenital ichthyosis with trichothiodystrophy). Eur J Pediatr 1984;141: 147–152

Kousseff BG. Collodion baby, sign of Tay syndrome. Pediatrics 1991;87:571–574

Lehmann AR, Arlett CF, Broughton BC, et al. Trichothiodystrophy, a human DNA repair disorder with heterogeneity in the cellular response to ultraviolet light. Cancer Res 1988;48:6090–6096

Motley RJ, Finlay AY. A patient with Tay's syndrome. Pediatr Dermatol 1989;6:202–205

Tay CH. Ichthyosiform erythroderma, hair shaft abnormalities, and mental and growth retardation. Arch Dermatol 1971;104:4–13

REFSUM DISEASE

Synonyms

- heredopathia atactica polyneuritiformis
- DOC 11

Skin

ichthyosis vulgaris–like eruption of variable severity

insidious onset, often in childhood, but as late as fourth or fifth decade

palmoplantar keratoderma

melanocytic nevi may be yellow due to presence of lipids

Non-Skin

ocular findings include retinitis pigmentosa (one of the earliest signs), night blindness, concentric constriction of visual fields, and pupillary abnormalities

neurologic changes include cerebellar ataxia, chronic peripheral polyneuritis with weakness, wasting and sensory loss, bilateral sensorineural deafness, and anosmia; intelligence is normal

cardiomyopathy

multiple epiphyseal dysplasia

Genetics

AR

Pathophysiology

phytanic acid oxidase deficiency; patients unable to metabolize plant-derived phytanic acid to alpha-hydroxyphytanic acid

excess phytanic acid replaces the normal fatty acid constituents of the epidermis

Laboratory Data

histopathology: compact hyperkeratosis with reduced to absent granular layer; keratinocytes may be vacuolated and contain lipid droplets

increased protein in cerebrospinal fluid

electrocardiographic and electroencephalographic abnormalities reported

Prognosis

phytanic acid–free diet or plasma exchanges may be beneficial

Discussion

infantile Refsum disease, a peroxisomal deficiency disorder (in addition to phytanic acid oxidase deficiency), has no cutaneous manifestations and should not be confused with Refsum disease

REFERENCES

McK 266500

Davies MG, Marks R, Dykes PJ, Reynolds D. Epidermal abnormalities in Refsum's disease. Br J Dermatol 1977;97:401–406

Flament-Durand J, Noel P, Rutsaert J, et al. A case of Refsum's disease: clinical, pathological, ultrastructural, and biochemical study. Pathol Eur 1971;6:172–191

Gibberd FB, Billimoria JD, Page NGR, Retsas S. Heredopathia atactica polyneuritiformis (Refsum's disease) treated by diet and plasma exchange. Lancet 1979;1:575–578

Masters-Thomas A, Bailes J, Billimoria JD, et al. Heredopathia atactica polyneuritiformis (Refsum's disease): I. Clinical features and dietary management. J Hum Nutr 1980;34:245–250

Poulos A, Pollard AX, Michell JD, et al. Patterns of Refsum's disease: phytanic acid oxidase deficiency. Arch Dis Child 1984; 59:222–229

Talwar D, Swaiman KF. Peroxisomal disorders: a review of a recently recognized group of clinical entities. Clin Pediatr 1987;26:497–504

DORFMAN-CHANARIN SYNDROME

Synonyms

- ichthyosis and neutral lipid storage disease
- neutral lipid storage disease
- DOC 12

Skin

generalized scaling, including flexures and face, with mild erythroderma, greatly resembling nonbullous congenital ichthyosiform erythroderma; occasional ectropion

nail abnormalities reported

Non-Skin

neurologic abnormalities include neurosensory deafness, mental retardation, nystagmus, and ataxia

bilateral cataracts, myopathy with or without muscle weakness and hepatosplenomegaly

Genetics

AR

Pathophysiology

neutral lipid storage disorder, possibly a triglyceride-related nonlysosomal storage disorder, but the specific defect is unknown and serum triglyceride levels are normal

Laboratory Data

intracellular lipid vacuoles are present in most granulocytes, monocytes, and cells of the liver, muscle, central nervous system, and epidermis; a peripheral smear may be diagnostic in the proper clinical setting

heterozygous carriers also have lipid vacuoles in granulocytes and monocytes

ichthyosis may be due to abnormal structure and dispersion of lamellar bodies and resultant abnormal cohesion and desquamation of corneocytes

Discussion

although ichthyosis and lipid vacuoles in the basal layer of epidermis occur in both the Dorfman-Chanarin syndrome and Refsum disease, increased serum levels of phytanic acid in the latter distinguish the two diseases

REFERENCES

McK 275630

Dorfman ML, Hershko C, Eisenberg S, Sagher F. Ichthyosiform dermatosis with systemic lipidosis. Arch Dermatol 1974;110:261–266

Elias PM, Williams ML. Neutral lipid storage disease with ichthyosis: defective lamellar body contents and intracellular dispersion. Arch Dermatol 1985;121:1000–1008

Srebrnik A, Tur E, Perluk C, et al. Dorfman-Chanarin syndrome: a case report and a review. J Am Acad Dermatol 1987;17:801–808

Venencie PY, Armengaud D, Foldès C, et al. Ichthyosis and neutral lipid storage disease (Dorfman-Chanarin syndrome). Pediatr Dermatol 1988;5:173–177

Williams ML, Koch TK, O'Donnell JJ, et al. Ichthyosis and neutral lipid storage disease. Am J Med Genet 1985;20:711–726

SJÖGREN-LARSSON SYNDROME

Synonym

- DOC 10

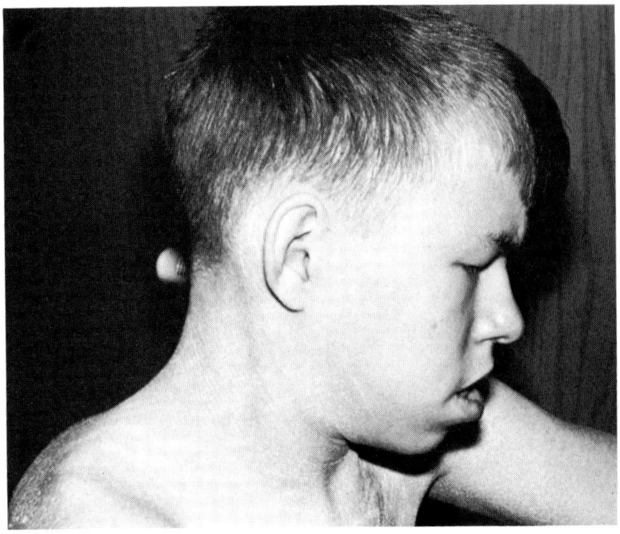

FIGURE 1–14
Ichthyosiform changes most pronounced on the neck and upper torso in a boy with Sjögren-Larsson syndrome.

Skin

see Figures 1–14 and 1–15

mild to moderate lamellar-like ichthyosis; present at birth or within first few months of life; becomes more pronounced in first year of life

generalized distribution, but most prominent on lower trunk, neck, and flexures; mild generalized erythema in some

mild to moderate palmoplantar hyperkeratosis

hair, nails, and sweat glands are normal

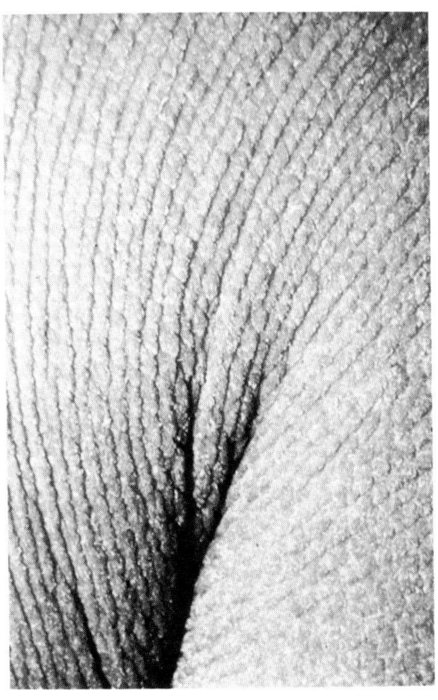

FIGURE 1–15
Close-up of skin of a patient with Sjögren-Larsson syndrome. Note the ridging of the scales and flexural involvement.

Non-Skin

usually, early severe mental retardation

other neurologic abnormalities include spastic diplegia or tetraplegia, which may be incapacitating; epilepsy occurs in one half of patients

eye abnormalities include atypical retinitis pigmentosa with "glistening dots" and "vitelliform" maculae resembling "sunny-side-up eggs" in about half of patients

short stature

Genetics

AR; most commonly seen in Sweden

Pathophysiology

fatty alcohol:nicotinamine adenine dinucleotide oxidoreductase activity is reduced; may be a primary enzymatic defect

Prognosis

total incapacitation and early mortality in some

improvement with restriction of dietary fat and supplementation with medium-chain triglycerides reported

REFERENCES

McK 270200

Jagell S, Gustavson K, Holmgren G. Sjögren-Larsson syndrome in Sweden: a clinical, genetic and epidemiological study. Clin Genet 1981;19:233–256

Jagell S, Lidén S. Ichthyosis in the Sjögren-Larsson syndrome. Clin Genet 1982; 21:243–252

Koone MD, Rizzo WB, Elias PM, et al. Ichthyosis, mental retardation, and asymptomatic spasticity: a new neurocutaneous syndrome with normal fatty alcohol: NAD+ oxidoreductase activity. Arch Dermatol 1990;126:1485–1490

Levisohn D, Dintiman B, Rizzo WB. Sjögren-Larsson syndrome: case reports. Pediatr Dermatol 1991;8:217–220

Rayner A, Lampert RP, Rennert OM. Familial ichthyosis, dwarfism, mental retardation, and renal disease. J Pediatr 1978;92:766–768

Rizzo WB, Dammann AL, Craft DA, et al. Sjögren-Larsson syndrome: inherited defect in the fatty alcohol cycle. J Pediatr 1989;115:228–234

X-LINKED DOMINANT CHONDRODYSPLASIA PUNCTATA

Synonyms

- Conradi disease
- Conradi-Hünermann syndrome
- DOC 17

Skin

widespread, ichthyosiform scaling eruption with characteristic whorled pattern on an erythematous background; present at birth (Fig. 1–16)

erythematous component clears early in life; ichthyosiform component may persist into adolescence or adulthood

occasional blotchy or striate hyperpigmentation, follicular atrophoderma, and scarring alopecia during childhood (Fig. 1–17)

erythroderma and ichthyosis may resolve; follicular atrophoderma and scarring alopecia persist

occasional palmoplantar keratoses

coarse and lusterless hair; sparse eyebrows and eyelashes; rare hair shaft defects

nail dystrophy and dental abnormalities reported

Non-Skin

abnormal craniofacies including frontal bossing, a flattened nasal bridge, malar hypoplasia ("flat-face"), and a high-arched palate (Fig. 1–18)

musculoskeletal abnormalities include asymmetrical thigh and upper extremity shortening, short stature, scoliosis, congenital hip dislocation, rib and vertebral anomalies, polydactyly, and flexion contractures of elbows and knees

ocular abnormalities including total or sectorial cataracts (in 50% to 75%; usually congenital and bilateral), optic atrophy, and microphthalmos; sectorial cataracts thought to be due to lyonization and analogous to patterned cutaneous lesions following Blaschko's lines

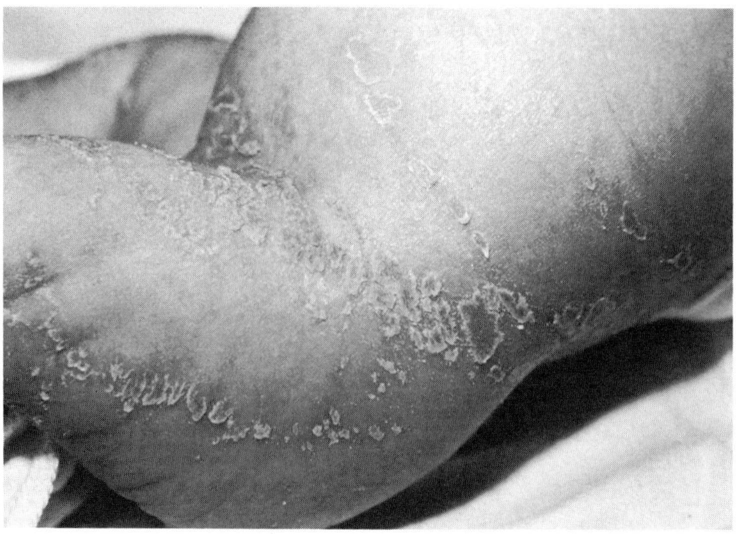

FIGURE 1–16
Patterned, egg shell–like, stuck-on scales following the lines of Blaschko in a patient with X-linked dominant chondrodysplasia punctata.

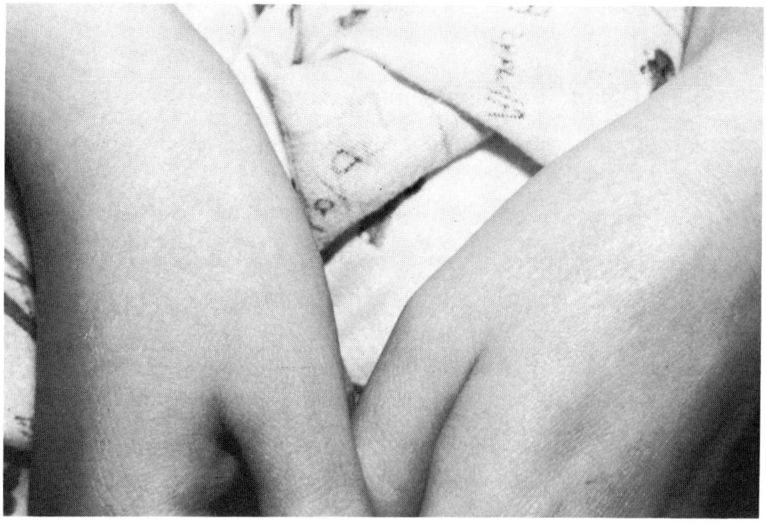

FIGURE 1–17
Follicular atrophoderma, a subtle cutaneous manifestation of X-linked dominant chondrodysplasia punctata, involving the arm and dorsum of the hand of a young girl.

Genetics

XLD; seen only in females

see discussion of AD, AR, and XLR forms of chondrodysplasia punctata

Pathophysiology

peroxisomal enzyme defect demonstrated, but not seen in all patients

FIGURE 1–18
Characteristic broad face with prominent forehead and markedly depressed nasal bridge in an infant with X-linked dominant chondrodysplasia punctata.

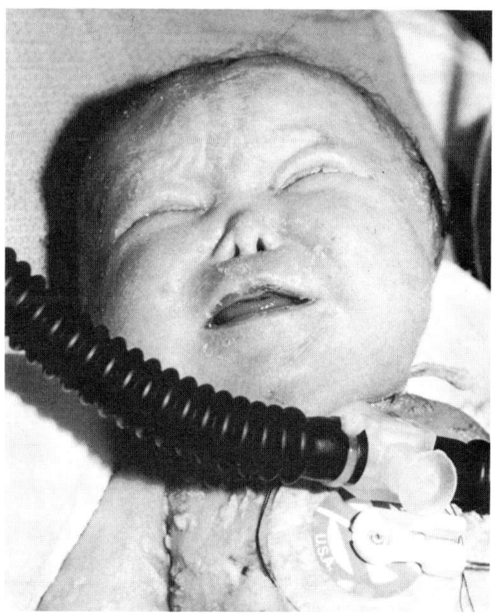

Laboratory Data

histopathology: basal layer hyperpigmentation and occasional needle-like calcium inclusions in epidermis

radiographs show widespread calcified stippling of cartilaginous epiphyses; detectable in utero or after birth but usually disappears within the first few months to years of life; disappearance of epiphyseal calcifications makes diagnosis more difficult in later years

Discussion

incomplete forms described (e.g., radiographic changes only or clinical changes only)

similar features (excepting skin changes) may be seen with maternal ingestion of coumarin during the first trimester

The nosologies of chondrodysplasia punctata and the Conradi-Hünermann syndrome are difficult. These diseases constitute a group of bone dysplasias with the common but variable findings of punctate epiphyseal calcification and abnormalities of eyes, skin, and other organs. The diseases are inherited in AD, AR, XLD, and XLR forms; the XLD form has the most prominent skin findings; the others are listed as variants (see later). Part of the difficulty in understanding these diseases is the inconsistent use of the term *chondrodysplasia punctata;* it has been used to refer to the radiographic changes alone (stippled calcification of the epiphyses), which are found in many different diseases, and as a descriptor for nomenclature for several of the individual diseases in this group.

REFERENCES

McK 302960

Crovato F, Rebora A. Acute skin manifestations of Conradi-Huenermann syndrome in a male adult. Arch Dermatol 1985;121: 1064–1065

Curry CJ, Magenis RE, Brown M, et al. Inherited chondrodysplasia punctata due to a deletion of the terminal short arm of an X chromosome. N Engl J Med 1984;311: 1010–1015

Hall JG, Pauli RM, Wilson KM. Maternal and fetal sequelae of anti-coagulant during pregnancy. Am J Med 1980;68:122–140

Happle R. X-linked dominant chondrodysplasia punctata: review of literature and report of a case. Hum Genet 1979;53:65–73

Happle R, Phillips RJ, Roessner A, et al. Homologous genes for X-linked chondrodysplasia punctata in man and mouse. Hum Genet 1983;63:24–27

Hosenfeld D, Wiedemann HR. Chondrodysplasia punctata in an adult recognized as vitamin K antagonist embryopathy. Clin Genet 1989;35:376–381

Kalter DC, Atherton DJ, Clayton PT. X-linked dominant Conradi-Hünermann syndrome presenting as congenital erythroderma. J Am Acad Dermatol 1989;21:248–256

Paltzik RL, Ente G, Penzer PH, Goldblum LM. Conradi-Hünermann disease: case report and mini-review. Cutis 1982;29:174–180

Prendiville JS, Zaparackas ZG, Esterly NB. Normal peroxisomal function and absent skeletal manifestations in Conradi-Hünermann syndrome. Arch Dermatol 1991;127: 539–542

Silengo MC, Luzzatti L, Silverman FN. Clinical and genetic aspects of Conradi-Hünermann disease: a report of three familial cases and review of the literature. J Pediatr 1980;97:911–917

CHONDRODYSPLASIA PUNCTATA, AD FORM

milder skeletal disease (dysplasia involves epiphyses only); better prognosis relative to other genetic forms of chondrodysplasia punctata

mostly reported as sporadic; may reflect a spontaneous mutation

---

McK 118650
Sheffield LJ, Danks DM, Mayne V, et al. Chondrodysplasia punctata: 23 cases of a mild and relatively common variety. J Pediatr 1976;89:916–923

CHONDROPLASIA PUNCTATA, AR FORM (CHONDRODYSPLASIA PUNCTATA II; CHONDRODYSPLASIA PUNCTATA, RHIZOMELIC DWARF TYPE)

mild widespread scaling and erythema in some; no follicular atrophoderma or patterned ichthyotic changes

severe musculoskeletal abnormalities include abnormal bone formation (metaphyseal and epiphyseal dysplasia), short bilateral proximal limbs, contractures, and abnormal facies

microcephaly, spasticity, severe psychomotor retardation, and failure to thrive

cataracts

peroxisomal enzyme defect

death in first year of life

McK 215100
Hoefler G, Hoefler S, Wattiers P, et al. Biochemical abnormalities in rhizomelic chondrodysplasia punctata. J Pediatr 1988;112:726–733

CHONDRODYSPLASIA PUNCTATA, X-LINKED RECESSIVE FORM

ichthyosis described in some families

musculoskeletal abnormalities include short stature and distal phalangeal hypoplasia

hypoplastic nares

mental retardation

failure to thrive

McK 302950
Curry CJR, Magers RE, Brown M, et al. Inherited chondrodysplasia punctata due to a deletion of the terminal short arm of an X chromosome. N Engl J Med 1984;311: 1010–1015

RUD SYNDROME

This entity is included for completeness only, since most authorities agree that Rud syndrome probably does not exist as a distinct entity; case reports probably represent other disorders.

McK 308200
Marxmiller J, Trenkle I, Ashwal S. Rud syndrome revisited: ichthyosis, mental retardation, epilepsy and hypogonadism. Dev Med Child Neurol 1985;27:335–343
Münke M, Kruse K, Goos M, et al. Genetic heterogeneity of the ichthyosis, hypogonadism, mental retardation, and epilepsy syndrome: clinical and biochemical investigations on two patients with Rud syndrome and review of the literature. Eur J Pediatr 1983;141:8–13

KERATITIS-ICHTHYOSIS-DEAFNESS SYNDROME

Synonyms

- KID syndrome
- ichthyosiform erythroderma–deafness-keratitis
- Wilson-Grayson-Pieroni syndrome
- Senter syndrome
- DOC 15

Skin

widely distributed, sharply circumscribed, erythematous, and thickened plaques, described as "leathery," "grainy," or "rugal"; present at birth

hyperkeratosis of the palms and soles with typical reticulated, stippled or moth-eaten pattern of surface elevations and depressions (Fig. 1–19)

characteristic perioral furrowing

occasional marked spiny follicular hyperkeratosis on the extremities and head (Fig. 1–20)

increased incidence of cutaneous bacterial and fungal infections and mucocutaneous squamous cell carcinoma; however, specific immune defect not yet identified

occasional hypohidrosis

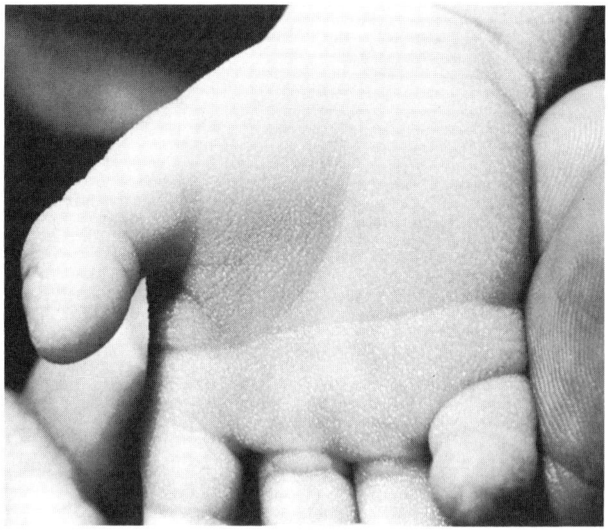

FIGURE 1–19
Reticulated hyperkeratosis of the palm, characteristic of patients with keratitis-ichthyosis-deafness syndrome.

hypotrichosis of scalp, eyelashes, and eyebrows; complete alopecia may result by age 2 years

aplastic or hypoplastic nails at birth; subsequently may be dystrophic

Non-Skin

photophobia and vascularized keratitis in early childhood

congenital sensorineural hearing loss (usually not entirely deaf) present from birth

increased incidence of otitis externa and otitis media

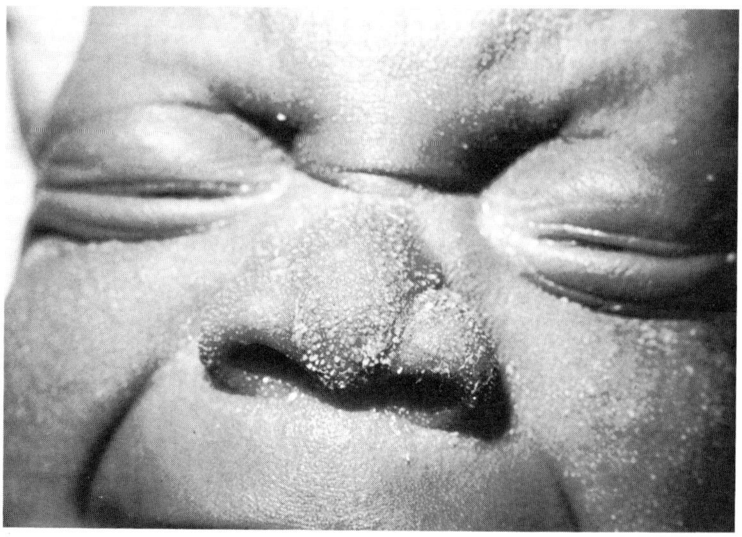

FIGURE 1–20
Multiple spiny follicular plugs over the nose of a newborn with keratitis-ichthyosis-deafness syndrome.

short stature, flexion contractures of the elbows and knees, and tight Achilles tendons

occasional dental abnormalities, including increased caries

Genetics

probably AD but most cases sporadic; AR kindreds also reported

Laboratory Data

histopathologic findings include basket-weave hyperkeratosis and follicular and occasional eccrine ostial plugging

Prognosis

retinoid therapy may worsen ophthalmic condition

Discussion

the use of the term *ichthyosis* is challenged by some authors, since the hyperkeratosis is not manifested as prominent fish-like scaling

REFERENCES

McK 148210
McK 242150 (AR form)
Grob JJ, Breton A, Bonafe JL, et al. Keratitis, ichthyosis, and deafness (KID) syndrome: vertical transmission and death from multiple squamous cell carcinomas. Arch Dermatol 1987;123:777–782
Harms M, Gilardi S, Levy PM, et al. KID syndrome (keratitis, ichthyosis, and deafness) and chronic mucocutaneous candidiasis: case report and review of the literature. Pediatr Dermatol 1984;2:1–7
Jurecka W, Aberer E, Mainitz M, et al. Keratitis, ichthyosis, and deafness syndrome with glycogen storage. Arch Dermatol 1985;121:799–801
Madariaga J, Fromowitz F, Phillips M, Hoover HCJ. Squamous cell carcinoma in congenital ichthyosis with deafness and keratitis: a case report and review of the literature. Cancer 1986;57:2026–2029
McGrae JD Jr. Keratitis, ichthyosis, and deafness (KID) syndrome. Int J Dermatol 1990; 29:89–93
Nazzaro V, Blanchet-Bardon C, Lorette G, Civatte J. Familial occurrence of KID (keratitis, ichthyosis, deafness) syndrome: case reports of a mother and daughter. J Am Acad Dermatol 1990;23:385–388
Skinner BA, Greist MC, Norins AL. The keratitis, ichthyosis, and deafness (KID) syndrome. Arch Dermatol 1981;117:285–289

FAMILIAL CONTINUAL SKIN PEELING

Synonyms

- peeling skin syndrome
- continual peeling skin syndrome
- DOC 21

Skin

there appear to be two presentations of familial skin peeling (see Laboratory Data for histopathologic differences):

- noninflammatory type:

  generalized desquamation, sparing palms and soles, usually beginning at birth or in infancy, or up to early second decade; may be pruritic

  hyperpigmentation may be noted, but lesions are usually without inflammatory changes; that is, there is no erythema or vesiculation

- inflammatory type:

  contrasting or additional features include generalized scaling erythematous plaques with rare vesiculation and hair that is easy to pull out

  worsens in summer

Genetics

probably AR

Pathophysiology

both proliferation hyperkeratosis and retention hyperkeratosis have been postulated as pathophysiologic mechanisms

Laboratory Data

histopathology: noninflammatory type shows intracorneal or subcorneal split; inflammatory type shows intracorneal or subcorneal split with additional hyperkeratosis, psoriasiform epidermal hyperplasia, and dermal inflammation

intercellular electron-dense globular deposits in stratum corneum reported, probably of lipid origin

Prognosis

persists lifelong

Discussion

superficial peeling of skin may appear similar to epidermolysis bullosa simplex superficialis (see Chapter 2)

REFERENCES

McK 270300

Abdel-Hafez K, Safer AM, Selim MM, Rehak A. Familial continual skin peeling. Dermatologica 1983;166:23–31

Dicken CH. Peeling skin syndrome. [Letter]. J Am Acad Dermatol 1985;13:158–160

Hacham-Zadeh S, Holubar K. Skin peeling syndrome in a Kurdish family. Arch Dermatol 1985;121:545–546

Levy SB, Goldsmith LA. The peeling skin syndrome. J Am Acad Dermatol 1982;7:606–613

Mevorah B, Frenk E, Saurat JH, Siegenthaler G. Peeling skin syndrome: a clinical, ultrastructural and biochemical study. Br J Dermatol 1987;116:117–125

Silverman AK, Ellis CN, Beals TF, et al. Continual skin peeling syndrome: an electron microscopic study. Arch Dermatol 1986;122:71–75

ERYTHROKERATODERMIA VARIABILIS

Synonyms

- Mendes da Costa syndrome
- keratosis rubra figurata
- DOC 18

Skin

both hyperkeratotic and erythrodermic components are seen; the former consist of persistent circinate, polycyclic plaques on the extremities, buttocks, and face and are separate or superimposed on erythrodermic patches of varying size, shape, and number; erythrodermic areas are transient, lasting hours to days (Figs. 1–21 and 1–22)

disease onset is usually after birth, occasionally at birth

hyperkeratotic lesions tend to increase in size until puberty, while erythrodermic lesions may diminish or disappear at puberty

Genetics

AD

Prognosis

course is chronic

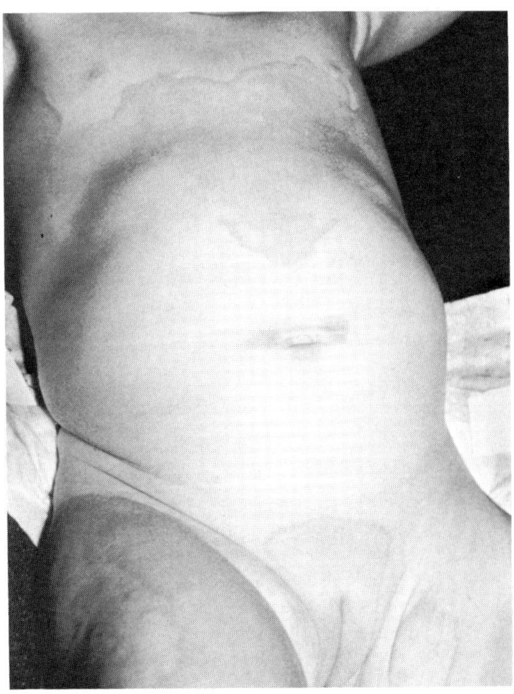

FIGURE 1–21
Erythrokeratodermia variabilis. Sharply demarcated plaques of yellow-red hyperkeratosis with a figurate border involving the torso, pubic area, and thighs.

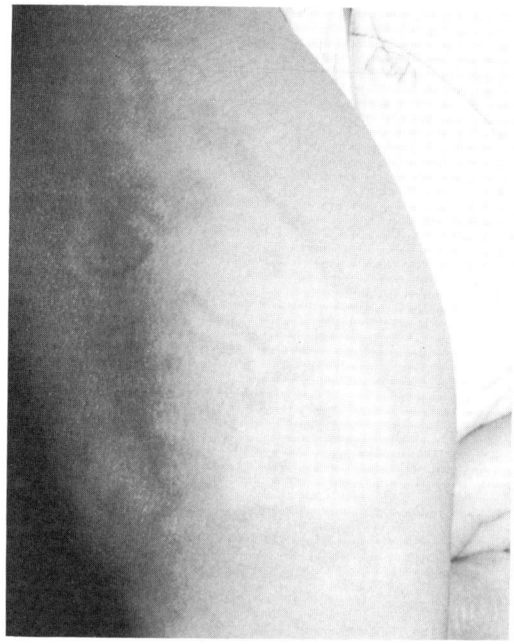

FIGURE 1–22
Erythrokeratodermia variabilis. Same patient as in Figure 1–21. Large hyperkeratotic plaque with figurate borders and areas of sparing on the thigh.

Discussion

some authors distinguish several variants (see below)

REFERENCES

McK 133200

Bond MJ, Donelan P, Fenske N. Erythrokeratodermia variabilis in a patient followed through the first year of life. Cutis 1982;30:633–637

Brown J, Kierland RR. Erythrokeratodermia variabilis. Arch Dermatol 1966;93:194–201

Cram DL. Erythrokeratoderma variabilis and variable circinate erythrokeratodermas. Arch Dermatol 1970;101:68–73

Gewirtzman GB, Winkler NW, Dobson RL. Erythrokeratodermia variabilis: a family study. Arch Dermatol 1978;114:259–261

Kelly LJ, Kocsard E. Congenital ichthyosis with erythema annulare centrifugum: a new form of ichthyosis affecting 12 members of a family of 31 in 5 generations. Dermatologica 1971;140:75–83

Luy JT, Jacobs AH, Nickoloff BJ. A child with erythematous and hyperkeratotic patches: erythrokeratodermia variabilis. Arch Dermatol 1988;124:1271–1272

Vakilzadeh F, Rose I. Erythrokeratodermia anularis migrans: eine neue Genodermatose? Hautarzt 1991;42:634–637

Vandersteen PR, Muller SD. Erythrokeratodermia variabilis: an enzyme, histochemical and ultrastructural study. Arch Dermatol 1971;103:362–370

ERYTHROKERATODERMIA WITH ATAXIA (DOC 23; GIROUX-BARBEAU SYNDROME)

acral papulosquamous plaques appearing shortly after birth, usually disappearing by adulthood

lesions may reappear in association with ataxia, dysarthria, nystagmus, and other neurologic signs

AD

McK 133190
Giroux JM, Barbeau A. Erythrokeratodermia with ataxia. Arch Dermatol 1972;106:183–188
Williams ML. A new look at the ichthyoses: disorders of lipid metabolism. Pediatr Dermatol 1986;3:476–486

CHIME SYNDROME

acronym for colobomata, heart defects, ichthyosiform dermatosis, mental retardation and ear defects; see Figures 1–23 and 1–24

migratory ichthyosiform dermatosis

defective dentition

bilateral retinal colobomas, distinctive craniofacies, broad second toe, seizures, conductive hearing loss, mental retardation, and congenital heart defects

probable AR

McK 280000
Zunich J, Esterly NB, Holbrook KA, et al. Congenital migratory ichthyosiform dermatosis with neurologic and ophthalmologic abnormalities. Arch Dermatol 1985;121: 1149–1156
Zunich J, Esterly NB, Kaye CI. Autosomal recessive transmission of neuroectodermal syndrome. [Letter]. Arch Dermatol 1988; 124:1188–1189
Zunich J, Kaye CI. Additional case report of new neuroectodermal syndrome. Am J Med Genet 1984;17:707–710

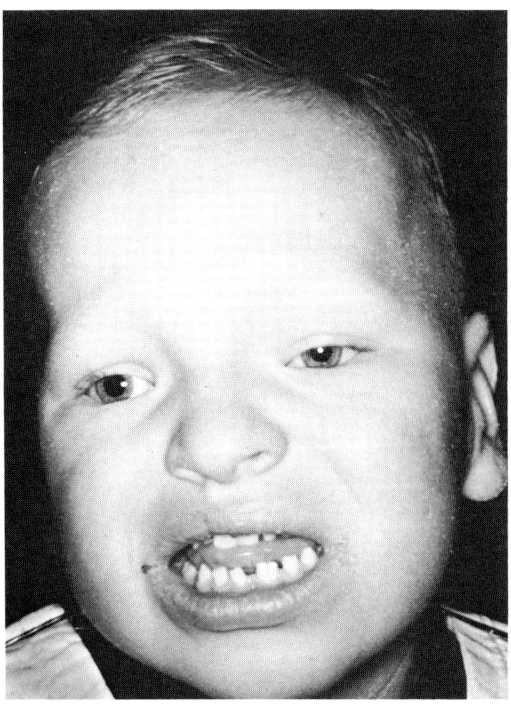

FIGURE 1–23
Characteristic facies of CHIME syndrome. Anomalous dentition and lamellar scaling of the cheeks.

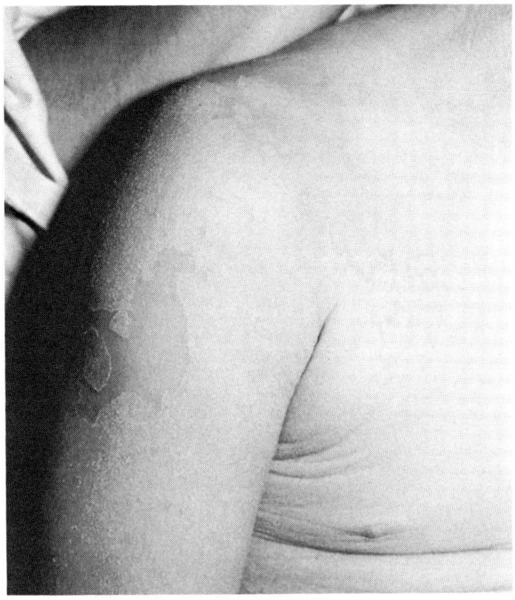

FIGURE 1–24
CHIME syndrome. Same patient as in Figure 1–23. A sharply demarcated scaly eruption with figurate borders is on the chest, shoulder, and arm. This eruption was migratory, with the pattern changing from week to week.

ERYTHROKERATODERMIA WITH DEAFNESS

skin findings as in erythrokeratodermia variabilis

retarded physical growth, neuropathy, and bilateral talipes due to neuropathy

AD

Beare JM, Nevin NC, Froggatt P, et al. Atypical erythrokeratodermia with deafness, physical retardation and peripheral neuropathy. Br J Dermatol 1972;87:308–314

Lamprecht A, Goecke T, Anton-Lamprecht I, Küster W. Progressive erythrokeratodermia and cochlear hearing impairment: a case report and review of the literature. Int J Pediatr Otorhinolaryngol 1988;15: 279–289

Schnyder VW, Wissler H, Wendt G. Eine weitere Form von atypischer Erythrokeratodermie mit Schwerborigkeit und cerebraler Schadigung. Helv Paediatr Acta 1968;23:220–230

ERYTHROKERATODERMIA EN COCARDES (DEGOS SYNDROME)

circinate erythematous lesions with central hyperkeratosis or scaling (resemble cockades or rosettes, hence "en cocardes") on buttocks, shoulder girdle, and legs, with onset in early childhood

lesions fade after a few weeks, except for hyperkeratotic lesions on knees and legs, but recur at irregular intervals

AD

Degos R, Delzant O, Morival H. Erytheme desquamatif en plaques, congenital et familial (genodermatose nouvelle?). Bull Soc Fr Derm Syph 1947;7:442
Griffiths WAD, Leigh IM, Marks R. Disorders of keratinization. In: Champion RH, Burton JL, Ebling FJG, eds. Textbook of Dermatology. Oxford, Blackwell Scientific Publications, 1992:1350

ERYTHROKERATOLYSIS HIEMALIS (DOC 19)

erythematous plaques on palms and soles with characteristic scaling; trunk and limbs may have symmetrical erythematous figurate lesions

full-thickness stratum corneum scale on lesions peels centrifugally in 2-month cycles, mostly in winter months, hence the term *hiemalis*

AD

histopatology: advancing edge shows necrosis of keratinocytes, absence of granular layer and parakeratosis

seen only in a limited population of South African Boers

McK 148370
Findlay GH, Morrison JG. Erythrokeratolysis hiemalis—keratolytic winter erythema or "Oudtshoorn skin": a new epidermal genodermatosis with its histological features. Br J Dermatol 1978;98:491–495

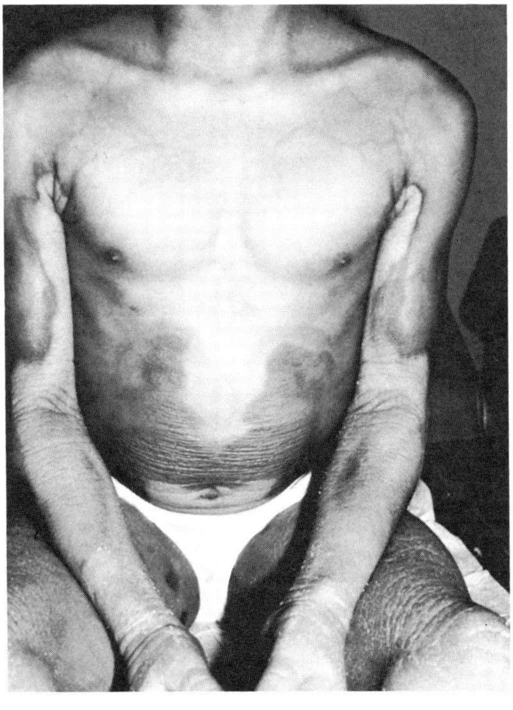

FIGURE 1–25
Symmetrical progressive erythrokeratodermia. Symmetrical hyperkeratotic plaques with erythema and figurate borders involving the arms, anterior torso, and portions of the legs.

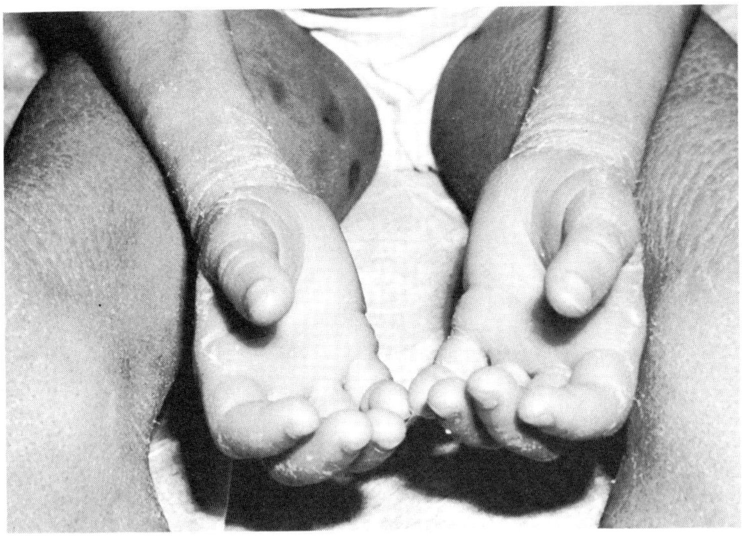

FIGURE 1–26
Symmetrical progressive erythrokeratodermia. Extreme hyperkeratosis of the palms with yellow discoloration.

SYMMETRICAL PROGRESSIVE ERYTHROKERATODERMIA (DOC 20; PROGRESSIVE SYMMETRICAL ERYTHROKERATODERMIA; GOTTRON SYNDROME)

symmetrical, well-defined, keratotic plaques on erythematous bases on the extremities (knees, elbows, feet, dorsa of hands and fingers, and shins), buttocks, and occasionally face, palms, and soles (Figs. 1–25 and 1–26)

onset usually in infancy or early childhood, rarely in adulthood

lesions usually most severe at puberty, but then may regress

symmetrical and fixed nature of lesions often striking, especially in comparison with those of erythrokeratodermia variabilis

AD with incomplete penetrance and variable expressivity; some sporadic and possible AR cases also reported

Nazzaro V, Blanchet-Bardon C. Progressive symmetric erythrokeratodermia: histological and ultrastructural study of patient before and after treatment with etretinate. Arch Dermatol 1986;122:434–440

Nir M, Tanzer F. Progressive symmetric erythrokeratodermia. Dermatologica 1978;156: 268–273

Rodriguez-Pichardo A, Garcia-Bravo B, Sanchez-Pedreño P, et al. Progressive symmetric erythrokeratodermia. [Letter]. J Am Acad Dermatol 1988;19:129–130

Ruiz-Maldonado R, Tamayo L, del Castillo V, et al. Erythrokeratodermia progressiva symmetrica: report of 10 cases. Dermatologica 1982;164:133–141

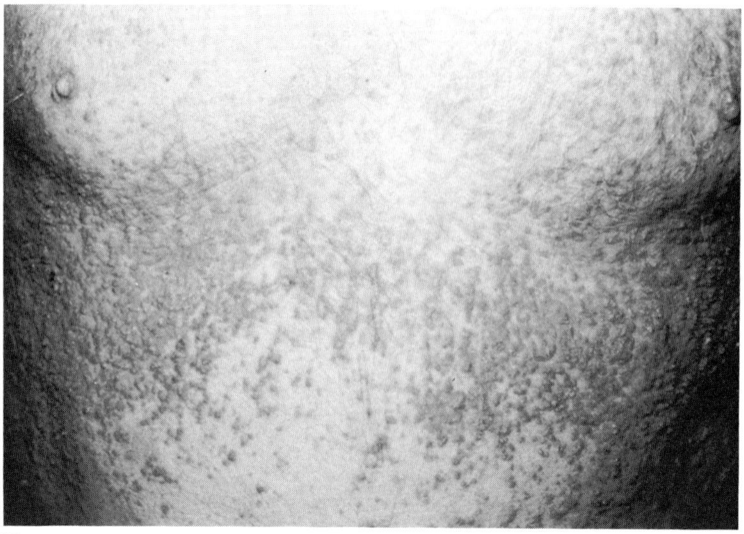

FIGURE 1–27
Darier disease. "Greasy" keratotic papules in a symmetrical distribution on the torso. (Courtesy of Benjamin K. Fisher, MD, Toronto, Ontario)

Darier Disease

Synonyms

- DOC 22
- keratosis follicularis
- Darier-White disease

Skin

skin-colored, yellow-brown, or brown "greasy" keratotic papules on the face (often the first finding), scalp, chest, back, extremities, and skin

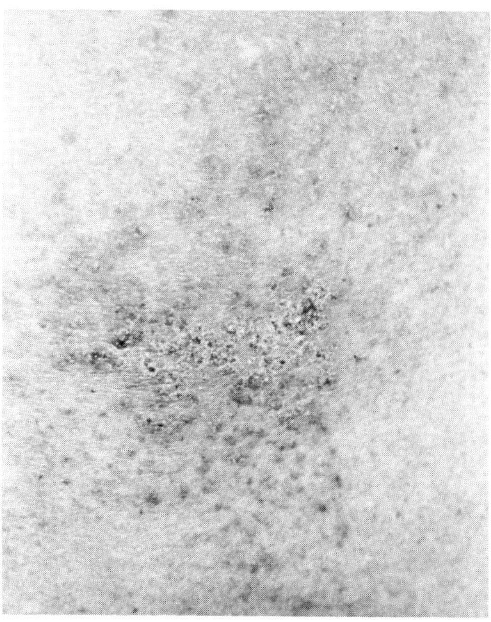

FIGURE 1–28
A closer view of Darier disease showing the development of numerous follicular lesions.

folds, especially in a seborrheic distribution; coalescence of papules may produce warty, vegetative, malodorous plaques, especially in flexures (Figs. 1–27 and 1–28)

skin changes are usually found in childhood, but may first manifest as late as the seventh decade

keratotic papules on dorsa of hands and feet (cf. similar lesions in acrokeratosis verruciformis of Hopf) (Fig. 1–29)

punctate palmoplantar keratoses or minute pits; rarely, diffuse yellow palmoplantar keratoderma

hypopigmented macules (leukoderma) on the trunk and limbs

increased incidence of chronic pyogenic infections

sunlight may exacerbate cutaneous eruption (Koebner phenomenon)

mucous membrane abnormalities include small papules, sometimes "cobblestoned," involving oral mucosa; pharyngeal, esophageal, laryngeal, vulval, vaginal, and rectal mucosae may also be involved; occasional gingival hypertrophy

rare scalp involvement may result in permanent alopecia

red, gray, or white longitudinal streaks or ridging of nails; distal V-shaped notching of distal end of the nail plate; subungual hyperkeratosis (Fig. 1–30)

Non-Skin

rare mental deficiency, epilepsy, and small stature

Genetics

AD; spontaneous mutations common

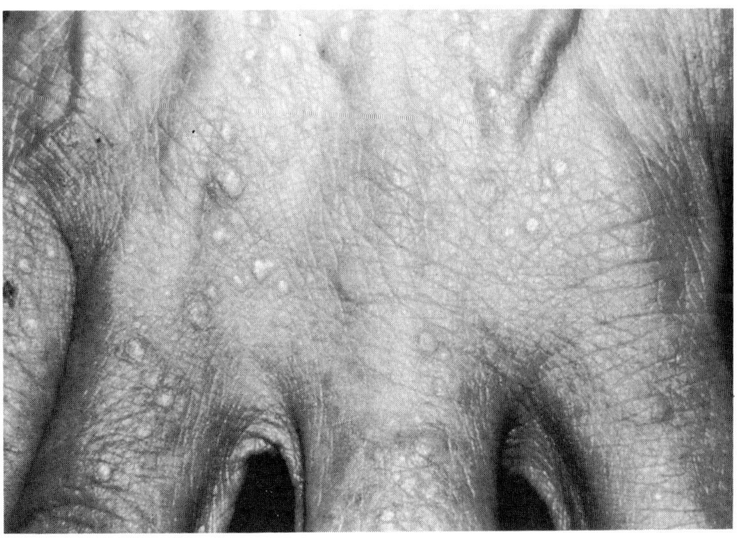

FIGURE 1–29
Many tiny acral verrucous papules. This is known as acrokeratosis verruciformis. It is seen in Darier disease and as an isolated syndrome.

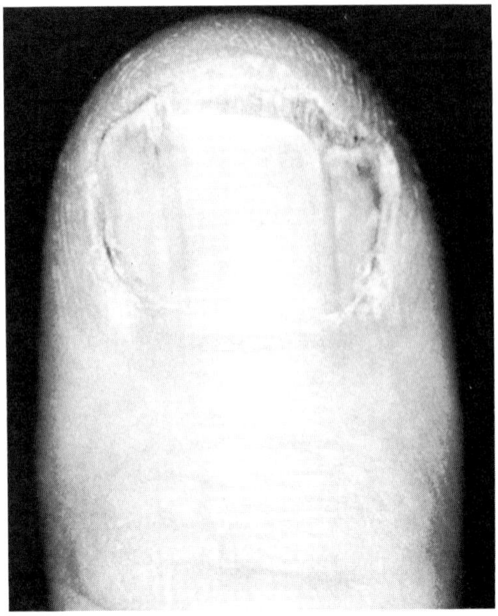

FIGURE 1–30
Nail dystrophy of Darier disease. Note the longitudinal streaks and the V-shaped notching of the distal edge of the nail plate. (Courtesy of Edward A. Krull, MD, Detroit, Michigan)

Laboratory Data

histopathology: acantholytic dyskeratosis (corps ronds, grains, and suprabasal clefts and lacunae; hyperkeratosis, acanthosis, and papillomatosis)

Prognosis

as in many widespread dermatoses, patients have an increased incidence of Kaposi's varicelliform eruption

good response to retinoids (etretinate more than isotretinoin); systemic antibiotics beneficial during flares

surgical excision may be helpful in hyperkeratotic variants

Discussion

linear or zosteriform cases reported, but these may represent epidermal nevi with acantholytic dyskeratosis; vesiculobullous variant also described

REFERENCES

McK 124200

Beck AL Jr, Finocchio AF, White JP. Darier's disease: a kindred with a large number of cases. Br J Dermatol 1977;97:335–339

Burge SM, Wilkinson JD. Darier-White disease: a review of the clinical features in 163 patients. J Am Acad Dermatol 1992; 27:40–50

Ferris T, Lamey PJ, Rennie JS. Darier's disease: oral features and genetic aspects. Br Dent J 1990;168:71–73

Munro CS. The phenotype of Darier's disease: penetrance and expressivity in adults and children. Br J Dermatol 1992;127:126–130

Peck GL, Kraemer KH, Wetzel B, et al. Cornifying Darier's disease—a unique variant. Arch Dermatol 1976;112:495–503

Peck GL, Yoder FW. Treatment of lamellar ichthyosis and other keratinising dermatoses with an oral synthetic retinoid. Lancet 1976;2:1172–1174

Ackrokeratosis Verruciformis

Synonym

- acrokeratosis verruciformis of Hopf

Skin

flat, wart-like or lichenoid papules on dorsa of hands and feet; extensor aspects of fingers, wrists, forearms and knees may be involved (see Fig. 1–29)

onset at birth or early childhood

occasional punctate keratoses of palms and soles

white, thickened, and ridged nails in some

Genetics

AD

Laboratory Data

histopathology: hyperorthokeratosis, acanthosis, papillomatosis ("church spires"), and prominent hypergranulosis; may have acantholysis, corps ronds, and grains as in Darier disease

Discussion

some authors consider acrokeratosis verruciformis a forme fruste of keratosis follicularis, with which it has been associated in some cases

REFERENCES

McK 101900
Niedelman ML, McKusick VA. Acrokeratosis verruciformis (Hopf): a follow-up study. Arch Dermatol 1962;86:779–782
Panja RK. Acrokeratosis verruciformis (Hopf)—a clinical entity? Br J Dermatol 1977;96:643–652
Schueller WA. Acrokeratosis verruciformis of Hopf. Arch Dermatol 1972;106:81–83

VAN DEN BOSCH SYNDROME

acrokeratosis verruciformis with anhidrosis, skeletal deformities, mental deficiency, and choroideremia

XLR

McK 314500
Van den Bosch J. A new syndrome in three generations of a Dutch family. Ophthalmologica 1959;137:422–423

Hyperkeratosis Lenticularis Perstans

Synonym

- Flegel disease

Skin

hyperkeratotic papules on legs and feet; may involve other areas of body; pinpoint depressions of the palms and soles are common (Fig. 1–31)

variable onset, usually in fourth to seventh decades

lesions progressive; do not remit

very rarely involves the oral mucosa

Genetics

AD

more common in women

Laboratory Data

histopathology: distinctive pattern of hyperkeratosis overlying epidermal atrophy and focal lichenoid infiltrate

electron microscopy: lamellar granules may be abnormal

Discussion

high incidence of cutaneous carcinoma (not arising in keratoses) in one family

FIGURE 1–31
Hyperkeratosis lenticularis perstans. Multiple hyperkeratotic papules with surrounding erythema. (Courtesy of Benjamin K. Fisher, MD, Toronto, Ontario)

REFERENCES

McK 144150

Beveridge GW, Langlands AO. Familial hyperkeratosis lenticularis perstans associated with tumours of the skin. Br J Dermatol 1973;88:453–458

Fathy S, Azadeh B. Hyperkeratosis lenticularis perstans. Int J Dermatol 1988;27:120–121

Flegel H. Hyperkeratosis lenticularis perstans. Hautarzt 1958;9:362–364

Pearson LH, Smith JGJ, Chalker DK. Hyperkeratosis lenticularis perstans (Flegel's disease): case report and literature review. J Am Acad Dermatol 1987;16:190–195

Price ML, Jones EW, MacDonald DM. A clinicopathological study of Flegel's disease (hyperkeratosis lenticularis perstans). Br J Dermatol 1987;116:681–691

Tidman MJ, Price ML, MacDonald DM. Lamellar bodies in hyperkeratosis lenticularis perstans. J Cutan Pathol 1987;14:207–211

Kyrle Disease

Synonym

- hyperkeratosis follicularis et parafollicularis in cutem penetrans

Skin

brownish red follicular and nonfollicular papules measuring 0.5 to 1.5 cm with central keratotic "cone-shaped" plugs found most commonly on the lower extremities (Fig. 1–32); in order of decreasing frequency, the upper extremities, head, neck, dorsa of feet, trunk, buttocks, and breasts may be involved; the palms, soles, and mucosae are not affected

the papules may coalesce into polycyclic verrucous plaques, especially on extensor extremities, while linear arrangements are more typical on ankles and in the antecubital and popliteal fossae

onset is usually in the third to seventh decades

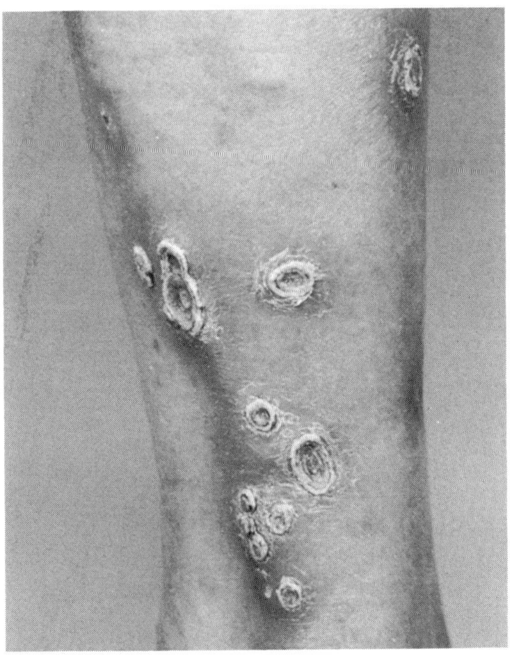

FIGURE 1–32
Kyrle disease. Multiple keratotic papules with characteristic central plugs distributed over the lower extremity. (Courtesy of Benjamin K. Fisher, MD, Toronto, Ontario)

Non-Skin

incidence of diabetes mellitus may be more common than in the general population

Genetics

although most cases are sporadic, AD cases reported

Laboratory Data

histopathology: epidermal invagination with keratotic plug containing parakeratotic column and basophilic debris; invaginations occur at both follicular and extrafollicular sites with occasional sites of penetration into dermis

Prognosis

persistent

Discussion

one of the perforating disorders

similar lesions occur in patients with chronic renal failure on hemodialysis

REFERENCES

McK 149500

Abele DC, Dobson RL. Hyperkeratosis penetrans (Kyrle's disease): report of a case in a Negro with autopsy findings. Arch Dermatol 1961;83:277–283

Carter VH, Constantine VS. Kyrle's disease: I. Clinical findings in five cases and review of literature. Arch Dermatol 1968;97:624–632

Constantine VS, Carter VH. Kyrle's disease: II. Histopathologic findings in five cases and review of the literature. Arch Dermatol 1968;97:633–639

Cunningham SR, Walsh M, Mathews R, et al. Kyrle's disease. J Am Acad Dermatol 1987;16:117–123

Reactive Perforating Collagenosis

Skin

umbilicated keratotic papules 5 to 10 mm in size in areas of trauma (prominent Koebner phenomenon), mostly on extremities (Fig. 1–33); onset in infancy and childhood

individual lesions involute within about 2 months, but new lesions continue to appear

Genetics

AR; some cases are AD

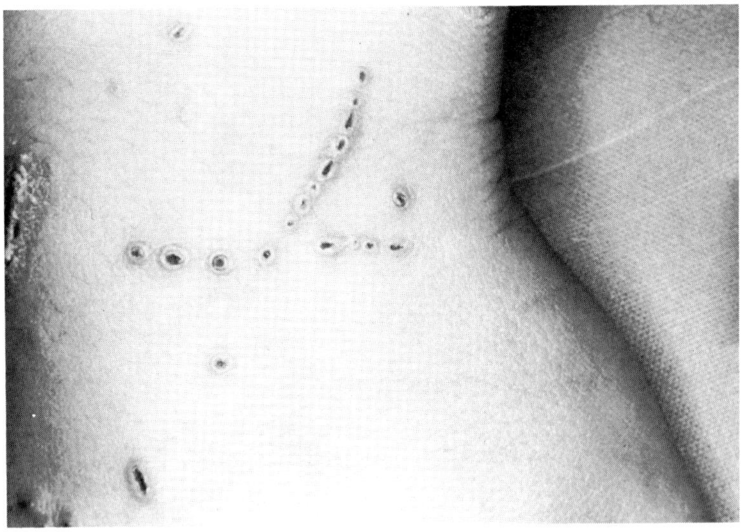

FIGURE 1–33
Reactive perforating collagenosis. Umbilicated hyperkeratotic papules, some in linear array, on the limb of a child. (Courtesy of Benjamin K. Fisher, MD, Toronto, Ontario)

Laboratory Data

histopathology: cup-shaped epidermal invagination with central perforation; necrobiotic basophilic bundles of collagen in dermis underlying and within epidermal perforation

Discussion

one of the perforating disorders

- *collagenoma perforans verruciforme*

  a variant form of reactive perforating collagenosis with verrucous lesions of reactive perforating collagenosis occurring in intertriginous areas as a single episode resulting from pronounced trauma; elastic fibers partially preserved in the central plug, unlike in reactive perforating collagenosis

  acquired

REFERENCES

McK 216700

Beck HI, Brandrup F, Hagdrup HK, et al. Adult, acquired reactive perforating collagenosis: report of a case including ultrastructural findings. J Cutan Pathol 1988; 15:124–128

Kanan MW. Familial reactive perforating collagenosis and intolerance to cold. Br J Dermatol 1974;91:405–414

Nair BK, Sarojini PA, Basheer AM, Nair CH. Reactive perforating collagenosis. Br J Dermatol 1974;91:399–403

Nyfors A, Mehregan AH. Reactive perforating collagenosis (Mehregan): report of two new cases and review of literature. Acta Derm Venereol 1973;53:375–380

Patterson JW. The perforating disorders. [Review]. J Am Acad Dermatol 1984;10:561–581

Elastosis Perforans Serpiginosa

Synonym

- Lutz disease

Skin

keratotic papules, 2 to 5 mm in size, in annular or serpiginous distribution, most commonly on nape and sides of neck (Fig. 1–34); may also involve upper extremities, face, lower extremities, or trunk

onset usually in second decade; most patients have onset before the fourth decade

lesions commonly scar when they resolve

Non-Skin

congenital cataracts and mental retardation reported

Genetics

most cases are sporadic, but AD, AR, and familial cases also reported (see discussion for disease associations)

Laboratory Data

histopathology: necrotic elastic fibers and other debris discharged through a complex epidermal sinus tract

electron microscopy: in penicillamine-induced elastosis perforans serpiginosa, elastic fibers show sac-like protuberances from their edges likened in appearance to "twigs of a bramble bush"

Prognosis

new lesions slowly appear as others resolve; overall eruption is persistent

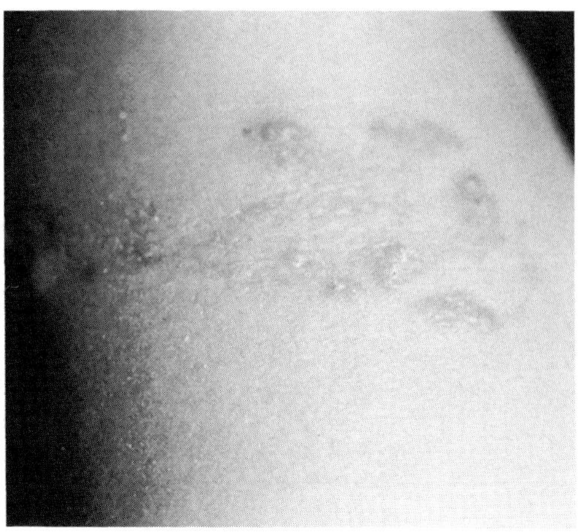

FIGURE 1–34
Elastosis perforans serpiginosa. This lesion shows several protuberant nodules amid an overall annular pattern.

Discussion

more than 25% of cases are associated with heritable disorders, usually of connective tissue, including Down syndrome, Marfan syndrome, osteogenesis imperfecta, Ehlers-Danlos syndrome, pseudoxanthoma elasticum, and Rothmund-Thomson syndrome

some authors classify elastosis perforans serpiginosa into three varieties: idiopathic, reactive (e.g., associated with connective tissue disorders), and drug-induced (e.g., in patients on penicillamine therapy, most often in patients with Wilson disease)

REFERENCES

McK 130100

Ayala F, Donofrio P. Elastosis perforans serpiginosa: report of a family. Dermatologica 1983;166:32–37

Bergman R, Friedman-Birnbaum R, Ludatscher R, et al. An ultrastructural study of the reactive type of elastosis perforans serpiginosa. [Letter]. Arch Dermatol 1987; 123:1127–1129

Langeveld-Wildschut EG, Toonstra J, van Vloten WA, Beemer FA. Familial elastosis perforans serpiginosa. Arch Dermatol 1993; 129:205–207

Rapini RP, Herbert AA, Drucker CR. Acquired perforating dermatosis: evidence for combined transepidermal elimination of both collagen and elastic fibers. Arch Dermatol 1989;125:1074–1078

Schamroth JM, Kellen P, Grieve TP. Elastosis perforans serpiginosa in a patient with renal disease. Arch Dermatol 1986;122:82–84

Woerdeman MJ, Bour DJH, Bijlsma JB. Elastosis perforans serpiginosa: report of a family with a chromosomal investigation. Arch Dermatol 1965;92:559–560

Follicular Syndromes With Atrophy and Inflammation

ATROPHODERMA VERMICULATUM

Synonyms

- honeycomb atrophy
- atrophoderma reticulatum
- folliculitis ulerythematosa reticulata

Skin

erythematous papules with follicular plugging; symmetrically distributed over cheeks, preauricular areas, and forehead; upper lip, chin, and ears may also be involved (Fig. 1–35)

onset is usually from 3 to 12 years of age, but presence at birth has been reported

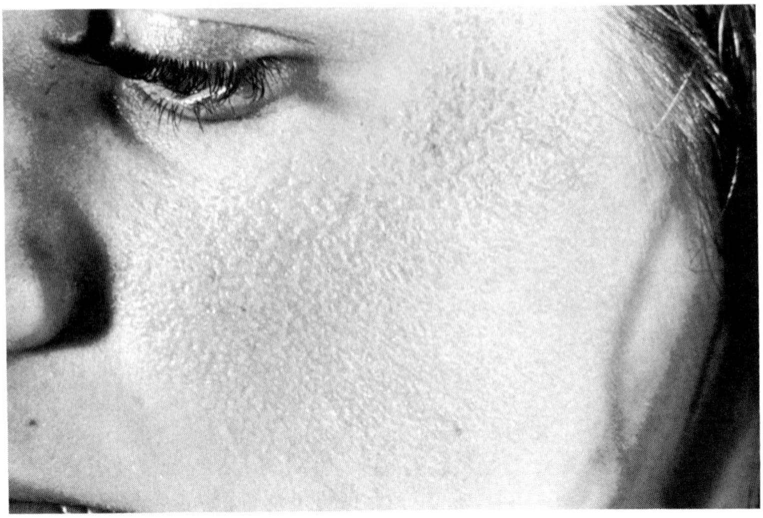

FIGURE 1–35
Atrophoderma vermiculatum. There are both erythema of the cheeks and numerous tiny patulous follicles. (Courtesy of Helmut Kerl, MD, Graz, Austria)

lesions subsequently develop follicular atrophy and pit-like depressions, resulting in a honeycomb, reticular, or worm-eaten appearance; occasional milia and telangiectases

keratosis pilaris elsewhere on body

Genetics

AD in some cases, but most are sporadic

Prognosis

inflammatory lesions frequently resolve spontaneously; dermabrasion may improve the appearance of scarring

Discussion

reports of coexistence with other cutaneous and internal (e.g., renal and central nervous system) abnormalities

chloracne, an acquired condition, may have scarring resembling atrophoderma vermiculatum, especially in many cases of dioxin-induced chloracne (e.g., in the Seveso, Italy, accident)

REFERENCES

McK 209700

Arrieta E, Milgram SY. Honeycomb atrophy on the right cheek: folliculitis ulerythematosa reticulata (atrophoderma vermiculatum). Arch Dermatol 1988;124:1101

Barron DR, Hirsch AL, Buchbinder L, et al. Folliculitis ulerythematosus reticulata: a report of four cases and brief review of the literature. Pediatr Dermatol 1987;4:85–89

Frosch PJ, Brumage MR, Schuster PC, Bersch A. Atrophoderma vermiculatum: case reports and review. J Am Acad Dermatol 1988;18:538–542

KERATOSIS FOLLICULARIS SPINULOSA DECALVANS

Synonyms

- DOC 24
- keratosis pilaris decalvans

Skin

spiny, follicular, noninflammatory keratoses; onset in infancy

initially involves face; during infancy or childhood may spread to scalp, dorsa of hands and fingers, trunk, and limbs

lesions resolve with follicular atrophy and milia formation; red-brown hyperpigmentation with telangiectases develops on cheeks and brows

characteristic patchy, scarring alopecia of eyebrows and scalp develops in late childhood or adolescence; may resemble ophiasis

occasional palmoplantar keratoderma

normal nails and teeth

Non-Skin

photophobia

occasional conjunctivitis, corneal opacities, and corneal vascularization due to trauma from hyperkeratotic eyelids

Genetics

XLD or XLR inheritance proposed for certain pedigrees

usually less severe in females

Discussion

may resemble atrichia with papular lesions or keratosis-ichthyosis-deafness syndrome

REFERENCES

McK 308800

Kuokkanen K. Keratosis follicularis spinulosa decalvans in a family from northern Finland. Acta Derm Venereol 1971;51:146–150

Rand R, Baden HP. Keratosis follicularis spinulosa decalvans: report of two cases and literature review. Arch Dermatol 1983;119:22–26

Van Osch LDM, Oranje AP, Keukens FM, et al. Keratosis follicularis spinulosa decalvans: a family study of seven male cases and six female carriers. J Med Genet 1992;29:36–40

ICHTHYOSIS FOLLICULARIS WITH ALOPECIA AND PHOTOPHOBIA

see Figure 1–36

onset at birth

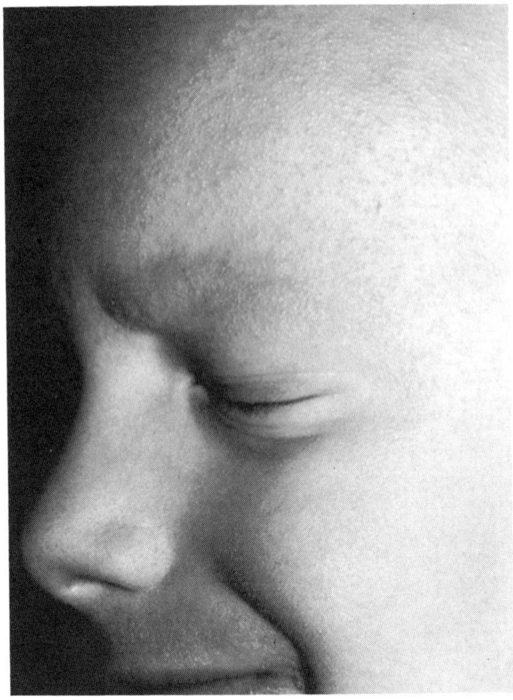

FIGURE 1–36
Ichthyosis follicularis with alopecia and photophobia. Numerous spiny follicular papules distributed over the forehead and lateral face associated with sparseness of the eyebrows.

thought by some to be a synonym of keratosis follicularis spinulosa decalvans, but ichthyosis follicularis with alopecia and photophobia has different onset and lacks follicular scarring, palmoplantar hyperkeratoses, telangiectases, and hyperpigmentation; also, alopecia is generalized rather than patchy

possibly XLR

histopathology: normal granular layer; accentuation of hyperkeratosis at follicular orifices

"follicular ichthyosis" described by Hazell and Marks may be a distinct syndrome, but some authors consider it to be the cutaneous manifestations of ichthyosis follicularis with alopecia and photophobia

McK 308205
Eramo LR, Esterly NB, Zieserl EJ, et al. Ichthyosis follicularis with alopecia and photophobia. Arch Dermatol 1985;121:1167–1174
Hazell M, Marks, R. Follicular ichthyosis. Br J Dermatol 1984;111:101–109
Rothe MJ, Weiss DS, Dubner BH, et al. Ichthyosis follicularis in two girls: an autosomal dominant disorder. Pediatr Dermatol 1990; 7:287–292
Traupe H: The Ichthyoses: A Guide to Clinical Diagnosis, Genetic Counseling and Therapy. Berlin, Springer Verlag, 1989:203–206
Zeligman I, Fleisher TL. Ichthyosis follicularis. Arch Dermatol 1959;80:413–420

ULERYTHEMA OPHRYOGENES

Synonyms

- keratosis pilaris atrophicans faciei

- keratosis pilaris rubra atrophicans faciei
- KPAF
- keratosis pilaris of Brocq
- folliculitis rubra

Skin

erythema of lateral third of eyebrows with or without follicular papules and plugging; onset at birth or early infancy (Fig. 1–37)

followed by gradual medial extension along eyebrows, development of alopecia, and atrophy of affected areas

may progress to cheeks and forehead

keratosis pilaris of extensor extremities

Non-Skin

may be associated with atopy or mental retardation

previous reports of associated renal disease and diabetes mellitus have been refuted

Genetics

AD in some; unclear inheritance in other cases

Discussion

some distinguish the synonyms by initial involvement on the cheeks in keratosis pilaris rubra atrophicans faciei and in the eyebrows in ulerythema ophryogenes

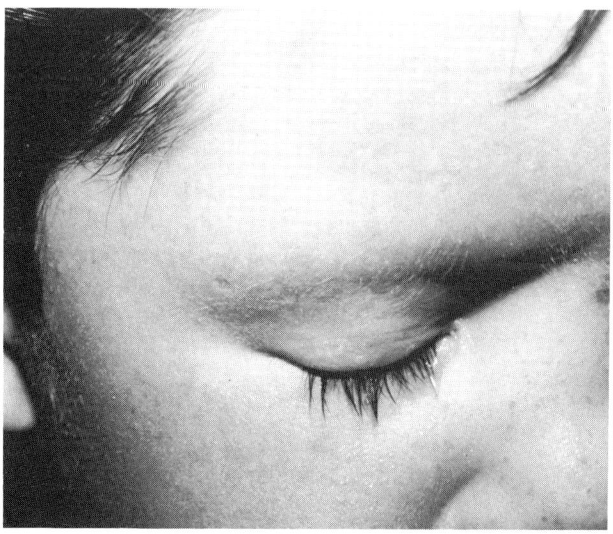

FIGURE 1–37
Ulerythema ophryogenes. Erythema, pitted scarring, follicular papules, and sparseness of the eyebrows in a patient with Noonan syndrome.

REFERENCES

Burnett JW, Schwartz MF, Berberian BJ. Ulerythema ophryogenes with multiple congenital anomalies. J Am Acad Dermatol 1988;18:437–440

Davenport DE. Ulerythema ophryogenes: review and report of a case: discussion of relationship to certain other skin disorders and association with internal abnormalities. Arch Dermatol 1964;89:74–80

Neild VS, Pegum JS, Wells RS. The association of keratosis pilaris atrophicans and woolly hair, with and without Noonan's syndrome. Br J Dermatol 1984;110:357–362

Pierini DO, Pierini AM. Keratosis pilaris atrophicans faciei (ulerythema ophryogenes): a cutaneous marker in the Noonan syndrome. Br J Dermatol 1979;100:409–416

FAMILIAL DYSKERATOTIC COMEDONES

Synonym

- familial comedones

Skin

up to thousands of comedones on almost all areas of body, generally sparing the scalp, mucous membranes, palms, and soles; usually asymptomatic, occasionally pruritic

lesions are first noted on the face, usually at 10 to 15 years of age

inflammatory acne lesions may coexist

Genetics

AD; males are more severely affected than females

Laboratory Data

histopathology: foci of dyskeratosis and acantholysis in base of the epidermal invaginations; occasional poorly formed corps ronds

REFERENCES

McK 120450

Carneiro SJC, Dickson JE, Knox JM. Familial dyskeratotic comedones. Arch Dermatol 1972;105:249–251

Hall JR, Holder W, Knox JM, et al. Familial dyskeratotic comedones: a report of three cases and review of the literature. J Am Acad Dermatol 1987;17:808–814

Harper KE, Spielvogel RL. Nevus comedonicus of the palm and wrist: case report with review of five previously reported cases. J Am Acad Dermatol 1985;12:185–188

Leppard BJ. Familial dyskeratotic comedones. Clin Exp Dermatol 1982;7:329–332

MULTIPLE MINUTE DIGITATE HYPERKERATOSIS

hundreds of asymptomatic, nonfollicular, keratotic, spiny or flat papules 1 to 3 mm in size, usually on back and chest

onset in second or third decade

AD

Balus L, Donati P, Amantea A, et al. Multiple minute digitate hyperkeratosis. J Am Acad Dermatol 1988;18:431–436

Palmoplantar Keratodermas

There are many types of palmoplantar keratodermas, and many classification schemes. Classification by etiology divides them into primary and secondary types, and classification by clinical presentation divides them into diffuse and punctate types. Extension of hyperkeratosis beyond the palmar or plantar surfaces onto the lateral or dorsal surfaces is called a "transgrediens" pattern. Most forms of palmoplantar keratoderma are inherited as an autosomal dominant trait, and many of the forms are represented by single pedigrees. In some pedigrees, isolated palmar or plantar involvement is seen. Numerous isolated cases of palmoplantar keratoderma have been associated with a spectrum of abnormalities of ectodermal or mesodermal origin (e.g., acanthosis nigricans, congenital deafness, hypothyroidism or hyperthyroidism, onychomadesis, and vitiligo), some of which are listed in the abbreviated entries section at the end of the chapter.

Clarke DB. Keratotic lesions of the palms and soles. J Assoc Milit Dermatol 1975;1:50–56
Sybert VP, Dale BA, Holbrook KA. Palmar-plantar keratoderma: a clinical, ultrastructural, and biochemical study. J Am Acad Dermatol 1988;18:75–86

DIFFUSE PALMOPLANTAR KERATODERMA

Synonym

- Unna-Thost syndrome

Skin

sharply circumscribed palmoplantar hyperkeratosis and flexural digit skin thickening; dorsal digits and knees may be also be involved (Figs. 1–38 and 1–39)

onset usually at age 3 to 12 months, rarely as late as adolescence

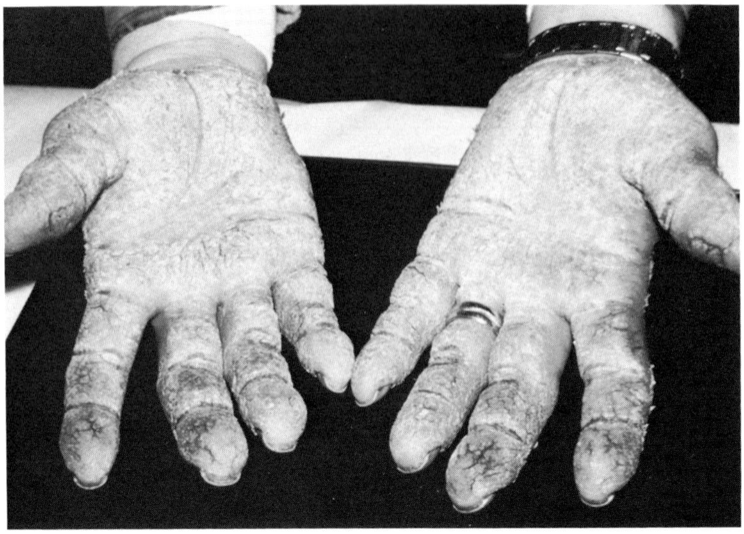

FIGURE 1–38
Diffuse palmoplantar keratoderma (Unna-Thost syndrome). Marked hyperkeratosis of the palms and volar aspects of the fingers with deep fissures in some areas.

keratoderma increases gradually, peaks in second and third decades; lesions persistent throughout life; worse in winter

hyperhidrosis of affected areas may develop

high prevalence of dermatophyte infections, which may result in painful fissuring

hair and teeth normal

nails may be dystrophic

Genetics

AD

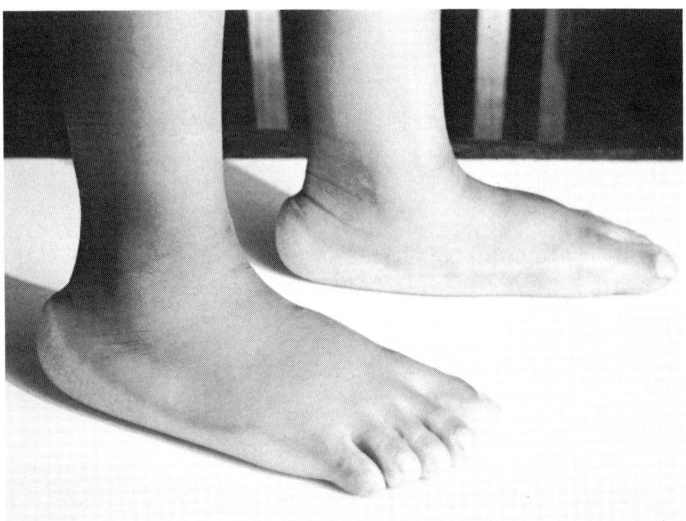

FIGURE 1–39
Diffuse palmoplantar keratoderma (Unna-Thost syndrome). Keratoderma of the soles with a sharp line of demarcation on the lateral aspect of the feet. This child's father was similarly affected.

REFERENCES

McK 148400
Bergström C. Keratodermia palmaris et plantaris. Nord Med 1967;78:155–156
Nielsen PG. Two different clinical and genetic forms of hereditary palmoplantar keratoderma in the northernmost county of Sweden. Clin Genet 1985;28:361–366
Sybert VP, Dale BA, Holbrook KA. Palmar-plantar keratoderma: a clinical, ultrastructural, and biochemical study. J Am Acad Dermatol 1988;18:75–86

HEREDITARY EPIDERMOLYTIC PALMOPLANTAR KERATODERMA (EPIDERMOLYTIC PALMOPLANTAR KERATODERMA, VORNER TYPE)

palmoplantar keratoderma present at birth or in early life; clinically very similar to Unna-Thost diffuse palmoplantar keratoderma

AD

histopathology: findings of epidermolytic hyperkeratosis (hyperkeratosis and vacuolar changes in upper layers of the stratum malpighii with clumped keratohyaline granules)

one of the most common forms of palmoplantar keratoderma

McK 144200
Camisa C, Williams H. Epidermolytic variant of hereditary palmoplantar keratoderma. Br J Dermatol 1985;112:221–225
Kanitakis J, Tsoitis G, Kanitakis C. Hereditary epidermolytic palmoplantar keratoderma (Vorner type): report of a familial case and review of the literature. J Am Acad Dermatol 1987;17:414–422
Kuster W, Becker A. Indication for the identity of palmoplantar type Unna-Thost with type Vorner. Acta Derm Venereol 1992; 72:120–122
Moriwaki S, Tanaka T, Horiguchi Y, et al. Epidermolytic hereditary palmoplantar keratoderma: histologic, ultrastructural, protein-chemical, and DNA analyses in two patients. Arch Dermatol 1988;124:555–559
Thomas JR III, Greene SL, Su WP. Epidermolytic palmoplantar keratoderma. Int J Dermatol 1984;23:652–655

GREITHER SYNDROME

progressive palmoplantar keratoderma, with extension to sides and dorsal surfaces of hands and feet (transgrediens pattern)

arms and legs may be involved; may progress until fourth decade

AD

some consider it a severe form of diffuse palmoplantar keratoderma

Greither A. Keratosis extremitatum hereditaria progrediens mit dominantem Erbgang. Hautarzt 1952;3:198–203
Kansky A, Arzensek J. Is palmoplantar keratoderma of Greither's type a separate nosologic entity? Dermatologica 1979;158: 244–248

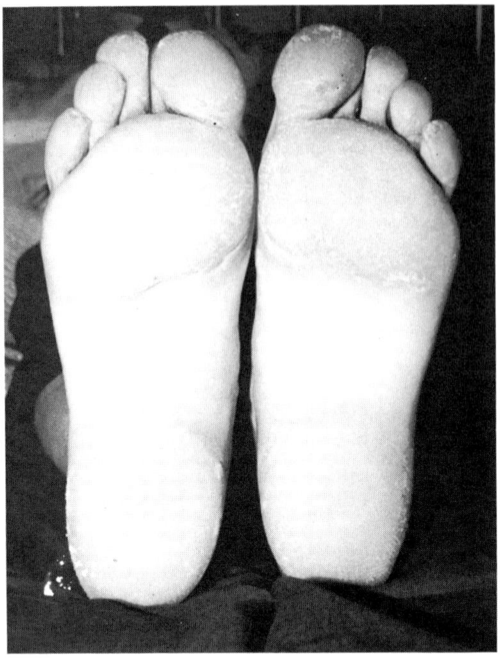

FIGURE 1–40
Howel-Evans syndrome. The striking symmetrical keratoderma is seen. (Courtesy of Dr. Peter Harper, Cardiff, Wales)

HOWEL-EVANS SYNDROME

palmoplantar keratoderma appears in first or second decade (Fig. 1–40)

development of esophageal and buccal leukokeratosis by the end of the second decade of life, followed by carcinoma of the esophagus in most by the seventh decade (Fig. 1–41)

AD

in contrast, patients with acquired palmoplantar keratoderma due to malignancy (a paraneoplastic phenomenon) are usually much older when the keratoderma has its onset

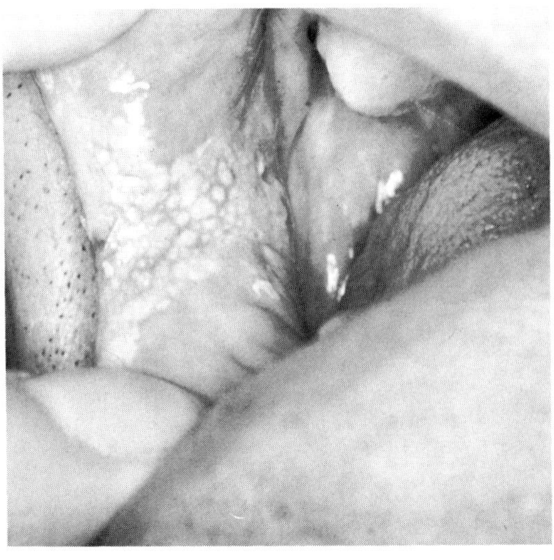

FIGURE 1–41
Leukokeratosis of buccal mucosa is often the first finding in Howel-Evans syndrome. (Courtesy of Dr. William Tyldesley, Liverpool, England)

McK 148500
Howel-Evans W, McConnell RB, Clarke CA, Sheppard PM. Carcinoma of the oesophagus with keratosis palmaris et plantaris (tylosis): a study of two families. Q J Med 1958;27:413–429
O'Mahony MY, Ellis JP, Hellier M, et al. Familial tylosis and carcinoma of the oesophagus. J R Soc Med 1984;77:514–517
Shine I, Allison PR. Carcinoma of the oesophagus with tylosis (keratosis palmaris et plantaris). Lancet 1966;1:951–953

KERATODERMA HEREDITARIA MUTILANS

Synonym

- Vohwinkel syndrome

Skin

diffuse palmoplantar keratoderma with a honeycomb appearance; onset in infancy

typical "starfish-shaped" keratoses appear on the dorsa of hands and feet, while linear keratotic lesions are present on elbows and knees

fingers become spindle-shaped, resembling the changes in acrosclerosis

around second decade, constricting keratotic bands form distal to the proximal phalanx of fingrs and toes; may cause autoamputation

occasional diffuse alopecia

Non-Skin

occasional neurosensory deafness

spastic paraplegia and myopathy reported

Genetics

AD; rarely AR

Prognosis

retinoids may cause dramatic improvement and prevent disability

REFERENCES

McK 124500
Gibbs RC, Frank SB. Keratoma hereditaria mutilans (Vohwinkel). Arch Dermatol 1966;94:619–625
Rivers JK, Duke EE, Justus DW. Etretinate: management of keratoma hereditaria mutilans in four family members. J Am Acad Dermatol 1985;13:43–49

MAL DE MELEDA

Synonym

- keratoderma palmoplantaris transgrediens

Skin

palmoplantar hyperkeratosis develops over base of erythema, followed by transgrediens spread onto dorsa of fingers and toes and flexures of wrists (Fig. 1–42)

lesions subsequently extend beyond digits onto dorsa of hands and feet, forearms, elbows, legs, and knees

rarely, hyperkeratotic plaques are found on trunk, in axillae, or periorally

persistent erythema of angles of mouth is typical

occasional local hyperhidrosis and fissuring

mucous membrane abnormalities include oral white plaques

hair and teeth are normal

nail abnormalities include koilonychia and subungual hyperkeratosis

Non-Skin

physical retardation, mental retardation, and electroencephalographic abnormalities

Genetics

AR

most patients are descendents of inhabitants of the island of Meleda in Dalmatia, where the original cases were described

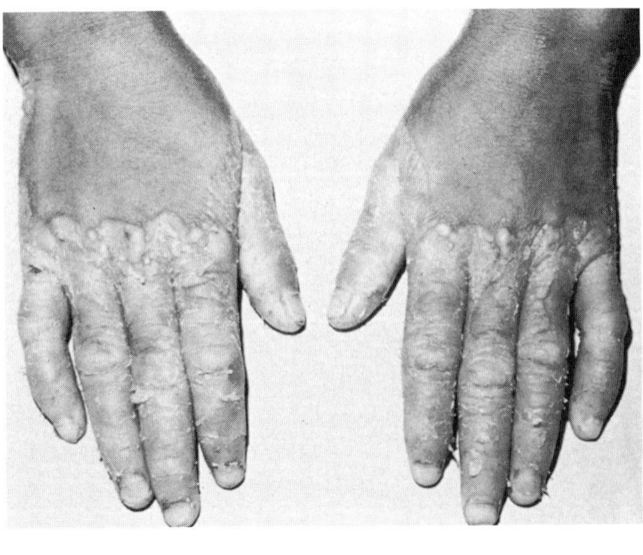

FIGURE 1–42
Mal de Meleda. Hyperkeratosis on the dorsum of the fingers and over the metacarpophalangeal joints. (Courtesy of Benjamin K. Fisher, MD, Toronto, Ontario)

Prognosis

wide range of severity; most patients with early onset have severe disease

tends to worsen until adolescence, then stabilizes; rare cases of complete remission are reported

REFERENCES

McK 248300

Franceschetti AT, Reinhart V, Schnyder UW. La maladie de Meleda. J Genet Hum 1972;20:267–296

Jee SH, Lee YY, Wu YC, et al. Report of a family with mal de Meleda in Taiwan: a clinical, histopathological and immunological study. Dermatologica 1985;171:30–37

Niles HD, Klumpp MM. Mal de Meleda: review of the literature and report of four cases. Arch Dermatol Syph 1939;39:409–421

PAPILLON-LEFÈVRE SYNDROME

Synonym

- keratosis palmoplantaris with periodontal disease

Skin

erythematous palmoplantar keratoderma appearing in childhood; rarely at birth

soles more severely involved than palms

plaques may extend onto dorsa of fingers, toes, hands, elbows, legs, and knees

keratoderma worse in winter

malodorous palmoplantar hyperhidrosis

increased incidence of infections including furunculosis

occasional sparse hair

nail abnormalities including ridging, onychogryposis, and koilonychia

normal eruption of deciduous teeth followed by dystrophic changes of surrounding alveolar processes around 4 to 5 years of age; results in severe gingivitis, destruction of periodontal ligaments, and tooth loss

periodontal disease usually simultaneous with skin changes; gingivae and skin lesions improve after teeth are shed

eruption of permanent teeth accompanied by similar sequelae, resulting in complete loss of permanent teeth except the third molars by the middle of the second decade

Genetics

AR

Laboratory Data

radiographs may show calcification of falx cerebri, choroid plexus, and tentorial attachments, but significance of this finding is unclear

Prognosis

keratoderma, after shedding of teeth, is mild but persistent

retention of teeth achieved in patients on continuous systemic retinoid therapy

REFERENCES

McK 245000

Gelmetti C, Nazzaro V, Cerri D, et al. Long-term preservation of permanent teeth in a patient with Papillon-Lefèvre syndrome treated with etretinate. Pediatr Dermatol 1989;6:222–625

Gorlin RJ, Sedano H, Anderson VE. The syndrome of palmar-plantar hyperkeratosis and premature periodontal destruction of the teeth: a clinical and genetic analysis of the Papillon-Lefèvre syndrome. Pediatrics 1964;65:895–907

Haneke E, Hornstein OP, Lex C. Increased susceptibility to infection in the Papillon-Lefèvre syndrome. Dermatologica 1975; 150:283–286

Haneke E. The Papillon-Lefèvre syndrome: keratosis palmoplantaris with periodontopathy: report of a case and review of the cases in the literature. Hum Genet 1979;51:1–35

Nguyen TQ, Greer KE, Fisher GBJ, et al. Papillon-Lefèvre syndrome: report of two patients treated successfully with isotretinoin. J Am Acad Dermatol 1986;15:46–49

SCHÖPF-SCHULZ-PASSARGE SYNDROME

dental abnormalities including hypodontia in childhood

palmoplantar keratoderma

eyelid cysts

hypotrichosis

nail dysplasia

AR

Font RL, Seabury SM, Scharrer MC. Apocrine hidrocystomas of the lids, hypodontia, palmar-plantar hyperkeratosis and onychodystrophy. Arch Ophthalmol 1986;104: 1811–1813

Monk BE, Pieris S, Soni V. Schöpf-Schulz-Passarge syndrome. Br J Dermatol 1992; 127:33–35

Nordin H, Mansson T, Svensson A. Familial occurrence of eccrine tumours in a family with ectodermal dysplasia. Acta Derm Venereol 1988;68:523–530

Schöpf E, Schulz HJ, Passarge E. Syndrome of cystic eyelids, palmo-plantar keratosis, hypodontia and hypotrichosis as a possible autosomal recessive trait. Birth Defects 1971;7:219–221

OLMSTED SYNDROME (CONGENITAL PALMOPLANTAR AND PERIORIFICIAL KERATODERMA)

sharply circumscribed palmoplantar and periorificial (mouth, nose, genitalia, and anus) keratoderma appearing in early childhood; keratotic papules may also be present elsewhere

other abnormalities include alopecia universalis, nail and tooth anomalies, joint laxity, and flexion contractures leading to constriction or autoamputation

mode of inheritance unknown

Atherton DJ, Sutton C, Jones BM. Mutilating palmoplantar keratoderma with periorificial keratotic plaques (Olmsted's syndrome). Br J Dermatol 1990;122:245–252

Hauber I, Frantzmann Y, Anton-Lamprecht I, et al. Olmsted syndrome. Hautarzt 1993; 44:394–400.

Poulin Y, Perry HO, Muller SA. Olmsted syndrome: congenital palmoplantar and periorificial keratoderma. J Am Acad Dermatol 1984;10:600–610

FOCAL PALMOPLANTAR AND ORAL MUCOSA HYPERKERATOSIS SYNDROME

progressive hyperkeratosis of weight- or pressure-bearing surfaces of palms and soles in early childhood

hyperkeratosis of gingivae and other oral mucosae

AD

McK 148730

Laskaris G, Vareltzidis A, Avgerinou G. Focal palmoplantar and oral mucosa hyperkeratosis syndrome: a report concerning five members of a family. Oral Surg 1980; 50:250–253

Young WG, Newcomb GM, Daley TJ. Focal palmoplantar and gingival hyperkeratosis syndrome: report of a family, with cytologic, ultrastructural, and histochemical findings. Oral Surg 1982;53:473–482

PUNCTATE PALMOPLANTAR KERATODERMA

Synonym

- keratosis palmaris et plantaris punctata

Skin

keratotic papules on palms, soles, and volar surface of fingers and toes; papules number from few to hundreds (Fig. 1–43)

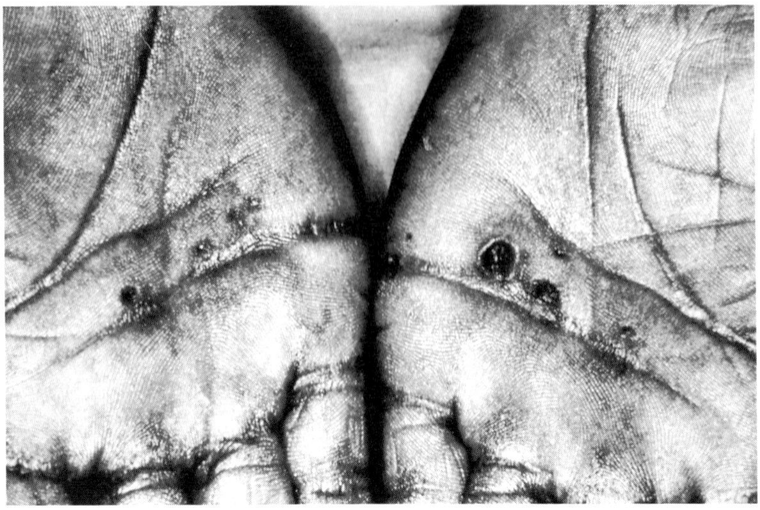

FIGURE 1–43
Punctate palmoplantar keratoderma. Variably sized keratotic papules on the palms.

insidious onset, usually from mid second to fourth decades

papules asymptomatic but tend to increase in size and number

occasional hyperhidrosis

nail abnormalities include dystrophy, onychomadesis, and onychauxis

Non-Skin

occasional atopy

possible association with colon carcinoma reported

Genetics

AD; females appear to be less severely affected

Discussion

- *hereditary papulotranslucent acrokeratoderma*

  yellowish white translucent papules and plaques on hands and feet

  fine scalp hair

  atopy

  AD

  possible variant of punctate palmoplantar keratoderma

  McK 101840

REFERENCES

McK 148600

Bennion SD, Patterson JW. Keratosis punctata palmaris et plantaris and adenocarcinoma of the colon: a possible familial association of punctate keratoderma and gastrointestinal malignancy. J Am Acad Dermatol 1984;10:587–591

Buchanan RN. Keratosis punctata palmaris et plantaris. Arch Dermatol 1963;88:644–650

Onwukwe MF, Mihm MC Jr, Toda K. Hereditary papulotranslucent acrokeratoderma: a new variant of familial punctate keratoderma? Arch Dermatol 1973;108:108–110

Tezuka T. Keratosis punctata palmaris et plantaris: a morphological study on the relation to the epidermal sweat duct unit. Acta Derm Venereol 1976;56:105–110

KERATOTIC PITS OF THE PALMAR CREASES

keratotic pits of the flexion creases of the palms and fingers, occasionally involving the soles; onset in adulthood; rarely painful

probable AD, very common; blacks much more frequently affected than whites

Ortega M, Quintana J, Camacho F. Keratosis punctata of the palmar creases. J Am Acad Dermatol 1985;13:381–382

Rustad OJ, Vance JC. Punctate keratoses of the palms and soles and keratotic pits of the palmar creases. J Am Acad Dermatol 1990;22:468–476

ACROKERATOELASTOIDOSIS OF COSTA

Skin

asymptomatic, small, firm, shiny smooth papules on dorsa of the fingers (especially over joints) and on dorsal and lateral aspects of hands, wrists, feet, and sometimes shins (Fig. 1–44)

papules sometimes keratotic or umbilicated; often grouped or confluent

onset in first or second decade

hyperhidrosis and mild diffuse palmoplantar hyperkeratosis reported

Genetics

mostly sporadic; some cases AD

Laboratory Data

histopathology: marked hyperorthokeratosis, acanthosis, and coarse fragmentation and reduction of elastic fibers in reticular dermis

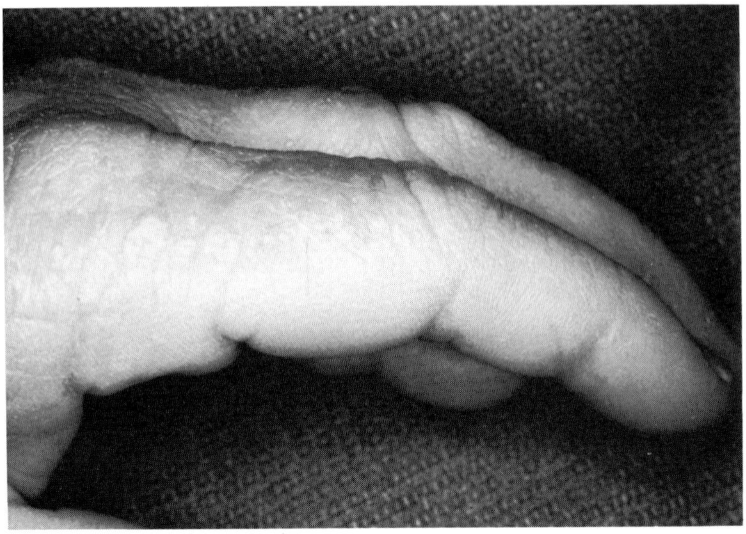

FIGURE 1–44
Acrokeratoelastoidosis of Costa. Firm, smooth papules on the lateral aspect of the index finger. (Courtesy of Benjamin K. Fisher, MD, Toronto, Ontario)

Discussion

cases of focal acral hyperkeratosis, keratoelastoides marginalis, and degenerative collagenous plaques have been described under the rubric of acrokeratoelastoidosis (see below)

- *keratoelastoides marginalis of the hands*

  asymptomatic, firm papules, sometimes linear, on medial and lateral aspects of hands and in first interdigital web space

  seen in older individuals, many of whom were white outdoor manual workers with long exposure to trauma and sunlight (thus the term *degenerative collagenous plaques of the hands* has been used)

  acquired

  in contrast to acrokeratoelastoidosis of Costa, histopathologically, there is actinic elastosis with thickening of collagen fibers, predominantly in upper dermis, but no elastic tissue changes

REFERENCES

McK 101850

Highet AS, Rook A, Anderson JR, et al. Acrokeratoelastoidosis. Br J Dermatol 1982; 106:337–344

Jordaan HF, Rossouw DJ. Digital papular calcific elastosis: a histopathological, histochemical and ultrastructural study of 20 patients. J Cutan Pathol 1990;17:358–370

Korc A, Hansen RC, Lynch PJ. Acrokeratoelastoidosis of Costa in North America: a report of two cases. J Am Acad Dermatol 1985;12:832–836

Ritchie EB, Williams HM, Jr. Degenerative collagenous plaques of the hands. Arch Dermatol 1966;93:202–203

FOCAL ACRAL HYPERKERATOSIS

pearly papules on lateral aspects of hands and feet

onset in first or second decade

thickening and hyperpigmentation over joints of fingers and toes

sporadic and possible AD cases reported

no elastic fiber abnormalities

Dowd PM, Harman RRM, Black MM. Focal acral hyperkeratosis. Br J Dermatol 1983;109:97–103

Ritchie EB, Williams HM, Jr. Degenerative collagenous plaques of the hands. Arch Dermatol 1966;93:202–203

Porokeratoses

The unifying feature of all of the porokeratoses is the cornoid lamella seen histopathologically. Exceptions and problems with this definition arise, as in any group of diseases based on a single histopathologic feature.

POROKERATOSIS OF MIBELLI

Skin

see Figure 1–45

centrifugally spreading keratotic papules coalescing to form annular plaques with furrowed, ridged borders; size ranges from millimeters to centimeters in diameter

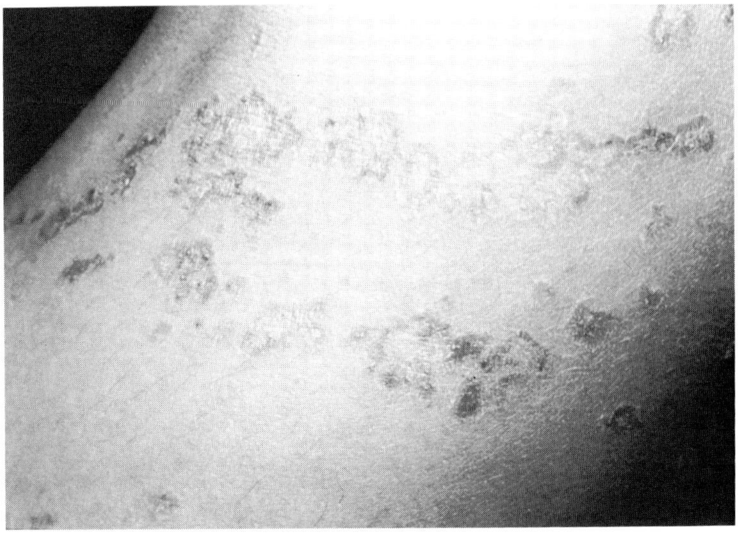

FIGURE 1–45
Porokeratosis of Mibelli. Keratotic papules with furrowed ridged borders coalescing and in linear array on the leg of a child.

onset usually in childhood, but papules may appear at any time

predilection for extremities; also face, neck, genitalia, and mucous membranes

lesions may expand slowly; atrophic scarring usually remains after lesions resolve

squamous cell carcinomas and, more rarely, basal cell carcinomas may arise in lesions

nails occasionally thickened, ridged, or split

mucous membranes rarely involved

Genetics

usually sporadic, but occasional AD cases reported

Laboratory Data

histopathology: keratin-filled, cup-shaped epidermal invagination with prominent cornoid lamella (parakeratotic column); granular layer absent under parakeratotic column

Prognosis

variable but chronic course

Discussion

rapid extension of lesions has followed immunosuppression; some authors suggest that lesions arise from an abnormal clone of cells unrestrained due to a deficient host immune response

- *linear porokeratosis*

unilateral linear coalescent keratotic papules on extremities (distal affected more than proximal), trunk, or face

onset at any age but most often in childhood

squamous cell carcinoma rarely develops in lesions

inheritance not established, probably sporadic

may resemble or overlap with linear epidermal nevus (including the presence of cornoid lamellae)

REFERENCES

McK 175800

Bloom D, Abramowitz EW. Porokeratosis of Mibelli: report of three cases in one family: histologic studies. Arch Dermatol Syphilol 1943;47:1–15

Commens CA, Shumack SP. Linear porokeratosis in two families with disseminated superficial actinic porokeratosis. Pediatr Dermatol 1987;4:209–214

Goldner R. Zosteriform porokeratosis of Mibelli. Arch Dermatol 1971;104:245–426

Helfman RJ, Poulos EG. Reticulated porokeratosis: a unique variant of porokeratosis. Arch Dermatol 1985;121:1542–1543

James WD, Rodman OG. Squamous cell carcinoma arising in porokeratosis of Mibelli. Int J Dermatol 1986;25:389–391
Lozinski AZ, Fisher BK, Walter JB, et al. Metastatic squamous cell carcinoma in linear porokeratosis of Mibelli. J Am Acad Dermatol 1987;16:448–451
Marghescu S, Anton LI, Melz RB. Disseminated bilateral hyperkeratotic variant of porokeratosis Mibelli. Arch Dermatol Res 1987;279:S38–S47
Mikhail GR, Wertheimer FW. Clinical variants of porokeratosis (Mibelli). Arch Dermatol 1968;98:124–131
Sarkany I. Porokeratosis Mibelli with basal cell epithelioma. Proc R Soc Med 1973;66:435–436
Scappaticci S, Lambiase S, Orecchia G, Fraccaro M. Clonal chromosome abnormalities with preferential involvement of chromosome 3 in patients with porokeratosis of Mibelli. Cancer Genet Cytogenet 1989;43:89–94

DISSEMINATED SUPERFICIAL ACTINIC POROKERATOSIS

Synonym

- DSAP

Skin

numerous (up to hundreds), small (size in millimeters), superficial, hyperkeratotic annular papules and plaques with minimally elevated borders

on sun-exposed areas, especially extensor extremities, of fair-skinned individuals in the third or fourth decade

palms, soles, and mucous membranes not involved

very rare development of squamous cell carcinoma in lesions

Genetics

AD; many sporadic cases reported

females reportedly affected more than males

Pathophysiology

experimentally induced by both UVA and UVB irradiation, most potent in combination

Laboratory Data

histopathology: cornoid lamellae less prominent than in Mibelli type (see under Porokeratosis of Mibelli)

Discussion

the most common form of porokeratosis

some cases are not limited to sun-exposed areas and are called disseminated superficial porokeratosis

REFERENCES

McK 175900

Anderson DE, Chernosky ME. Disseminated superficial actinic porokeratosis: genetic aspects. Arch Dermatol 1969;99:408–412

Brodkin RH, Rickert RR, Fuller FW, et al. Malignant disseminated porokeratosis. Arch Dermatol 1987;123:1521–1526

de Oliveira-Filho J, Cutin SL, Cuce LC. Disseminated superficial actinic porokeratosis in a black patient. Arch Dermatol 1986; 122:852–853

Dover JS, Phillips TJ, Burns DA, Krafchik BR. Disseminated superficial actinic porokeratosis: coexistence with other porokeratotic variants. Arch Dermatol 1986;122:887–889

Neumann RA, Knobler RM, Jurecka W, et al. Disseminated superficial actinic porokeratosis: experimental induction and exacerbation of skin lesions. J Am Acad Dermatol 1989;21:1182–1188

Pirozzi DJ, Rosenthal A. Disseminated superficial actinic porokeratosis: analysis of an affected family. Br J Dermatol 1976;95: 429–432

PUNCTATE PALMOPLANTAR POROKERATOSIS

Synonyms

- porokeratosis punctata, palmaris et plantaris
- punctate porokeratosis
- porokeratosis plantaris, palmaris et disseminata

Skin

multiple small keratotic papules resembling “spines of an old-fashioned music box” on palms and soles

onset usually in first to third decades; may spread symmetrically to sun-exposed and non–sun-exposed areas (e.g., extremities and trunk); rarely, nonpalmoplantar areas are first to be affected; mucous membranes rarely involved

Genetics

AD; about half of cases are sporadic

Laboratory Data

histopathology: no cornoid lamellae

Discussion

some argue that this is not a form of porokeratosis because of the absence of centrifugally expanding lesions, cornoid lamellae, and electron microscopic findings of vacuolar degeneration, tonofilament clumping, and vacuolar degeneration typical of porokeratosis; they suggest term “spiny keratoderma” of the palms and soles

sporadic cases tend to have a later age at onset

acquired solitary lesions especially on soles are extremely common

REFERENCES

McK 175850
McK 175860
Heierli-Forrer E. Zur Klinik und Genetik der hereditären papulösen Palmoplantarkeratosen. Dermatologica 1959;119:309–327
Himmselstein R, Lynfield YL. Punctate porokeratosis. Arch Dermatol 1984;120:263–264
Kondo S, Shimoura T, Hozumi Y, Aso K. Punctate porokeratotic keratoderma: some pathogenetic analyses of hyperproliferation and parakeratosis. Acta Derm Venereol 1990;70:478–482
Lestringant GG, Berge T. Porokeratosis punctata palmaris et plantaris: a new entity? Arch Dermatol 1989;125:816–819
Mandojana RM, Katz R, Rodman OG. Porokeratosis plantaris discreta. J Am Acad Dermatol 1984;10:679–682
Neumann RA, Knobler RM, Gebhart W. Unusual presentation of porokeratosis palmaris, plantaris et disseminata. J Am Acad Dermatol 1989;21:1131–1133
Sakas EL, Gentry RH. Porokeratosis punctata palmaris et plantaris (punctate porokeratosis): case report and literature review. J Am Acad Dermatol 1985;13:908–912
Schiff BL, Hughes D. Palmoplantar keratosis acuminata with facial sebaceous hyperplasia. Arch Dermatol 1974;109:86–87

Disorders of Cornification—Abbreviated Entries

ICHTHYOSIS-CHEEK-EYEBROW SYNDROME (ICE SYNDROME)

ichthyosis vulgaris–like eruption; "full" cheeks; sparse lateral eyebrows

craniofacial and musculoskeletal abnormalities

AD

McK 146720
Goodman RM, Sidransky E, Feinstein A. Ichthyosis-cheek-eyebrow syndrome (ICE [skin]). [Letter]. Clin Genet 1987;32:206
Sidransky E, Feinstein A, Goodman RM. Ichthyosis-cheek-eyebrow (ICE) syndrome: a new autosomal dominant disorder. Clin Genet 1987;31:137–142
Traupe H. What is the ichthyosis in the so-called ichthyosis-cheek-eyebrow (ICE) syndrome? [Letter]. Clin Genet 1987;32:418

AUTOSOMAL DOMINANT ICHTHYOSIS EXFOLIATIVA

generalized fine scaling sparing face

dark gray hyperkeratotic plaques on waist, dorsa of hands and feet, extensor and flexural surfaces of elbows and knees, and axillae; occasional superimposed blisters and subsequent erosions in these areas

in general, increased susceptibility of skin to blister spontaneously or secondary to minor trauma

onset at birth

AD

histopathology: features include hyperkeratosis, acanthosis, edema of cells of granular and spinous layers and occasional subcorneal split; no coarse keratohyaline granules

electron microscopy: no clumped tonofilaments

Vakilzadeh and Kolde distinguish this entity from both bullous congenital ichthyosiform erythroderma and ichthyosis bullosa of Siemens on clinical and ultrastructural grounds

Sahn and colleagues reported a similar-appearing entity that they called "annular epidermal ichthyosis"

Sahn EE, Weimer CE, Garen PD. Annular epidermolytic ichthyosis: a unique phenotype. J Am Acad Dermatol 1992;27:348–355

Vakilzadeh F, Kolde G. Autosomal dominant ichthyosis exfoliativa. Br J Dermatol 1991;124:191–194

SHWACHMAN SYNDROME

ichthyosiform and eczematous cutaneous lesions; variable asteatosis

skin infections

pancreatic insufficiency

bone abnormalities include rib anomalies, metaphyseal dysplasia, and short-limbed dwarfism

increased hematologic malignancies

bone marrow hypoplasia resulting in neutropenia and less commonly anemia and thrombocytopenia

otitis media and respiratory infections

psychomotor retardation

probably AR

defective neutrophil chemotaxis in heterozygotes

McK 260400

Goeteyn M, Oranje AP, Vuzevski VD, et al. Ichthyosis, exocrine pancreatic insufficiency, impaired neutrophil chemotaxis, growth retardation, and metaphyseal dysplasia (Shwachman syndrome): report of a case with extensive skin lesions (clinical, histological, and ultrastructural findings). Arch Dermatol 1991;127:225–230

Mortureux P, Taieb A, Bazeille JE, et al. Shwachman syndrome: a case report. Pediatr Dermatol 1992;9:57–61

CONGENITAL ICHTHYOSIFORM DERMATOSIS WITH LINEAR KERATOTIC FLEXURAL PAPULES AND SCLEROSING PALMOPLANTAR KERATODERMA

possibly AR

Pujol RM, Moreno A, Alomar A, et al. Congenital ichthyosiform dermatosis with linear keratotic flexural papules and sclerosing palmoplantar keratoderma. Arch Dermatol 1989;125;103–106

MILLER SYNDROME (DEFECTIVE NEUTROPHIL CHEMOTAXIS)

congenital ichthyosis characterized by generalized diffuse scaling with widespread superimposed red hyperkeratotic plaques

characteristic increase in *Trichophyton rubrum* infections

AD

neutrophils have abnormal response to chemotactic signal even though their number, morphology, and phagocytic and bacteriocidal abilities are normal

McK 162820

Koblenzer PJ, Miller ME. Lamellar ichthyosis, recurrent *Trichophyton rubrum* infections, familial abnormality of polymorphonuclear leukocytes. Arch Dermatol 1972;106:755–756

Miller ME, Norman ME, Koblenzer PJ, et al. A new familial defect of neutrophil movement. J Lab Clin Med 1973;82:1–8

Shelley ED, Shelley WB, Schafer RL. Generalized *Trichophyton rubrum* infection in congenital ichthyosiform erythroderma. J Am Acad Dermatol 1989;20:1133–1134

ORAL AND DIGITAL ANOMALIES WITH ICHTHYOSIS

generalized ichthyosis in infancy

redundant skin on neck and upper back

developmental delay

abnormal craniofacies

musculoskeletal abnormalities include joint contractures and hypoplastic digits

recurrent infections especially of lungs and gastrointestinal tract

probable AR

McK 258840
Clayton-Smith J, Donnai D. A new recessive syndrome of unusual facies, digital abnormalities, and ichthyosis. J Med Genet 1989;26:339–342

ICHTHYOSIS WITH ALOPECIA, ECLABIUM, ECTROPION, AND MENTAL RETARDATION

congenital lamellar-like ichthyosis with marked scalp involvement, alopecia, ectropion, eclabium, claw-like nails, spasticity, and mental retardation

no spastic diplegia or glistening fundal dots as in Sjögren-Larsson syndrome

AR

McK 242510
Jagell SF, Holmgren G, Hofer PA. Congenital ichthyosis with alopecia, eclabion, ectropion and mental retardation: a new genetic syndrome. Clin Genet 1987;31:102–108

ICHTHYOSIS, CEREBELLAR DEGENERATION, AND HEPATOSPLENOMEGALY

autosomal versus X-linked recessive

McK 242520
Dykes PJ, Marks R, Harper PS. A syndrome of ichthyosis, hepatosplenomegaly and cerebellar degeneration. Br J Dermatol 1979; 100:585–590

ICHTHYOSIS, MENTAL RETARDATION, DWARFISM, AND RENAL IMPAIRMENT

AR

McK 242530
Passwell JH, Goodman RM, Ziprkowski M, Cohen BE. Congenital ichthyosis, mental retardation, dwarfism and renal impairment: a new syndrome. Clin Genet 1975; 8:59–65

ICHTHYOSIS, SPLIT HAIRS, AND AMINOACIDURIA

AR

McK 242550
Yesudian P, Srinivas K. Ichthyosis with unusual hair shaft abnormalities in siblings. Br J Dermatol 1977;96:199–203

CORNEODERMATO-OSSEOUS SYNDROME (CDO SYNDROME)

palmoplantar keratoderma in first year of life; in addition, erythematous scaly plaques on knuckles, elbows, and knees

buccal mucosal leukokeratosis; nail and dental abnormalities

corneal dystrophy

premature birth, short stature, brachydactyly, and mental retardation

AD

McK 122440
Stern JK, Lubinsky MS, Durrie DS, Luckasen JR. Corneal changes, hyperkeratosis, short stature, brachydactyly, and premature birth: a new autosomal dominant syndrome. Am J Med Genet 1984;18:67–77

PALMOPLANTAR KERATODERMA WITH PARTIAL OR TOTAL ALOPECIA, HYPERHIDROSIS, AND TONGUE-SHAPED CORNEAL OPACITIES

probable AD

McK 122440
Zmegac ZJ, Sarajlic MV. A rare form of an inheritable palmar and plantar keratosis. Dermatologica 1964;130:40–52

DIFFUSE PALMOPLANTAR KERATODERMA ASSOCIATED WITH ACROCYANOSIS

possible AD

Nielsen PG. Diffuse palmoplantar keratoderma associated with acrocyanosis: a family study. Acta Derm Venereol 1989;69:156–161

LETHAL CONGENITAL ERYTHRODERMA

congenital exfoliative erythroderma resistant to treatment

failure to thrive

hypoalbuminemia

probable AR

death in first year of life

McK 227090

Shield JPH, Judge MR, Reardon W, et al. Lethal congenital erythroderma: a newly recognised genetic disorder. Clin Genet 1992;41:273–277

PALMOPLANTAR KERATODERMA, NORRBOTTEN TYPE

rare, severe form of diffuse palmoplantar keratoderma in northern Sweden

AR

McK 244850

Gamborg Nielsen P. Two different clinical and genetic forms of hereditary palmoplantar keratoderma in the northernmost country of Sweden. Clin Genet 1985;28:361–366

Kastl I, Anton-Lamprecht, Gamborg Nielsen P. Hereditary palmoplantar keratosis of the Gamborg Nielsen type. Arch Dermatol Res 1990;282:363–370

ANKYLOSING VERTEBRAL HYPEROSTOSIS WITH TYLOSIS

punctate keratoderma of palms and soles

AD

McK 106400

Beardwell A. Familial ankylosing vertebral hyperostosis with tylosis. Ann Rheum Dis 1969;28:518–523

PALMOPLANTAR KERATODERMA WITH CLINODACTYLY

AD

McK 148520
Anderson IF, Klintworth GK. Hypovitaminosis-A in a family with tylosis and clinodactyly. Br Med J 1961;1:1293–1297
Hernandez A, Aguirre-Negrete MG, Gonzalez-Mendoza A, et al. Autosomal dominant keratosis palmaris et plantaris with clinodactyly. Birth Defects 1982;18(3B):207–210

PALMOPLANTAR KERATODERMA WITH DEAFNESS

Onset from infancy to late childhood of variable palmoplantar keratoderma

deafness

AR

McK 148350
Bitici OO. Familial hereditary progressive sensorineural hearing loss with keratosis palmaris and plantaris. J Laryngol Otol 1975;89:1143–1146
Hatamochi A, Nakagawa S, Ueki H, et al. Diffuse palmoplantar keratoderma with deafness. Arch Dermatol 1982;118:605–607
Sharland M, Bleach NR, Goberdhan PD, Patton MA. Autosomal dominant palmoplantar hyperkeratosis and sensorineural deafness in three generations. J Med Genet 1992;29:50–522
Verbov J. Palmoplantar hyperkeratosis and deafness. J Med Genet 1992;29:440

BRUNAUER SYNDROME

keratosis palmoplantaris striata associated with mental retardation, defective enamel formation, and hyperhidrosis

AD

Brunauer SR. Zur Vererbung des keratomas hereditarium palmare et plantare. Acta Derm Venereol 1923;4:489
Ortega M, Quintana J, Camacho F. Keratosis palmoplantar striata (Brunauer-Fuhs type). Acta Derm Venereol 1982;63:273–275

PALMOPLANTAR KERATODERMA, NAIL DYSTROPHY, AND HEREDITARY MOTOR AND SENSORY NEUROPATHY

AD

nail dystrophy was not seen in kindreds reported by Powell and colleagues and Rabbiosi and associates; there is extensive genetic heterogeneity among the palmoplantar keratodermas and the hereditary motor and sensory neuropathies

McK 148360

Powell FC, Venencie PY, Gordon H, Winkelmann RK. Keratoderma and spastic paralysis. Br J Dermatol 1983;109:589–596

Rabbiosi G, Borroni G, Pinelli P, et al. Palmoplantar keratoderma and Charcot-Marie-Tooth disease. Arch Dermatol 1980; 116: 789–790

Tolmie JL, Wilcox DE, McWilliam R, et al. Palmoplantar keratoderma, nail dystrophy, and hereditary motor and sensory neuropathy: an autosomal dominant trait. J Med Genet 1988;25:754–757

MENTAL RETARDATION, SPASTIC PARAPLEGIA, AND PALMOPLANTAR HYPERKERATOSIS

XLR

McK 309560

Fitzsimmons JS, Fitzsimmons EM, McLachlan JI, Gilbert GB. Four brothers with mental retardation, spastic paraplegia and palmoplantar hyperkeratosis: a new syndrome? Clin Genet 1983;23:329–335

HYPOPIGMENTATION WITH PUNCTATE KERATODERMA

diffuse, irregularly speckled hypopigmented macules with onset in infancy, with subsequent development of palmoplantar keratoses

AD

Cole LA. Hypopigmentation with punctate keratosis of the palms and soles. Arch Dermatol 1976;112:998–1000

Pratt SB, Griffin TB, Stretcher GS. Hypopigmentation with punctate keratosis of the palms and soles. [Letter]. Arch Dermatol 1977;113:689

HEREDITARY PAINFUL CALLOSITIES (KERATOSIS PALMOPLANTARIS NUMMULARIS)

round hyperkeratotic papules and plaques on plantar feet and toes at sites of pressure points

onset in early childhood to mid teens

minimal involvement of hands and when present related to manual labor

subungual keratoses

nail dystrophy

AD

McK 114140
Roth W, Penneys NS, Fawcett N. Hereditary painful callosities. Arch Dermatol 1978;114: 591–592
Wachters DHJ, Frensdorf EL, Hausman R, van Dijk E. Keratosis palmoplantaris nummularis ("hereditary painful callosities"): clinical and histopathologic aspects. J Am Acad Dermatol 1983;9:204–209

KERATOSIS PALMOPLANTARIS PAPULOSA (KERATODERMIA PALMOPLANTARIS PAPULOSA BUSCHKE-FISCHER-BRAUER)

hyperkeratotic yellowish papules and plaques on volar surfaces of hands and feet

onset in late teens or adulthood

AD

McK 148600
Heierli-Forrer E. Zur Klinik und Genetik der hereditären papulösen palmoplantar keratosen. Dermatologica 1959;119:309–327
Salamon T, Stolic V, Lazovic-Tepavac O, et al. Peculiar findings in a family with keratodermia palmoplantare papulosa Buschke-Fischer-Brauer. Hum Genet 1982;60:14–19

KERATOSIS PALMOPLANTARIS STRIATA

palmoplantar keratoderma with a variable linear pattern, often extending from palm to fingers; usually less evident on soles

onset usually in second or third decade; may be related to trauma

AD; may be genetically heterogeneous

some authors consider it in the middle of the spectrum between diffuse palmoplantar keratoderma and punctate palmoplantar keratoderma

McK 148700
Bologna EI. Durch vier Generationenen dominant vererblich geschlechtsgebundene Keratosis palmaris striata (linearia). Dermatol Wochenschr 1966;152:446–457
Clarke DB. Keratotic lesions of the palms and soles. J Milit Dermatol 1975;1:50–56
De Villez RL. Unilateral striate palmarplantar keratoderma. Cutis 1972;10:506–507

KERATOSIS PALMOPLANTARIS WITH PERIODONTOSIS AND ONYCHOGRYPOSIS

congenital palmoplantar hyperkeratosis, onychogryposis, periodontosis, arachnodactyly, pes planus, and acro-osteolysis

probable AR

seen in a small community of Jews from Cochin, India

McK 245010

Puliyel JM, Sridharan Iyer KS. A syndrome of keratosis palmo-plantaris congenita, pes planus, onychogryphosis, periodontosis, arachnodactyly and a peculiar acro-osteolysis. Br J Dermatol 1986;115:243–248

ACRAL KERATODERMA

diffuse and striate hyperkeratotic papules and plaques on distal extremities, elbows, and knees

onset in infancy or adolescence

occasional pseudoainhum

possibly AR

Nesbitt LT, Rothschild H, Ichinose H, et al. Acral keratoderma. Arch Dermatol 1975; 111:763–768

PALMOPLANTAR HYPERKERATOSIS, SHORT STATURE, FACIAL DYSMORPHISM, AND HYPODONTIA

AD

Seow WK. Palmoplantar hyperkeratosis with short stature, facial dysmorphism, and hypodontia—a new syndrome? case report. Pediatr Dent 19898;11:145–150

LACTATE DEHYDROGENASE M-SUBUNIT DEFICIENCY

nonpruritic follicular papules and erythematous plaques with scaly edges on extensor surfaces of extremities; starts in childhood and improves after puberty

myoglobinuria and myoglobinemia with muscle rigidity after strenuous exercise

AR

reported only in Japanese patients

McK 150000
Nazzari G, Crovato F. Annually recurring acroerythema and hereditary lactate dehydrogenase M-subunit deficiency. J Am Acad Dermatol 1992;27:262–263
Takayasu S, Fujiwara S, Waki T. Hereditary lactate dehydrogenase M-subunit deficiency: lactate dehydrogenase activity in skin lesions and in hair follicles. J Am Acad Dermatol 1991;24:339–342
Yoshikuni K, Tagami H, Yamada M, et al. Erythematosquamous skin lesions in hereditary lactate dehydrogenase M-subunit deficiency. Arch Dermatol 1986;122:1420–1424

ALOPECIA, KERATOSIS PILARIS, CATARACTS, AND PSORIASIS

AD

Apell ML, Sherertz EF. A kindred with alopecia, keratosis pilaris, cataracts, and psoriasis. J Am Acad Dermatol 1987;16:89–95

CHAPTER

2

Bullous Disorders

The epidermolysis bullosas, or mechanobullous disorders, are considered in this chapter as are other hereditary syndromes in which blistering is a major or minor feature. Many diseases described elsewhere in this book also have blistering as an integral finding; however, the presence of more distinctive features influenced our arbitrary decision to include them in other chapters. Obvious examples are the porphyrias, which appear in Chapter 15 on metabolic disorders, and Kindler syndrome, which is included in Chapter 3 on poikilodermatous disorders.

Epidermolysis Bullosa: Classification and General Comments

Epidermolysis bullosa (EB) refers to a group of inherited mechanobullous disorders characterized by skin fragility (Table 2–1). The diseases have been classified by cutaneous findings, associated clinical features, and pedigree information, but identification of the level of cleavage by ultrastructural studies or immunofluorescence mapping is currently most definitive. Clinically, in addition to mucocutaneous blisters and increased skin fragility, areas of congenital localized absence of skin may be seen in all forms of EB and in themselves are not indicative of a more severe type of EB.

In general, there are three main types of EB, reflecting three cleavage levels in the region of the basement membrane zone:

1. EB simplex: cleavage in the lower epidermis
2. Junctional EB: cleavage in the lamina lucida
3. Dystrophic EB: cleavage below the lamina densa

We use the following classification, which is derived from that of the Subcommittee on Diagnosis and Classification of the National Epidermolysis Bullosa Registry. New types and variants continue to be described. Significant changes in nomenclature and categorization will most likely occur once spe-

TABLE 2–1
EPIDERMOLYSIS BULLOSA SIMPLEX (EBS)

Type	Inheritance	Skin	Hair, Nails, Teeth	Non-Skin	Histopathology
Epidermolysis Bullosa, Simplex (EBS), Localized					
EBS of hands and feet (Weber-Cockayne variant)	AD	Trauma-induced blisters, usually hands and feet; onset usually in infancy to early childhood; palmoplantar hyperhidrosis; nonscarring			Cytolysis of basal cells, perhaps higher than EBS-Koebner; minimal dyskeratosis
EBS with anodontia/ hypodontia (Kallin syndrome)	AR	Acral blistering in first year of life	Hair: alopecia with brittle hair Nails: dystrophic Teeth: anodontia/ hypodontia	Oral erosions; myopia; hearing loss	Intraepidermal blister; not well characterized
Epidermolysis Bullosa Simplex, Generalized					
EBS, Koebner variant	AD	Blisters, erosions present at birth or shortly after; nonscarring; plantar calluses common	Hair: normal Nails: rarely dystrophic Teeth: normal	Mild oral and nasopharyngeal involvement	Cytolysis of basal cells; minimal dyskeratosis
EBS herpetiformis (Dowling-Meara variant)	AD	Herpetiform blisters especially acrally, present at birth; may heal with milia; palmoplantar hyperkeratosis in childhood	Hair: normal Nails: dystrophic Teeth: natal teeth; anodontia	Oral blisters	Cytolysis of basal cells; secondary dyskeratosis; prominent clumping of tonofilaments

EBS with mottled pigmentation with or without keratoderma	AD	Widespread blisters, rarely herpetic or annular; onset at birth or in early infancy; post-blistering and idiopathic pigmentation; blistering improves with age, pigmentation worsens; punctate keratoderma on palms, diffuse on plantar surfaces	Hair: normal Nails: thickened Teeth: carious	Oral lesions early in life	Cytolysis of basal cells
EBS superficialis	AD	Widespread blisters at birth or in infancy; scarring, milia, and atrophy common	Hair: normal Nails: onychogryphosis Teeth: normal	Oral erosions common; occasional conjunctival vesiculation	
EBS, Ogna variant	AD	Acral blistering due to trauma with bruising elsewhere; onset in early childhood	Hair: normal Nails: dystrophic Teeth: normal		Cytolysis of basal cells
EBS with or without associated neuromuscular disease (latter also called EBS letalis)	AR	Generalized or extremity erosions and blisters at birth or in early infancy	Hair: scarring alopecia Nails: dystrophy Teeth: defective enamel rarely	Oral ulcerations; anemia and growth retardation; congenital myasthenia gravis and muscular dystrophy; most patients have died of unexplained causes, gastrointestinal obstruction, septicemia	Cytolysis of basal cells
EBS, Mendes da Costa variant	XLR	Acral blistering especially early in life with reticulate hyperpigmentation and atrophy	Hair: alopecia Nails: normal Teeth: normal	Microcephaly	Cytolysis of basal cells

cific gene defects are identified. For example, epidermolysis bullosa simplex has been linked to mutations in genes encoding keratins 5 and 14 located on chromosomes 12g and 17g, respectively.

I. Epidermolysis Bullosa Simplex (EBS)
   1. EBS, localized forms
      a. EBS of hands and feet (Weber-Cockayne variant)
      b. EBS with anodontia/hypodontia (Kallin syndrome)
   2. EBS, generalized forms
      a. EBS, Koebner variant
      b. EBS herpetiformis (Dowling-Meara variant)
      c. EBS with mottled pigmentation with or without keratoderma
      d. EBS superficialis
      e. EBS, Ogna variant
      f. EBS with or without associated neuromuscular disease (also called EBS letalis)
      g. EBS, Mendes da Costa variant

II. Junctional Epidermolysis Bullosa (JEB)
   1. JEB, localized forms
      a. JEB, inversa
      b. JEB, acral (JEB minimus)
      c. JEB, progressiva (neurotropica) variant
      d. JEB, late-onset, localized, and mental retardation
   2. JEB, generalized forms
      a. JEB, gravis (Herlitz variant)
      b. JEB, mitis (non-Herlitz variant; generalized atrophic benign EB)
      c. Cicatricial junctional EB

III. Dystrophic Epidermolysis Bullosa (DEB)
   1. DEB, localized forms
      a. DEB, inversa
      b. DEB, acral (DEB minimus)
      c. DEB, pretibial
      d. DEB, centripetal
   2. DEB, generalized forms, autosomal dominant (dominant dystrophic EB [DDEB])
      a. DDEB, albopapuloidea (Pasini variant)
      b. DDEB, hyperplasique (Cockayne-Touraine variant)
      c. Transient bullous dermolysis of the newborn
   3. DEB, generalized forms, autosomal recessive (recessive dystrophic EB [RDEB])
      a. RDEB, gravis (Hallopeau-Siemens variant)
      b. RDEB, mitis

It is impossible to accurately identify the level of cleavage on routine light microscopy. Occasionally one can see lower epidermal cytolysis in forms of EB simplex or dermal vacuoles in dystrophic variants, but most often one is confronted with a minimally inflammatory subepidermal blister with considerable artifact. Either transmission electron microscopy or immunofluorescence mapping (using antibodies against bullous pemphigoid antigen, laminin, type IV collagen, and other antigens) are needed to identify the level of separation. A recent spontaneous lesion or an erythematous papule induced by mild local trauma should be studied. Sometimes immunofluorescence mapping or electron microscopy can be done on fetal skin biopsy specimens obtained from fetuses at risk, but it is a difficult technique and not universally available.

Allman S, Haynes L, MacKinnon P, Atherton DJ. Nutrition in dystrophic epidermolysis bullosa. Pediatr Dermatol 1992;9:231–238.
Bauer EA, Cooper TW. Therapeutic considerations in recessive dystrophic epidermolysis bullosa. Arch Dermatol 1981;117:529–530
Bauer EA, Kim YH, Woodley DT, et al. Epidermolysis bullosa: recent advances in understanding pathogenetic mechanisms. Curr Probl Dermatol 1992; IV(3):104–119
Epstein EH Jr. Molecular genetics of epidermolysis bullosa. Science 1992;256:799–804
Fine JD. Changing clinical and laboratory concepts in inherited epidermolysis bullosa. [Review]. Arch Dermatol 1988;124:523–526
Fine JD, Bauer EA, Briggaman RA, et al. Revised clinical and laboratory criteria for subtypes of inherited epidermolysis bullosa: a consensus report by the Subcommittee on Diagnosis and Classification of the National Epidermolysis Bullosa Registry. J Am Acad Dermatol 1991;24:119–135
Gedde-Dahl T Jr. Epidermolysis Bullosa: A Clinical, Genetic and Epidemiologic Study. Baltimore, Johns Hopkins University Press, 1971
Gedde-Dahl T. Sixteen types of epidermolysis bullosa. Acta Derm Venereol 1981; 95 (suppl):74–87
Kanzler MH, Smoller B, Woodley DT. Congenital localized absence of the skin as a manifestation of epidermolysis bullosa. Arch Dermatol 1992;128:1087–1090
Lin AN, Carter DM. Epidermolysis Bullosa: Basic and Clinical Aspects. New York, Springer-Verlag, 1992
Pearson RW. Clinicopathologic types of epidermolysis bullosa and their nondermatological complications. [Review]. Arch Dermatol 1988;124:718–725

Epidermolysis Bullosa Simplex

EPIDERMOLYSIS BULLOSA SIMPLEX OF HANDS AND FEET

Synonym

- epidermolysis bullosa simplex of Weber-Cockayne

Skin

recurrent trauma-induced blisters of hands and feet usually first appearing in childhood but may begin at any time from infancy to adulthood (Fig. 2–1); lesions heal without scarring

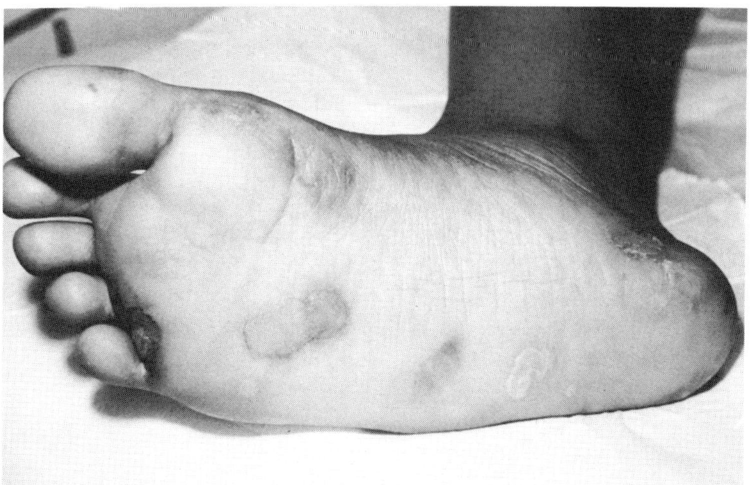

FIGURE 2–1
Epidermolysis bullosa simplex of the hands and feet (Weber-Cockayne syndrome). Several intact and eroded blisters are on the sole.

worse in warm weather; some patients have blisters only during summer

palmoplantar hyperhidrosis

nail dystrophy rare; normal teeth and oral mucosa

association with macular amyloidosis reported

Genetics

AD

Pathophysiology

abnormal epidermal glycosylation reported

Discussion

as noted in the discussion of EBS, Koebner variant, kindreds may also include individuals with more generalized lesions

besides this entity, other forms of EBS with onset in infancy or early childhood rather than at birth are EBS Ogna, macular dystrophic epidermolysis bullosa of Mendes da Costa, EBS superficialis, and EBS with anodontia/hypodontia (Kallin syndrome)

REFERENCES

McK 131800

Fine JD, Johnson L, Wright T, et al. Epidermolysis bullosa simplex: identification of a kindred with autosomal recessive transmission of the Weber-Cockayne variety. Pediatr Dermatol 1989;6:1–5

Haneke E, Anton-Lamprecht I. Ultrastructure of blister formation in epidermolysis bullosa hereditaria: V. Epidermolysis bullosa simplex localisata type Weber-Cockayne. J Invest Dermatol 1982;78:219–223

Kantor GR, Kasick JM, Bergfeld WF, et al. Epidermolysis bullosa of the Weber-Cockayne type with macular amyloidosis. Cleve Clin Q 1985;52:425–428

Niemi KM, Sommer H, Kero M, et al. Epidermolysis bullosa simplex associated with muscular dystrophy with recessive inheritance. Arch Dermatol 1988;124:551–554

Readett MD. Localized epidermolysis bullosa. Br J Med 1961;1:1510–1511

EPIDERMOLYSIS BULLOSA SIMPLEX WITH ANODONTIA/HYPODONTIA (KALLIN SYNDROME)

onset of acral blisters in first year of life (not at birth)

erosions of oral mucosa

sparse brittle scalp hair in infancy or childhood; becomes normal in second decade

nail dystrophy

hypodontia and anodontia

myopia and hearing loss

AR

Gamborg-Nielsen P, Sjolund E. Epidermolysis bullosa simplex localisata associated with anodontia, hair and nail disorders: a new syndrome. Acta Derm Venereol 1985; 65:526–530

EPIDERMOLYSIS BULLOSA SIMPLEX, KOEBNER VARIANT

Skin

generalized tense blisters induced by trivial trauma; extremities have greatest area of involvement

onset at birth, infancy, or early childhood

lesions heal without scarring

some infants born with localized absence of skin

occasional palmoplantar keratoderma

worse in warm weather

rare oral mucosal involvement

nail dystrophy rarely

Genetics

AD

Pathophysiology

mutations in keratin 14 gene

Prognosis

tends to improve with age, especially following puberty

Discussion

kindreds in which most affected members have generalized lesions, as in the Koebner variant of EBS, may also include individuals with more localized lesions (as in EBS of Weber-Cockayne) and vice versa, thus underscoring the close relationship between the Koebner and Cockayne-Weber variants of EBS, the two most common forms of EBS

REFERENCES

McK 131900

Bonifas JM, Rothman AL, Epstein EH Jr. Epidermolysis bullosa simplex: evidence in two families for keratin gene abnormalities. Science 1991;254:1202–1205

Coulombe PA, Hutton ME, Vassar R, Fuchs E.

A function for keratins and a common thread among different types of epidermolysis bullosa simplex diseases. J Cell Biol 1991;115:1661–1674
Fine JD, Bauer EA, Briggaman RA, et al. Revised clinical and laboratory criteria for subtypes of inherited epidermolysis bullosa: a consensus report by the Subcommittee on Diagnosis and Classification of the National Epidermolysis Bullosa Registry. J Am Acad Dermatol 1991;24:119–135
Humphries MM, Sheils D, Lawler M, et al. Epidermolysis bullosa: evidence for linkage to genetic markers on chromosome 1 in a family with the autosomal dominant simplex form. Genomics 1990;7:377–381
Mulley JC, Nicholls CM, Propert DN, Turner T, Sutherland GR. Genetic linkage analysis of epidermolysis bullosa simplex, Koebner type. Am J Med Genet 1984;19:573–577

EPIDERMOLYSIS BULLOSA SIMPLEX HERPETIFORMIS

Synonym

- epidermolysis bullosa simplex, Dowling-Meara type

Skin

severe, widespread blistering with prominent acral involvement (Figs. 2–2 and 2–3); occasional involvement of oral cavity; onset at birth

after first few months of life, frequent palmoplantar lesions and characteristic herpetiform (grouped) blisters on trunk and limbs

blisters may heal with milia formation but no scarring

palmoplantar keratoderma appears late in first decade and may be disabling (Fig. 2–4)

some born with localized absence of skin

disease is reputed to improve during febrile illnesses and not worsen with warm weather, but exceptions to both patterns reported; condition improves in late childhood

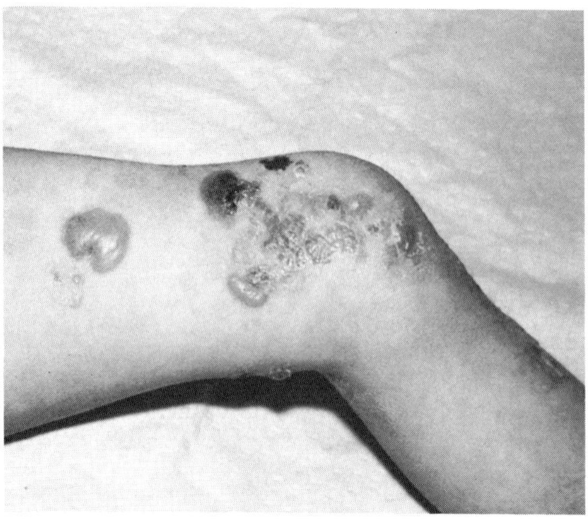

FIGURE 2–2
Multiple intact blisters and crusted plaques are grouped around the knee of this child with epidermolysis bullosa simplex herpetiformis (Dowling-Meara syndrome).

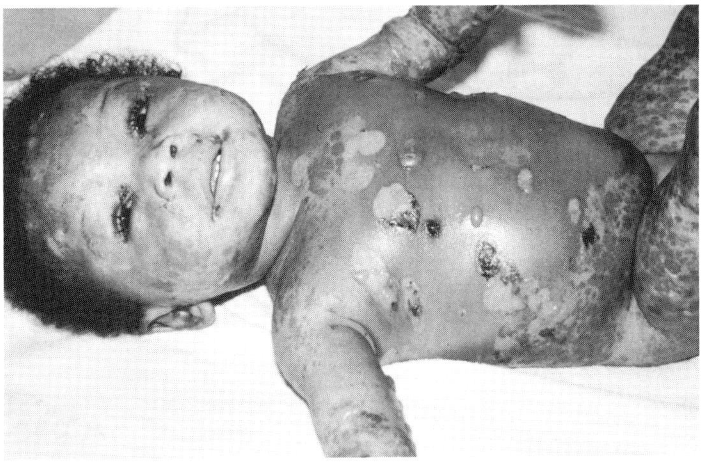

FIGURE 2–3
Multiple intact blisters, erosions, and areas of dyspigmentation widely scattered over the entire body of this infant with epidermolysis bullosa simplex herpetiformis (Dowling-Meara syndrome).

onychomadesis may occur, but nails regrow normally

dental abnormalities include natal teeth and anodontia

Genetics

AD

Laboratory Data

electron microscopy: clumping of tonofilaments (both typical round clumping and whisk-type clumping reported) in basal cells; clefts form adjacent to hemidesmosomes before cytolysis

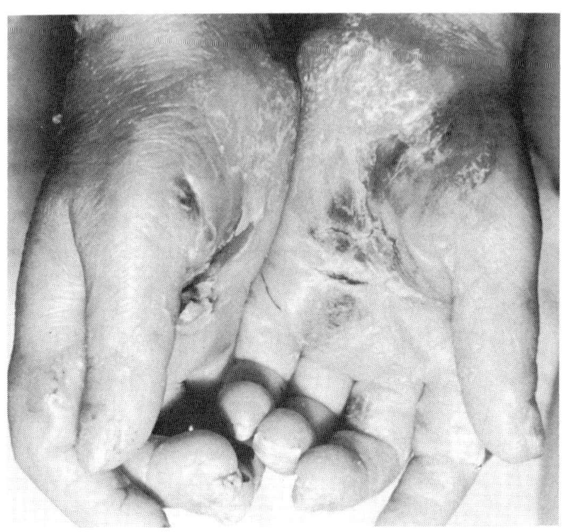

FIGURE 2–4
Keratoderma of the palms and nail dystrophy in a patient with epidermolysis bullosa simplex herpetiformis (Dowling-Meara syndrome).

REFERENCES

McK 131760
Buchbinder LH, Lucky AW, Ballard E, et al. Severe infantile epidermolysis bullosa simplex: Dowling-Meara type. Arch Dermatol 1986;122:190–198
Hacham-Zadeh S, Rappersberger K, Livshin R, et al. Epidermolysis bullosa herpetiformis Dowling-Meara in a large family. J Am Acad Dermatol 1988;18:702–706
Kitajima Y, Jokura Y, Yaoita H. Epidermolysis bullosa simplex, Dowling-Meara type: a report of two cases with different types of tonofilament clumping. Br J Dermatol 1993;128:79–85
McGrath JA, Ishida-Yamamota A, Tidman MJ, et al. Epidermolysis bullosa simplex (Dowling-Meara): a clinicopathological review. Br J Dermatol 1992;126:421–430
Tidman MJ, Eady RA, Leigh IM, et al. Keratin expression in epidermolysis bullosa simplex (Dowling-Meara). Acta Derm Venereol 1988;68:15–20

EPIDERMOLYSIS BULLOSA SIMPLEX WITH MOTTLED PIGMENTATION WITH OR WITHOUT KERATODERMA

skin findings as in generalized or localized EBS, but with mottled hyperpigmentation and hypopigmentation mainly on the trunk and extremities that develops in childhood; pigmentary changes may fade with time

rare herpetiform or annular lesions

with age, blistering may become less frequent or cease

mild atrophic areas occasionally seen

palmoplantar keratoderma in some

occasional nail dystrophy

carious teeth reported, which may be due to poor hygiene because of frequent mucosal blisters or erosions

AD

McK 131960
Bruckner-Tuderman L, Vogel A, Ruegger S, et al. Epidermolysis bullosa simplex with mottled pigmentation. J Am Acad Dermatol 1989;21:425–432
Fischer T, Gedde-Dahl T Jr. Epidermolysis bullosa simplex and mottled pigmentation: a new dominant syndrome: I. Clinical and histological features. Clin Genet 1979; 15:228–238
Medenica ML, Fenske NA, Espinoza CG. Epidermolysis bullosa herpetiformis with mottled pigmentation and an unusual punctate keratoderma. Arch Dermatol 1986; 122:900–908

EPIDERMOLYSIS BULLOSA SIMPLEX SUPERFICIALIS

generalized blisters, milia, atrophic scarring and nail dystrophy; erosions of oral and occasionally ocular mucosa

onset at birth or within first 2 years of life

spares palms and soles

AD

histopathology: clefting usually subcorneal, occasionally in lower third of stratum malpighii

differs from peeling skin syndrome (see main entry) principally by presence of blisters and absence of continued exfoliation

Fine JD, Johnson L, Wright T. Epidermolysis bullosa simplex superficialis: a new variant of epidermolysis bullosa characterized by subcorneal skin cleavage mimicking peeling skin syndrome. Arch Dermatol 1989;125:633–638

EPIDERMOLYSIS BULLOSA SIMPLEX, OGNA VARIANT

hemorrhagic and serous blisters, primarily on extremities; onset in early childhood

worse in warm weather

easy bruisability

onychogryphosis

AD

described in patients living in or around Ogna, Norway

genetically linked with erythrocyte glutamic-pyruvic transaminase (GPT) locus

McK 131950
Gedde-Dahl T Jr. Epidermolysis Bullosa: A Clinical, Genetic and Epidemiologic Study. Baltimore, Johns Hopkins University Press, 1971
Olaisen B, Gedde-Dahl T Jr. GPT–epidermolysis bullosa simplex (EBS Ogna) linkage in man. Hum Hered 1973;23:189–196

EPIDERMOLYSIS BULLOSA SIMPLEX WITH OR WITHOUT ASSOCIATED NEUROMUSCULAR DISEASE

erosions present at birth and are widespread early in life; later, blisters mostly acral in distribution

cutaneous scarring and atrophy, including scarring alopecia of scalp mild oral erosions

nail dystrophy

tooth enamel defects, rarely

anemia and growth retardation

neuromuscular disease in some (e.g., muscular dystrophy or myasthenia gravis)

gastrointestinal obstruction

septicemia

AR

most patients have died of unexplained causes

this variant is termed *epidermolysis bullosa simplex letalis* when neuromuscular disease is present

McK 226670

Fine JD, Stenn J, Johnson L, et al. Autosomal recessive epidermolysis bullosa simplex: generalized phenotypic features suggestive of junctional or dystrophic epidermolysis bullosa, and association with neuromuscular diseases. Arch Dermatol 1989;125:931–938

Kletter G, Evans OB, Lee JA, et al. Congenital muscular dystrophy and epidermolysis bullosa simplex. J Pediatr 1989;114:104–107

Niemi KM, Sommer H, Kero M, et al. Epidermolysis bullosa simplex associated with muscular dystrophy with recessive inheritance. Arch Dermatol 1988;124:551–554

Salih MAM, Lake BD, El Hag MA, Atherton DJ. Lethal epidermolytic epidermolysis bullosa: a new autosomal recessive type of epidermolysis bullosa. Br J Dermatol 1985;113:135–143

EPIDERMOLYSIS BULLOSA SIMPLEX, MENDES DA COSTA VARIANT (MACULAR DYSTROPHIC EPIDERMOLYSIS BULLOSA OF MENDES DA COSTA)

tense blisters on trunk and extremities; onset in infancy

reticulated hyperpigmentation and macular atrophy develop on face and extremities

alopecia of scalp

microcephaly

occasional mental retardation

XLR; only males are affected

shortened life expectancy reported

McK 302000

Fine JD, Bauer EA, Briggaman RA, et al. Revised clinical and laboratory criteria for subtypes of inherited epidermolysis bullosa: a consensus report by the Subcommittee on Diagnosis and Classification of the National Epidermolysis Bullosa Registry. J Am Acad Dermatol 1991;24:119–135

Mendes da Costa S, Van der Valk JW. Typus maculatus der bullosen hereditaren Dystrophie. Arch Dermatol Syphilol 1908; 91:1–8

Junctional Epidermolysis Bullosa

JUNCTIONAL EPIDERMOLYSIS BULLOSA INVERSA (EPIDERMOLYSIS BULLOSA ATROPHICANS INVERSA)

generalized neonatal blistering

blisters resolve after 3 to 5 months but recur in childhood, most severely in body folds

healing leaves characteristic atrophic white ("albostriate") streaks on trunk

occasional mild mucosal involvement

occasional nail dystrophy or loss

tooth enamel defects reported

AR

Fine JD, Bauer EA, Briggaman RA, et al. Revised clinical and laboratory criteria for subtypes of inherited epidermolysis bullosa: a consensus report by the Subcommittee on Diagnosis and Classification of the National Epidermolysis Bullosa Registry. J Am Acad Dermatol 1991;24:119–135

JUNCTIONAL EPIDERMOLYSIS BULLOSA, ACRAL (JUNCTIONAL EPIDERMOLYSIS BULLOSA MINIMUS)

blisters on hands and lower extremities; onset at birth

worse in warm weather

erosions of oral and nasal mucosa

nail abnormalities

tooth enamel hypoplasia

AR

TABLE 2–2
JUNCTIONAL EPIDERMOLYSIS BULLOSA (JEB)

Type	Inheritance	Skin	Hair, Nails, Teeth	Non-Skin	Histopathology
Junctional Epidermolysis Bullosa Localized					
JEB inversa	AR	Blisters at birth or early infancy, often widespread, but later concentrated in axillae, groin ("inverse" distribution); heal with atrophy	Hair: normal Nails: dystrophy or absence Teeth: "dysplastic"	Corneal erosions; oral, esophageal, and anal erosions	Subepidermal separation Electron microscopy: lamina lucida split with alteration of hemidesmosomes
JEB, acral (JEB minimus)	AR	Acral blistering from birth with scarring; atrophy	Hair: normal Nails: absent Teeth: enamel hypoplasia	Nasal, oral ulcerations	Subepidermal separation Electron microscopy: lamina lucida split with alterations of hemidesmosomes
JEB, progressiva variant (JEB neurotropica)	AR	Delayed onset; children 5 to 8 years old with acral blisters and atrophy; fingers have contractures	Hair: normal Nails: dystrophic or absent, often first sign Teeth: enamel hypoplasia	Oral blisters and loss of tongue markings; hearing loss; mild finger contractures	Subepidermal separation Electron microscopy: lamina lucida split with deposition of amorphous material
JEB, late-onset localized type with mental retardation	?AR	Blisters late first decade on legs, hands, and forearms	Hair: normal Nails: dystrophy Teeth: enamel defects	Mental retardation, subluxation of ocular lenses, craniofacial abnormalities	Subepidermal separation Electron microscopy; lamina plucida split with alteration of hemidesmosomes
Junctional Epidermolysis Bullosa, Generalized					
JEB gravis (Herlitz variant)	AR	Congenital erosions and deeper defects; generalized blisters with scarring and atrophy; perioral vegetating lesions characteristic	Hair: infrequent scarring alopecia Nails: dystrophic or absent Teeth: characteristic pitted enamel hypoplasia, hypodontia, and caries	All mucosae involved (nasal, oral, pharyngeal, esophageal, anal); also pyloric atresia, renal collecting system abnormalities, anemia, growth retardation, early death	Subepidermal separation Electron microscopy: lamina lucida split with alterations of hemidesmosomes
JEB mitis (non-Herlitz variant; generalized atrophic benign EB)	AR	Generalized erosions with focal scarring and atrophy	Hair: infrequent scarring alopecia Nails: dystrophic or absent Teeth: pitted enamel hypoplasia, hypodontia, and caries	Mucosa as in JEB gravis but less severe and not with internal abnormalities; normal growth; patients live into adulthood	Subepidermal separation Electron microscopy: lamina lucida split with alterations of hemidesmosomes
Cicatricial JEB	AR	Generalized blisters from birth, worse acrally; scarring occurs and "mitten" hands with contractures develop	Hair: scarring alopecia Nails: normal Teeth: dystrophic	Similar to JEB mitis with severe mucosal involvement and some internal disease; anemia; renal disease; "mitten" deformities of hands and feet	Subepidermal separation Electron microscopy: lamina lucida split with alteration of hemidesmosomes

Fine JD, Bauer EA, Briggaman RA, et al. Revised clinical and laboratory criteria for subtypes of inherited epidermolysis bullosa: a consensus report by the Subcommittee on Diagnosis and Classification of the National Epidermolysis Bullosa Registry. J Am Acad Dermatol 1991;24:119–135

JUNCTIONAL EPIDERMOLYSIS BULLOSA, PROGRESSIVA VARIANT (JEB NEUROTROPICA)

trauma-induced blisters of extremities and oral mucosa occurring in mid to late first decade

healing with progressive and diffuse skin atrophy

thickened palmar skin

oral blisters and loss of tongue papillae

nail dystrophy or loss, often first sign

"dysplastic" teeth

finger contractures

hearing loss

AR

worsens with age

McK 226500
Haber RM, Hanna W. Epidermolysis bullosa progressiva. J Am Acad Dermatol 1987; 16:195–200

LATE-ONSET LOCALIZED JUNCTIONAL EPIDERMOLYSIS BULLOSA AND MENTAL RETARDATION

blisters occurring on anterior aspect of the legs and, less commonly, on dorsa of hands and forearms in late first decade; increased blistering in warm weather

dystrophic toenails

defective dental enamel

mental retardation

subluxation of ocular lenses

craniofacial abnormalities include cleft palate, short midface and philtrum, prognathism, and thin vermilion border of the upper lip

possible AR

light and electron microscopy findings show junctional form of EB

McK 226440
Nakar S, Ingber A, Kremer I, et al. Late-onset localized junctional epidermolysis bullosa and mental retardation: a distinct autosomal recessive syndrome. Am J Med Genet 1992;43:776–779

JUNCTIONAL EPIDERMOLYSIS BULLOSA, GRAVIS

Synonyms

- junctional epidermolysis bullosa of Herlitz
- epidermolysis bullosa letalis

Skin

mostly generalized, nonscarring, clear or hemorrhagic blisters at birth; hands and feet usually spared

blisters may rupture and leave large denuded areas, especially on trunk and extremities (Fig. 2–5)

persistent plaques of granulation tissue in perioral and other areas are characteristic

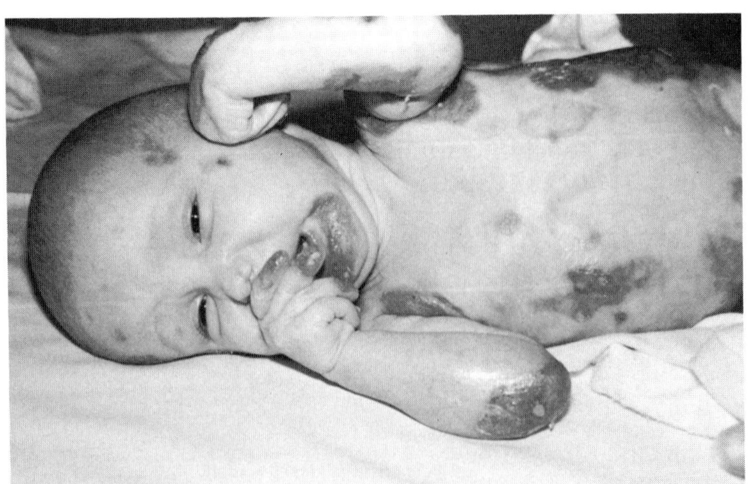

FIGURE 2–5
Widespread erosions particularly at pressure points and in the perioral area in an infant with junctional epidermolysis bullosa, gravis type.

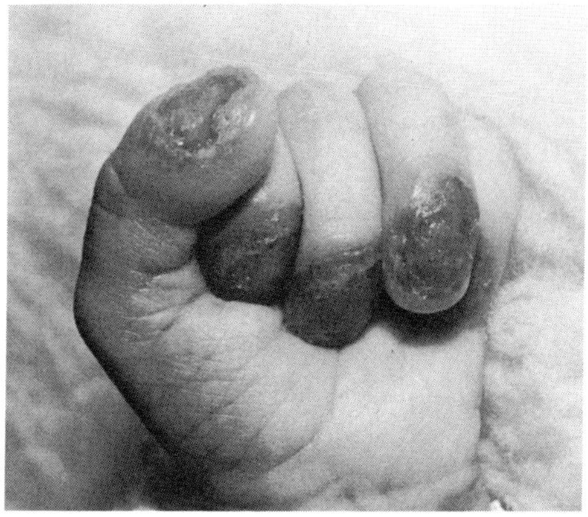

FIGURE 2–6
Newborn with junctional epidermolysis bullosa, gravis type. The terminal phalanges have a bulbous appearance. Nail plates are absent; erosions and granulation tissue involve entire nail units.

some born with areas of congenital absence of skin

mucosal lesions common and may involve all sites, including oral, ocular, genital, gastrointestinal, and respiratory tracts

scalp lesions common but only occasional scarring alopecia

milia not seen except when secondary infection of lesions leads to scarring and/or milia formation

paronychia (a hallmark of the neonatal period), dystrophy, or anonychia may develop (Fig. 2–6)

dental abnormalities include pitted enamel hypoplasia

Non-Skin

blistering of gastrointestinal and respiratory tracts

secondary growth retardation is common, due in part to continual protein loss from skin wounds

anemia of iron deficiency and/or chronic disease

occasional congenital pyloric atresia (see Discussion)

rare genitourinary disease

Genetics

AR

Laboratory Data

electron microscopy: blister formation in lamina lucida, with laminin in the floor and bullous pemphigoid antigen in the roof; hemidesmosomes may be abnormal and reduced in number

absence of staining with the following anti–basement membrane antibodies in the more severe forms of JEB: anti-hemidesmosomal antigens (BM-600/nicein [GB3]; AA3) and anti–anchoring filament–associated antigens (19-DEJ-1) prenatal diagnosis possible: fetal skin biopsy specimens show decreased staining on direct immunofluorescence with antibody to GB3

Prognosis

prognosis no longer uniformly fatal; therefore, *letalis* term is inappropriate

mortality frequently due to sepsis

Discussion

junctional epidermolysis bullosa with pyloric atresia distinguished by some as a separate entity (McK 226730)

junctional EB, disentis type, has been described as an "adult form" of JEB gravis; may be allelic with JEB gravis (McK 226650)

REFERENCES

McK 226700

McK 226730

Bergenholtz A, Olsson O. Epidermolysis bullosa hereditaria: I. Epidermolysis bullosa hereditaria letalis: a survey of the literature and report of 11 cases. Acta Derm Venereol 1968;48:220–241

Berger TG, Detlefs RL, Donatucci CF. Junctional epidermolysis bullosa, pyloric atresia, and genitourinary disease. Pediatr Dermatol 1986;3:130–134

Bull MJ, Norins AL, Weaver DD, et al. Epidermolysis bullosa–pyloric atresia: an autosomal recessive syndrome. Am J Dis Child 1983;137:449–451

Fine JD, Bauer EA, Briggaman RA, et al. Revised clinical and laboratory criteria for subtypes of inherited epidermolysis bullosa: a consensus report by the Subcommittee on Diagnosis and Classification of the National Epidermolysis Bullosa Registry. J Am Acad Dermatol 1991;24:119–135

Hausser I, Anton-Lamprecht I, Gustavii B. Prenatal diagnosis of junctional epidermolysis bullosa Herlitz type. [Letter]. Lancet 1989;2:1035–1036

Heagerty AH, Eady RA, Kennedy AR, et al. Rapid prenatal diagnosis of epidermolysis bullosa letalis using GB3 monoclonal antibody. Br J Dermatol 1987;117:271–275

Heagerty AH, Kennedy AR, Leigh IM, et al. Identification of an epidermal basement membrane defect in recessive forms of dystrophic epidermolysis bullosa by LH 7:2 monoclonal antibody: use in diagnosis. Br J Dermatol 1986;115:125–131

Kennedy AR, Heagerty AH, Ortonne JP, et al. Abnormal binding of an anti-amnion antibody to epidermal basement membrane provides a novel diagnostic probe for junctional epidermolysis bullosa. Br J Dermatol 1985;113:651–659

Lestringant GG, Akel SR, Qayed KI. The pyloric atresia-junctional epidermolysis bullosa syndrome. Arch Dermatol 1992; 128:1083–1086

Nazzaro V, Nicolini U, De Luca L, et al. Prenatal diagnosis of junctional epidermolysis bullosa associated with pyloric atresia. J Med Genet 1990;27:244–248

JUNCTIONAL EPIDERMOLYSIS BULLOSA, MITIS (JEB, NON-HERLITZ VARIANT; GENERALIZED ATROPHIC BENIGN EPIDERMOLYSIS BULLOSA; EPIDERMOLYSIS BULLOSA ATROPHICANS GENERALISATA MITIS; NONLETHAL JUNCTIONAL EPIDERMOLYSIS BULLOSA)

generalized blistering, frequently present at birth

blistering heals with atrophy; worse in warm weather

milia and granulation tissue not seen

oral involvement mild

alopecia (rarely scarring) and atrophy of scalp may be prominent; variable alopecia of axillae, pubes, eyelashes, and eyebrows

occasional nail dystrophy and tooth enamel defects

AR

histopathologic and electron microscopic findings are the same as in JEB gravis

absence or reduction of staining with the following anti–basement membrane antibodies: anti-hemidesmosome BM-600/nicein (GB3)

disease improves with age; overall prognosis is good

may be difficult to distinguish from JEB gravis in early infancy; however, growth is normal and anemia is not seen

Foldes C, Wallach D, Aubiniere E, et al. Generalized atrophic benign form of junctional epidermolysis bullosa. Dermatologica 1988; 176:83–90

Hacham ZS. Benign junctional epidermolysis bullosa in three related Moroccan families. [Letter]. J Am Acad Dermatol 1986;14: 508–509

Heagerty AHM, Tidman MJ, Bor S, Eady RAJ. Non-lethal junctional epidermolysis bullosa in two adult sisters. J R Soc Med 1985;78:32–33

Hintner H, Wolff K. Generalized atrophic benign epidermolysis bullosa. Arch Dermatol 1982;118:375–384

Paller AS, Fine JD, Kaplan S, et al. The generalized atrophic benign form of junctional epidermolysis bullosa: experience with four patients in the United States. Arch Dermatol 1986;122:704–710; see Arch Dermatol 1986;122:1297 for erratum

CICATRICIAL JUNCTIONAL EPIDERMOLYSIS BULLOSA

generalized blisters of skin and oral, nasal, esophageal, and laryngeal mucosae

present at birth

blisters heal with scarring and atrophy; stenosis of anterior nares characteristic

scarring alopecia of scalp

dental abnormalities including increased caries and enamel hypoplasia

mitten deformities of hands and feet

anemia and renal disease reported

AR

Haber RM, Hanna W, Ramsay CA, et al. Cicatricial junctional epidermolysis bullosa. J Am Acad Dermatol 1985;12:836–844

Dystrophic Epidermolysis Bullosa

DYSTROPHIC EPIDERMOLYSIS BULLOSA (DEB), INVERSA (EPIDERMOLYSIS BULLOSA DYSTROPHICA INVERSA OF GEDDE-DAHL)

generalized blisters; onset at birth or early infancy

later in life, blisters are predominantly intertriginous and/or flexural (i.e., in an "inverse" distribution)

oral and esophageal blistering severe, similar to recessive dystrophic EB gravis (Hallopeau-Siemens); ankyloglossia

blisters heal with superficial atropic scars but milia are absent

occasional scarring alopecia of scalp

nail and tooth dystrophy

stature and development are otherwise normal

corneal erosions

AR

intermittent and mild compared with recessive dystrophic EB gravis (Hallopeau-Siemens)

McK 226450
Pearson RW, Paller AS. Dermolytic (dystrophic) epidermolysis bullosa inversa. Arch Dermatol 1988;124:544–547

DYSTROPHIC EPIDERMOLYSIS BULLOSA, ACRAL (DYSTROPHIC EPIDERMOLYSIS BULLOSA MINIMUS)

acral blisters in early childhood

nail dystrophy

AD

possible milder variant of Cockayne-Touraine DEB

Fine JD, Bauer EA, Briggaman RA, et al. Revised clinical and laboratory criteria for subtypes of inherited epidermolysis bullosa: a consensus report by the Subcommittee on Diagnosis and Classification of the National Epidermolysis Bullosa Registry. J Am Acad Dermatol 1991;24:119–135

DYSTROPHIC EPIDERMOLYSIS BULLOSA, PRETIBIAL

blistering of dorsa of feet and pretibial areas; onset usually in mid childhood through adulthood, occasionally as early as infancy

blisters heal with scarring and atrophy

AD

other affected family members have either pretibial EB alone or other forms of dominant DEB (e.g., DDEB Cockayne-Touraine or DDEB Pasini), of which this disease may be a variant

Furue M, Ando I, Inoue Y, et al. Pretibial epidermolysis bullosa: successful therapy with a skin graft. Arch Dermatol 1986; 122:310–313

Garcia-Perez A, Carapeto FJ. Pretibial epidermolysis bullosa: report of two families and review of the literature. Dermatologica 1975;150:122–128

Lichtenwald DJ, Hanna W, Sauder DN, et al. Pretibial epidermolysis bullosa: report of a case. J Am Acad Dermatol 1990;22:346–350

DYSTROPHIC EPIDERMOLYSIS BULLOSA, CENTRIPETAL

acral blisters at birth with progressive centripetal progression that heal with scarring, milia, and atrophy

nail dystrophy

contractures, acral deformities, growth retardation, and mucosal lesions not seen

may be a variant of dominant DEB

Fine JD, Osment LS, Gay S. Dystrophic epidermolysis bullosa: a new variant characterized by progressive symmetrical centripetal involvement with scarring. Arch Dermatol 1985;121:1014–1017

DOMINANT DYSTROPHIC EPIDERMOLYSIS BULLOSA, ALBOPAPULOIDEA (DYSTROPHIC EPIDERMOLYSIS BULLOSA OF PASINI)

generalized cutaneous blistering at birth; mild oral and esophageal involvement; more extensive than in the Cockayne-Touraine type, and mucosal involvement more common

blisters heal with atrophic scarring and milia

TABLE 2–3
DYSTROPHIC EPIDERMOLYSIS BULLOSA

Type	Inheritance	Skin	Hair, Nails, Teeth	Non-Skin	Histopathology
Dominant Dystrophic Epidermolysis Bullosa (DDEB), Localized					
DDEB, inversa	AR	Blisters and erosions at birth; axilla, groin, and neck most affected	Hair: scarring alopecia may be seen Nails: normal Teeth: mild "dystrophy," hypodontia, and caries	Oral mucosal and esophageal involvement is severe compared with the skin; tongue is bound down; keratitis	Separation beneath basal lamina; anchoring fibrils abnormal, also in adjacent skin
DDEB, acral (DDEB minimus)	AD	Mild acral blistering early childhood, later, occasional blistering with nail dystrophy	Hair: normal Nails: dystrophic Teeth: normal		Separation beneath basal lamina, anchoring fibrils abnormal; adjacent skin has normal anchoring fibrils
DDEB, pretibial	AD	Blisters that heal with scarring of dorsal feet, pretibial areas	Hair: normal Nails: normal Teeth: normal		Separation beneath basal lamina, anchoring fibrils abnormal; adjacent skin has normal anchoring fibrils
DDEB, centripetal		Acral blisters at birth with progressive centripetal involvement	Hair: normal Nails: dystrophic or absent Teeth: normal		
Dominant Dystrophic Epidermolysis Bullosa, Generalized					
DDEB, albopapuloidea (Pasini variant)	AD	Blisters and erosions at birth commonly with milia, scarring, and atrophy; later, hypopigmented and papular (albopapuloid) scars mainly acrally but not pathognomonic; rarely, patients develop squamous cell carcinoma	Hair: normal Nails: dystrophic or absent Teeth: normal		Separation beneath basal lamina; adjacent skin has normal anchoring fibrils

DDEB, hyperplasique (Cockayne-Touraine variant)	AD	Generalized and acral blisters at birth commonly with milia, scarring, and atrophy; rarely, patients develop squamous cell carcinoma	Hair: normal Nails: dystrophic or absent Teeth: normal	Keratitis may occur; oral ulcers rare; esophageal stenosis	Separation beneath basal lamina; anchoring fibrils decreased in number and poorly developed, even in adjacent normal skin
Transient bullous dermolysis of the newborn	AD; ?AR	Generalized blisters with marked acral involvement at birth; patient clinically normal by 1 year of age	Hair: normal Nails: usually normal Teeth: normal		Separation beneath basal lamina; anchoring fibrils abnormal
Recessive Dystrophic Epidermolysis Bullosa (RDEB), Generalized					
RDEB, gravis (Hallopeau-Siemens variant)	AR	Blisters and erosions at birth; severe scarring with milia and atrophy; "mitten" deformities of hands and feet and significant risk for squamous cell carcinoma	Hair: scarring alopecia Nails: absent Teeth: dystrophic	Keratitis common; severe widespread mucosal involvement; esophageal stenosis; severe anemia and growth retardation; failure to thrive; increased mortality (childhood and early adulthood)	Separation beneath basal lamina; anchoring fibrils reduced in number and poorly developed, also in adjacent skin
RBED, mitis	AR	Generalized blisters at birth; scarring, milia, and atrophy present	Hair: normal Nails: dystrophic or absent Teeth: normal	Mild oral erosions	

albopapuloid lesions (papular scars) appear on trunk at puberty, either spontaneously or in areas of healing blisters

nail dystrophy

cutaneous squamous cell carcinoma in some

occasional growth retardation and musculoskeletal deformities

AD

increased urinary excretion of chondroitin sulfate

electron microscopy: abnormal anchoring fibrils in all skin (cf. Cockayne-Touraine variant, in which abnormalities are only in blistered skin)

McK 131750

Anton-Lamprecht I, Hashimoto I. Epidermolysis bullosa dystrophica dominans (Pasini): a primary structural defect of the anchoring fibrils. Hum Genet 1976;32:69–76

DOMINANT DYSTROPHIC EPIDERMOLYSIS BULLOSA, HYPERPLASIQUE

Synonym

- epidermolysis bullosa dystrophica of Cockayne-Touraine

Skin

trauma-induced blisters, mostly on extremities, rarely widespread (Fig. 2–7); onset at birth

blisters heal with milia and scarring, which is usually atrophic

some infants born with localized absence of skin

erosions and blisters occasionally involve conjunctival and corneal mucosa, rarely the oropharynx, esophagus, or larynx; esophageal stenosis may develop

palmoplantar hyperhidrosis is common, but keratoderma occurs only occasionally

rarely, cutaneous squamous cell carcinoma develops

hair and teeth are normal

nail dystrophy or loss may occur

Genetics

AD

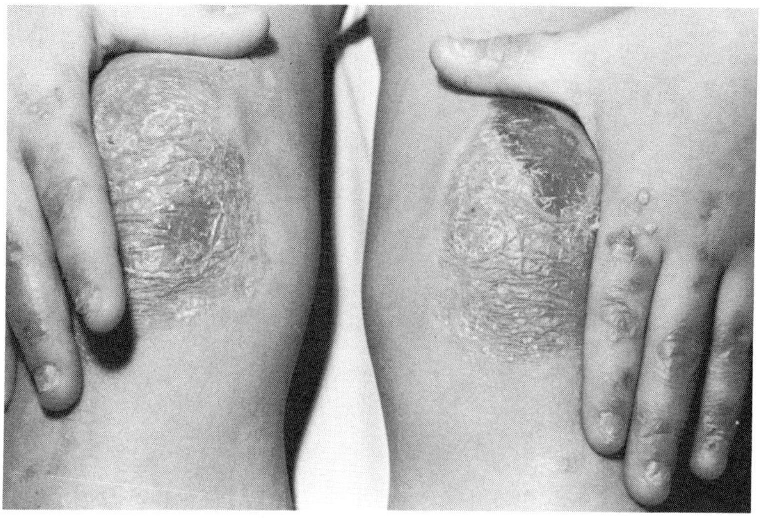

FIGURE 2–7
Healing erosions, atrophic scars, nail dystrophy, and multiple milia in a child with dominant dystrophic epidermolysis bullosa.

Pathophysiology

genetic linkage to type VII collagen gene reported in families with dominant dystrophic EB

Laboratory Data

electron microscopy: separation is beneath basal lamina; decreased or rudimentary anchoring fibrils in blister-prone skin only (cf. albopapuloid Pasini variant, in which anchoring fibrils are abnormal in all skin)

Prognosis

normal life expectancy

Discussion

rare kindreds with dermolytic EB and palmoplantar keratoderma are distinguished by some researchers as belonging to a separate genetic entity, but others believe it is a chance occurrence of two autosomal dominant traits, possibly in linkage dysequilibrium

REFERENCES

Bouwes-Bavinck JN, van Haeringen A, Ruiter D, et al. Autosomal dominant epidermolysis bullosa dystrophica: are the Cockayne-Touraine, the Pasini and the Bart types different expressions of the same mutant gene? Clin Genet 1987;31:416–424

DeRaeve L, DeDobbeleer G, Song M, et al. Dominant dystrophic epidermolysis bullosa of Cockayne-Touraine in father and son: clinical and ultrastructural similarities. Dermatologica 1988;176:91–94

Fine JD, Eady RA, Levy ML, et al. Prenatal diagnosis of dominant and recessive dystrophic epidermolysis bullosa: application and limitations in the use of KF-1 and LH 7:2 monoclonal antibodies and immuno-

fluorescence mapping technique. J Invest Dermatol 1988;91:465–471
Kero M. Epidermolysis bullosa in Finland: clinical features, morphology and relation to collagen metabolism. Acta Derm Venereol Suppl 1984;110:1–51
Puig L, Moreno A, Noguera X, et al. Dominant dystrophic epidermolysis bullosa with keratosis punctata. [Letter]. J Am Acad Dermatol 1986;15:1289–1291
Schwartz RA, Birnkrant AP, Rubenstein DJ, et al. Squamous cell carcinoma in dominant type epidermolysis bullosa dystrophica. Cancer 1981;47:615–620

TRANSIENT BULLOUS DERMOLYSIS OF THE NEWBORN (CONGENITAL SELF-HEALING [TRANSIENT] MECHANOBULLOUS DERMATOSIS)

generalized blistering of skin and mucous membranes at birth or in early infancy, lasting only a few months

milia and minimal scarring and atrophy present

nail dystrophy uncommon

AD; possible AR

subbasal lamina split on electron microscopy

probably a mild form of dominant dystrophic EB

McK 131705
Fisher GBJ, Greer KE, Cooper PH. Congenital self-healing (transient) mechanobullous dermatosis. [Review]. Arch Dermatol 1988; 124:240–243
Hashimoto K, Burk JD, Bale GF, et al. Transient bullous dermolysis of the newborn: two additional cases. J Am Acad Dermatol 1989;21:708–713
Hashimoto K, Matsumoto M, Iacobelli D. Transient bullous dermolysis of the newborn. Arch Dermatol 1985;121:1429–1438

RECESSIVE DYSTROPHIC EPIDERMOLYSIS BULLOSA (RDEB), GRAVIS

Synonym

- epidermolysis bullosa dystrophica of Hallopeau-Siemens

Skin

generalized flaccid hemorrhagic blisters, especially in areas of trauma (Fig. 2–8)

onset at birth or in infancy, rarely later

blisters heal with marked scarring and atrophy; scarring may fuse digits together into “mitten” hands and feet and cause severe contractures (Fig. 2–9)

milia common, especially on ears, extensor extremities, dorsa of hands and fingers

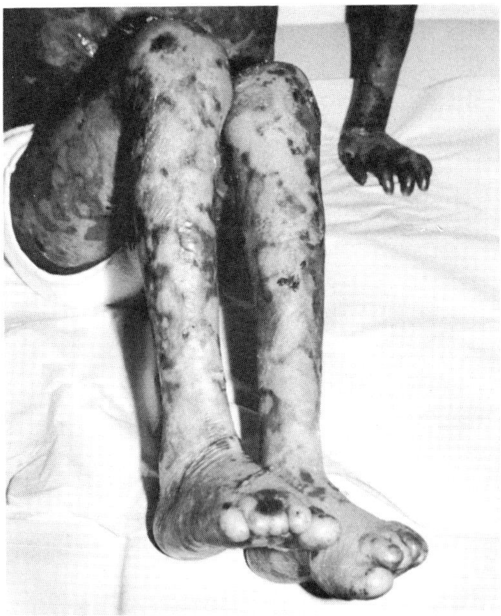

FIGURE 2–8
Extensive erosions and a few intact bullae on the torso and limbs of a child with recessive dystrophic epidermolysis bullosa.

palmoplantar hyperhidrosis

some born with localized absence of skin

severe blistering and erosions of oropharynx; may complicate feeding

mucosal scarring may obliterate gingivolabial sulcus or cause ankyloglossia

squamous cell carcinoma of affected areas may develop (Fig. 2–10)

scant scalp and body hair; occasional cicatricial alopecia of scalp

nail dystrophy or anonychia; may be noted at birth

dental abnormalities include cone-shaped teeth, early caries, and decreased size and number of teeth

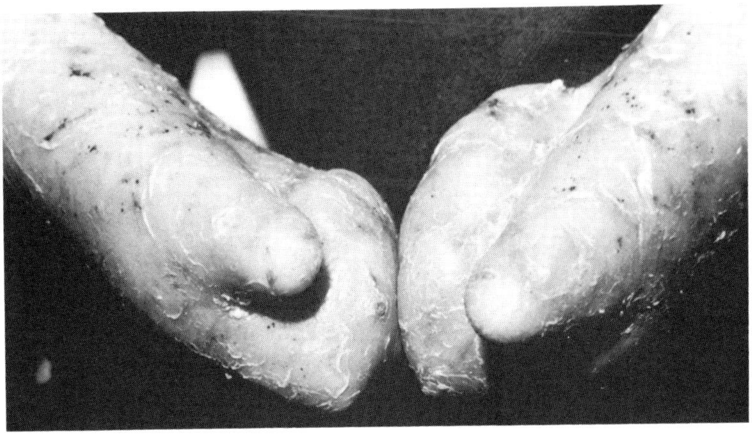

FIGURE 2–9
Mitten-hand deformity in a patient with recessive dystrophic epidermolysis bullosa.

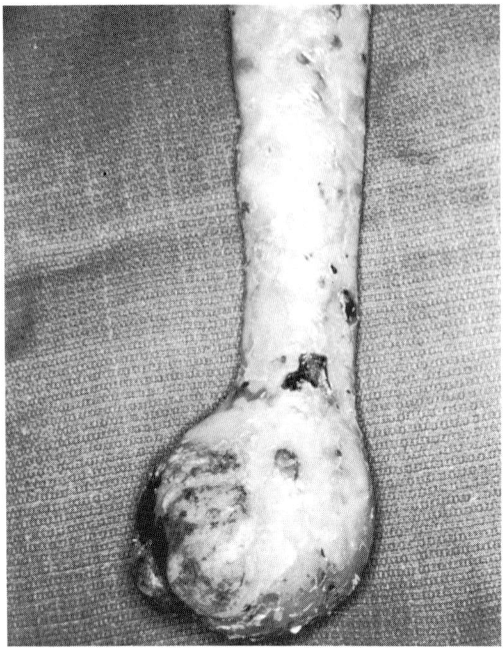

FIGURE 2–10
Squamous cell carcinoma developing in a mitten-hand deformity of a patient with recessive dystrophic epidermolysis bullosa. (Courtesy of Benjamin K. Fisher, MD, Toronto, Ontario)

Non-Skin

laryngeal and esophageal involvement may result in scarring and stenoses; malnutrition with growth retardation and/or aspiration pneumonitis may follow

eye abnormalities include cicatricial ectropion, scarring of lacrimal ducts, corneal erosions and opacification, and loss of vision

Genetics

AR

Pathophysiology

abnormalities in anchoring fibrils (see under Laboratory Data) may be due to mutations in the type VII collagen gene and/or due to excessive degradation by increased amounts of collagenase

Laboratory Data

electron microscopy: blister below basal lamina; diminished or absent anchoring fibrils

absence or reduction of staining with the following anti–basement membrane antibodies: anti–type VII collagen (LH 7:2; L3d); anti–lamina densa antigen (KF-1); anti–anchoring fibril epitopes (AF-1, AF-2); anti–chondroitin-6-sulfate proteoglycan (CSPG)

Prognosis

life expectancy may be shortened; causes of death include infectious pneumonitis, aspiration pneumonia, sepsis, malignancy (squamous cell carcinoma may develop from scars or mucosal leukoplakia from third decade onward), and secondary amyloidosis

REFERENCES

Bruckner-Tuderman L, Niemi KM, Kero M, et al. Type VII collagen is expressed but anchoring fibrils are defective in dystrophic epidermolysis bullosa inversa. Br J Dermatol 1990;122:383–390

Fine JD, Bauer EA, Briggaman RA, et al. Revised clinical and laboratory criteria for subtypes of inherited epidermolysis bullosa: a consensus report by the Subcommittee on Diagnosis and Classification of the National Epidermolysis Bullosa Registry. J Am Acad Dermatol 1991;24:119–135

Gryboski JD, Touloukian R, Campanella RA. Gastrointestinal manifestations of epidermolysis bullosa in children. Arch Dermatol 1988;124:746–752

Keefe M, Wakeel RA, Dick DC. Death from metastatic, cutaneous, squamous cell carcinoma in autosomal recessive dystrophic epidermolysis bullosa despite permanent inpatient care. Dermatologica 1988;177:180–184

Mann JF, Zeier M, Zilow E, et al. The spectrum of renal involvement in epidermolysis bullosa dystrophica hereditaria: report of two cases. Am J Kidney Dis 1988;11:437–441

Reed WB, College J Jr, Francis MJO, et al. Epidermolysis bullosa dystrophica with epidermal neoplasms. Arch Dermatol 1974;110:894–902

Yi S, Naito M, Takahashi K, et al. Complicating systemic amyloidosis in dystrophic epidermolysis bullosa, recessive type. Pathology 1988;20:184–187

RECESSIVE DYSTROPHIC EPIDERMOLYSIS BULLOSA, MITIS

generalized blistering at birth; heals with milia, scarring, and atrophy, mostly confined to sites of trauma

mucous membranes generally spared; occasional mild erosions

occasional nail dystrophy or loss

AR

phenotypically resembles generalized DDEB; mild end of spectrum of RDEB, with RDEB gravis (Hallopeau-Siemens) at the severe end

Fine JD, Bauer EA, Briggaman RA, et al. Revised clinical and laboratory criteria for subtypes of inherited epidermolysis bullosa: a consensus report by the Subcommittee on Diagnosis and Classification of the National Epidermolysis Bullosa Registry. J Am Acad Dermatol 1991;24:119–135

Other Bullous Disorders

BART SYNDROME

trauma-induced blisters of skin and oral mucosa noted at birth; blisters cease in infancy or childhood and are usually nonscarring

some infants born with localized absence of skin, especially on lower extremities; may be eroded blisters

nail dystrophy and onychomadesis

AD

on electron microscopy, split below the lamina densa

initially classified as a variant of EBS, but nail dystrophy, occasional scarring, and electron microscopic and immunofluorescent studies suggest it may be a variant of dominant dystrophic EB; electron microscopy was not done in Bart's original series, so type of EB is not known in that series

considerable confusion exists since the term *Bart syndrome* has been applied to the association of many types of EB with congenital localized absence of skin (so-called aplasia cutis–like lesions); ultrastructural studies indicate that lesions of congenital localized absence of skin are simply a manifestation of EB originating in utero

cases in which lesions cease after infancy probably include instances of congenital self-healing mechanobullous dermatosis

McK 132000

Bart BJ, Gorlin RJ, Anderson VE, et al. Congenital localized absence of skin and associated abnormalities resembling epidermolysis bullosa: a new syndrome. Arch Dermatol 1966;93:296–304

Butler DF, Berger TG, James WD, et al. Bart's syndrome: microscopic, ultrastructural, and immunofluorescent mapping features. Pediatr Dermatol 1986;3:113–118

Kanzler MH, Smoller B, Woodley DT. Congenital localized absence of the skin as a manifestation of epidermolysis bullosa. Arch Dermatol 1992;128:1087–1090

Smith SZ, Cram DL. A mechanobullous disease of the newborn: Bart's syndrome. Arch Dermatol 1978;114:81–84

Wojnarowska FT, Eady RA, Wells RS. Dystrophic epidermolysis bullosa presenting with congenital localized absence of skin: report of four cases. Br J Dermatol 1983;108:477–483

EPIDERMOLYSIS BULLOSA ACQUISITA

an acquired mechanobullous condition with blistering, scarring, and milia

wide spectrum of severity

often confused with hereditary epidermolysis bullosa, especially dystrophic forms

onset from childhood to adulthood

antibodies to type VII collagen demonstrated

Burke WA, Briggaman RA, Gammon WR. Epidermolysis bullosa acquisita in a patient with multiple endocrinopathies syndrome. Arch Dermatol 1986;122:187–189

Gammon WR, Briggaman RA, Woodley DT, et al. Epidermolysis bullosa acquisita: a pemphigoid-like disease. J Am Acad Dermatol 1984;11:820–832

McCuaig CC, Chan LS, Woodley DT, et al. Epidermolysis bullosa acquisita in childhood. Differentiation from hereditary epidermolysis bullosa. Arch Dermatol 1989;125:944–949

ACRODERMATITIS ENTEROPATHICA

Synonyms

- Danbolt-Closs syndrome
- Brandt syndrome

Skin

vesicles and bullae followed by formation of erythematous psoriasiform plaques distributed symmetrically around mucocutaneous orifices, occiput, and distal extremities (Figs. 2–11 through 2–13); lesions are not due to antecedent trauma

onset ranges from first month to 10 years of age, with most cases occurring in infancy, often during weaning (resumption of breast feeding improves the condition)

lesions usually heal without scarring

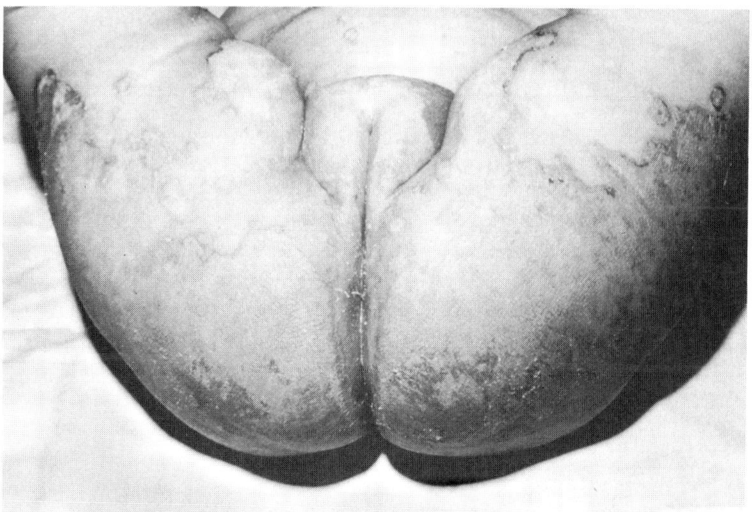

FIGURE 2–11
Sharply demarcated erythematous scaly eruption in the diaper area of an infant with acrodermatitis enteropathica. (Courtesy of Benjamin K. Fisher, MD, Toronto, Ontario)

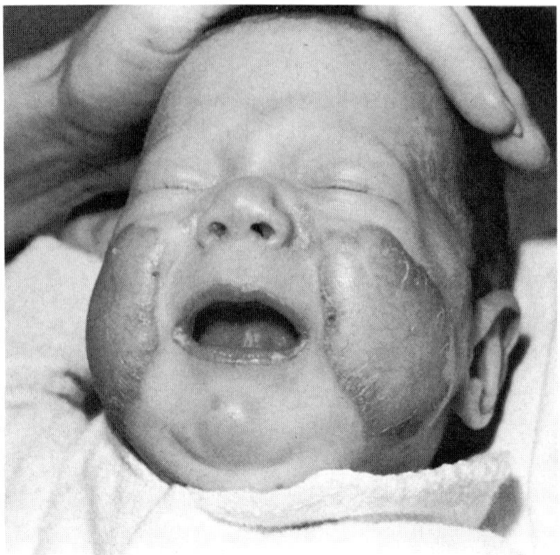

FIGURE 2–12
Psoriasiform dermatitis involving both cheeks, the paranasal skin, and the lips of an infant with acquired zinc deficiency, a disease with skin manifestations very similar in appearance to acrodermatitis enteropathica.

secondary impetiginization or colonization with *Candida* species common

perioral fissuring and angular cheilitis

blistering may involve oral mucosa, especially tongue and buccal surfaces

total or partial alopecia of scalp, eyebrows, and eyelashes is common early in disease, usually following the onset of dermatitis

nail dystrophy and paronychia common; occasionally, nails are shed

Non-Skin

intermittent diarrhea, often mucoid, is prominent

other gastrointestinal findings include abdominal pain and marked anorexia

failure to thrive and developmental retardation results

apathy, behavioral difficulties, mood changes, and other psychiatric symptoms are common

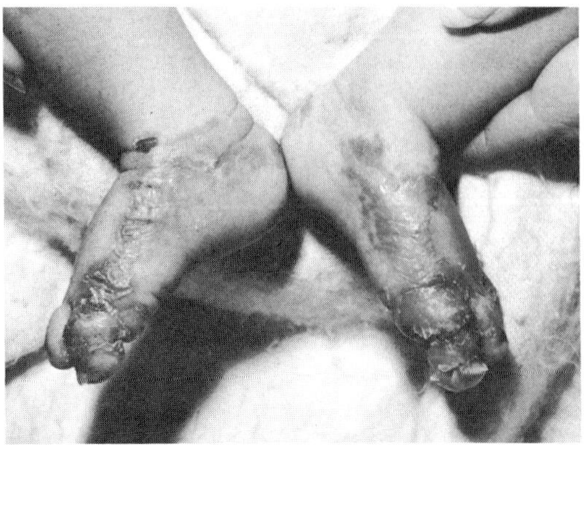

FIGURE 2–13
Same infant as in Figure 2–12. Bilateral symmetrical deeply erythematous, scaly plaques involving the medial ankles and dorsa of the feet and toes in association with nail dystrophy.

ocular mucosa may be involved, causing blepharoconjunctivitis and photophobia

Genetics

AR

Pathophysiology

low serum zinc levels in most, probably due to an intestinal absorption defect

Laboratory Data

for accurate serum zinc measurements, blood must be drawn and stored in zinc-free system

decreased serum alkaline phosphatase levels

impaired cell-mediated immunity and defective neutrophil chemotaxis reported

Paneth cell abnormalities may be demonstrated by electron microscopy of small bowel biopsy specimens

Prognosis

elemental zinc therapy (2 mg/kg/day) rapidly controls the disease; in the past, death in untreated patients was common

improvement with age is commonly reported, especially in adolesence

Discussion

variability in symptomatology (e.g., absence of diarrhea) may make diagnosis difficult

some patients have serum zinc levels in the normal range; response to zinc therapy and electron microscopic findings of small bowel biopsy help establish the diagnosis

interpretation of serum zinc levels is often difficult; diurnal variation or contamination from sources including zinc-coated needles may cause inconsistent determinations

■ *acquired zinc deficiency:*

may resemble acrodermatitis enteropathica; occurs in premature infants who receive inadequate zinc in hyperalimentation, breast-fed infants of mothers whose breast milk is low in zinc, and infants with severe diarrhea and malabsorption

other causes of zinc deficiency include penicillamine therapy and malnutrition states such as alcoholism, anorexia nervosa, overzealous or fad dieting, and total parenteral nutrition

REFERENCES

McK 201100

Bronson DM, Barsky R, Barsky S. Acrodermatitis enteropathica. J Am Acad Dermatol 1983;9:140–144

Bye AME, Goodfellow A, Atherton DJ. Transient zinc deficiency in a full-term breast-fed infant of normal birth weight. Pediatr Dermatol 1985;2:308–311

Fraker PJ, Jardieu P, Cook J. Zinc deficiency and immune function. Arch Dermatol 1987;123:1699–1701

Graves K, Kestenbaum T, Kalivas J. Hereditary acrodermatitis enteropathica in an adult. Arch Dermatol 1980;116:562–564

Kenny F, Sriram K, Hammond JB. Clinical zinc deficiency during adequate enteral nutrition. J Am Coll Nutr 1989;8:83–85

Lee MG, Hong KT, Kim JJ. Transient symptomatic zinc deficiency in a full term breast-fed infant. J Am Acad Dermatol 1990; 23:375–379

Mack D, Koletzko B, Cunnane S, et al. Acrodermatitis enteropathica with normal serum zinc levels: diagnostic value of small bowel biopsy and essential fatty acid determination. Gut 1989;30:1426–1429

Margileth AM. Acrodermatitis enteropathica: case report and review of literature. Am J Dis Child 1963;105:101–107

Nelder KH, Hambridge KM. Zinc therapy of acrodermatitis enteropathica. N Engl J Med 1975;292:879–882

Prasad AS. Clinical manifestations of zinc deficiency. Annu Rev Nutr 1985;5:341–363

Van Wouwe JP. Clinical and laboratory diagnosis of acrodermatitis enteropathica. Eur J Pediatr 1989;149:2–8

West BL, Anderson PC. Alcohol and acquired acrodermatitis enteropathica. [Letter]. J Am Acad Dermatol 1986;15:1305

HAILEY-HAILEY DISEASE

Synonym

- familial benign chronic pemphigus

Skin

easily ruptured flaccid bullae and vesicles leaving moist erosions and crusts (Figs. 2–14 and 2–15); bases of lesions may be erythematous or noninflamed; secondary impetiginization very common

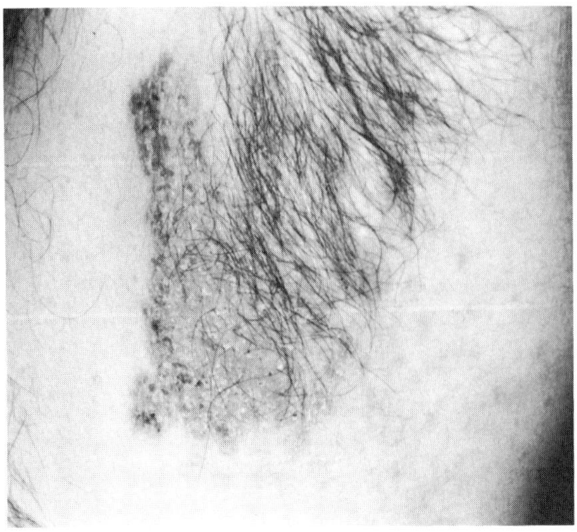

FIGURE 2–14
Hailey-Hailey disease. Eroded velvety plaques are often seen in the armpit, a frequent site of involvement. Secondary infection is common.

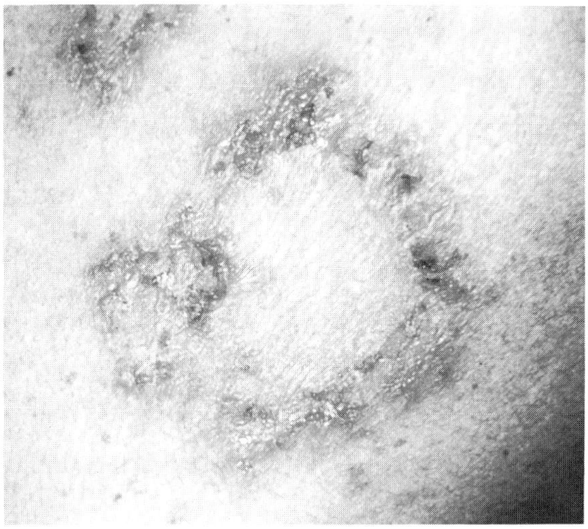

FIGURE 2–15
Annular lesions are often seen in Hailey-Hailey disease.

usually seen in intertriginous, flexural, and other areas subject to shearing forces; may rarely be seen on scalp, back, or thighs; Nikolsky's sign may be noted

onset is usually shortly after puberty, but lesions may not appear until middle or late adulthood

besides friction, precipitating phenomena include sweating, infection, freezing, and ultraviolet irradiation

intertriginous plaques may become verrucous

rarely, oral, esophageal, and ocular mucosae are involved; lesions heal without scarring

disease worsens in the summer; rare malignant degeneration of lesions reported

disease severity and frequency decrease with age; remissions lasting several years may occur

Genetics

AD

Laboratory Data

histopathology: "dilapidated brick wall" acantholysis of epidermal cells is considered characteristic, but a pattern indistinguishable from that in pemphigus vulgaris may also be seen

Prognosis

most patients respond to topical corticosteroids and oral antibiotics; in severe cases, oral corticosteroids are used

superficial ablation (down to papillary dermis) of affected skin (e.g., electrodesiccation, dermabrasion, or laser treatment) may be beneficial

Discussion

variants include localized disease such as warty, hyperkeratotic lesions on legs or papular lesions of the anogenital areas

REFERENCES

McK 169600

Brownstein MH. Acantholytic acanthoma. J Am Acad Dermatol 1988;19:783–786

Burge SM. Hailey-Hailey disease: the clinical features, response to treatment and prognosis. Br J Dermatol 1992;126:275–282

Chun SI, Whang KC, Su WP. Squamous cell carcinoma arising in Hailey-Hailey disease. J Cutan Pathol 1988;15:234–237

Don PC, Carney PS, Lynch WS, et al. Carbon dioxide laser abrasion: a new approach to management of familial benign chronic pemphigus (Hailey-Hailey disease). J Dermatol Surg Oncol 1987;13:1187–1194

Hailey H, Hailey H. Familial benign chronic pemphigus: report of 13 cases in 4 generations of a family and report of 9 additional cases in 4 generations of a family. Arch Dermatol Syphilol 1939;39:679–685

Langenberg A, Berger TG, Cardelli M, et al. Genital benign chronic pemphigus (Hailey-Hailey disease) presenting as condylomas. J Am Acad Dermatol 1992;26:951–955

Menz P, Jackson IT, Connolly S. Surgical control of Hailey-Hailey disease. Br J Plast Surg 1987;40:557–561

Quitadamo MJ, Spencer SK. Surgical management of Hailey-Hailey disease. J Am Acad Dermatol 1991;25:342–343

Steffen CG. Familial benign chronic pemphigus. Am J Dermatopathol 1987;9:58–73

Zachariae H. Dermabrasion of Hailey-Hailey disease and Darier's disease. J Am Acad Dermatol 1992;27:136

CHAPTER

3

Poikilodermatous Disorders

Poikiloderma is defined as a skin disorder with the following features:

1. Diffuse atrophy
2. Telangiectases
3. Leukomelanoderma (hyperpigmentation and hypopigmentation, often in a speckled pattern)

A patient must have two of the three criteria to qualify.

Congenital poikilodermas are further characterized by

- early appearance
- familial occurrence
- associated malformations

Two classifications of the congenital poikilodermas are presented in Tables 3–1 and 3–2. The first, a simple schema proposed by Marghescu, consists

TABLE 3–1
CONGENITAL POIKILODERMAS: AN OVERVIEW

Syndrome	Inheritance	Cataracts	Leukoplakia	Blisters	Keratoses	Sclerosis
Rothmund	AR	+	−	−	−	−
Thomson	AR	−	−	−	−	−
Dyskeratosis congenita	XLR	−	+	−	−	−
Kindler	Probable AR	−	−	+	−	−
Hereditary acrokeratotic poikiloderma	AD	−	−	−	+	−
Hereditary sclerosing poikiloderma	AD	−	−	−	−	+

+, Present; −, absent.

Note: Marghescu splits Rothmund-Thomson syndrome into separate syndromes. Rothmund syndrome is characterized by ophthalmologic findings (e.g., cataracts), while Thomson syndrome mainfests poikiloderma and bony abnormalities. In the text, we have combined these into Rothmund-Thomson syndrome.

Modified from Marghescu D. Kongenitale Poikilodermien. Z Hautkrankheit 1989:64, 167–169.

TABLE 3–2
POIKILODERMATOUS DISORDERS

Syndrome	Inheritance	Bullae	Photosensitivity	Poikiloderma	Acral Keratoses	Eczematous Dermatitis	Nail Changes	Mucous Membrane Lesions
Dyskeratosis congenita	XLR, AD; possible AR	+/–	–	+	–	–	+	+
Kindler syndrome	Probable AR	Acral	+/–	Widespread with atrophy	+/–	+/–	+/–	+/–
Hereditary acrokeratotic poikiloderma	AD	Acral	–	Accentuated in flexures; spares face	+	+	–	–
Hereditary sclerosing poikiloderma	AD	–	–	Accentuated in flexures	–	–	Clubbing	–
Rothmund-Thomson (poikiloderma congenitale)	AR	Light-exposed skin	+/–	Photo distribution	+/–	–	+/–	–
Xeroderma pigmentosum	AR	+/–	+	Photo distribution	–	–	–	+/–
Bloom syndrome	AR	+/–	+	Photo distribution	+	–	–	–
Cockayne syndrome	AR	–	+	Photo distribution	–	–	–	–
Werner syndrome	AR	–	Acral accentuation	–	+	–	+/–	–
Franceschetti-Jadassohn syndrome	AD	–	–	+	–	–	–	–
Dermatopathia pigmentosa reticularis	AD	+	–	–	+	–	+	–

+, Present; –, absent; +/–, reported occasionally.

Modified from Forman AB, Prendiville JS, Esterly NB, et al. Kindler syndrome: report of two cases and review of the literature. Pediatr Dermatol 1989;6:91–101; and Dintiman B, Burgdorf WHC. Poikiloderma. In: Demis DJ, Thiers BH, Smith EB, Burgdorf WHC, eds. Clinical Dermatology. Philadelphia, JB Lippincott, 1991.

of six disorders; in this classification the Rothmund-Thomson syndrome has been split into separate entities, a somewhat unconventional viewpoint. Table 3–2 represents a more extensive listing of the congenital poikilodermas. Because the clinical findings are so variable in these disorders, some entities in which poikiloderma is a less prominent finding are included elsewhere in the book, such as in Chapter 4 on premature aging syndromes since poikilodermatous skin often has an aged appearance.

Dintiman B, Burgdorf WHC. Poikiloderma. In: Demis DJ, Thiers BH, Smith EB, Burgdorf WHC, eds. Clinical Dermatology. Philadelphia, JB Lippincott, 1991

Marghescu S. Kongenitale Poikilodermien. Z Hautkrankheit 1989;64:167–169

DYSKERATOSIS CONGENITA

Synonym

- Zinsser-Cole-Engman syndrome

Skin

ulceration of oral mucosa (Fig. 3–1); onset most frequently in mid first decade

leukokeratotic plaques then develop in oral mucosa and genitourinary and gastrointestinal tracts; strictures of esophagus, anus, ureters, and urethra may result

malignant degeneration of mucosal leukokeratosis is common; onset from third decade onward

nail dystrophy with fingers affected more than toes (Fig. 3–2); rarely, anonychia results; onset usually between mid first and second decades; may be the initial sign of the disease

poikiloderma, primarily hypopigmentation and hyperpigmentation, develops on face, neck, upper chest, and flexures (e.g., groin) and later becomes more generalized (Fig. 3–3); may appear at same time as nail changes or 2 to 3 years later; usually reaches full extent of severity after 3 to 5 years

later, atrophy and cyanosis of hands, feet, elbows, and knees develop, resembling acrodermatitis chronica atrophicans

palms and soles are frequently hyperkeratotic and moist, whereas other skin is dry; rarely, blisters develop

hair sparse to normal

dental abnormalities include early caries, tooth loss, and periodontal disease

occasional purpura due to aplastic anemia

macular amyloidosis reported

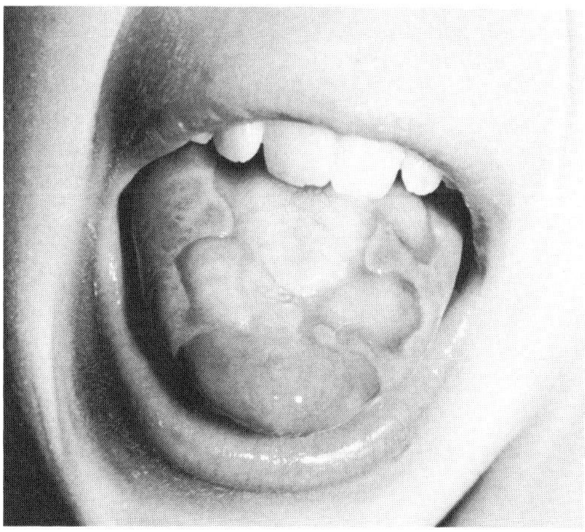

FIGURE 3–1
Multiple large coalescing ulcers on the tongue of a boy with dyskeratosis congenita.

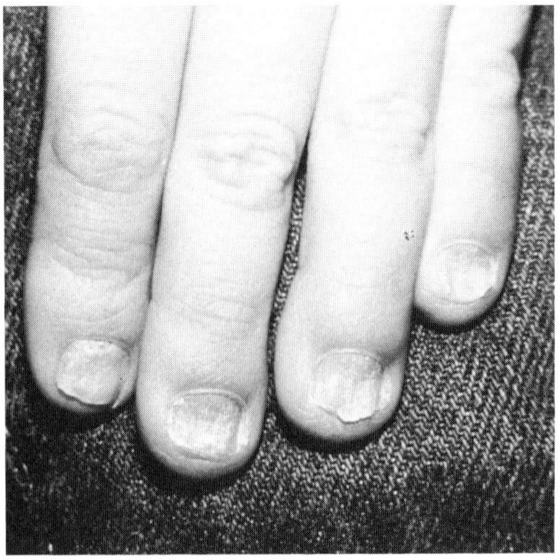

FIGURE 3–2
Nail dystrophy in a boy with dyskeratosis congenita. Koilonychia, onychorrhexis, and onychoschizia are seen.

Non-Skin

aplastic anemia in about 50% of patients by end of third decade; may evolve into pancytopenia

ocular abnormalities include bullous conjunctivitis, loss of eyelashes, and lacrimal duct atresia causing continuous tearing

splenomegaly

hypogonadism in about 40%

small stature in some

Genetics

XLR; AR (McK 224230) and AD (McK 127550) cases reported

male to female ratio: 8:1

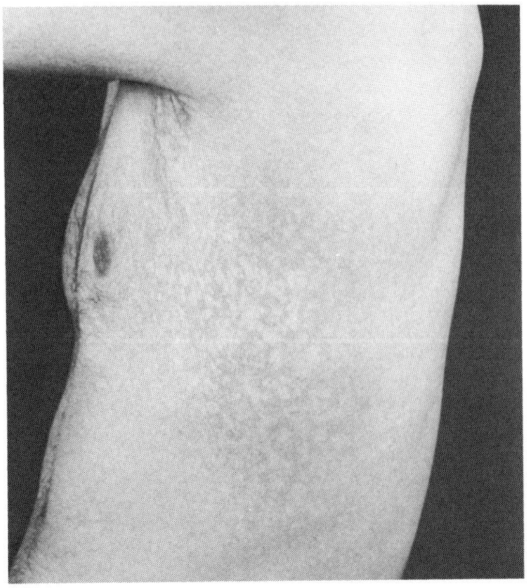

FIGURE 3–3
Poikilodermatous change on the trunk of a young man with dyskeratosis congenita. (Courtesy of Edward A. Krull, MD, Detroit, Michigan)

Pathophysiology

increased chromosomal breaks and rearrangements reported

possible increase in sister chromatid exchanges

Laboratory Data

radiographs rarely show intracranial calcifications

Prognosis

decreased life expectancy due to aplastic anemia (resulting in hemorrhage or infection) or malignancy (arising in mucosal lesions)

bone marrow transplantation may be helpful

regression of mucosal plaques with retinoids reported

Discussion

incomplete expression may be seen (e.g., poikiloderma and nail dystrophy without leukokeratosis)

chronic graft-versus-host disease (GVHD) may mimic dyskeratosis congenita (both have similar poikiloderma, white plaques on mucous membranes, and nail dystrophy); further complicating the issue is that dyskeratosis congenita patients may develop GVHD following bone marrow transplantation

- *dyskeratosis congenita, Scoggins type*

  the eponym for an autosomal dominant form of dyskeratosis congenita

- *familial pigmentation with dystrophy of the nails*

  may be a form fruste of dyskeratosis congenita

REFERENCES

McK 305000

McK 127550-McK 224230

Connor JM, Teague RH. Dyskeratosis congenita: report of a large kindred. Br J Dermatol 1981;105:321–325

Dodd HJ, Devereux S, Sarkany I. Dyskeratosis congenita with pancytopenia. Clin Exp Dermatol 1985;10:73–78

Esterly NB. Nail dystrophy in dyskeratosis congenita and chronic graft-vs-host disease. [Letter]. Arch Dermatol 1986;122:506–507

Ling NS, Fenske NA, Julius RL, et al. Dyskeratosis congenita in a girl simulating chronic graft-vs-host disease. Arch Dermatol 1985;121:1424–1428

Llistosella E, Moreno A, de Moragas JM. Dyskeratosis congenita with macular cutaneous amyloid deposits. Arch Dermatol 1984;120:1381–1382

Moon-Adams D, Slatkin MH. Familial pigmentation with dystrophy of the nails. Arch Dermatol 1955;71:591–598

Ogden GR, Connor E, Chisholm DM. Dyskeratosis congenita: report of a case and review of the literature. Oral Surg 1988;65:586–591

Pai GS, Morgan S, Whetsell C. Etiologic heterogeneity in dyskeratosis congenita. Am J Med Genet 1989;32:63–66

Phillips RJ, Judge M, Webb D, Harper JI. Dyskeratosis congenita: delay in diagnosis and successful treatment of pancytopenia by bone marrow transplantation. Br J Dermatol 1992;127:278–280

Sirinavin C, Trowbridge AA. Dyskeratosis congenita: clinical features and genetic aspects. Report of a family and review of the literature. J Med Genet 1975;12:339–354

Steier W, Van Voolen GA, Selmanowitz VJ. Dyskeratosis congenita: relationship to Fanconi's anemia. Blood 1972;39:510–521

FANCONI ANEMIA

Synonym

- Fanconi pancytopenia

Skin

in most patients, generalized hyperpigmentation, most prominent on non–sun-exposed skin, especially the lower trunk and flexures, including the axillae, groin, popliteal and antecubital fossae, and neck; oral mucosa not involved

scattered over the areas of diffuse hyperpigmentation are guttate hypopigmented and hyperpigmented macules

onset of pigmentary changes about mid to late first decade; usually precedes anemia by many years but may follow

café-au-lait macules in some

Non-Skin

severe pancytopenia, usually manifesting in second half of first decade

rudimentary thumbs and aplasia of the radii

short stature with slender build, short broad hands, and tapering fingers

frequent microcephaly

mental retardation

hypogonadism

increased incidence of malignancies including acute leukemia and hepatocellular carcinoma

Genetics

AR; possible multiple allelism

at least two complementation groups exist

Laboratory Data

spontaneous and clastogen-induced chromosomal breakage

deficient ability to excise ultraviolet light–induced pyrimidine dimers

prenatal diagnosis possible by detecting clastogen-induced chromosomal breakage in amniotic fluid cells

Prognosis

poor prognosis due to aplastic anemia; death commonly follows diagnosis of anemia within 3 years

anabolic steroids or bone marrow transplantation may improve survival

high incidence of leukemia in patients and family members

Discussion

reports of increased incidence of squamous cell carcinoma of mucosae may not be reliable, since some cases were confused with dyskeratosis congenita

one study reported increased incidence of genitourinary and distal limb malformations among heterozygotes

otherwise unaffected siblings may have hematologic abnormalities

incidence of leukemia may be increased in family members

- *thrombocytopenia and absent radius syndrome*

  thrombocytopenia most severe in early infancy; occasional ecchymoses and purpura

  absence or hypoplasia of the radii, often associated with defects of hands and lower extremities

  AR

  death due to gastrointestinal or cerebral hemorrhage common

  prognosis improves after 1 year of age

  some have considered this to be an abortive form of Fanconi pancytopenia

REFERENCES

McK 274000
McK 227650
McK 227660
Auerbach AD, Min Z, Ghosh R, et al. Clastogen-induced chromosomal breakage as a marker for first trimester prenatal diagnosis of Fanconi anemia. Hum Genet 1986; 73:86–88
Auerbach AD, Sagi M, Adler B. Fanconi anemia: prenatal diagnosis in 30 fetuses at risk. Pediatrics 1985;76:794–800
Cohen MM, Levy HP. Chromosome instability syndromes. Adv Hum Genet 1989;18:43–149
Fanconi G. Familial constitutional panmyelocytopathy, Fanconi's anemia (F.A.): I. Clinical aspects. Semin Hematol 1966;4:233–240
Hedberg VA, Lipton JM. Thrombocytopenia with absent radii: a review of 100 cases. Am J Pediatr Hematol Oncol 1988;10:51–64
Jacobs P, Karabus C. Fanconi's anemia: a family study with 20-year follow-up including associated breast pathology. Cancer 1984; 54:1850–1853
Shahidi NT. Fanconi anemia, dyskeratosis congenita, and WT syndrome. Am J Med Genet Suppl 1987;3:263–278
Welshimer K, Swift M. Congenital malformations and developmental disabilities in ataxia-telangiectasia, Fanconi anemia, and xeroderma pigmentosum families. Am J Hum Genet 1982;34:781–793

KINDLER SYNDROME

Skin

blisters, mostly acral, following minor trauma; onset at birth or early infancy

decrease in blistering with age

diffuse poikiloderma initially limited to sun-exposed areas, later spreading elsewhere, develops after 1 year of age (Fig. 3–4); persists into adulthood

mild to severe photosensitivity

palmoplantar keratoderma

cutaneous atrophy may be widespread but is most prominent on dorsa of hands and feet; mild proximal webbing of digits develops (Fig. 3–5)

occasional gingival hypertrophy, fragility, and hemorrhage

other reported mucosal involvement includes anal, esophageal, and urethral stenoses as well as leukokeratosis

nail dystrophy

Genetics

probable AR

Laboratory Data

histopathology: intraepidermal and subepidermal bullae

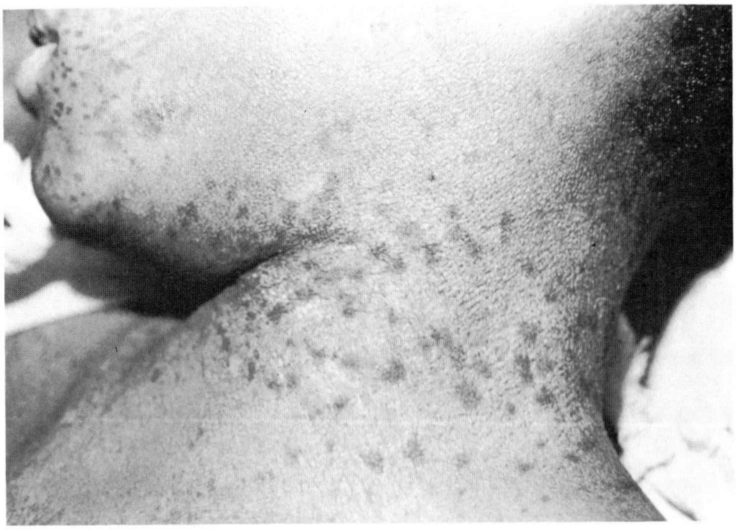

FIGURE 3–4
Characteristic dyspigmentation of the neck and submental area in a boy with Kindler syndrome. The skin is also telangiectatic and somewhat atrophic.

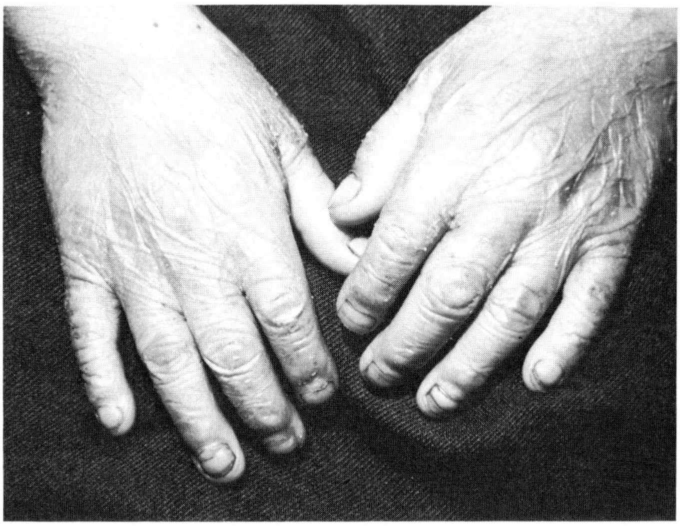

FIGURE 3–5
Poikiloderma and proximal webbing of the digits in a child with Kindler syndrome.

electron microscopy: cleavage planes in the basal layer, lamina lucida, and sub–lamina densa

REFERENCES

McK 173650

Bordas X, Palou J, Capdevila JM, et al. Kindler's syndrome: report of a case. J Am Acad Dermatol 1982;6:263–265

Forman AB, Prendiville JS, Esterly NB, et al. Kindler syndrome: report of two cases and review of the literature. Pediatr Dermatol 1989;6:91–101

Hovnanian A, Blanchet-Bardon C, de Prost Y. Poikiloderma of Theresa Kindler: report of a case with ultrastructural study and review of the literature. Pediatr Dermatol 1989;6:82–90

Kindler T. Congenital poikiloderma with traumatic bulla formation and progressive cutaneous atrophy. Br J Dermatol 1954; 66:104–111

HEREDITARY ACROKERATOTIC POIKILODERMA (DOWLING SYNDROME; POIKILODERMA WITH KERATOSES; GREITHER SYNDROME; WEARY SYNDROME)

vesicles or vesiculopustules of hands and feet arise in early infancy, peak by age 9 months, and then gradually remit

widespread, eczematous dermatitis develops several months after the blisters, gradually resolving by age 5

poikiloderma with striate and reticulate atrophy subsequently forms, most pronounced in flexural areas, minimally involving acral skin; eyelids always involved, but otherwise face, scalp, and ears are spared; dyschromia is prominent

persistent keratotic papules on hands, feet, elbows, and knees appearing in first 5 years of life

photosensitivity is absent

AD; minor differences may be seen between pedigrees

Draznin MB, Esterly NB, Fretzin DF. Congenital poikiloderma with features of hereditary acrokeratotic poikiloderma. Arch Dermatol 1978;114:1207–1210

Larregue M, Prigent F, Lorette G, et al. [Bullous and hereditary Weary-Kindler's acrokeratotic poikiloderma.] Ann Dermatol Venereol 1981;108:69–76

Weary PE, Manley WF Jr, Graham GF. Hereditary acrokeratotic poikiloderma. Arch Dermatol 1971;103:409–422

HEREDITARY SCLEROSING POIKILODERMA

normal at birth

progressive development of widespread poikiloderma before age 4 years, most prominent in flexures but sparing scalp, ears, and face except for eyebrows (Fig. 3–6)

progressive development of reticulated, occasionally linear, hyperkeratotic and sclerotic bands 1 to 2 mm wide that are accentuated in the flexures

sclerosis of the palms, volar fingers, and, to a lesser extent, the soles

clubbing of digits reported

AD

do not confuse with hereditary acrokeratotic poikiloderma

McK 173700

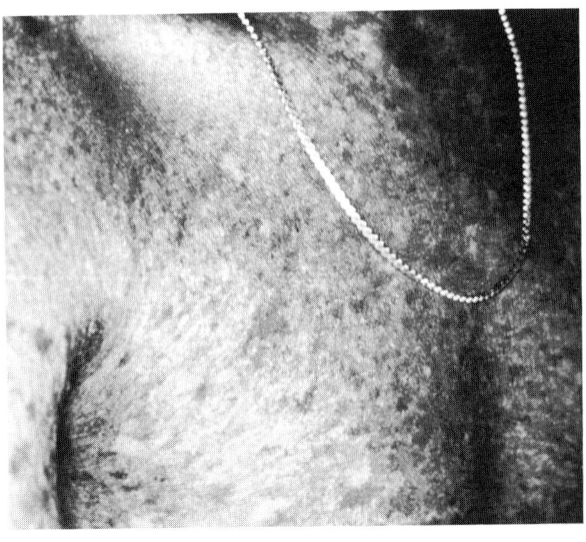

FIGURE 3–6
This 12-year-old boy with hereditary sclerosing poikiloderma has mild hypopigmentation and hyperpigmentation.

REFERENCES

Greer KE, Weary PE, Nagy R, Robinow M. Hereditary sclerosing poikiloderma. Int J Dermatol 1978;17:316–322

Weary PE, Hsu YT, Richardson DR, et al. Hereditary sclerosing poikiloderma: report of two families with an unusual and distinctive genodermatosis. Arch Dermatol 1969; 100:413–422

ROTHMUND-THOMSON SYNDROME

Synonym

- poikiloderma congenitale

Skin

diffuse erythema, often reticular, and edema usually of the face and ears; hands and feet are next most commonly involved, followed by arms, legs, and buttocks (Color Fig. 3–1)

erythema usually appears a few months after birth, but rarely at birth or as late as 2 years of age

photosensitivity in one third of children, usually decreasing with age; exposure to ultraviolet light may result in blistering

varying combinations of atrophy, telangiectasia, hypopigmentation and hyperpigmentation develop subsequent to the erythema and progress for several years after which the lesions stabilize; non–sun-exposed areas (e.g., trunk) may be involved, in which hyperpigmentation may be the sole finding

keratoses, mostly on the distal extremities, develop in about one fourth of patients, usually from adolescence onward; occasionally may transform into squamous cell carcinoma

occasional elastosis perforans serpiginosa

sparse scalp, eyelash, and eyebrow hair in more than 50%; pubic and axillary hair may also be sparse

occasional nail dystrophy

no mucous membrane involvement (cf. dyskeratosis congenita); occasional dental abnormalities

Non-Skin

skeletal abnormalities include short stature, radial hypoplasia or aplasia, syndactyly, small hands; possible increased incidence of osteogenic sarcoma

cataracts develop in about half of patients, usually before age 7 years; initially unilateral, but eventually bilateral, resulting in blindness abnormal craniofacies with depressed nasal bridge

mental development usually normal

hypogonadism and decreased fertility in adults

Genetics

AR

male to female ratio: about 1:2

Prognosis

usually progressive in infancy

life expectancy normal

Discussion

some clinicians distinguish Rothmund syndrome by the presence of cataracts and Thomson syndrome by findings of bony defects primarily

REFERENCES

McK 268400

Berg E, Chuang TY, Cripps D. Rothmund-Thomson syndrome: a case report, phototesting, and literature review. J Am Acad Dermatol 1987;17:332–338

Collins P, Barnes L, McCabe M. Poikiloderma congenitale: case report and review of the literature. Pediatr Dermatol 1991;8:58–60

Dick DC, Morley WN, Watson JT. Rothmund-Thomson syndrome and osteogenic sarcoma. Clin Exp Dermatol 1982;7:119–123

Kirkham TH, Werner EB. The ophthalmic manifestations of Rothmund's syndrome. Can J Ophthalmol 1975;10:1–14

Moss C. Rothmund-Thomson syndrome: a report of two patients and a review of the literature. Br J Dermatol 1990;122:821–829

Nanda A, Kanwar AJ, Kapoor MM, et al. Rothmund-Thomson syndrome in two siblings. Pediatr Dermatol 1989;6:325–328

Roth DE, Campisano LC, Callen JP, et al. Rothmund-Thomson syndrome: a case report. Pediatr Dermatol 1989;6:321–324

Rothmund A. Uber Kataracte in Verbindung mit einer eigentum-lichen Hautdegeneration. Graefes Arch Ophthalmol 1868; 14:159–182

Shinya A, Nishigori C, Moriwaki S, et al. A case of Rothmund-Thomson syndrome with reduced DNA repair capacity. Arch Dermatol 1993;129:332–336

Shuttleworth D, Marks R. Epidermal dysplasia and skeletal deformity in congenital poikiloderma (Rothmund-Thomson syndrome). Br J Dermatol 1987;117:377–384

Starr DG, McClure JP, Connor JM. Nondermatological complications and genetic aspects of the Rothmund-Thomson syndrome. Clin Genet 1985;27:102–104

Vennos EM, Collins M, James WD. Rothmund-Thomson syndrome: review of the world literature. J Am Acad Dermatol 1992; 27:750–762

GLOMERULONEPHRITIS, SPARSE HAIR, AND TELANGIECTASES

telangiectases on cheeks, elbows, and dorsal fingers

sparse scalp hair, eyebrows, and eyelashes

membranoproliferative glomerulonephritis

AD

McK 137940

Proesmans W, Legius E, Van Herck K, Van Damme B. Cutaneous telangiectasia, sparse hair and membranoproliferative glomerulonephritis: a new case of a newly recognized entity. Pediatr Nephrol 1989; 3:162–165

Sherwood MC, Pincott JR, Goodwin FJ, Dillon MJ. Dominantly inherited glomerulonephritis and an unusual skin disease. Arch Dis Child 1987;62:1278–1280

Xeroderma Pigmentosum: General Comments

Xeroderma pigmentosum (XP) refers to a group of diseases caused by abnormalities in the repair mechanisms of deoxyribonucleic acid (DNA). These diseases are characterized by congenital marked photosensitivity and the sequelae of marked ultraviolet (UV) light–induced damage, including cutaneous carcinomas and melanomas. XP consists of at least seven complementation groups (A through G; groups H and I were retracted) and additional variants (Table 3–3). Fibroblasts from patients with XP are studied for the rate of induced unscheduled DNA synthesis after UV exposure and the UV dose required to reduce fibroblast colony-forming ability in vitro. Clinicians encountering children with unusual photosensitivity should consider the diagnosis of

TABLE 3–3
XERODERMA PIGMENTOSUM COMPLEMENTATION GROUPS

Complementation Group	Neurologic Findings	% of Normal DNA Repair	Comments
A (McK 278700)	+	2–5	Most common and most severe (mostly DeSanctis-Cacchione patients)
B (McK 133510)	+	3–7	Very rare; association with Cockayne syndrome reported
C (McK 278720)	−	5–20	Second most common
D (McK 278730)	+ develop later than in group A	25–50	May be the same as some cases of PIBI[D]S syndrome
E (McK 278740)	−	40–50	Mild; rare
F (McK 278760)	−	18	Mild; very rare; Japanese
G (McK 278780)	+/−	<2	Very rare; clinically heterogeneous
H (McK 278790)	+	30	Very rare; association with Cockayne syndrome; group H withdrawn and reassigned to group D
I (McK 278810)	+	15–40	Withdrawn; shown to be group C

Reference: Cleaver JE, Kraemer KH. Xeroderma pigmentosum. In: Scriver CR, Beaudet AL, Sly WS, Valle D, eds. Metabolic Basis of Inherited Disease. 6th ed. New York, McGraw-Hill, 1989:2949–2971.

XP and consult with expert laboratories to facilitate evaluation. If the disease can be identified early, sunscreens and other life-style modifications may be extremely effective in delaying or preventing the sequelae of UV light–induced damage, including cutaneous carcinomas. However, avoidance of UV light will not ameliorate neurologic abnormalities.

Skin

photosensitivity is usually the first manifestation; appears in first year of life

ephelides are another early manifestation; usually appear on sun-exposed areas during first or second year of life; darken and spread to less exposed areas, including oral and ocular mucosae

early in life, blisters and persistent erythema may develop following moderate sun exposure

rarely, skin changes do not occur until second decade

skin becomes atrophic, and punctate and stellate telangiectases appear; with development of hypopigmentation and hyperpigmentation, poikiloderma results (Figs. 3–7 and 3–8)

benign and malignant tumors occur subsequently and intercurrently, most frequently basal and squamous cell carcinomas (Fig. 3–9), but also melanomas (latter constitute 5% of all malignancies and are often multiple), keratoacanthomas, sarcomas, fibromas, fibrosarcomas, angiomas, and angiosarcomas

tumors may develop on any sun-exposed area (e.g., even the tip of the tongue, on which squamous cell carcinoma has been reported); first tumor usually occurs in first decade of life

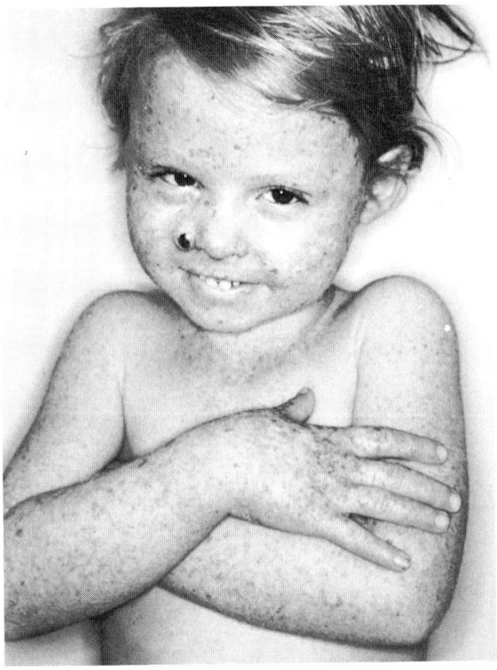

FIGURE 3–7
Widespread cutaneous changes of atrophy, numerous ephelides, and telangiectases in a child with xeroderma pigmentosum. Note the crusted tumor lateral to the nose. (Courtesy of Benjamin K. Fisher, MD, Toronto, Ontario)

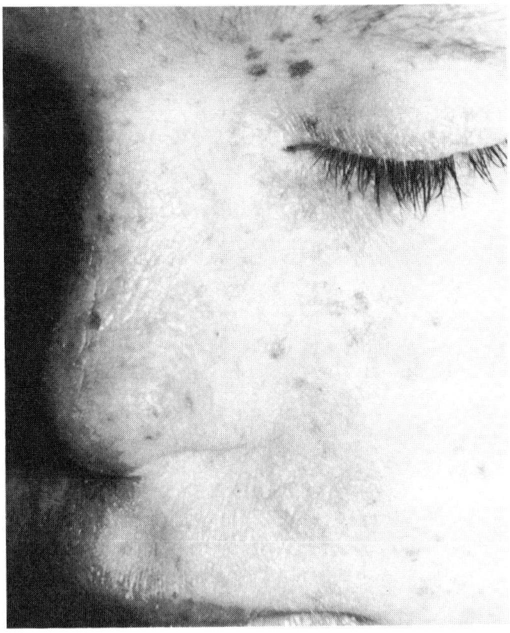

FIGURE 3–8
Close-up of the facial skin of a child with xeroderma pigmentosum showing telangiectasia, atrophy, multiple ephelides, and several pearly papules. On biopsy the papules were identified as squamous cell carcinomas.

Non-Skin

ocular abnormalities in 40%, including actinic conjunctivitis with extreme photophobia early in life (may be first sign); later, blepharitis, symblepharon, and corneal opacities develop

mental deficiency and neurologic abnormalities occur in about one fifth of all patients; presence unrelated to severity of skin findings, except in the DeSanctis-Cacchione syndrome, in which skin findings are always severe

neurologic abnormalities include spastic-ataxic gait, athetoid movements, speech disturbances, pyramidal and extrapyramidal signs

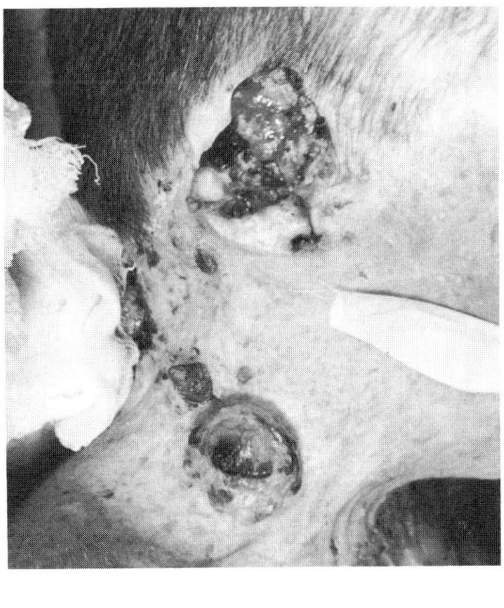

FIGURE 3–9
Multiple ulcerated squamous cell carcinomas in a patient with xeroderma pigmentosum.

increased incidence of internal neoplasms in reported patients, including leukemia, and lung and central nervous system tumors

Genetics

with all forms of XP presented in the text, inheritance is AR; however, AD inheritance has been reported

the existence of many complementation groups (see later) indicates the heterogeneous nature of the molecular defects in this disorder

Pathophysiology

inability to repair UV light–induced DNA damage, especially from light in 280- to 310-nm range

pyrimidine dimers, most commonly thymine-thymine, are frequent UV light–induced DNA change

at least seven genetic complementation groups have been identified thus far (designated A through G), each with a different defect in DNA repair

severity of disease does not correlate with the severity of the DNA repair abnormality

unlike UV light–induced damage, x-ray–induced damage is repaired normally

Laboratory Data

prenatal diagnosis may be possible by detecting abnormalities in DNA repair (usually unscheduled DNA synthesis) after irradiation of cultured amniotic fluid fibroblasts with UV light

Prognosis

death is usually due to malignancy (often from metastases of cutaneous carcinomas); many patients die in first 2 decades of life

reports of improved survival with early and diligent sun protection

oral retinoids used prophylactically may decrease the incidence of skin cancer

Discussion

heterozygotes usually have normal excision repair of DNA and few, if any, clinical features (e.g., marked freckling in heterozygous siblings has been reported)

complementation groups A and C and XP variant are the most common forms

complementation group B has been associated with Cockayne syndrome

REFERENCES

Anderson T, Begg M. Xeroderma pigmentosum of mild type. Br J Dermatol 1950;62:402–407

Cohen MM, Levy HP. Chromosome instability syndromes. Adv Hum Genet 1989;18:43–149

Fujiwara Y, Matsumoto A, Ichihashi M, et al. Heritable disorders of DNA repair: xeroderma pigmentosum and Fanconi's anemia. Curr Probl Dermatol 1987;17:182–198

Imray FP, Hockey A, Relf W, et al. Sensitivity to ultraviolet radiation in a dominantly inherited form of xeroderma pigmentosum. J Med Genet 1986;23:72–78

Jung EG, Bantle K. Xeroderma pigmentosum and pigmented xerodermoid. Birth Defects 1971;7:125–128

Jung EG. Xeroderma pigmentosum. Int J Dermatol 1986;25:629–633

Kondo S, Mamada A, Miyamoto C, et al. Late onset of skin cancers in 2 xeroderma pigmentosum group F siblings and a review of 30 Japanese xeroderma pigmentosum patients in groups D, E and F. Photodermatol 1989;6:89–95

Kondo S, Satoh Y, Kuroki T. Reduced levels of UV-induced unscheduled DNA synthesis in epidermal keratinocytes of patients with xeroderma pigmentosum and correlation with development of skin neoplasms. Cancer Res 1989;49:1927–1930

Kraemer KH, Lee MM, Scotto J. Xeroderma pigmentosum: cutaneous, ocular, and neurologic abnormalities in 830 published cases. Arch Dermatol 1987;123:241–250

Lambert WC. Genetic diseases associated with DNA and chromosomal instability. Dermatol Clin 1987;5:85–108

Lambert WC. Xeroderma pigmentosum. N J Med 1989;86:383–386

Lynch HT, Frichot BC III, Lynch JF. Cancer control in xeroderma pigmentosum. Arch Dermatol 1977;113:193–195

Parshad R, Sanford KK, Kraemer KH, et al. Carrier detection in xeroderma pigmentosum. J Clin Invest 1990;85:135–138

Yamamura K, Ichihashi M, Hiramoto T, et al. Clinical and photobiological characteristics of xeroderma pigmentosum complementation group F: a review of cases from Japan. Br J Dermatol 1989;121:471–480

XERODERMA PIGMENTOSUM, COMPLEMENTATION GROUP A

severe and early appearance of skin cancers, especially basal cell carcinomas

neurologic abnormalities tend to develop in early to mid first decade and vary from mild to severe (see DeSanctis-Cacchione syndrome); absence of neurologic findings reported

includes most patients with DeSanctis-Cacchione syndrome

defective gene localized to chromosome 9 q

McK 278700

DESANCTIS-CACCHIONE SYNDROME (XERODERMIC IDIOCY)

form of complementation group A XP with early onset of severe skin findings and mental retardation, microcephaly, dwarfism, neurologic abnormalities (including ataxia and deafness), shortening of the Achilles tendon, and hypogonadism

McK 278800

Roytta M, Anttinen A. Xeroderma pigmentosum with neurological abnormalities: a clinical and neuropathological study. Acta Neurol Scand 1986;73:191–199

Reed WB, Sugarman GI, Mathis RA. DeSanctis-Cacchione syndrome: a case report with autopsy findings. Arch Dermatol 1977;113:1561–1563

XERODERMA PIGMENTOSUM, COMPLEMENTATION GROUP B

clinical and cytobiologic characteristics of both XP and Cockayne syndrome

defective gene localized to chromosome 2 q

McK 133510

Robbins JH, Kraemer KH, Lutzner MA, et al. Xeroderma pigmentosum: an inherited disease with sun sensitivity, multiple cutaneous neoplasms, and abnormal DNA repair. Ann Intern Med 1974;80:221–248

Lehmann AR. Three complementation groups in Cockayne syndrome. Mutat Res 1982; 106:347–356

XERODERMA PIGMENTOSUM, COMPLEMENTATION GROUP C

cutaneous findings, skin cancers typical of XP, but neurologic abnormalities absent in almost all cases

largest group of XP in Europe and United States

defective gene localized to chromosome 19 q

McK 278720

Wade MH, Plotnick H. Xeroderma pigmentosum and squamous cell carcinoma of the tongue: identification of two black patients as members of complementation group C. J Am Acad Dermatol 1985;12:515–521

XERODERMA PIGMENTOSUM, COMPLEMENTATION GROUP D

trichothiodystrophy reported in addition to typical cutaneous manifestations of XP

neurologic abnormalities usually seen but with later onset than in complementation group A; at least one case without neurologic abnormalities reported

the ERCC2 DNA repair gene corrects the defect in XP complementation group D cells (localized to chromosome 19 q)

may be the same as some cases of PIBI[D]S syndrome (see under Trichothiodystrophy in Chapter 9); in addition, some patients with trichothiodystropy and photosensitivity may have the same repair abnormalities as in XP complementation group D but do not develop the skin cancers

McK 278730
Flejter WL, McDaniel LD, Johns D, et al. Correction of xeroderma pigmentosum complementation group D mutant cell phenotypes by chromosome and gene transfer: involvement of the human ERCC2 DNA repair gene. Proc Natl Acad Sci USA 1992;89: 261–265
Ichihashi M, Yamamura K, Hiramoto T, Fujiwara Y. No apparent neurologic defect in a patient with xeroderma pigmentosum complementation group D. Arch Dermatol 1988;124:256–260
Rebora A, Crovato F. PIBI(D)S syndrome—trichothiodystrophy with xeroderma pigmentosum (group D) mutation. J Am Acad Dermatol 1987;16:940–947

XERODERMA PIGMENTOSUM, COMPLEMENTATION GROUP E

mild skin symptoms; decreased incidence and late onset of skin cancers (particularly basal cell carcinoma) compared with other groups (e.g., complementation group A)

no neurologic abnormalities

McK 278740
Kondo S, Fukuro S, Mamada A, et al. Assignment of three patients with xeroderma pigmentosum to complementation group E and their characteristics. J Invest Dermatol 1988;90:152–157

XERODERMA PIGMENTOSUM, COMPLEMENTATION GROUP F

mild skin findings; skin cancers uncommon and onset is in adulthood

no ocular or neuropsychiatric findings in patients in several series

almost all patients in Japan

mild clinical manifestations and late onset, despite low DNA repair capacity reported

McK 278760
Norris PG, Hawk JL, Avery JA, et al. Xeroderma pigmentosum complementation group F in a non-Japanese patient. J Am Acad Dermatol 1988;18:1185–1188
Yamamura K, Ichihashi M, Hiramoto T, et al. Clinical and photobiological characteristics of xeroderma pigmentosum complementation group F: a review of cases from Japan. Br J Dermatol 1989;121:471–480

XERODERMA PIGMENTOSUM, COMPLEMENTATION GROUP G

mild skin findings

no neurologic sequelae reported

defective gene localized to chromosome 13 q

McK 278780
Norris PG, Hawk JLM, Avery JA, Giannelli F. Xeroderma pigmentosum complementation group G: report of two cases. Br J Dermatol 1987;116:861–866

XERODERMA PIGMENTOSUM, COMPLEMENTATION GROUP H

patient has findings of both XP and Cockayne syndrome

group H has been reassigned to group D

McK 278730
Robbins JH. Xeroderma pigmentosum complementation group is withdrawn and reassigned to group D. Hum Genet 1991;88:242

XERODERMA PIGMENTOSUM, COMPLEMENTATION GROUP I

this designation has been withdrawn because study of this line of cells showed that it actually belonged to complementation group C

McK 278810
Bootsma D, Keijzer W, Jung EG, Bohnert E. Xeroderma pigmentosum complementation group XP-I withdrawn. Mutat Res 1989;218:149–151

XERODERMA PIGMENTOSUM VARIANT (XP VARIANT)

similar clinically to XP but with normal replication repair

high incidence of skin cancers, comparable to that seen in group A, but commonly of much later onset

neurologic and other systemic abnormalities are usually not seen

DNA excision repair is normal in contrast to markedly reduced levels in other XP complementation groups

however, depression of DNA synthesis after exposure to UV light and replication of DNA after UV irradiation in abnormally short fragments demonstrated although the exact defect or defects are not known, other DNA repair pathways are abnormal (e.g., post-replication repair)

erythema response normal

probably represents a heterogeneous group of disorders with variable onset and severity of disease; the exact delineation between XP variant and pigmented xerodermoid, if any, is not clear; pigmented xerodermoid may be analogous to late-onset forms of XP variant

McK 278750

Cleaver JE. Similar defects in DNA repair and replication in the pigmented xerodermoid and the xeroderma pigmentosum variants. Carcinogenesis 1980;1:647–655

Fischer E, Jung EG, Cleaver JE. Pigmented xerodermoid and XP-variants. [Letter]. Arch Dermatol Res 1980;269:329–330

Hessel A, Siegle RJ, Mitchell DL, Cleaver JE. Xeroderma pigmentosum variant with multisystem involvement. Arch Dermatol 1992;128:1233–1237

Hofmann H, Jung EG, Schnyder UW. Pigmented xerodermoid: first report of a family. Bull Cancer 1978;65:347–350

Jung EG. Xeroderma pigmentosum. Int J Dermatol 1986;25:629–633

Kraemer KH, Lee MM, Scotto J. Xeroderma pigmentosum: cutaneous, ocular, and neurologic abnormalities in 830 published cases. Arch Dermatol 1987;123:241–250

BLOOM SYNDROME

Synonym

- congenital telangiectatic erythema

Skin

erythematous, telangiectatic plaques on face (usually in a “butterfly” distribution), neck, and frequently on the forearms and dorsa of hands (see Color Fig. 3–2); intensity of erythema fades after puberty

telangiectases may appear on dorsa of hands, ears, flanks, and buttocks

photosensitivity usually develops within first two summers of life and diminishes with age

with age, facial skin becomes atrophic

café-au-lait macules in over 50% of patients in addition to hypopigmented macules and patches on the trunk and extremities

marked fissuring of vermilion of lips; may be preceded by blisters

Non-Skin

see Figure 3–10

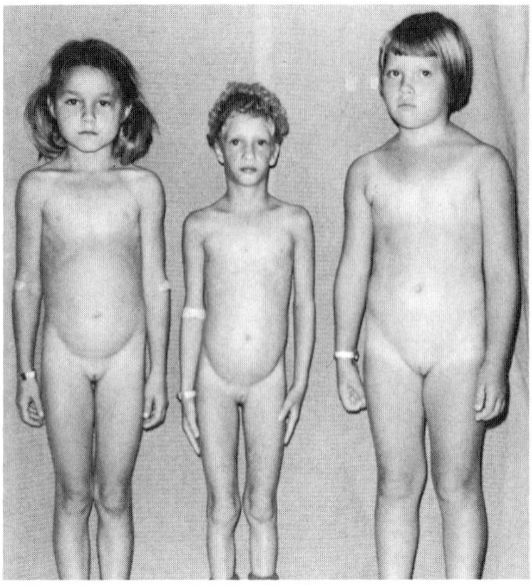

FIGURE 3–10
A girl with Bloom syndrome *(center)* shown with two other girls of the same age. Note the small stature, facial eruption, distinctive facies, and dolichocephaly. (Courtesy of Benjamin K. Fisher, MD, Toronto, Ontario)

severe prenatal and postnatal growth retardation

normal intelligence

craniofacial abnormalities producing a distinctive appearance include dolichocephaly, a small, narrow face, and long nose

skeletal defects include clinodactyly and syndactyly

testicular atrophy is common, and male patients are characteristically sterile

other abnormalities include high-pitched voice and hypospadias

increased occurrence of malignancies including leukemia, lymphoma, and carcinoma (especially of the gastrointestinal tract)

Genetics

AR

most frequent among Ashkenazi Jews, but reported among many other ethnic groups

Laboratory Data

10-fold increase in spontaneous sister chromatid exchanges in cultured lymphocytes; this finding is pathognomonic for Bloom syndrome

increased chromosomal breaks and rearrangements (quadriradial configuration is characteristic); cultured cells have increased sensitivity to ultraviolet light

heterozygotes do not have increased chromosomal breakage

prenatal diagnosis by detection of high number of sister chromatid exchanges in amniotic fluid cells

decreased serum IgA, IgG, and IgM levels

Prognosis

decreased life expectancy due to increased incidence of severe bacterial infections (usually involving respiratory or gastrointestinal systems) and malignancies

REFERENCES

McK 210900

Bloom D. The syndrome of congenital telangiectatic erythema and stunted growth. J Pediatr 1966;68:103–113

German J, Bloom D, Passarge E. Bloom's syndrome: XI. Progress report for 1983. Clin Genet 1984;25:166–174

German J, Bloom D, Passarge E. Bloom's syndrome: V. Surveillance for cancer in affected families. Clin Genet 1977;12:162–168

German J. Genetical and clinical observations in the first twenty-seven patients. Am J Hum Genet 1969;21:196–227

Gretzula JC, Hevia O, Weber PJ. Bloom's syndrome. J Am Acad Dermatol 1987;17:479–488

Nicotera TM, Notaro J, Notaro S, et al. Elevated superoxide dismutase in Bloom's syndrome: a genetic condition of oxidative stress. Cancer Res 1989;49:5239–5243

Oono T, Arata J, Fukuma A, et al. Bloom's syndrome with dimorphism of sister chromatid exchanges in phytohemagglutinin-stimulated lymphocytes. [Letter]. Arch Dermatol 1987;123:988–990

Takemiya M, Shiraishi S, Teramoto T, et al. Bloom's syndrome with porokeratosis of Mibelli and multiple cancers of the skin, lung and colon. Clin Genet 1987;31:35–44

DUBOWITZ SYNDROME

erythema and scaling of face and extremities in infancy

sparse scalp and eyebrow hair, often blond

delayed eruption of teeth

prenatal and postnatal growth retardation

occasional mild mental retardation

craniofacial abnormalities producing a "sad clown" face include microcephaly, telecanthus, eyelid ptosis, blepharophimosis, broad nasal tip, cleft palate, bifid uvula, micrognathia, and prominent ears

high-pitched, hoarse voice

AR

McK 223370

Dubowitz V. Familial low birthweight dwarfism with an unusual facies and a skin eruption. J Med Genet 1965;2:12–17

Kuster W, Majewski F. The Dubowitz syndrome. Eur J Pediatr 1986;144:574–578

Wilroy RS Jr, Tipton RE, Summitt RL. The Dubowitz syndrome. Am J Med Genet 1978;2:275–284

Poikilodermatous Disorders—Abbreviated Entries

CUTANEOUS PHOTOSENSITIVITY AND COLITIS, LETHAL

inheritance is probably AR

McK 219095

Labrune P, Huguet P, Alagille D, Odievre M. Familial cutaneous photosensitivity and colitis with lethal outcome. J Med Genet 1991;28:114–116

FAMILIAL SPASTIC PARAPLEGIA, NEUROPATHY, AND POIKILODERMA

inheritance is AD

McK 182815

Antinolo G, Nieto M, Borrego S, et al. Familial spastic paraplegia with neuropathy and poikiloderma: a new syndrome? Clin Genet 1992;41:281–284

CHAPTER

4

Premature Aging Syndromes

No disease exists that truly represents an acceleration of the normal aging process, but there are a number of disorders in which patients appear wizened or aged. Such progeroid syndromes may have the following cutaneous features (Gilchrest, 1984):

- *atrophy*
- *hyperpigmentation or hypopigmentation*
- *wrinkling*
- *loss of subcutaneous fat*
- *graying of hair; hair loss*

Mental retardation is usually not a feature.

In one review, Martin (1982) identified 162 diseases with premature aging or progeroid features. We have included only selected disorders here. Others are covered elsewhere in the book. The characteristics of the major premature aging syndromes are summarized in Table 4–1.

REFERENCES

Brown WT. Premature aging syndromes. Curr Probl Dermatol 1987;17:152–165

Gilchrest BA. Skin and Aging Processes. Boca Raton, FL, CRC Press, 1984:57–66

Martin GM. Genetic syndromes in man with potential relevance to the pathobiology of aging. In: Bergsma D, Harrison DE, eds. Genetic Effects of Aging. New York, Alan R. Liss, The National Foundation–March of Dimes, 1978

Martin GM. Syndromes of accelerated aging. NCI Monogr 1982;60:241–247

TABLE 4–1
SELECTED DISEASES WITH THE APPEARANCE OF PREMATURE AGING

Disease	Inheritance	Onset	Life Span	Skin	Poikiloderma	Stature	Systemic Findings	Secondary Sexual Development	Hair	Cataracts
Progeria	?; possible AR and AD cases reported	Infancy	Death in second decade	Atrophy; sclerosis	+	Small	Atherosclerosis; severe heart disease	↓↓	Fine, gray, sparse	None
Cockayne syndrome	AR	Early childhood	Reduced	Atrophy; photosensitivity	+	Small	Mental retardation; optic atrophy; deafness; ↓ joint mobility; peripheral neuropathy	↓	Normal	None
Werner syndrome	AR	Adolescence	Reduced	Atrophy; ulcers; subcutaneous calcification	+	Small	Atherosclerosis; heart disease	↓	Gray, sparse	Present
Acrogeria	mostly sporadic; AD, AR reported	Birth	Normal	Atrophy of distal limbs	+	None	Normal	Normal	None	
Metageria	?; possibly AR	Birth	Reduced	Atrophy; ulcers	+	Tall	Diabetes; atherosclerosis	Normal	Fine	None

↓, Decreased; ↓↓, markedly decreased.
Modified from Gilkes JJH, Sharvill DE, Wells RS. The premature ageing syndromes: report of eight cases and description of a new entity named metageria. Br J Dermatol 1974;91:243–262.

PROGERIA

Synonym

- Hutchinson-Gilford syndrome

Skin

scleroderma-like skin changes of torso and upper thighs; onset at birth or in early infancy

finely wrinkled and/or atrophic skin and gradual loss of subcutaneous tissue and muscle develop by age 2 years

mottled hyperpigmentation of sun-exposed areas develops in childhood, described by some as "poikilodermatous"

superficial veins become more visible, especially over scalp and thighs

hair is gray, fine, fuzzy, and sparse, usually an early manifestation; the scalp is always involved and sometimes shows complete alopecia; eyebrows and eyelashes are similarly affected

occasional midfacial cyanosis from birth to early childhood

keloid-like nodules reported on arms and hands

nail changes include yellowish discoloration, thinning, and brittleness

dental abnormalities include delayed eruption

Non-Skin

normal intelligence

cardiovascular disease is the major cause of morbidity and mortality, including atherosclerosis, cardiomegaly, myocardial infarction, hypertension, congestive heart failure, and stroke

myocardial infarction or stroke occurs as early as 7 to 8 years of age

weight and height are normal or slightly decreased at birth, but by age 6 months the height and especially the weight percentiles for age begin to decline

sexual maturation does not usually occur

features creating a "plucked bird" facies include small ears without earlobes, thin beak-like nose, and scalp alopecia

facial hypoplasia results in "hydrocephalic" appearance and prominent eyes

other craniofacial findings include frontal and parietal bossing, open anterior fontanelle, thin calvarium, poor mastoid development, and frequent absence of frontal sinuses

musculoskeletal changes include coxa valga (a constant finding), joint stiffness (e.g., mild flexion of the knees resulting in a wide-gaited "horse-riding" habitus), aseptic necrosis of femoral head, hip dislocation, thin chest and limbs, and acro-osteolysis

protuberant abdomen

high-pitched voice

Genetics

inheritance unclear; AR inheritance in some kindreds, while other cases may represent new mutations with AD inheritance

occurs mostly in whites

very rare; one in 8 million live births

Laboratory Data

radiographs show widespread degenerative changes of bone demonstrable in first or second year of life, including osteoporosis, attenuated cortices, widened metaphyses, distal resorption of phalanges, and facial bone hypoplasia

Prognosis

average age at death is 13 years, 80% due to myocardial infarctions or congestive heart failure

Discussion

features commonly associated with aging that are not seen in progeria include increased cataracts, amyloid deposition, and cancer

REFERENCES

McK 176670

Badame AJ. Progeria. [Review]. Arch Dermatol 1989;125:540–544

Brown WT, Kieras FJ, Houck GE Jr, et al. A comparison of adult and childhood progerias: Werner syndrome and Hutchinson-Gilford progeria syndrome. Adv Exp Med Biol 1985;190:229–244

DeBusk FL. The Hutchinson-Gilford progeria syndrome: report of 4 cases and review of the literature. J Pediatr 1972;80:697–724

Gillar PJ, Kaye CI, McCourt JW. Progressive early dermatologic changes in Hutchinson-Gilford progeria syndrome. Pediatr Dermatol 1991;8:199–206

Hutchinson J. Congenital absence of hair and mammary glands with atrophic condition of the skin and its appendages in a boy whose mother had been almost totally bald from alopecia areata from age six. Medicochir Trans 1886;69:473–477

Jimbow K, Kobayashi H, Ishii M, et al. Scar and keloidlike lesions in progeria: an electron-microscopic and immunohistochemical study. Arch Dermatol 1988;124:1261–1266

Khalifa MM. Hutchinson-Gilford progeria syndrome: report of a Libyan family and evidence of autosomal recessive inheritance. Clin Genet 1989;35:125–132

Maciel AT. Evidence for autosomal recessive inheritance of progeria (Hutchinson-Gilford). Am J Med Genet 1988;31:483–487

Parkash H, Sidhu SS, Raghavan R, Deshmukh RN. Hutchinson-Gilford progeria: familial occurrence. Am J Med Genet 1990;36:431–433

COCKAYNE SYNDROME

Skin

malar erythema appearing in second year of life, aggravated by sunlight; onset occasionally earlier

diffuse pigmentation, atrophic scarring, and loss of subcutaneous fat of face eventually results

light sensitivity decreases with age

skin of extremities is shiny and tense with subcutaneous atrophy; rarely, subcutaneous tissue is thickened near larger joints

increased cold sensitivity with acrocyanosis

occasional generalized hypohidrosis

hair usually normal but sometimes sparse or gray

dental abnormalities include caries and hypoplastic or absent teeth

Non-Skin

mental retardation

birth weight is normal, but severe growth retardation apparent in early life ("cachectic dwarfism")

microcephaly, sunken eyes, thin nose, and prognathism give an appearance of premature senility or "bird-like" facies

disproportionately long extremities and enlarged hands and feet result in a "bird-like" or "Mickey Mouse" appearance

frequent retinal pigmentary degeneration, optic atrophy, and cataracts, causing blindness; occasional corneal dystrophy

progressive sensorineural hearing loss

other neurologic abnormalities include central and peripheral nervous system demyelination, coarse tremor, and unsteady gait

other skeletal abnormalities include kyphoscoliosis, flexion contractures, and skull thickening

cryptorchidism or small testes in about one third of males; small breasts and oligomenorrhea reported

early atherosclerosis may develop, as in progeria

Genetics

AR

slight male predominance

three complementation groups described

Pathophysiology

cellular hypersensitivity to ultraviolet (UV) light (UV light–treated fibroblasts have decreased survival); fibroblast survival after x-ray exposure is normal

UV light exposure increases frequency of spontaneous sister chromatid exchanges, but otherwise sister chromatid exchanges are normal

Laboratory Data

impaired renal function

radiographs: skull thickening and calcification of falx cerebri, cerebrum, basal ganglia, and cerebellum

prenatal diagnosis possible; abnormal colony-forming ability of amniotic fluid cells following UV irradiation

Prognosis

increased skin cancers and pigmentary changes as seen in xeroderma pigmentosum do not occur, except that xeroderma pigmentosum complementation group B has been associated with Cockayne syndrome

survival beyond the second decade is unusual; death usually occurs in second decade from inanition or respiratory tract infections

severe neurologic dysfunction from birth

congenital structural eye abnormalities and cataracts within first 3 years of life associated with severe disease and earlier death

REFERENCES

McK 216400

McK 216410 (complementation group II); McK 216411 (complementation group III)

Greenhaw GA, Hebert A, Duke-Woodside ME, et al. Xeroderma pigmentosum and Cockayne syndrome: overlapping clinical and biochemical phenotypes. Am J Hum Genet 1992;50:677–689

Lehmann AR. Three complementation groups in Cockayne syndrome. Mutat Res 1982;106:347–356

Lehmann AR, Francis AJ, Giannelli F. Prenatal diagnosis of Cockayne's syndrome. Lancet 1985;1:486–488

Lehmann AR, Norris PG. DNA repair and cancer: speculations based on studies with xeroderma pigmentosum, Cockayne's syndrome and trichothiodystrophy. Carcinogenesis 1989;10:1353–1356

Mayne LV, Lehmann AR. Failure of RNA synthesis to recover after UV irradiation: an early defect in cells from individuals with Cockayne's syndrome and xeroderma pigmentosum. Cancer Res 1982;42:1473–1478

Nance MA, Berry SA. Cockayne syndrome: review of 140 cases. Am J Med Genet 1992;42:68–84

Otsuka F, Robbins JH. The Cockayne syndrome—an inherited multisystem disorder with cutaneous photosensitivity and defective repair of DNA: comparison with xeroderma pigmentosum. Am J Dermatopathol 1985;7:387–392

Schmickel RD, Chu EH, Trosko JE, et al. Cockayne syndrome: a cellular sensitivity to ultraviolet light. Pediatrics 1977;60:135–139

Seguin LR, Tarone RE, Liao KH, et al. Ultraviolet light–induced chromosomal aberrations in cultured cells from Cockayne syndrome and complementation group C xeroderma pigmentosum patients: lack of correlation with cancer susceptibility. Am J Hum Genet 1988;42:468–475

WERNER SYNDROME

Synonyms

- progeria of the adult
- scleroderma and cataracts syndrome
- dyshormonal dermatosis
- pangeria

Skin

premature canities of the temples in mid second decade, with subsequent alopecia and graying of scalp hair, eyebrows, facial hair, and pubic hair (Fig. 4–1)

atrophy of skin, subcutis, and, to varying degrees, the muscles of the face and extremities develops in late second to early third decade; distal extremities are the most severely involved

atrophy of oral mucosa reported

skin may appear shiny, smooth and bound down, giving a sclerodermoid appearance

mottled hyperpigmentation and telangiectases on face, neck, and extremities

calluses develop over bony pressure points and the soles, where subcutaneous tissue is already diminished

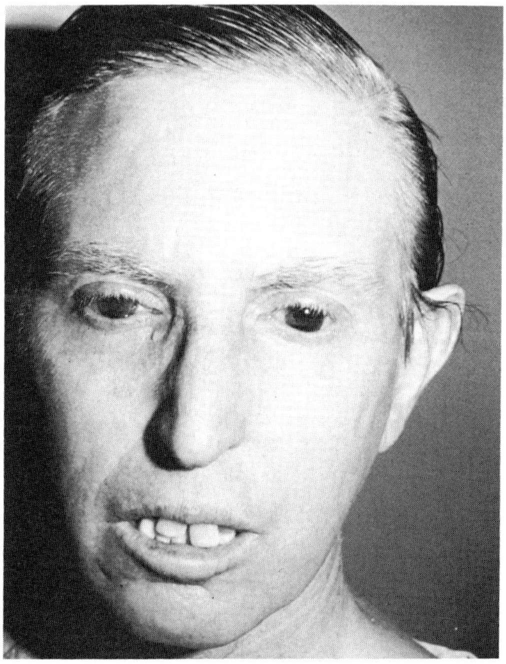

FIGURE 4–1
Werner syndrome. Premature graying of the scalp hair, eyebrows, and eyelashes. Characteristic facies including small mouth, receding chin, and beak-like nose and atrophy and telangiectasia of the facial skin. (Courtesy of Benjamin K. Fisher, MD, Toronto, Ontario)

skin ulcers secondary to ischemia may develop over pressure and nonpressure areas (e.g., over Achilles tendon); occasional acral gangrene

nails may be brittle, atrophic, or absent

Non-Skin

normal until adolescence, then growth retardation manifests

craniofacial abnormalities contributing to "bird-like" facies include small mouth, receding chin, and beak-shaped nose

vocal cord abnormalities and a high-pitched voice

ocular findings include bilateral cataracts of posterior lens (juvenile type; star-like opacities) that occur in late third or early fourth decade

musculoskeletal abnormalities include spindle-shaped extremities, pes plana, ankylosis, sclerodactyly, hyporeflexia of the Achilles tendons, and almost invariably osteoporosis

in addition, there are calcification of ligaments, tendons, synovia, and adjacent subcutaneous tissue, especially of extremities, aorta, and large arteries

hypogonadism with decreased libido

latent or overt diabetes mellitus in more than 50% of cases

malignancy, most commonly sarcomas, in about 10%

Genetics

AR

Laboratory Data

increased hyaluronic acid in urine

poor growth and decreased life span of cultured skin fibroblasts

increased chromosomal breaks, both spontaneous and clastogen induced; sister chromatid exchanges are normal

Prognosis

death by fifth decade due to myocardial infarction, stroke, or malignancy

REFERENCES

McK 277700

Bauer EA, Silverman N, Busiek D, et al. Diminished response of Werner's syndrome fibroblasts to growth factors PDGF and FGF. Science 1986;234:1240–1243

Epstein CJ, Martin GM, Motulsky AG. Werner's syndrome; caricature of aging: a genetic model for the study of degenerative diseases. Trans Assoc Am Physicians 1965;78:73–81

Frenkel G. Schleimhautatrophie unter besonderer Beruecksichtigung des Werner-Syndroms. Dtsch Zahnaerztl Z 1970;25:1026–1039

Gawkrodger DJ, Priestley GC, Vijayalaxmi, et al. Werner's syndrome: biochemical and cy-

togenetic studies. Arch Dermatol 1985; 121:636–641
Gebhart E, Bauer R, Raub U, et al. Spontaneous and induced chromosomal instability in Werner syndrome. Hum Genet 1988;80:135–139
Goto M, Tanimoto K, Horiuchi Y, Sasazuki T. Family analysis of Werner's syndrome: a survey of 42 Japanese families with a review of the literature. Clin Genet 1981;19:8–15
Hrabko RP, Milgrom H, Schwartz RA. Werner's syndrome with associated malignant neoplasms. Arch Dermatol 1982;118:106–108

STORM SYNDROME (CALCIFIC CARDIAC VALVULAR DEGENERATION WITH PREMATURE AGING; WERNER-LIKE SYNDROME)

thinning of scalp hair, eyebrows, and eyelashes in adolescence

tightening of skin of face and dorsal hands; wrinkling of palmar skin

progressive calcific cardiac valvular degeneration beginning in childhood

joint abnormalities and intestinal fat malabsorption

AD

differences from Werner syndrome include absence of scleroderma-like cutaneous changes and cataracts and pattern of inheritance

McK 185069
Weisman HF, Gaither NS, Moore J, et al. The Storm syndrome: a new, pleiotropic, autosomal dominant disorder affecting connective tissue. [Abstract]. Am J Hum Genet 1989;45(suppl):A67

FAMILIAL MANDIBULOACRAL DYSPLASIA

mottled hyperpigmentation and atrophy of skin of hands and feet; mottled hyperpigmentation may also involve trunk and extremities

sparse scalp hair by third decade

occasional plantar hyperkeratosis

occasional calcinosis cutis

broad, brittle nails reported

loss of teeth during adolescence

pointed nose and prominent eyes

short stature

acro-osteolysis of hands and feet resulting in short, club-shaped terminal phalanges

other bony abnormalities include mandibular hypoplasia, delayed cranial suture closure and dysplastic clavicles

probable AR

may be confused with Werner syndrome or acrogeria

McK 248370
Gorlin RJ, Cohen MM Jr, Levin LS. Syndromes affecting bone: other skeletal disorders. In: Syndromes of the Head and Neck. 3rd ed. New York, Oxford University Press, 1990:266–267
Mensing H, Schaeg G, Burck U, Meigel W. Werner-Syndrom-artige Erkrankung bei drei Brudern. Hautarzt 1982;33:542–547
Zina AM, Cravario A, Bundino S. Familial mandibuloacral dysplasia. Br J Dermatol 1981;105:719–723

FLYNN-AIRD SYNDROME

atrophy of skin and subcutis of shins and dorsa of feet; frequent skin ulceration, especially of ankles

sparse scalp hair

dental caries

bilateral sensorineural deafness in nearly all; almost always the first symptom; onset in first or second decade

ocular abnormalities include myopia, bilateral cataracts, atypical retinitis pigmentosa, and blindness

skeletal deformities include kyphoscoliosis

neurologic abnormalities include mental retardation, epilepsy, dementia, and peripheral neuritis

AD

electroencephalogram: dysrhythmias

life span is normal

McK 136300
Flynn P, Aird RB. A neuroectodermal syndrome of dominant inheritance. J Neurol Sci 1965;2:161–182

ACROGERIA

Synonym

- Gottron syndrome

Skin

thin, wrinkled skin due to cutaneous and subcutaneous atrophy, most prominently on the distal extremities with onset at or shortly after birth

prominence of veins because of cutaneous atrophy

mottled hyperpigmentation and telangiectases on the upper trunk and extremities

easy bruisability and abnormal scarring of skin reported

normal hair

nail abnormalities include onychogryphosis, koilonychia, and atrophy

Non-Skin

craniofacial abnormalities contributing to a "pinched" facies include prominent eyes, hollow cheeks, beaked nose, and thin lips

low birth weight

short stature; hands and feet may be small

Genetics

mostly sporadic; rare AR and AD cases reported

most patients are female

Prognosis

life expectancy and general health are normal

Discussion

features including normal hair and lack of cataracts distinguish this disease from progeria and Werner syndrome

REFERENCES

McK 201200

de Groot WP, Tafelkruyer J, Woerdeman MJ. Familial acrogeria (Gottron). Br J Dermatol 1980;103:213–223

Ho A, White SJ, Rasmussen JE. Skeletal abnormalities of acrogeria, a progeroid syndrome. Skeletal Radiol 1987;16:463–468

Pope FM, Nicholls AC, Jones PM, et al. EDS IV (acrogeria): new autosomal dominant and recessive types. J R Soc Med 1980;73:180–186

METAGERIA

generalized decrease in subcutaneous fat from infancy

fine, thin scalp hair

around puberty, development of diffuse mottled hyperpigmentation and telangiectases on neck, trunk, and extremities

peripheral vasospasm resulting in ulceration and gangrene

thin face, prominent eyes, and beaked nose

diabetes mellitus in second or third decade

inheritance not established; possible AR

possible decreased life span

Gilkes JJH, Sharvill DE, Wells RS. The premature ageing syndromes: report of eight cases and description of a new entity named metageria. Br J Dermatol 1974; 91:243–262

NEONATAL PROGEROID SYNDROME OF WIEDEMANN-RAUTENSTRAUCH

sparse hair and prominent veins of the scalp at birth

generalized decrease in subcutaneous fat

atrophic nails and dental abnormalities

entropion

craniofacial abnormalities include beaked nose, malar hypoplasia, widened anterior fontanelle, and small mouth

intrauterine growth retardation and physical and mental retardation

probable AR

McK 264090

Devos EA, Leroy JG, Frijns JP, Van den Berghe H. The Wiedemann-Rautenstrauch or neonatal progeroid syndrome: report of a patient with consanguineous parents. Eur J Pediatr 1981;136:245–248

Rudin C, Thommen L, Fliegel C, et al. The neonatal pseudo-hydrocephalic progeroid syndrome (Wiedemann-Rautenstrauch): report of a new patient and review of the literature. Eur J Pediatr 1988;147:433–438

Toriello HV. Wiedemann-Rautenstrauch syndrome. J Med Genet 1990;27:256–257

Wiedemann HR. An unidentified neonatal progeroid syndrome: follow-up report. Eur J Pediatr 1979; 130:65–70

OSTEODYSPLASTIC GERODERMA (WALT DISNEY DWARFISM)

lax, wrinkled, senile appearance of skin, especially over face and hands, at birth

normal hair

"sad" facies with drooping eyelids and jowls (Fig. 4–2)

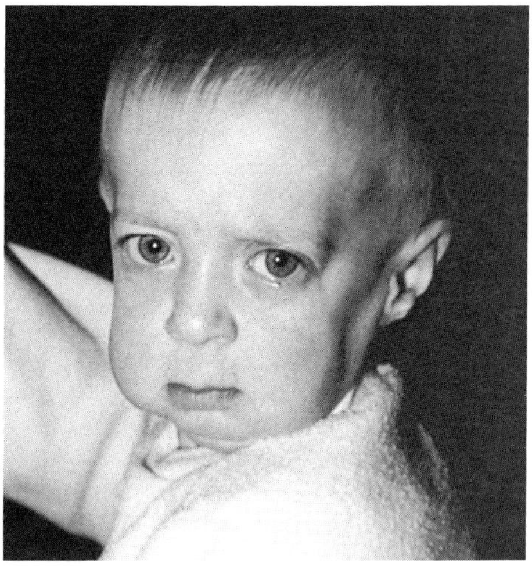

FIGURE 4–2
Osteodysplastic geroderma, otherwise known as "Walt Disney dwarfism." Affected children have a "sad" facies with drooping eyelids and jowls due to skin laxity. (Courtesy of Neil S. Goldberg, MD, Valhalla, New York)

musculoskeletal abnormalities include short stature, joint laxity, pes planus, generalized osteoporosis, pathologic fractures, and skeletal malformations

skin biopsy may show fragmented elastic fibers

McK 231070

Hunter AGW. Is geroderma osteodysplastica underdiagnosed? J Med Genet 1988; 25:854–857

Hunter AGW, Martsolf JT, Baker CG, Reed MH. Geroderma osteodysplastica: a report of two affected families. Hum Genet 1978;40:311–324

Lisker R, Hernandez A, Martinez-Lavin M, et al. Gerodermia osteodysplastica hereditaria: report of three affected brothers and literature review. Am J Med Genet 1979;3:389–395

SCLEROATROPHIC AND KERATOTIC DERMATOSIS OF LIMBS (SCLEROATROPHIC SYNDROME OF HURIEZ)

diffuse atrophic fibrosis ("scleroatrophy") of limbs, predominantly hands

sclerodactyly

palmar, and occasionally plantar, keratoderma present at birth; progresses throughout childhood

palmar hypohidrosis reported

nail hypoplasia and white discoloration

squamous cell carcinoma frequently develops in atrophic skin

AD

McK 181600

Fischer S. La génodermatose scleroatrophiante et keratodermique des extrémités (au sujet de trois nouveaux cas familiaux). Ann Dermatol Venereol 1978;105:1079–1082

Huriez C, Deminatti M, Agache P, Mennecier M. A propos de 28 cas d'épidermolyse bulleuse dans 11 familles dont une famille etudiée du point d'une génétique, sans mise en evidence de linkage. Bull Soc Fr Derm Syph 1968;75:750–755

Patrizi A, Di Lernia V, Patrone P. Palmoplantar keratoderma with sclerodactyly (Huriez syndrome). J Am Acad Dermatol 1992;26:855–857

PROGEROID SHORT STATURE WITH PIGMENTED NEVI

multiple pigmented papules on face and trunk

occasional fine sparse scalp hair

dental abnormalities

low birth weight

short stature

bird-like facies with small chin, prominent forehead, and decreased facial fat gives prematurely aged appearance

mental retardation

hepatomegaly

inheritance unknown

McK 176690

Baraitser M, Insley J, Winter RM. A recognisable short stature syndrome with premature aging and pigmented naevi. J Med Genet 1988;25:53–56

Mulvihill JJ, Smith DW. Another disorder with prenatal shortness of stature and premature aging. Birth Defects 1975;11:368–371

Shephard MK. An unidentified syndrome with abnormality of skin and hair. Birth Defects 1971;7:353–354

Premature Aging Syndrome—Abbreviated Entry

GRANDDAD SYNDROME

acronym for Growth Retardation, Aged facies, Normal Development, Decreased subcutaneous fat, Autosomal Dominant inheritance

thin or absent scalp hair

AD

McK 138920
Marion RW, Goldberg RB, Young RS, et al. The GRANDDAD syndrome: a disorder combining growth delay, "aged facies," normal development, and deficiency of subcutaneous fat. [Abstract]. Am J Hum Genet 1989;45(suppl):A53

CHAPTER

5

Disorders of Hypopigmentation

Syndromes in which decreased cutaneous pigmentation is either the primary or a major clinical feature are considered in this section. These disorders are caused by different abnormalities in the pathway of melanin production. For example, the albinisms are caused by defects in the enzyme tyrosinase while piebaldism and related disorders are associated with an absence of melanocytes in depigmented areas.

Some diseases in this chapter overlap clinically with the poikilodermatous disorders. Likewise, decreased pigmentation may be an important manifestation of other inherited disorders presented elsewhere in the book, such as pigment dilution in phenylketonuria.

HYPOMELANOSIS OF ITO

Synonym

- incontinentia pigmenti achromians

Skin

asymmetrical hypopigmented macular whorls, streaks, and patches ("marble cake" pattern), unilateral or bilateral (Fig. 5–1); follows Blaschko's lines and located anywhere on body except scalp, palms, soles, and mucous membranes

may appear at birth, infancy, or in childhood

dental abnormalities reported

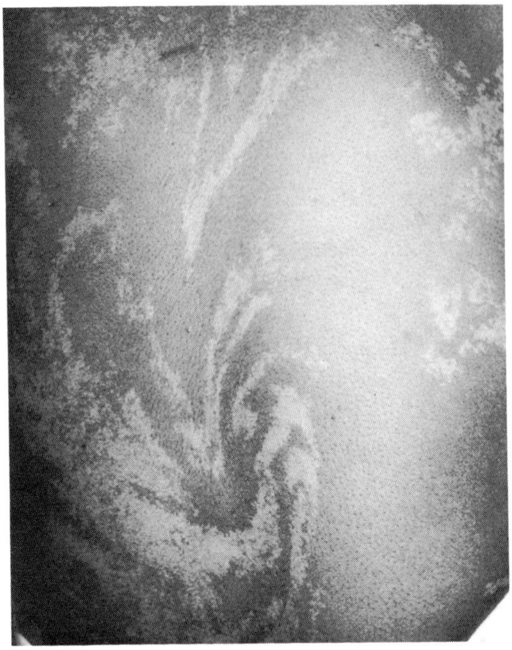

FIGURE 5–1
Patterned hypopigmented macules and patches following the lines of Blaschko on the back of a patient with widespread lesions of hypomelanosis of Ito.

Non-Skin

at least 50% have extracutaneous abnormalities

developmental delay

ophthalmologic abnormalities include strabismus and cataracts

skeletal abnormalities include scoliosis and asymmetry of limbs

central nervous system abnormalities include seizures, mental retardation, and deafness

Genetics

sporadic; rare reports of familial cases challenged

thought by some to be due to a heterogeneous group of disorders that results from chromosomal mosaicism or chimerism, either of which results in the presence of two genetically different cell lines in the individual

association with chromosomal translocation involving Xp11 reported

male to female ratio: 2:1

Laboratory Data

histopathology: decreased epidermal melanocytes and melanin in hypopigmented areas

Discussion

lesions of nevus depigmentosus (systematized depigmented nevi) are congenital hypopigmented macules present from birth that do not change and are due to a melanosome transfer defect; localized hypomelanosis of Ito (latter not necessarily at birth) can occasionally be confused with nevus depigmentosus clinically

REFERENCES

McK 146150

Donnai D, Read AP, McKeown C, Andrews T. Hypomelanosis of Ito: a manifestation of mosaicism or chimerism. J Med Genet 1988;25:809–818

Glover MT, Brett EM, Atherton DJ. Hypomelanosis of Ito: spectrum of the disease. J Pediatr 1989;115:75–80

Ito M. Studies of melanin: XI. Incontinentia pigmenti achromians: a singular case of nevus depigmentosus systematicus bilateralis. Tokoku J Exp Med 1952;55:57–59

Lungarotti MS, Martello C, Calabro A, Baldari F, Mariotti G. Hypomelanosis of Ito associated with chromosomal translocation involving Xp11. Am J Med Genet 1991;40:447–448

Montagna P, Procaccianti G, Galli G, et al. Familial hypomelanosis of Ito. Eur Neurol 1991;31:345–347

Moss C, Burn J. Genetic counselling in hypomelanosis of Ito: case report and review. Clin Genet 1988;34:109–115

Ortonne J, Mosher DB, Fitzpatrick TB. Vitiligo and Other Hypomelanoses of Hair and Skin. New York, Plenum Medical Book, 1983

Ruiz-Maldonado R, Toussaint S, Tamayo L, et al. Hypomelanosis of Ito: diagnostic criteria and report of 41 cases. Pediatr Dermatol 1992;9:1–10

Schwartz MF Jr, Esterly NB, Fretzin DF, et al. Hypomelanosis of Ito (incontinentia pigmenti achromians): a neurocutaneous syndrome. J Pediatr 1977;90:236–240

Sybert VA, Pagon RA, Donian M, Bradley CM. Pigmentary abnormalities and mosaicism for chromosomal aberration: association with clinical features similar to hypomelanosis of Ito. J Pediatr 1990;116:581–586

Sybert VA. Hypomelanosis of Ito. Pediatr Dermatol 1990;7:74–76

Albinism and Albinoidism

Albinism is a heterogeneous group of heritable disorders of the melanocyte pigmentary system. Its manifestations are the sequelae caused by decreased melanin pigment produced by melanocytes, abnormal development of certain structures of the central nervous system, and other defects. Tissues containing melanocytes include the skin, hair, eyes, and central nervous system.

In oculocutaneous albinism (OCA), skin and hair coloration varies from pure white to shades of blond, brown, and red, usually from birth. Cutaneous photosensitivity is almost always present. Eye involvement is constant and varies in severity depending on the type of OCA, but in general there are hypoplasia of the fovea, translucent irides, photophobia, nystagmus, decreased visual acuity, and absence of binocular vision.

In ocular albinism (OA), the eye is the principal site of involvement but the skin may show varying degrees of hypopigmentation; thus, clinically, OA may overlap with OCA. Deafness and other extracutaneous ectodermal abnormalities can be seen in some forms of OCA and OA.

In albinoidism, there is hypomelanosis without nystagmus, photophobia, and decreased visual acuity.

Many of the clinical descriptions of patients with diseases presented in this chapter are race dependent; in general, the findings listed are for white patients. However, similarly affected individuals of dark-skinned races may have more pigmentation.

Most types of OCA are inherited as autosomal recessive traits. OA is

TABLE 5–1
OCULOCUTANEOUS ALBINISMS

Type	Inheritance	Skin Color	Hair Color	Tanning Ability	Nystagmus	Iris Pigment	Hair Bulb Pigmentation in Tyrosine	Nevi or Freckles	Comments
IA (McK 203100) Tyrosinase negative	AF	Pink	White	None	+ + + +	None	–	–	
IB (McK 203100) Yellow mutant	AR	Cream	Yellow-red	Slight	+/+ + +	Cartwheel	–/+	+	
IC Platinum	AR	Pink	Off-white	None	+ + + +	Central, or cartwheel	+	+/–	
II (McK 203200) Tyrosinase positive	AR	Cream	Yellow-tan	None	+ +/+ + +	Central, peripheral, or cartwheel	+ + + +	+	
III (McK 203280) Minimal	AR	Pink	White-yellow	None	+ + + +	Central or peripheral	?	–	
IV (McK 203290) Brown	AR	Light tan	Beige	Present	+/+ +	Cartwheel	–/+	+/–	Africans
V (McK 278400) Rufous	AR	Red-brown	Red	?	–/+ +	Slight	+ + + +	+	Africans
VIA (McK 203300) Hermansky-Pudlak syndrome	AR	Cream-gray	White-brown		+/+ + +	None to cartwheel	+	+	Abnormal platelets; ceroid inclusions
VIB (McK 214500) Chédiak-Higashi syndrome	AR	Pink	Steel-gray		–/+ +	Cartwheel to normal	+ + + +	+	Giant lysosomal storage
VII Autosomal dominant oculocutaneous albinism	AD	Cream	White to cream		+ +/+ + +	None to cartwheel	+ + + +	+	

Data from Witkop CJ Jr, Quevedo WC Jr, Fitzpatrick TB, King RA. Albinism. In: Scriver CR, Beaudet AL, Sly WS, Valle D, eds. The Metabolic Basis of Inherited Disease. 6th ed. New York, McGraw-Hill, 1989: 2905–2947; and Mosher DB, Fitzpatrick TB, Ortonne JP, Hori Y. Disorders of pigmentation. In: Fitzpatrick TB, Eisen AZ, Wolff K, Freedberg IM, Austen KF, eds. Dermatology in General Medicine. New York, McGraw-Hill, 1987: 794–876.

usually inherited as an X-linked recessive trait, but autosomal recessive and dominant cases have also been reported.

Incubation of hair bulbs in tyrosine produces no pigment in tyrosinase-negative OCA and its variants (types IA, IB and IC; see Table 5–1). In most other forms of albinism, some pigmentation is produced. This test has been used to distinguish patients with different types of albinism (e.g., tyrosinase-positive OCA, tyrosinase-negative OCA, and their variants). However, because of the overlap of results among individual patients with different types of albinism, the hair bulb test is not regarded as entirely reliable. In addition, because of phenotypical overlap, the distinction between OCA (autosomal recessive) and OA (mostly X-linked recessive) may not be clear. Some have proposed to simply use the terms *autosomal recessive albinism* and *X-linked recessive albinism,* rather than make distinctions based on variable phenotype and hair bulb test results. Identification of genes for the different types of albinism will help to clarify classification.

REFERENCES

Ortonne J, Mosher DB, Fitzpatrick TB. Vitiligo and Other Hypomelanoses of Hair and Skin. New York, Plenum Medical Book Company, 1983

Witkop CJ Jr. Inherited disorders of pigmentation. Clin Dermatol 1985;3:70–134

Witkop CJ Jr, Quevedo WC Jr, Fitzpatrick TB, King RA. Albinism. In: Scriver CR, Beaudet AL, Sly WS, Valle D, eds. The Metabolic Basis of Inherited Disease. 6th ed. New York, McGraw-Hill, 1989:2905–2947

TYROSINASE-NEGATIVE OCULOCUTANEOUS ALBINISM

Synonym

- albinism type IA, ty-neg

Skin

see Color Figure 5–1

absence of skin, hair, and eye pigmentation; onset at birth

skin is pink to red, may be xerotic, and does not tan; patients of darker races may have pigmented macules

mucosae are depigmented

hypohidrosis

hair is fine, silky, flaxen, and yellow-white

Non-Skin

severe, rapid, and pendular nystagmus, often congenital

pink iris in light-skinned races and light blue iris in dark-skinned races

retinal red reflex present; absence of fundal pigment

severe photophobia, with blinking and lacrimation

abnormally developed fovea centralis

poor visual acuity; most patients are legally blind and myopic

intelligence may be below normal; this is often blamed on visual problems

increased susceptibility to pyogenic infections

delayed menses and decreased fertility

Genetics

AR

tyrosinase gene encoded on chromosome 11 q

Laboratory Data

melanocytes morphologically normal, with stage I to II melanosomes

no pigment on incubation of hair bulb in tyrosine

Prognosis

condition persistent; does not improve

actinic damage and sequelae may be severe: increased sunburns, solar elastosis, actinic keratoses, and cutaneous malignancies (basal and squamous cell carcinomas); dysplastic nevi and melanomas also reported

life expectancy may be decreased

REFERENCES

McK 203100

Pehamberger H, Honigsmann H, Wolff K. Dysplastic nevus syndrome with multiple primary amelanotic melanomas in oculocutaneous albinism. J Am Acad Dermatol 1984;11:731–735

Witkop CJ Jr, Quevedo WC Jr, Fitzpatrick TB, King RA. Albinism. In Scriver CR, Beaudet AL, Sly WS, Valle D, eds. The Metabolic Basis of Inherited Disease. 6th ed. New York, McGraw-Hill, 1989:2905–2947

YELLOW MUTANT ALBINISM (ALBINISM TYPE IB, YM; AMISH ALBINISM; XANTHOUS ALBINISM)

white skin at birth; exposed skin may tan and pigmented nevi may develop

white hair at birth that becomes yellow to yellow-red or brown around 6 months of age

mild to moderate nystagmus

iris may be pink at birth but blue in infancy; darkens with age

retinal red reflex present; minimal fundal pigment, may increase with age

mild to moderate photophobia

visual acuity initially the same as tyrosinase-negative albinism but improves with age

AR

some pigment may be present in hair bulbs, but pigment does not increase with tyrosine incubation alone; minimal increase in pigment (pheomelanin) results when L-cysteine is added

yellow mutant albinism is an allelic variant of tyrosinase-negative OCA; they are indistinguishable at birth

Hu F, Hanifin JM, Prescott GH, et al. Yellow mutant albinism: cytochemical, ultrastructural, and genetic characterization suggesting multiple allelism. Am J Hum Genet 1980;32:387–395

Nance WE, Jackson CE, Witkop CJ Jr. Amish albinism: a distinctive autosomal recessive phenotype. Am J Hum Genet 1970;22:579–586

PLATINUM OCULOCUTANEOUS ALBINISM (ALBINISM TYPE IC, PT)

pink to red skin

metallic-cream to platinum hair; not stark white

gray to blue iris but no fundal pigmentation

retinal red reflex present

severe nystagmus

severe photophobia

visual acuity as in tyrosinase-negative OCA

AR

none to little pigment on incubation of hair bulbs in tyrosine

may be the same as minimal pigment disease (see main entry)

Witkop CJ Jr, Quevedo WC Jr, Fitzpatrick TB, King RA. Albinism. In: Scriver CR, Beaudet AL, Sly WS, Valle D, eds. The Metabolic Basis of Inherited Disease. 6th ed. New York, McGraw-Hill, 1989:2905–2947

TYROSINASE-POSITIVE OCULOCUTANEOUS ALBINISM

Synonym

- albinism type II, ty-pos

Skin

see Color Figure 5–2

onset at birth

pink-white to cream skin; lightly pigmented nevi in some

white, yellow, or red hair; darkens with age

the clinical appearance may resemble tyrosinase-negative albinism early in life, but increased pigment in skin, hair, and eyes may be seen with age

Non-Skin

moderate nystagmus

blue, yellow, or brown iris; darker in patients of dark-skinned races; may darken with age

retinal red reflex present; may be absent in patients of dark-skinned races

none to little fundal pigment (more pigment with age)

moderate photophobia (less than tyrosinase-negative OCA)

markedly decreased visual acuity but in general better than in patients with tyrosinase-negative OCA; may improve with age

Genetics

AR

Laboratory Data

pigment produced on incubation of hair bulbs in tyrosine

Discussion

most common type of albinism in North Americans, Chinese, and Native Americans

REFERENCES

McK 203200

Akiyama M, Shimizu H, Sugiura M, Nishikawa T. Do pigmented naevi in albinism provide evidence of tyrosinase positivity? Br J Dermatol 1992;127:649–653

Levin DL, Roth DE, Muhlbauer JE. Sporadic dysplastic nevus syndrome in a tyrosinase-positive oculocutaneous albino. J Am Acad Dermatol 1988;19:393–396

Witkop CJ Jr, Niswander JD, Bergsma DR, et al. Tyrosinase positive oculocutaneous albinism among the Zuni and the Brandywine triracial isolate: biochemical and clinical characteristics and fertility. Am J Phys Anthropol 1972;36:397–405

MINIMAL PIGMENT DISEASE (ALBINISM TYPE III)

patients are hypopigmented and do not tan

minimal amounts of pigment develop in the iris in childhood

AR

may be the same as platinum OCA (see main entry)

McK 203280

King RA, Wirtschafter JD, Olds DP, Brumbaugh J. Minimal pigment: a new type of oculocutaneous albinism. Clin Genet 1986;29:42–50

BROWN OCULOCUTANEOUS ALBINISM (ALBINISM TYPE IV)

cream to light brown skin; moderate tanning on exposure to sunlight

beige to light brown hair

blue to hazel to light brown iris and mild to moderate fundal pigment in adults

retinal red reflex present but may be absent in adults

moderate nystagmus

mild photophobia and mild decrease in visual acuity

AR

pigment produced on incubation of hair bulbs in tyrosine

patients with brown OCA are darker than patients with tyrosinase-positive albinism at birth, but they do not increase pigmentation with age nor do they tan as well

seen in Africans, black Americans, and New Guineans

McK 203290

King RA, Lewis RA, Townsend D, et al. Brown oculocutaneous albinism: clinical, ophthalmological, and biochemical characterization. Ophthalmology 1985;92:1496–1505

King RA, Rich SS. Segregation analysis of brown oculocutaneous albinism. Clin Genet 1986;29:496–501

RUFOUS OCULOCUTANEOUS ALBINISM (ALBINISM TYPE V; XANTHISM)

reddish brown ("rufous") skin

mahogany red to deep red hair

reddish brown to brown iris and moderate fundal pigment

mild nystagmus

mild photophobia and mildly to moderately decreased visual acuity

AR

seen in Africans and New Guineans

McK 278400

Barnicot NA. Human pigmentation. Man 1957;57:114–120

Pearson KD, Nettleship E, Usher CH. A Monograph on Albinism in Man. Series VI, VIII, IX, parts I, II and IV. London, Cambridge University Press, 1911–1913

Witkop CJ Jr, Quevedo WC Jr, Fitzpatrick TB, King RA. Albinism. In: Scriver CR, Beaudet AL, Sly WS, Valle D, eds. The Metabolic Basis of Inherited Disease. 6th ed. New York, McGraw-Hill, 1989:2905–2947

HERMANSKY-PUDLAK SYNDROME

Synonym

- albinism type VIA, HPS

Skin

see Figures 5–2 and 5–3

creamy-gray to light normal skin (race dependent: darker in more darkly pigmented races); pigment increases with age

white to red-brown hair; race dependent

rarely, papules may develop on palate

Non-Skin

blue-gray to brown iris; race dependent

retinal red reflex present in light-skinned races, but absent in dark-skinned races

none to little fundal pigment in adulthood

mild to moderate nystagmus

mild to severe photophobia

decreased to normal visual acuity

hemorrhagic diathesis due to storage pool platelet defect with manifestations including easy bruisability, epistaxis, and excessive bleeding (e.g., prolonged hemorrhage after tooth extraction or childbirth); worsened by use of aspirin

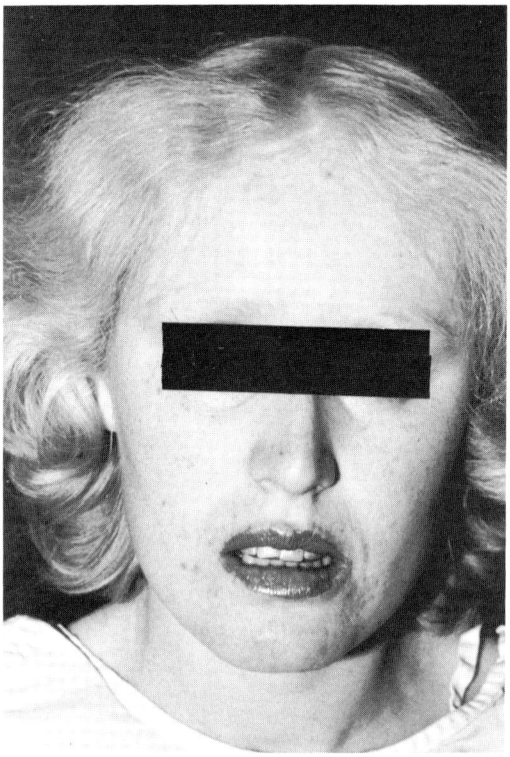

FIGURE 5–2
This Puerto Rican woman with Hermansky-Pudlak syndrome had hypopigmentation, blond hair, and a prominent red reflex.

pulmonary fibrosis, frequently severe, with restrictive lung disease may occur by third decade

ulcerative, granulomatous colitis in one third of patients

occasional renal and cardiac failure

recurrent infections including pharyngitis and tonsillitis

Genetics

AR

more common in Puerto Ricans

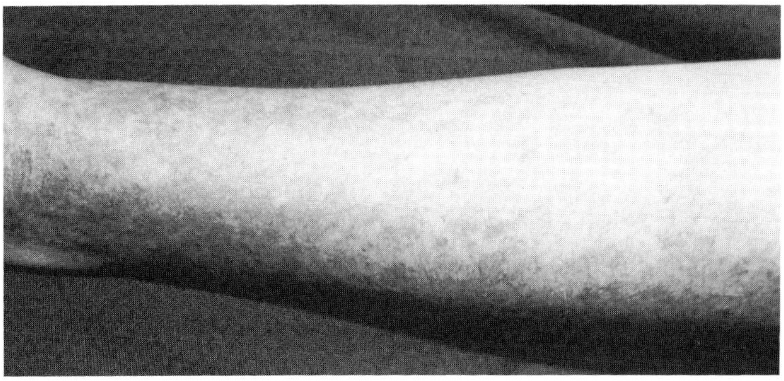

FIGURE 5–3
The same patient as in Figure 5–2 shows mild pigmentation of the lower extremity, demonstrating that patients with Hermansky-Pudlak syndrome have the ability to develop some pigment.

Laboratory Data

melanocytes are tyrosinase positive and are decreased in number; macromelanosomes are characteristic

ceroid inclusions in cells of the monocyte-phagocytic system and numerous viscera

pulmonary fibrosis (frequently severe) may be seen in chest radiographs of patients older than 30 years old

platelet defects, including deficient dense bodies and abnormal aggregation

fluorescent microscopy of urinary sediment shows orange-red fluorescent cytoplasmic granules

Prognosis

patients should avoid aspirin and related products

Discussion

Chédiak-Higashi syndrome (see main entry) also has pigmentary abnormalities and inclusion bodies, but the inclusion bodies in Chédiak-Higashi syndrome are in all leukocytes and not just in monocytes

REFERENCES

McK 203300

DePinho RA, Kaplan KL. The Hermansky-Pudlak syndrome: report of three cases and review of pathophysiology and management considerations. Medicine (Baltimore) 1985;64:192–202

Kinnear PE, Tuddenham EG. Albinism with haemorrhagic diathesis: Hermansky-Pudlak syndrome. Br J Ophthalmol 1985; 69:904–908

Schachne JP, Glaser N, Lee SH, et al. Hermansky-Pudlak syndrome: case report and clinicopathologic review. J Am Acad Dermatol 1990;22:926–932

Schallreuter KU, Witkop CJ Jr. Thioredoxin reductase activity in Hermansky-Pudlak syndrome: a method for identification of putative heterozygotes. J Invest Dermatol 1988;90:372–377

Schinella RA, Greco MA, Garay SM, et al. Hermansky-Pudlak syndrome: a clinicopathologic study. Hum Pathol 1985;16:366–376

Shanahan F, Rolph L, King R, et al. Hermansky-Pudlak syndrome: an immunologic assessment of 15 cases. Am J Med 1988; 85:823–828

Witkop CJ Jr, Krumwiede M, Sedano H, et al. Reliability of absent platelet dense bodies as a diagnostic criterion for Hermansky-Pudlak syndrome. Am J Hematol 1987; 26:305–311

CHÉDIAK-HIGASHI SYNDROME

Synonyms

- albinism type VIB
- anomalous panleukocytic granulation
- Steinbrinck-Higashi syndrome
- Aleutian mink disease

Skin

see Color Figure 5–3

pigmentary dilution of skin; race dependent; multiple scattered nevi and ephelides common

blond to dark brown hair; may be silvery

hyperhidrosis

superficial pyodermas to deep subcutaneous abscesses and ulcers (especially due to staphylococcal and streptococcal group A organisms); frequently heal with gaping, atrophic scars

oral ulcerations and gingivitis

occasional dental abnormalities include caries and periodontal disease

Non-Skin

retinal red reflex present; diminishes after 5 years of age

blue to dark brown iris and mild to moderate fundal pigment

none to moderate photophobia and nystagmus (horizontal)

mildly to severely decreased visual acuity; occasional papilledema

neurologic abnormalities caused by progressive neurologic deterioration include clumsiness, abnormal gait, dysesthesias, epilepsy, and cranial and peripheral neuropathies; may develop in mid first decade

recurrent bacterial (especially staphylococcal and streptococcal), viral and fungal infections of the skin and respiratory tract present in late first decade

85% of patients develop an "accelerated phase," usually following the appearance of neurologic manifestations; features include anemia, thrombocytopenia, and neutropenia followed by fever, adenopathy, hepatosplenomegaly, jaundice, aphthae, and gingivitis; usually results in death

Genetics

AR

Pathophysiology

pigmentary dilution results from a reduced number of large melanin complexes in keratinocytes

failure of degranulation of large, peroxidase-rich granules in leukocytes

Laboratory Data

giant, azurophilic lysosome-like inclusions in all leukocytes is pathognomonic; also seen in cells of mucosa, hair shaft, skin, iris, nerves, and multiple viscera cellular inclusions may also be seen in the leukocytes of clinically normal heterozygous relatives

neutropenia; impaired neutrophil chemotaxis and killing ability

abnormal natural killer cell activity

histopathology: large melanin granules in skin and hair shafts

electron microscopy: giant melanosomes in melanocytes

Prognosis

most die in the first decade owing to hemorrhage, pneumonia, or septicemia

patients who survive into the second or third decades frequently die of hematologic malignancies, usually associated with the accelerated phase

successful bone marrow transplantation reported

Discussion

some speculate that the "accelerated phase" of Chédiak-Higashi syndrome is a reactive process that may be a variant of the virus-associated hemophagocytic syndrome, while others view this as a neoplastic process

Hermansky-Pudlak syndrome (see main entry) also has pigmentary abnormalities and inclusion bodies, which, however, are located in monocytes, not granulocytes

REFERENCES

McK 214500

Anderson LL, Paller AS, Malpass D, et al. Chédiak-Higashi syndrome in a black child. Pediatr Dermatol 1992;9:31–36

Barak Y, Nir E. Chédiak-Higashi syndrome. Am J Pediatr Hematol Oncol 1987;9:42–55

Rubin C, Burke B, McKenna RW, et al. The accelerated phase of Chédiak-Higashi syndrome: an expression of the virus-associated hemophagocytic syndrome? Cancer 1985;56:524–530

Siccardi AG, Bianchi E, Calligari A, et al. A new familial defect in neutrophil bactericidal activity. Helv Paediatr Acta 1978; 33:401–412

Stolz W, Graubner U, Gerstmeier J, et al. Chédiak-Higashi syndrome approaches in diagnosis and treatment. Curr Probl Dermatol 1989;18:93–100

GRISCELLI SYNDROME (CHÉDIAK-HIGASHI–LIKE SYNDROME; PAID [PARTIAL ALBINISM IMMUNODEFICIENCY] SYNDROME)

silvery gray hair of scalp, eyebrows, and eyelashes with large hair shaft pigment inclusions (larger than in Chédiak-Higashi syndrome) at birth

fair complexion with scattered areas of depigmentation

multiple immunodeficiencies and frequent pyogenic infections hepatosplenomegaly and lymphadenopathy

central nervous system demyelination and atrophy

probable AR

neutrophils morphologically normal (no giant granule inclusions)

McK 214450

Brismar J, Harfi HA. Partial albinism with immunodeficiency: a rare syndrome with prominent posterior fossa white matter changes. Am J Neuroradiol 1992;13:387–393

Griscelli C, Durandy A, Guy-Grand D, et al. A syndrome associating partial albinism and immunodeficiency. Am J Med 1978; 65:691–702

NEUROECTODERMAL MELANOLYSOSOMAL DISEASE (ELEJALDE SYNDROME)

generalized hypopigmentation

silver hair with abnormal melanolysosomes in cells including melanocytes and keratinocytes

severe neurologic abnormalities including seizures and severe psychomotor retardation

probable AR

hair shaft pigment inclusions are larger than in Chédiak-Higashi syndrome

relationship to Chédiak-Higashi syndrome unclear

McK 256710

Elejalde BR, Holguin J, Valencia A, et al. Mutations affecting pigmentation in man: I. Neuroectodermal melanolysosomal disease. Am J Med Genet 1979;3:65–80

AUTOSOMAL DOMINANT OCULOCUTANEOUS ALBINISM (ALBINISM TYPE VII)

skin color is white to light cream; pigmented nevi may be seen

white hair; may have slight red tints

irides gray to gray-blue with marked translucency

nystagmus and photophobia similar to tyrosinase-positive albinism

AD

normal melanocyte numbers and melanosome structure

Frenk E, Calame A. Hypopigmentation oculo-cutanée familiar à transmision dominante d'un trouble de la formation des melanosomes. Schweiz Med Wochenschr 1977; 107:1964

Witkop CJ Jr, Quevedo WC Jr, Fitzpatrick TB, King RA. Albinism. In: Scriver CR, Beaudet AL, Sly WS, Valle D, eds. The Metabolic Basis of Inherited Disease. 6th ed. New York, McGraw-Hill, 1989:2905–2947

OCULAR ALBINISM (OA)

only ocular pigmentation is consistently abnormal; different types are listed below.

X-LINKED OCULAR ALBINISM OF NETTLESHIP-FALLS (XOAN; VOGT OCULAR ALBINISM)

decreased ocular pigmentation (blue to light-green fundus)

nystagmus, severe photophobia, strabismus, severely decreased visual acuity, and foveal hypoplasia

XLR

melanin macroglobules found in normal skin

the most common OA

female heterozygotes display mosaic pigmentation pattern of the retina due to Lyon inactivation

McK 300500

Cortin P, Tremblay M, Lemagne JM. X-linked ocular albinism: relative value of skin biopsy, iris transillumination and funduscopy in identifying affected males and carriers. Can J Ophthalmol 1981;16:121–123

X-LINKED OCULAR ALBINISM WITH SENSORINEURAL DEAFNESS (WINSHIP OCULAR ALBINISM)

ocular albinism and sensorineural deafness

XLR

melanin macroglobules are found in normal skin

McK 300650
Winship I, Gericke G, Beighton P. X-linked inheritance of ocular albinism with late-onset sensorineural deafness. Am J Med Genet 1984;19:797–803

AUTOSOMAL RECESSIVE OCULAR ALBINISM (AROA)

ocular albinism

AR

McK 203310
O'Donnell FEJ, King RA, Green WR, et al. Autosomal recessively inherited ocular albinism: a new form of ocular albinism affecting females as severely as males. Arch Ophthalmol 1978;96:1621–1625

AUTOSOMAL DOMINANT OCULAR ALBINISM (OCULAR ALBINISM WITH SENSORINEURAL DEAFNESS; ADOA)

multiple cutaneous pigmented macules

ocular albinism

congenital vestibular deafness and vestibular abnormalities

AD

melanin macroglobules found in pigmented macules

McK 103470
Lewis RA. Ocular albinism and deafness. Am J Hum Genet 1978;30:57A

Albinoidism

Albinoidisms are inherited hypomelanotic conditions lacking nystagmus, diaphanous irides, photophobia, and decreased visual acuity. All forms of albinism may have anomalous optic tracts, but these pathways are normal in albinoid conditions. Piebaldism is a condition in which portions of the hair and skin are hypopigmented from birth.

OCULOCUTANEOUS ALBINOIDISM (DOMINANT ALBINOIDISM; LEUCISM; CUTANEOUS ALBINISM)

pink to pink-white skin

white to light blond hair

no nystagmus

blue iris and punctate pigmentation of the fundus

retinal red reflex absent

no photophobia and normal visual acuity

AD

actinic damage of skin is similar to OCA

although some reports refer to this entity as albinism, it is distinguished from albinism by nearly normal eye findings

McK 126070

King RA. Autosomal dominant oculocutaneous albinism with a mild phenotype. [Abstract]. Hum Genet 1979;31:75A

Witkop CJ Jr, Quevedo WC Jr, Fitzpatrick TB, King RA. Albinism. In: Scriver CR, Beaudet AL, Sly WS, Valle D, eds. The Metabolic Basis of Inherited Disease. 6th ed. New York, McGraw-Hill, 1989:2905–2947

Witkop CJ Jr. Depigmentations of the general and oral tissues and their genetic foundations. Ala J Med Sci 1979;16:330–333

TIETZ SYNDROME

variant of albinoidism with absence of eyebrows and deaf-mutism

AD

McK 103500

Reed WB, Stone VM, Boder E, Ziprkowski L. Pigmentary disorders in association with congenital deafness. Arch Dermatol 1967;95:176–186

Tietz W. A syndrome of deaf-mutism associated with albinism showing dominant autosomal inheritance. Am J Hum Genet 1963;15:259–264

BLACK LOCKS-ALBINISM-DEAFNESS SYNDROME (BADS)

white skin with brown macules

white hair with pigmented locks

red reflex present in children and adults

gray-blue irides but no fundal pigment

severe photophobia and nystagmus and poor visual acuity

sensorineural deafness

AR

no melanocytes in white hair and skin, but melanocytes are present in pigmented hair and skin; not a true albinism owing to absence of melanocytes

McK 227010
O'Doherty NJ, Gorlin RJ. The ermine phenotype: pigmentary–hearing loss heterogeneity. Am J Med Genet 1988;30:945–952
Witkop CJ Jr, Quevedo WC Jr, Fitzpatrick TB, King RA. Albinism. In: Scriver CR, Beaudet AL, Sly WS, Valle D, eds. The Metabolic Basis of Inherited Disease. 6th ed. New York, McGraw-Hill, 1989:2905–2947

CROSS-McKUSICK-BREEN SYNDROME

Synonyms

- Cross syndrome
- oculocerebral syndrome with hypopigmentation
- gingival fibromatosis, hypopigmentation, microphthalmia, oligophrenia, and athetosis

Skin

hypopigmented skin

hypopigmented hair; a few dark strands may develop

gingival fibromatosis; lips may protrude

Non-Skin

microphthalmos, cataracts, and corneal clouding

gray-blue iris

severe nystagmus and blindness

neurologic abnormalities including severe mental retardation, athetosis, spasticity, developmental defects, and high-pitched cry

Genetics

AR

seen in Amish kindreds; very rare

Laboratory Data

histopathology: decreased melanocytes; tyrosinase positive

REFERENCES

McK 257800
Castle DJ, Jenkins T, Shawinsky AA. The oculocerebral syndrome in association with generalized hypopigmentation: a case report. S Afr Med J 1989;76:35–36
Fryns JP, Dereymaeker AM, Heremans G, et al. Oculocerebral syndrome with hypopigmentation (Cross syndrome): report of two siblings born to consanguineous parents. Clin Genet 1988;34:81–84
Lerone M, Pessagno A, Taccone A, et al. Oculocerebral syndrome with hypopigmentation (Cross syndrome): report of a new case. Clin Genet 1992;41:87–89

OCULOCEREBRAL HYPOPIGMENTATION SYNDROME OF PREUS

generalized cutaneous hypopigmentation

craniofacial abnormalities include dolichocephaly and high-arched palate

syndactyly

psychomotor retardation

ocular abnormalities include nystagmus, pale translucent irides, photophobia, and cataracts; albinoid ocular fundi

McK 257790
Patton MA, Baraitser M, Heagerty AHM, Eady RAJ. An oculocerebral hypopigmentation syndrome: a case report with clinical, histochemical, and ultrastructural findings. J Med Genet 1987;24:118–122
Preus M, Fraser FC, Wigglesworth JW. An oculocerebral hypopigmentation syndrome. J Genet Hum 1983;31:323–328

PIEBALDISM

Synonyms

- congenital vitiligo
- congenital leukoderma
- partial albinism

Skin

white forelock with underlying triangular or diamond-shaped area of depigmented skin (Fig. 5–4); present at birth

additionally, depigmented areas may symmetrically involve forehead, medial eyebrows, eyelashes, anterior chest and abdomen, flanks, medial thighs, and legs (Fig. 5–5)

rarely, hands, wrists, feet, ankles, and midline of the back involved

characteristic hyperpigmented macules in depigmented areas and in normal skin

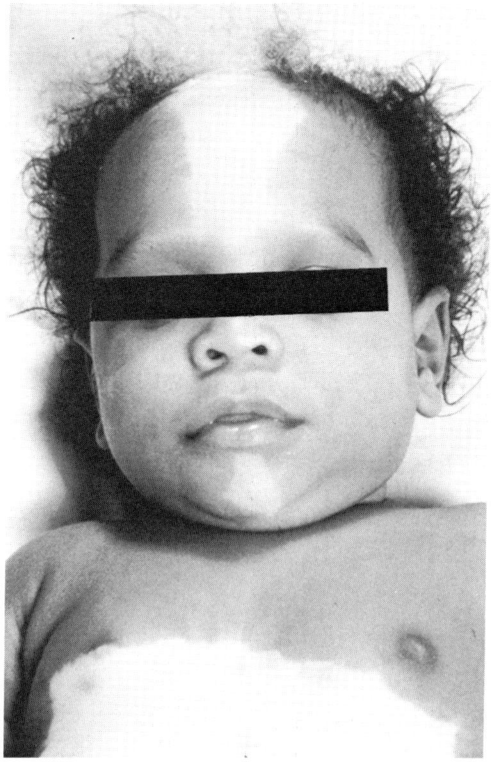

FIGURE 5–4
Piebaldism. White forelock with midfacial pigment loss on the forehead and chin. Another patch of depigmented skin with characteristic pigmented macules within the depigmented area is apparent on the torso.

Non-Skin

normal mental and physical development

Genetics

AD

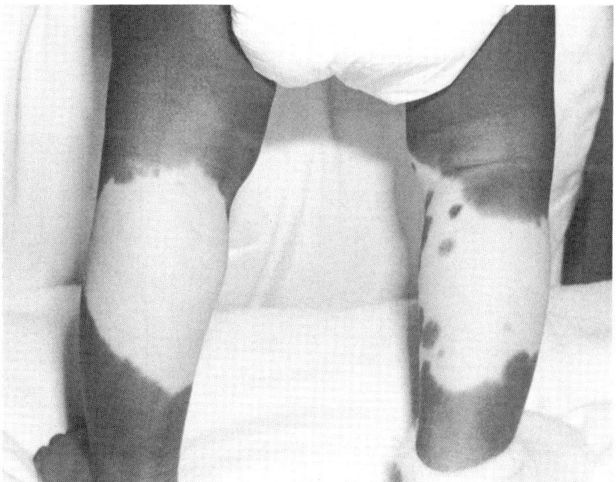

FIGURE 5–5
Lower legs of a child with piebaldism showing depigmented symmetrical patches within which are several normally pigmented macules.

Pathophysiology

mutations of the c-KIT (mast/stem cell growth factor receptor) proto-oncogene (mapped to chromosome 4q) are implicated in the molecular pathogenesis of human piebaldism

Laboratory Data

histopathology: absence of melanocytes in depigmented areas

Prognosis

depigmentation persists; general health is good

Discussion

about 10% of cases involve skin alone and do not include a white forelock

- *Vogt-Koyanagi-Harada syndrome:*

  leukoderma, poliosis, and alopecia

  meningeal signs, bilateral uveitis, and dysacousia or deafness

  acquired; believed to be postviral in etiology

REFERENCES

McK 172800

Barnes L. Vitiligo and the Vogt-Koyanagi-Harada syndrome. Dermatol Clin 1988;6:229–239

Fleischman RA, Saltman DL, Stastny V, Zneimer S. Deletion of the c-*kit* protooncogene in the human developmental defect piebald trait. J Natl Acad Sci USA 1991; 88(23):10885–10889

Hulten MA, Honeyman MM, Mayne AJ, et al. Homozygosity in piebald trait. J Med Genet 1987;24:568–571

Jimbow M, Jimbow K. Pigmentary disorders in oriental skin. Clin Dermatol 1989;7:11–27

Kaplan P, de Chaderevian JP. Piebaldism-Waardenburg syndrome: histopathologic evidence for a neural crest syndrome. Am J Med Genet 1988;31:679–688

Nordlund JJ, Albert D, Forget B, et al. Halo nevi and the Vogt-Koyanagi-Harada syndrome: manifestations of vitiligo. Arch Dermatol 1980;116:690–692

Ortonne JP. Piebaldism, Waardenburg's syndrome, and related disorders: "neural crest depigmentation syndromes"? Dermatol Clin 1988;6:205–216

Pierard GE, Franchimont C, Lapiere M. Six generations of piebaldism. Dermatologica 1979;158:184

Spritz RA, Holmes SA, Ramesar R, et al. Mutations of the KIT (mast/stem cell growth factor receptor) proto-oncogene account for a continuous range of phenotypes in human piebaldism. Am J Hum Genet 1992;51(5):1058–1065

Winship I, Young K, Martell R, et al. Piebaldism: an autonomous autosomal dominant entity. Clin Genet 1991;39:330–337

CONGENITAL POLIOSIS (CONGENITAL CANITIES)

white locks of hair, usually present at birth, sometimes delayed until puberty

central or lateral frontal scalp most commonly involved

AD

the equivalent of piebaldism confined to the hair; very rare

Froggatt P. An outline, with bibliography of human piebaldism and white forelock. Ir J Med Sci 1959;398:86–94

Ortonne J, Mosher DB, Fitzpatrick TB. Vitiligo and Other Hypomelanoses of Hair and Skin. New York, Plenum Medical Book Company, 1983:320–321

WAARDENBURG SYNDROME

Skin

midline white forelock with underlying depigmented skin; almost always present at birth

additionally, poliosis of scalp, eyebrows, and eyelashes as well as variably distributed hypopigmented cutaneous macules may appear

Non-Skin

bilateral (sometimes unilateral) hearing loss in about 25% of patients; severity varies

dystopia canthorum (lateral displacement of medial canthi); causes false appearance of convergent squint

broadened nasal root with hypertrichosis of medial portion of eyebrows, sometimes resulting in synophrys

depigmentation of the iris causes partial or total heterochromia iridis with blue replacing the normal color (Color Fig. 5–4); sometimes bilateral

depigmentation of ocular fundus parallel to that of the iris

lateral displacement of lower lacrimal puncta; superior puncta are normal

blepharophimosis

clefting of lip and/or palate and face; protuberant lower lip

possible higher incidence of Hirschsprung disease

Genetics

AD; gene mutation localized to chromosome 2q

Pathophysiology

melanocytes absent from depigmented skin

Discussion

some authors distinguish type I and type II of Waardenburg syndrome, in which the former shows dystopia canthorum while the latter does not but has a higher incidence of deafness

the white forelock may pigment early in life, only to later become prematurely gray or white

the cutaneous manifestations of Waardenburg syndrome are identical to piebaldism

REFERENCES

McK 193500
McK 193510
Mallory SB, Wiener E, Nordlund JJ. Waardenburg's syndrome with Hirschsprung's disease: a neural crest defect. Pediatr Dermatol 1986;3:119–124
Omenn GS, McKusick VA. The association of Waardenburg syndrome and Hirschsprung megacolon. Am J Med Genet 1979;3:217–223
Preus M, Linstrom C, Polomeno RC, et al. Waardenburg syndrome: penetrance of major signs. Am J Med Genet 1983; 15:383–388
Winship I, Beighton P. Phenotypic discriminants in the Waardenburg syndrome. Clin Genet 1992;41:181–188

KLEIN-WAARDENBURG SYNDROME

some consider this to be a distinct entity comprising the usual features of Waardenburg syndrome along with other features including bilateral upper limb anomalies and microcephaly

AD

McK 148820
Klein D. Historical background and evidence for dominant inheritance of the Klein-Waardenburg syndrome (type III). Am J Med Genet 1983;14:231–239
Sheffer R, Zlotogora J. Autosomal dominant inheritance of Klein-Waardenburg syndrome. Am J Med Genet 1992;42:320–322

WAARDENBURG-SHAW SYNDROME

white forelock, eyebrows and eyelashes; onset in infancy

isochromia iridis

Hirschsprung disease

AR, or possibly the same AD entity as Waardenburg syndrome with pleiotropic effects mimicking AR inheritance

McK 277580

Badner JA, Chakravarti A. Waardenburg syndrome and Hirschsprung disease: evidence for pleiotropic effects of a single dominant gene. Am J Med Genet 1990;35:100–104

Mallory SB, Wiener E, Nordlund JJ. Waardenburg's syndrome with Hirschsprung's disease: a neural crest defect. Pediatr Dermatol 1986;3:119–124

Shah KN, Dalal SJ, Desai MP, et al. White forelock pigmentary disorder of irides and long segment Hirschsprung disease: possible variant of Waardenburg syndrome. J Pediatr 1981;99:432–435

ZIPRKOWSKI-MARGOLIS SYNDROME (PARTIAL ALBINISM AND DEAFNESS)

depigmentation of skin and hair at birth with areas of hyperpigmentation, especially over sacrum

deaf-mutism

heterochromia iridis

XLR

melanocytes are present in biopsies of hypochromic skin

McK 300700

Margolis E. A new hereditary syndrome: sex-linked deaf-mutism associated with total albinism. Acta Genet Statist Med 1962; 12:12–19

Ortonne J, Mosher DB, Fitzpatrick TB. Vitiligo and Other Hypomelanoses of Hair and Skin. New York, Plenum Medical Book Company, 1983:373–374

Ziprkowski L, Krakowski A, Adam A, et al. Partial albinism and deaf-mutism due to a recessive sex-linked gene. Arch Dermatol 1962;86:530–539

WOOLF SYNDROME (PIEBALDISM WITH DEAFNESS)

generalized, large, irregular patches of hypopigmentation of skin

deaf mutism

blue irides

XLR

McKusick does not distinguish this entity from Ziprkowski-Margolis syndrome (see main entry)

McK 300700
Ortonne J, Mosher DB, Fitzpatrick TB. Vitiligo and Other Hypomelanoses of Hair and Skin. New York, Plenum Medical Book Company, 1983:369–372
Woolf CM, Dolowitz DA, Aldous HE. Congenital deafness associated with piebaldness. Arch Otolaryngol 1965;82:244–250

ROZYCKI SYNDROME

depigmented patches of skin

congenital deafness

short stature, muscle wasting, and achalasia

AR

McK 221350
Rozycki DL, Ruben RJ, Rapin I, Spiro AJ. Autosomal recessive deafness associated with short stature, vitiligo muscle wasting and achalasia. Arch Otolaryngol 1971;93:194–197

HYPERHIDROSIS, PREMATURE GRAYING OF THE HAIR, AND PREMOLAR HYPODONTIA (BÖÖK SYNDROME; PREMOLAR APLASIA, PALMOPLANTAR HYPERHIDROSIS, AND CANITIES PREMATURA SYNDROME)

premature graying of scalp hair in first three decades; similar graying of axillary and pubic hair, eyebrows, and cilia in about one third of patients

skin pigmentation normal

palmoplantar hyperhidrosis in about two thirds of patients

premolars are partially absent in half of patients and completely absent in the other half

AD

abnormalities persist but general health is good

McK 112300
Böök JA. Clinical and genetic studies of hypodontia: I. Premolar aplasia, hyperhidrosis, and canities prematura; a new hereditary syndrome in man. Am J Hum Genet 1950;2:240–263

Disorders of Hypopigmentation—Abbreviated Entries

PROGRESSIVE SPASTIC PARAPARESIS, VITILIGO, PREMATURE GRAYING, AND DISTINCT FACIAL APPEARANCE

widespread depigmented patches of skin

gray scalp or body hair

café-au-lait macules and lentigines on trunk and extremities

spastic paraparesis or paraplegia

craniofacial abnormalities

AR

other families have been described with features including localized or widespread areas of cutaneous hypo- or depigmentation, gray scalp and body hair, spastic paraparesis or paraplegia, and possible AR inheritance (McK 270750)

McK 270680

Abdallat A, Davis SM, Farrage J, McDonald WI. Disordered pigmentation, spastic paraparesis and peripheral neuropathy in three siblings: a new neurocutaneous syndrome. J Neurol Neurosurg Psychiatry 1980;43:92–96

Lison M, Kornbrut B, Feinstein A, et al. Progressive spastic paraparesis, vitiligo, premature graying and distinct facial appearance: a new genetic syndrome in three sibs. Am J Med Genet 1981;9:351–357

Mukamel M, Weitz R, Metzker A, Varsano I. Spastic paraparesis, mental retardation and cutaneous pigmentation disorder: a new syndrome. Am J Dis Child 1985;139:1090–1092

Stewart RM, Tunell G, Ehle A. Familial spastic paraplegia, peroneal neuropathy, and crural hypopigmentation: a new neurocutaneous syndrome. Neurology 1981;31:754–757

OSTEOPATHIA STRIATA WITH PIGMENTARY DERMOPATHY INCLUDING WHITE FORELOCK

probable XLD

McK 311280

Whyte MP, Murphy WA. Osteopathia striata associated with familial dermopathy and white forelock: evidence for postnatal development of osteopathia striata. Am J Med Genet 1980;5:227–234

PIEBALD TRAIT WITH NEUROLOGIC DEFECTS

piebaldism, cerebellar ataxia, mental retardation, and deafness

AD

McK 172850
Telfer MA, Sugar M, Jaeger EA, Mulcahy J. Dominant piebald trait (white forelock and leukoderma) with neurological impairment. Am J Hum Genet 1971;23:383–389

SYMMETRICAL ACROLEUKOPATHY

depigmentation of periungual skin in infancy or childhood

possible AD

McK 102000
Sugai T, Saito T, Hamada T. Symmetric acroleukopathy in mother and daughter. Arch Dermatol 1965;92:172–173

OCCIPITAL WHITE LOCK OF HAIR

X-linked recessive

McK 310900
Pearson KD, Nettleship E, Usher CH. A Monograph on Albinism in Man. Cambridge, Drapers Company Research Memoirs, 1911–1913;1:255

PREMATURE CANITIES

gray hair appearing in childhood; condition progressive so that entire scalp hair is gray by third or fourth decade

eyebrows and eyelashes retain dark pigment, but axillary and pubic hair tend to gray

complex etiology; simple form is AD

McK 139100
Hare HJH. Premature whitening of hair. J Hered 1929;20:31–32

CHAPTER

6

Disorders of Hyperpigmentation

Syndromes in which increased cutaneous pigmentation is either the primary or a major clinical feature are considered in this section. They are grouped as nearly as possible by type of hyperpigmentation (e.g., patterned versus diffuse). Some diseases in this chapter have cutaneous features that overlap considerably with those of the poikilodermatous disorders. Pigmentary disturbances are also seen in many disorders of premature aging in addition to various disorders discussed in many other chapters of the book.

INCONTINENTIA PIGMENTI

Synonyms

- Bloch-Sulzberger syndrome
- Bloch-Siemens syndrome

Skin

four patterns or stages of lesions are seen and typically, but not always, evolve one after the other; onset is at birth or within first weeks of life:

1. *Inflammatory stage:* tense vesicles or bullae, usually with erythema and often in linear distribution, predominantly on extremities (Fig. 6–1); occurs in first few weeks of life
2. *Verrucous stage:* linear verrucous plaques with or without antecedent bullae, predominantly on extremities, in second to sixth weeks of life or later (Fig. 6–2); bullous and hypertrophic stages usually last only a few months

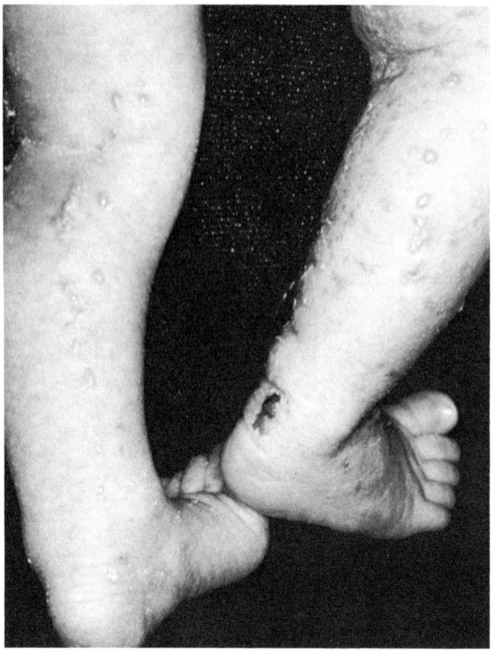

FIGURE 6–1
Vesicles in linear array on the legs of an infant with incontinentia pigmenti.

3. *Pigmentary stage:* reticulated, streaked, or whorled hyperpigmentation, most frequently manifesting during the third to sixth months of life (Fig. 6–3); hyperpigmentation follows lines of Blaschko and does not follow dermatomes or lines of skin cleavage; may cross midline; pigmentary stage lasts for years but may resolve
4. *Scarring stage:* hypopigmented scars devoid of hair and sweat glands, most apparent on legs

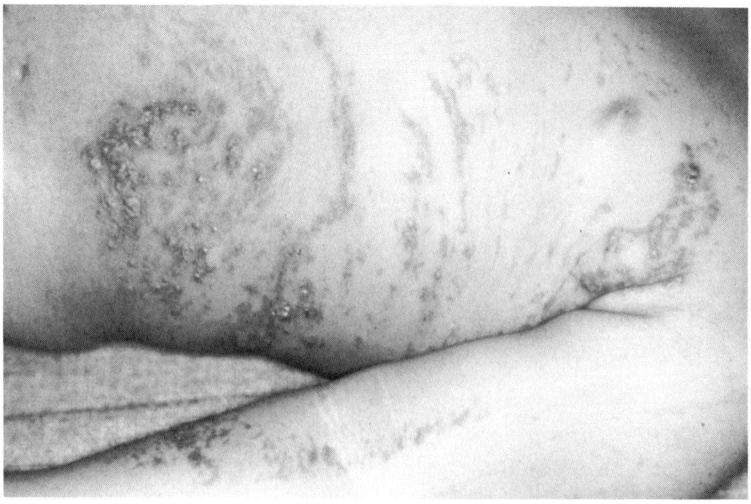

FIGURE 6–2
Whorled hyperpigmentation and warty lesions on the torso and arm of a girl with incontinentia pigmenti. (Courtesy of Benjamin K. Fisher, MD, Toronto, Ontario)

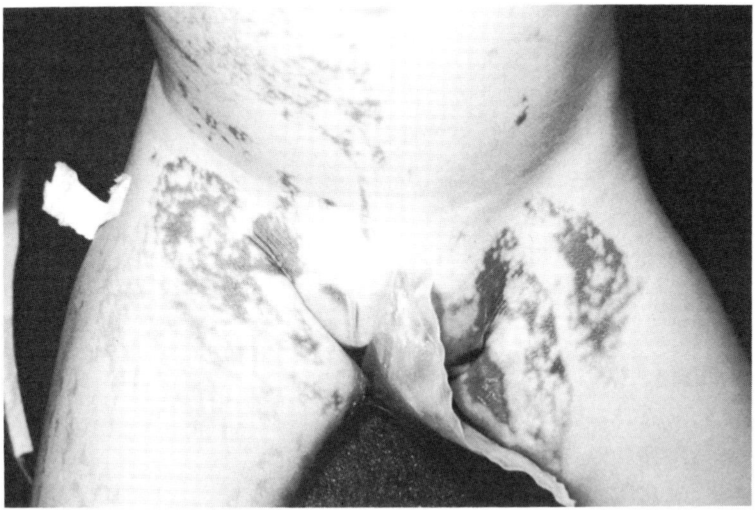

FIGURE 6–3
Extensive tan and dark brown reticulated hyperpigmented lesions on the torso and thighs of a girl with incontinentia pigmenti.

nail dystrophy in less than 10%; rare subungual keratotic tumors, usually developing in adolescence or adulthood and resolving spontaneously

occasional mild to severe alopecia

dental abnormalities in most, including anodontia, delayed eruption of deciduous teeth and peg-shaped teeth (Fig. 6–4)

Non-Skin

neurologic abnormalities in about one third of patients, including mental retardation, epilepsy, and hydrocephalus

ocular abnormalities in about 30% of patients include microphthalmos, strabismus, cataracts, optic atrophy, blindness, vascular abnormalities of retina, and a condition resembling retrolental fibroplasia

FIGURE 6–4
Partial anodontia and peg-shaped teeth in a girl with incontinentia pigmenti. This patient's mother was affected and also had anomalous dentition as well as sparse pigmentary lesions.

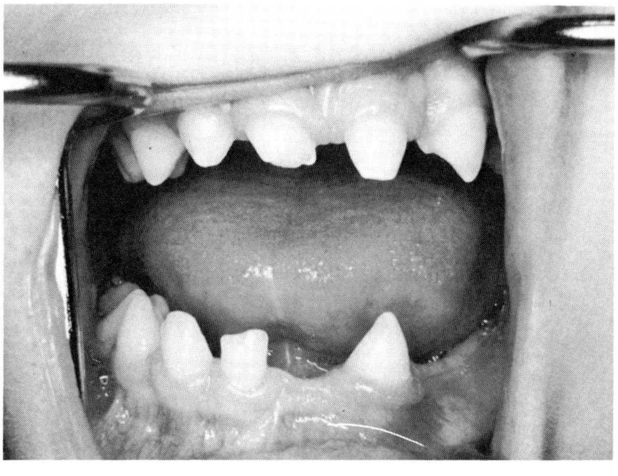

rarely, musculoskeletal and other developmental anomalies and microcephaly

Genetics

XLD

may be fatal in utero to males; affected males may represent new mutation in somatic cells (mosaicism)

male cases with Klinefelter syndrome (XXY) reported

Laboratory Data

histopathology:

inflammatory stage: epidermal and adnexal eosinophilic pustules with dyskeratosis

verrucous stage: epidermal acanthosis and necrotic keratinocytes; eosinophils may be seen in epidermis and dermal infiltrate

pigmentary stage: pigment incontinence is the typical histologic finding but may not be seen in older patients

scarred stage: fibrosis and lack of epidermal adnexa

leukocytosis and eosinophilia may occur in infancy

Prognosis

most patients have a normal life span; prognosis most related to degree of mental retardation, which is independent of skin involvement

Discussion

- *linear and whorled nevoid hypermelanosis:*

  asymmetrically distributed hyperpigmented whorls and streaks following Blaschko's lines

  resembles pigmentary stage of incontinentia pigmenti clinically but lacks pigment incontinence on histologic examination

  onset in first few weeks of life

  gradual progression during first 2 years of life, after which it stabilizes

  spares mucous membranes, palms, and soles

  not preceded by vesicular or hyperkeratotic lesions

  increased pigmentation of basal layer and possibly increased melanocytes

  many similar cases under different designations have been described

  sporadic

REFERENCES

McK 308300
Ashley JR, Burgdorf WHC. Incontinentia pigmenti: pigmentary changes independent of incontinence. J Cutan Pathol 1987;14:248–250
Carney RG Jr. Incontinentia pigmenti. Arch Dermatol 1976;112:535–542
Kalter DC, Griffiths WA, Atherton DJ. Linear and whorled nevoid hypermelanosis. J Acad Dermatol 1988;19:1037–1044
Mascaro JM, Palou J, Vives P. Painful subungual keratotic tumors in incontinentia pigmenti. J Am Acad Dermatol 1985;13:913–918
Moss C, Ince P. Anhidrotic and achromians lesions in incontinentia pigmenti. Br J Dermatol 1987;116:839–849
Pallotta R, Dalpra L. Chromosomal instability in incontinentia pigmenti: study of four families. Ann Genet 1988;31:27–31
Prendiville JS, Gorski JL, Stein CK, et al. Incontinentia pigmenti in a male infant with Klinefelter syndrome. J Am Acad Dermatol 1989;937–940
Rosenfeld SI, Smith ME. Ocular findings in incontinentia pigmenti. Ophthalmology 1985;92:543–546
Sefiani A, Abel S, Heuertz D, et al. The gene for incontinentia pigmenti is assigned to Xq28. Genomics 1989;4:427–429
Spallone A. Incontinentia pigmenti (Bloch-Sulzberger syndrome): seven case reports from one family. Br J Ophthalmol 1987;71:629–634

FRANCESCHETTI-JADASSOHN SYNDROME (NAEGELI SYNDROME)

reticulate gray to brown pigmentation of neck, upper trunk and limbs, especially flexures; onset in early childhood; no preceding inflammation or vesiculation

frequent punctate or diffuse palmoplantar keratoderma

hypohidrosis and poor heat tolerance (decreased number of eccrine sweat glands)

nail abnormalities include onycholysis and subungual hyperkeratosis

yellowish discoloration of tooth enamel

normal mental and physical development

AD; extremely rare

some have erroneously referred to this syndrome as "the male type of incontinentia pigmenti"

McK 161000
Person JR, Perry HO. Congenital poikiloderma with traumatic bulla formation, anhidrosis, and keratoderma. Acta Derm Venereol 1979;59:347–351
Sparrow GP, Samman PD, Wells RS. Hyperpigmentation and hypohidrosis. (The Naegeli-Franceschetti-Jadassohn syndrome): report of a family and review of the literature. Clin Exp Dermatol 1976;1:127–140

CARNEY SYNDROME

Synonyms

- spotty pigmentation, myxoma, endocrine overactivity syndrome
- NAME syndrome
- LAMB syndrome

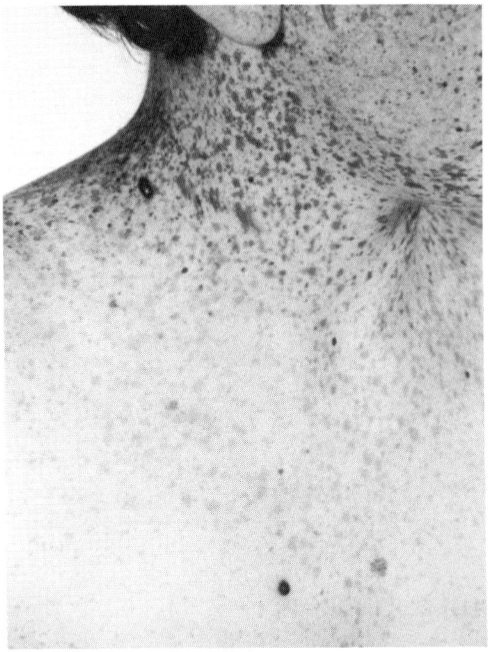

FIGURE 6–5
Carney syndrome. This patient has multiple lentigines, and at least two blue nevi are visible. (Courtesy of Dr. David Atherton, London, England; reprinted with permission from Atherton DJ, Pitcher DW, Wells RS, et al. A syndrome of various cutaneous pigmented lesions, myxoid neurofibromata and atrial myxoma: The NAME syndrome. Br J Dermatol 1980;103:421–429)

Skin

few to profuse mucocutaneous lentigines, ephelides, and blue nevi in over half of patients, mostly on the head and face, especially in the periocular and perinasal areas (Figs. 6–5 and 6–6)

lesions also noted on lips, conjunctivae, neck, trunk, distal extremities, and genitalia

onset from birth onward, usually before detection of cardiac myxomas

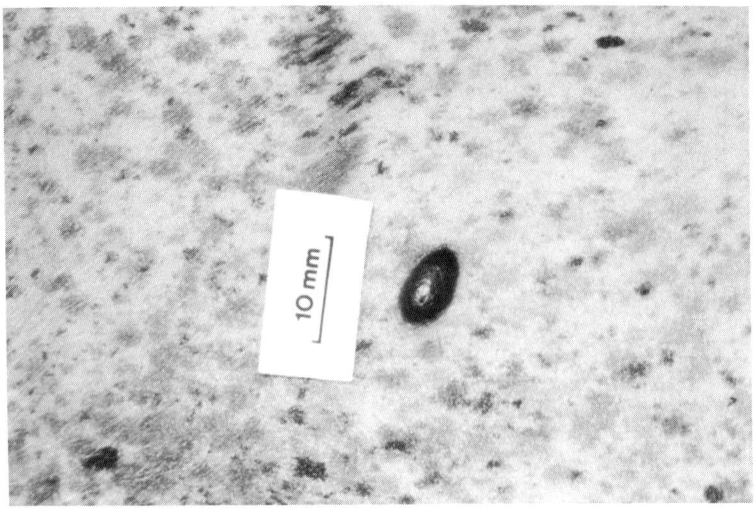

FIGURE 6–6
Carney syndrome. Close-up view of a large blue nevus as well as many lentigines. (Courtesy of Dr. David Atherton, London, England)

single or multiple papular or nodular flesh-colored cutaneous myxomas, usually less than 1 cm in diameter; myxomas most typically found on eyelids, ears, and nipples but may manifest anywhere, including mucosae

usual onset of cutaneous myxomas is in second decade but may be the only sign or the presenting sign of the disease

Non-Skin

cardiac myxomas in 75% of patients, detected from first through fifth decades; frequently multiple; may involve any chamber

myxoid fibroadenomas of the breast in about one fourth of patients

primary pigmented nodular adrenal hyperplasia, also known as ACTH-independent Cushing disease or antibody-mediated Cushing disease, found in almost half of patients; may cause Cushing syndrome, with onset usually in late first to early second decade; antibodies against adrenal ACTH receptors are thought to stimulate steroidogenesis

testicular tumors in about half of males, usually presenting in the second decade; characteristically bilateral; usually of the multicentric large cell calcifying Sertoli cell type

growth hormone–secreting pituitary tumors causing acromegaly or gigantism, with symptoms presenting in second or third decade

psammomatous melanotic schwannomas most commonly in peripheral nerve roots and gastrointestinal tract but also reported in skin

Genetics

AD

Prognosis

patients with two or more clinical features of the syndrome should have full evaluation, as should their first-degree relatives

Discussion

although listed as synonyms, the acronyms of NAME and LAMB do not always match the clinical findings in a particular patient, the disease being highly variable; therefore, the neutral designation of Carney syndrome is preferred

- *NAME syndrome:*

  an acronym for Nevi, Atrial myxoma, Myxoid tumors (neurofibromas), and Ephelides

- *LAMB syndrome:*

  an acronym for Lentigines, Atrial myxoma, Mucocutaneous myxoma (myxoid neurofibroma), and Blue nevi

REFERENCES

McK 160980

Atherton DJ, Pitcher DW, Wells RS, et al. A syndrome of various cutaneous pigmented lesions, myxoid neurofibromata and atrial myxoma: the NAME syndrome. Br J Dermatol 1980;103:421–429

Carney JA, Gordon H, Carpenter PC, et al. The complex of myxomas, spotty pigmentation, and endocrine overactivity. Medicine 1985;64:270–283

Carney JA, Headington JT, Su WP. Cutaneous myxomas: a major component of the complex of myxomas, spotty pigmentation, and endocrine overactivity. Arch Dermatol 1986;122:790–798

Carney JA. Psammomatous melanotic schwannoma: a distinctive, heritable tumor with special associations, including cardiac myxoma and the Cushing syndrome. Am J Surg Pathol 1990;14:206–222

Proppe KH, Scully RE. Large-cell calcifying Sertoli cell tumor of the testis. Am J Clin Pathol 1980;74:607–619

Rees JR, Ross FG, Keen G. Lentiginosis and left atrial myxoma. Br Heart J 1973; 35:874–876

Rhodes AR, Silverman RA, Harrist TJ, et al. Mucocutaneous lentigines, cardiomucocutaneous myxomas, and multiple blue nevi: the "LAMB" syndrome. J Am Acad Dermatol 1984;10:72–82

Utiger CA, Headington JT. Psammomatous melanotic schwannoma. Arch Dermatol 1993;129:202–204

Van Berkhout FT, Croughs RJM, Kater L, et al. Familial Cushing's syndrome due to nodular adrenocortical dysplasia: a putative receptor-antibody disease? Clin Endocrinol 1986;24:299–310

Young WF, Carney JA, Musa BU, et al. Familial Cushing's syndrome due to primary pigmented nodular adrenocortical disease: reinvestigation 50 years later. N Engl J Med 1989;321:1659–1678

FAMILIAL MULTIPLE BLUE NEVI

blue and blue-black nodules on face, trunk, extremities, and sclera from birth

AD

Blackford S, Roberts DL. Familial multiple blue naevi. Clin Exp Dermatol 1991; 16:308–309

MULTIPLE LENTIGINES SYNDROME

Synonyms

- LEOPARD syndrome
- progressive cardiomyopathic lentiginosis

Skin

lentigines, up to 5 mm in diameter, concentrated on neck and upper trunk; fewer on face, scalp, axillae, palms, soles, and genitalia (Figs. 6–7 and 6–8); other mucosae spared

appear at or shortly after birth; increase in number and pigmentation with age

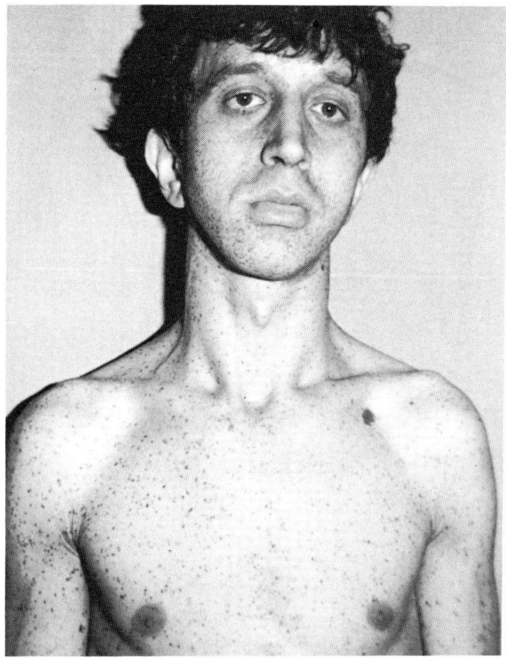

FIGURE 6–7
Multiple lentigines syndrome. Numerous lentigines scattered over the face, neck, torso, and arms. Note also the café-au-lait macule on the upper anterior left chest. (Courtesy of Benjamin K. Fisher, MD, Toronto, Ontario)

occasional café-au-lait macules

occasional koilonychia or white nails

Non-Skin

cardiac abnormalities include anatomic malformations (e.g., pulmonic stenosis) and conduction defects

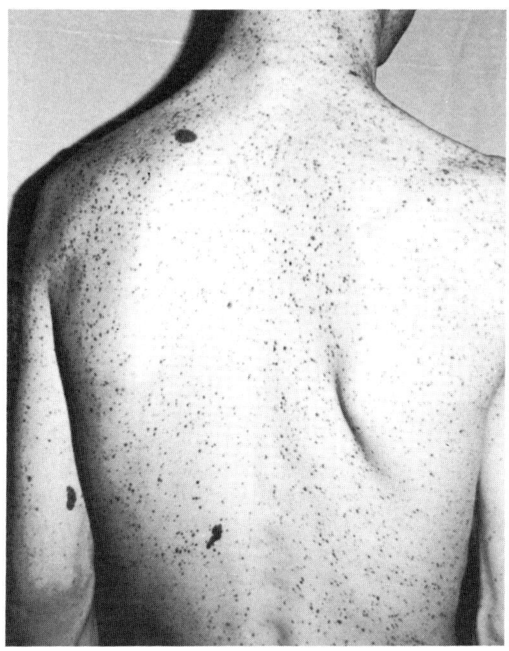

FIGURE 6–8
Multiple lentigines syndrome. Same patient as in Figure 6–7. A myriad of lentigines and three café-au-lait macules are seen. (Courtesy of Benjamin K. Fisher, MD, Toronto, Ontario)

retarded growth (below 25th percentile)

ocular hypertelorism

musculoskeletal abnormalities include pectus carinatum or excavatum and kyphoscoliosis

genitourinary abnormalities include cryptorchidism, gonadal hypoplasia, and hypospadias; delayed puberty is frequent

sensorineural deafness reported in about 25%, but true prevalence not known; onset usually in childhood but less commonly later on or rarely at birth

Genetics

AD

Laboratory Data

biopsy of pigmented cutaneous lesions is nondiagnostic, revealing lentigines or junctional melanocytic nevi

Prognosis

most patients lead normal lives, except those with symptomatic cardiac abnormalities, especially obstructive myopathy; surgery may be beneficial

Discussion

LEOPARD is an acronym for Lentigines, Electrocardiographic abnormalities, Ocular hypertelorism, Pulmonic stenosis, Abnormal genitalia, Retarded growth, and Deafness

markedly variable expressivity; few patients have all features of the syndrome, and some even lack lentigines

acquired lentiginosis may be seen in generalized, unilateral, centrofacial, and periorificial distributions

Moynahan syndrome is probably the same as multiple lentigines syndrome; emphasis on early appearance of pigmented macules

REFERENCES

McK 151100

Capute AJ, Rimoin DL, Konigsmark BW, et al. Congenital deafness and multiple lentigines. Arch Dermatol 1969;100:207–213

Gorlin RJ, Anderson RC, Blaw ME. Multiple lentigines syndrome. Am J Dis Child 1969;117:652–662

Moynahan EJ. Progressive cardiomyopathic lentiginosis: first report of autopsy findings in a recently recognized inheritable disorder (autosomal dominant). Proc R Soc Med 1970;63:448–451

Polani PE, Moynahan EJ. Progressive cardiomyopathic lentiginosis. Q J Med 1972; 41:205–225

Selmanowitz VJ, Orentreich N, Felsenstein

JM. Lentiginosis profusa syndrome (multiple lentigines syndrome). Arch Dermatol 1971;104:393–401
Seuanez H, Mane-Garzon F, Kolski R. Cardio-cutaneous syndrome (the "LEOPARD" syndrome): review of the literature and a new family. Clin Genet 1976;9:266–276
St. John Sutton MG, Tajik AJ, Giuliani ER, et al. Hypertrophic obstructive cardiomyopathy and lentiginosis: a little known neural ectodermal syndrome. Am J Cardiol 1981;47:214–217
Voron DA, Hatfield HH, Kalkhoff RK. Multiple lentigines syndrome: case report and review of the literature. Am J Med 1976;60:447–456

TOURAINE CENTROFACIAL LENTIGINOSIS

pigmented macules on malar areas and nose ("butterfly" distribution) and occasionally on forehead, eyelids, and upper lip

lesions appear in infancy and regress after first decade

mucosa spared

frequent central nervous system abnormalities, including oligophrenia and emotional instability

musculoskeletal abnormalities due to midline fusion defects (dysraphism) include high forehead, pectus excavatum, kyphosis, spina bifida, and umbilical herniae

AD; possible AR

McK 151000
Dociu I, Galaction-Nitelea O, Sirjita N, et al. Centrofacial lentiginosis. Br J Dermatol 1976;94:39–43
Touraine A. Lentiginose centro-faciale et dysplasies associées. Bull Soc Fr Derm Syph 1941;48:518–521

INHERITED PATTERNED LENTIGINOSIS IN BLACKS

numerous pigmented macules on face and lips (but not on oral mucosa) and, less frequently, on buttocks and extremities (Fig. 6–9)

onset in infancy or early childhood; lesions persist

no systemic abnormalities

AD

seen in light-skinned blacks, especially those with reddish brown hair

extremely common, regarded as normal in most instances

McK 151001
O'Neill JF, James WD. Inherited patterned lentiginosis in blacks. [Review]. Arch Dermatol 1989;125:1231–1235

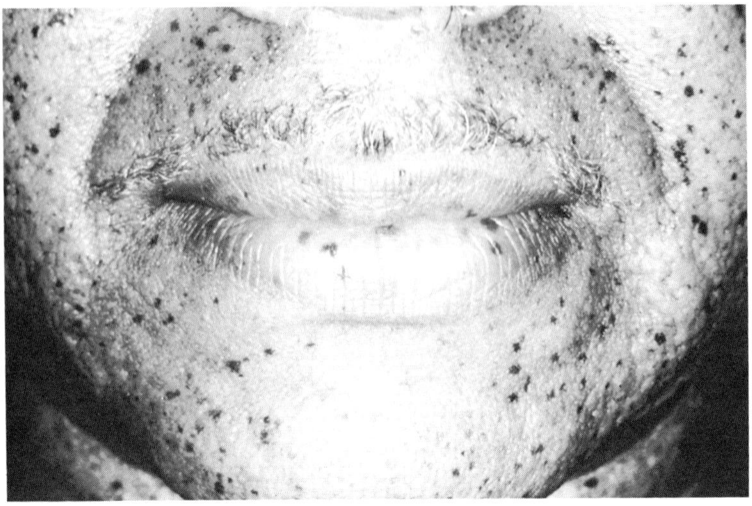

FIGURE 6–9
Inherited patterned lentiginosis in blacks. Young black man has numerous well-defined brown macules across the face. (Courtesy of William D. James, MD, Washington, DC)

PEUTZ-JEGHERS SYNDROME

Synonym

- generalized intestinal polyposis type II

Skin

brown macules and patches (1 to 12 mm), most frequently on the lips and buccal mucosa, less commonly on the gingiva and hard palate, and rarely on the tongue (Figs. 6–10 and 6–11)

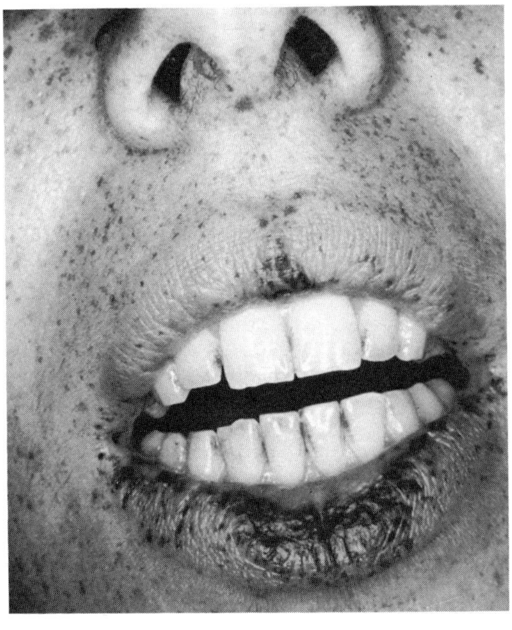

FIGURE 6–10
Peutz-Jeghers syndrome. Numerous hyperpigmented macules of the facial skin and oral mucosae, especially the lower lip. (Courtesy of Benjamin K. Fisher, MD, Toronto, Ontario)

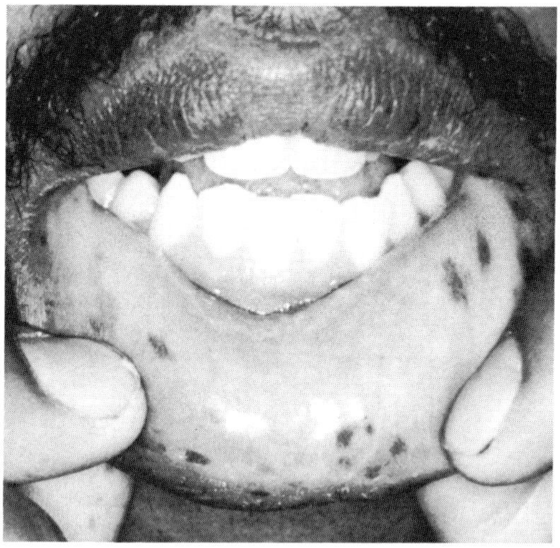

FIGURE 6–11
Pigmented macules on the oral vestibular mucosa of a black patient with Peutz-Jeghers syndrome.

onset may be at birth, but usually during infancy or childhood

nasal, genital, and rectal mucosae rarely involved

brown macules less than 1 mm on face, especially around mouth and nose, sometimes around eyes

brown, 1- to 3-mm macules are found on the volar surfaces of fingers and toes, rarely on hands and feet

cutaneous pigmentation tends to fade after puberty, but intraoral pigmentation persists

brown discoloration of nails

Non-Skin

polyps throughout entire gastrointestinal tract, but especially jejunum and ileum; also seen in nasopharynx, bronchi, urethra, bladder, ureters, and cervix

polyps usually hamartomatous, especially in small intestine

increased gastrointestinal carcinomas mainly of the colon and stomach; however, these generally arise from adenomatous rather than hamartomatous polyps

nongastrointestinal, benign and malignant neoplasms include multiple myeloma, ovarian and testicular tumors, and adenocarcinoma of the pancreas (100-fold increase over the general population reported), breast, and lung

although overall incidence of gastrointestinal and nongastrointestinal carcinoma reported as high as 48% (study by Giardello and colleagues [1987]), incidence of gastrointestinal carcinoma usually quoted at 2% to 3%

Genetics

AD

Laboratory Data

histopathology: increased epidermal melanin but normal number of melanocytes

occasional blood in stool and hypochromic anemia

Prognosis

intestinal symptoms and sequelae are frequent, especially recurrent intussusception, at any time but usually in second or third decade

Discussion

rarely, some family members have gastrointestinal polyposis without pigmentary abnormalities

two acquired conditions that may overlap clinically with Peutz-Jeghers syndrome are described below:

- *Cronkhite-Canada syndrome:*

  nail dystrophy and alopecia

  hyperpigmented macules of the face, upper and lower extremities, palms and soles; mucosa usually not involved

  gastrointestinal signs and symptoms include pain, diarrhea, hemorrhage, and broad-based inflammatory polyps of the stomach (most commonly) and small and large intestine

  most patients are older than 50 years of age at onset

  cutaneous findings usually follow the appearance of gastrointestinal symptoms and are important in diagnosis

  acquired

  McK 175500

- *Laugier-Hunziker syndrome:*

  hyperpigmented macules of the oral mucosa and lips

  longitudinal hyperpigmented streaks of nails

  onset in adulthood

  no gastrointestinal polyposis or other systemic findings

  acquired

REFERENCES

McK 175200

Baran R, Barriere H. Longitudinal melanonychia with spreading pigmentation in Laugier-Hunziker syndrome: a report of two cases. Br J Dermatol 1986;115:707–710

Burdick D, Prior JT. Peutz-Jeghers syndrome: a clinicopathologic study of a large family with a 27-year follow-up. Cancer 1982; 50:2139–2146

Burke AP, Sobin LH. The pathology of Cronkhite-Canada polyps: a comparison to juvenile polyposis. Am J Surg Pathol 1989;13:940–946

Daniel ES, Ludwig SL, Lewin KJ, et al. The

Cronkhite-Canada syndrome: an analysis of clinical and pathologic features and therapy in 55 patients. Medicine 1982; 61:293–309
Giardiello FM, Welsh SB, Hamilton SR, et al. Increased risk of cancer in the Peutz-Jeghers syndrome. N Engl J Med 1987; 316:1511–1514
Koch SE, LeBoit PE, Odom RB. Laugier-Hunziker syndrome. J Am Acad Dermatol 1987;16:431–434
Laugier P, Hunziker N. Pigmentation mélanique lenticulaire, essentielle, de la muqueuse jugale et des lévres. Arch Belg Dermatol Syphiligr 1970;26:391–399
McAllister AJ, Richards KF. Peutz-Jeghers syndrome: experience with twenty patients in five generations. Am J Surg 1977; 134:717–720
Nonomura A, Ohta G, Ibata T, et al. Cronkhite-Canada syndrome associated with sigmoid cancer: case report and review of 54 cases with the syndrome. Acta Pathol Jpn 1980;30:825–845

CANTU SYNDROME

pigmented macules of face, forehead, arms, and feet; onset in adolescence

palmoplantar hyperkeratosis

AD

McK 114620
Cantu JM, Sanchez-Corona J, Fragoso R, et al. A "new" autosomal dominant genodermatosis characterized by hyperpigmented spots and palmoplantar hyperkeratosis. Clin Genet 1978;14:165–168

McCUNE-ALBRIGHT POLYOSTOTIC FIBROUS DYSPLASIA

Synonyms

- McCune-Albright syndrome
- Albright syndrome

Skin

large brown patches, often with irregular, jagged borders; most commonly on trunk and extremities, but also on scalp, neck, and buttocks (Fig. 6–12); rarely, oral mucosa involved

onset usually in infancy or early childhood, occasionally at birth

pigmentation may follow lines of Blaschko and is often segmentally or linearly arranged in same distribution as osseous lesions

Non-Skin

bones affected with areas of patchy rarefaction, most frequently involving long bones of the lower limbs; the pelvis, clavicles, upper extremities, and bones of the hands and feet are also involved; enlargement of

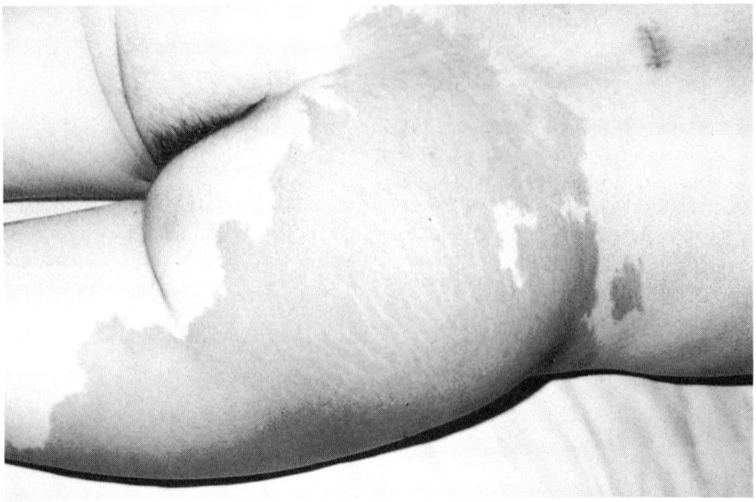

FIGURE 6–12
Sharply demarcated unilateral café-au-lait spot with irregular border involving the flank, buttock, and upper thigh in a patient with McCune-Albright syndrome. (Courtesy of Benjamin K. Fisher, MD, Toronto, Ontario)

bony pseudocysts stops after skeletal growth ceases; pathologic fractures are common in childhood

rarely, skull is involved, which may result in facial disfigurement, visual disturbances, hearing loss, and proptosis

skeletal features always present; may occur with or without skin or endocrine disease

rare fibrosarcomatous degeneration of bone lesions

endocrine abnormalities are multiple and due to autonomous function of endocrine glands

sexual precocity often, mostly in females (half are affected); may show abnormal vaginal bleeding as early as infancy; normal menstruation and fertility occur at usual time of puberty

other endocrinologic abnormalities include hyperthyroidism, hyperparathyroidism, hyperprolactinemia, hypersomatotropism, hypophosphatemia, and Cushing syndrome

Genetics

mostly sporadic; few familial cases reported

may be due to a lethal AD gene surviving in a mosaic state by somatic mutation; the distribution of skin and bone lesions along lines of Blaschko supports this theory

"sex-influenced autosomal dominant" inheritance has been postulated to explain mild disease expression in many affected males

Laboratory Data

histopathology: cutaneous macules show increased epidermal melanin

electron microscopy of skin: rarely, giant melanin macroglobules are present

histopathology of bone: poorly differentiated fibrous tissue with interspersed bony trabeculae

alkaline phosphatase level elevated in about one third of patients

Prognosis

life expectancy usually normal; however, those with severe disease early in life may have poorer prognosis

pathologic fractures may cause deformities or limb-length discrepancy

sexual precocity may be treatable with aromatase inhibitors (inhibit estrogen synthesis)

Discussion

although café-au-lait macules with a "coast of Maine" border are reputed to be characteristic of this disorder, this finding is not reliable; in general, the macules are larger, are less numerous, and tend to be linear or segmental as compared with those of neurofibromatosis, but the lesions may be indistinguishable

the incidence of simple polyostotic fibrous dysplasia is 30 to 40 times more common than the full syndrome (skin, bone, and endocrinologic abnormalities); additionally, bone and endocrine findings can occur in the absence of cutaneous lesions

if cutaneous lesions are absent, the syndrome is often not recognized until pathologic fractures occur

skin findings and bony cysts differentiate from other causes of precocious puberty

do not confuse with Albright hereditary osteodystrophy; they have the same eponym and both have endocrine and bone abnormalities; see main entry

REFERENCES

McK 174800

Albright F, Butler AM, Hampton AO, et al. Syndrome characterized by osteitis fibrosa disseminata, areas of pigmentation and endocrine dysfunction, with precocious puberty in females. N Engl J Med 1937;216:727–746

D'Armiento M, Reda G, Camagna A, Tardella L. McCune-Albright syndrome: evidence for autonomous multiendocrine hyperfunction. J Pediatr 1983;102:584–586

Happle R. Lethal genes surviving by mosaicism: a possible explanation for sporadic birth defects involving the skin. J Am Acad Dermatol 1987;16:899–906

Lee PA, Van Dop C, Migeon CJ. McCune-Albright syndrome: long-term follow-up. JAMA 1986;256:2980–2984

Mauras N, Blizzard AM. The McCune-Albright syndrome. Acta Endocrinol Suppl 1986; 279:207–217

Roth JG, Esterly NB. McCune-Albright syn-

drome with multiple bilateral café au lait spots. Pediatr Dermatol 1991;8:35–39
Rustin MH, Bunker CB, Gilkes JJ, et al. Polyostotic fibrous dysplasia associated with extensive linear epidermal naevi. Clin Exp Dermatol 1989;14:371–375

SILVER-RUSSELL SYNDROME (RUSSELL-SILVER SYNDROME)

café-au-lait macules in about 25%

short stature and low birth weight

skeletal asymmetry

small, incurved fifth finger

triangular facies

blue sclerae

abnormal sexual development

mostly sporadic; some familial cases reported

McK 270050
Duncan PA, Hall JG, Shapiro LR, Vibert BK. Three-generation dominant transmission of the Silver-Russell syndrome. Am J Med Genet 1990;35:245–250
Fuleihan DS, Der Kaloustian VM, Najjar SS. The Russell-Silver syndrome: report of three siblings. J Pediatr 1971;78:654–657

RETICULAR PIGMENTED ANOMALY OF THE FLEXURES (DOWLING-DEGOS DISEASE)

asymptomatic, symmetrical 2- to 5-mm brown macules, tending to become confluent in a reticular pattern, initially involving the flexures, inner thighs, groins, and genitalia; onset most frequent in the fourth decade

later, intergluteal and inframammary folds, neck, trunk, and arms may be involved

mucous membranes are not affected

mostly sporadic; AD cases reported

histopathology: lacy downward epithelial proliferations similar to some seborrheic keratoses; normal number of melanocytes

worsens with age

the nosology of Dowling-Degos disease is confusing; Kitamura's reticulate acropigmentation and Haber syndromes (see later) show some overlap in findings, especially histopathologically

Berth-Jones J, Graham-Brown RA. A family with Dowling-Degos disease showing features of Kitamura's reticulate acropigmentation. Br J Dermatol 1989;120:463–466
Brown WG. Reticulate pigmented anomaly of the flexures. Arch Dermatol 1982;118:490–493
Crovato F, Desirello G, Rebora A. Is Dowling-Degos disease the same disease as Kitamura's reticulate acropigmentation? Br J Dermatol 1983;109:105–110
Crovato F, Nazzari G, Rebora A. Dowling-Degos disease (reticulate pigmented anomaly of the flexures) is an autosomal dominant condition. Br J Dermatol 1983;108:473–476
Degos R, Ossipowski B. Dermatose pigmentaire reticulée des plis. Ann Dermatol Syphilol 1954;81:147–151
Rebora A, Crovato F. The spectrum of Dowling-Degos disease. Br J Dermatol 1984;110:627–630
Smith EL, Dowling GB, Wilson Jones E. Acquired axillary and inguinal pigmentation: an epidermal naevoid abnormality not to be confused with acanthosis nigricans. Br J Dermatol 1971;85:295–296
Wilson-Jones E, Grice K. Reticulate pigmented anomaly of the flexures. Arch Dermatol 1978;114:1150–1157

HABER SYNDROME

rosacea-like eruption of face, worse after sun exposure; onset in childhood; papules, pustules, scarring, and telangiectasia may follow erythema

reticulate keratotic plaques on trunks and limbs; onset following childhood

AD

histopathology: rosacea-like eruption reveals sebaceous hyperplasia and basaloid tumor islands that may mimic basal cell carcinoma; reticulate plaques show findings identical to those in Dowling-Degos disease

Binet O, Audefray D, Beltzer-Garelly E, Gauchy O, Cesarini JP. Le syndrome de Haber. Ann Dermatol Venereol 1986;113:43–50
Kikuchi I, Inoue S, Narita H, et al. The broad spectrum of Dowling-Degos disease, including Haber syndrome—a hereditary abnormal reactivity to stimulation, increasing with age? Case reports and management. J Dermatol 1983;10:361–375
Seiji M, Otaki N. Haber's syndrome: familial rosacea-like dermatosis with keratotic plaques and pitted scars. Arch Dermatol 1971;103:452–455

RETICULATE ACROPIGMENTATION OF KITAMURA

brown, slightly depressed macules up to 1 cm in size, arranged in a reticulated pattern on extensor hands and feet; onset in first or second decade

lesions gradually extend onto arms, legs, neck, lower face, eyelids, and upper trunk

pitting of the palms, described as "sloping," interrupts the normal dermatoglyphics; sometimes also involves volar fingers

mostly sporadic; AD cases also reported

Bajaj AK, Gupta SC. Reticulate acropigmentation of Kitamura: a report of two families. Dermatologica 1984;168:247–9
Crovato F, Rebora A. Reticulate pigmented anomaly of the flexures associating reticulate acropigmentation: one single entity. J Am Acad Dermatol 1986;14:359–361
Mizoguchi M, Kukita A. Behavior of melanocytes in reticulate acropigmentation of Kitamura. Arch Dermatol 1985;121:659–661
Sharma R, Sharma SC, Radotra BD, et al. Reticulate acropigmentation of Kitamura. Clin Exp Dermatol 1989;14:302–303
Woodley DT, Caro I, Wheeler CE Jr. Reticulate acropigmentation of Kitamura. Arch Dermatol 1979;115:760–761

Disorders of Hyperpigmentation—Abbreviated Entries

DYSCHROMATOSIS UNIVERSALIS HEREDITARIA

light to dark brown macules of variable shape separated by depigmented macules; may be widespread, sparing only palms and soles

begins in infancy or early childhood and stabilizes with age

no photosensitivity or atrophy

possible AD

occurs in Japanese

in infancy and childhood may resemble xeroderma pigmentosum; DNA repair studies may be needed to distinguish these entities

McK 127400

Hata S, Yokomi I. Density of dopa-positive melanocytes in dyschromatosis symmetrica hereditaria. Dermatologica 1985;171:27–29

DYSCHROMATOSIS SYMMETRICA HEREDITARIA (LEUKOPATHIA PUNCTATA ET RETICULARIS; ACROPIGMENTATIO SYMMETRICA)

localized form of dyschromatosis affecting face and acral areas

possible AD

possible variant of dyschromatosis universalis hereditaria

McK 127500

Satoh Y, Yoshida M. Clinical and photobiological differences between dyschromatosis symmetrica hereditaria and xeroderma pigmentosum. J Dermatol 1980;7:317–322
Suenaga M. Dyschromatosis universalis hereditaria in 5 generations. Tohoku J Exp Med 1952;55:373–376

HEREDITARY UNIVERSAL MELANOSIS (MELANOSIS UNIVERSALIS HEREDITARIA)

case reports of different patterns of hyperpigmentation are described, including diffuse, reticular, or confluent macules and patches

scattered hypopigmented macules occur within areas of hyperpigmentation

variable mucosal involvement

onset in infancy or early childhood

AD and possible AR cases reported

may be the same as cases of dyschromatosis reported in Japan

McK 155800

Leber R. Ueber eine Familie mit erblichem universellem Melanismus. Z Kinderheilkd 1936;58:142–147

Orth H. Ueber zwei Faelle von erblichem Melanismus. Arch Dermatol Syphilol 1929;158:95–97

Pegum JS. Diffuse pigmentation in brothers. Proc R Soc Med 1955;48:179–180

Wende GW, Bauckus HH. A hitherto undescribed generalized pigmentation of the skin appearing in infancy in brother and sister. J Cutan Dis 1919;37:685–701

SYMMETRICAL ACROPIGMENTATION OF DOHI

mottled patches of hyperpigmentation with areas of depigmentation on dorsa of hands and feet and occasionally elsewhere on limbs

onset in infancy or early childhood

probable AD

appears mostly in Japan

Bleehen SS, Ebling FJG, Champion RH. Disorders of skin colour. In: Champion RH, Burton JL, Ebling FJG, eds. Textbook of Dermatology. Oxford, Blackwell Scientific Publications, 1992:1561–1622

DERMATOPATHIA PIGMENTOSA RETICULARIS

macular hyperpigmentation, mostly of trunk, starting in infancy and becoming reticular

other reported findings include acral bullae, palmar keratoses with subsequent ainhum-like constrictions, nail hypoplasia, absent dermatoglyphics, and alopecia

inheritance unclear; AD cases reported

Heimer WL II, Brauner G, James WD. Dermatopathia pigmentosa reticularis: a report of a family demonstrating autosomal dominant inheritance. J Am Acad Dermatol 1992;26:298–301
Maso MJ, Schwartz RA, Lambert WC. Dermatopathia pigmentosa reticularis. Arch Dermatol 1990;126:935–939
van der Lugt L. Dermatopathia pigmentosa reticularis hyperkeratotica et mutilans. Dermatologica 1970;140:294–302

FAMILIAL PROGRESSIVE HYPERPIGMENTATION

widespread hyperpigmented macules and patches of both skin and mucous membranes

onset at birth or in early infancy

lesions increase in size and number with age but stabilize after puberty

probable AD

no pigment incontinence in skin biopsy specimens of hypopigmented lesions

clinical findings, inheritance pattern, and lack of pigment incontinence on histopathology help distinguish this disease from incontinentia pigmenti

McK 145250
Chernosky ME, Anderson DE, Change JP, et al. Familial progressive hyperpigmentation. Arch Dermatol 1971;103:581–591
Debao L, Ting L. Familial progressive hyperpigmentation: a family study in China. Br J Dermatol 1991;125:607

UNIVERSAL ACQUIRED MELANOSIS (CARBON BABY)

inheritance unclear; possible AR

Rebora A, Parodi A. Universal inherited melanodyschromatosis: a case of melanosis universalis hereditaria? [Letter]. Arch Dermatol 1989;125:1442–1443
Ruiz-Maldonado R, Tamayo L, Fernández-Diez J. Universal acquired melanosis. Arch Dermatol 1978;114:775–778

FAMILIAL PERIORBITAL HYPERPIGMENTATION

variable hyperpigmentation that may begin below lower eyelids; onset in early childhood

with age, spreads to upper eyelids and entire periorbital region

AD

histopathology: increased epidermal melanin; melanophages in dermis

McK 145100
Goodman RM, Belcher RW. Periorbital hyperpigmentation: an overlooked genetic disorder of pigmentation. Arch Dermatol 1969;100:169–174

FAMILIAL MELANOPATHY WITH GIGANTIC MELANOCYTES

diffuse brown hyperpigmentation of face, trunk and extremities; guttate hypopigmented macules within areas of hyperpigmentation

fair-colored scalp, eyebrow, and body hair

no endocrinologic abnormalities or mental retardation

AD

histopathology: increased numbers of enlarged, hypermelanotic melanocytes in basal layer of the epidermis and melanophages in papillary dermis; abnormal transfer of melanin to keratinocytes is postulated

no increase in incidence of malignant melanoma

El Darouti MA. Familial melanopathy with gigantic melanocytes. Am J Dermatopathol (Suppl) 1984;6:31–34

UNIVERSAL DYSCHROMATOSIS, SMALL STATURE, AND HIGH-TONE DEAFNESS

possible AR

Rycroft RJG, Calnan CD, Wells RS. Universal dyschromatosis, small stature and high-tone deafness. Clin Exp Dermatol 1977;2:45–48

FAMILIAL TRANSVERSE NASAL HYPERPIGMENTATION

AD

McK 161530

Pierce ER, Teneyck FD. Hereditary hyperpigmentation anomalies in blacks. J Hered 1974;65:157–159

CHAPTER 7

Tumors and Proliferative Disorders

The heritable cutaneous tumors include true neoplasias, hyperplasias, and various nevi. Multiple cutaneous tumors generally are inherited in an autosomal dominant fashion; however, each of these tumors may be seen more commonly as a solitary sporadic occurrence. In some of the syndromes, tumors in organs other than the skin represent a more serious aspect of the disorder but the cutaneous tumors may serve as markers to permit early indentification of affected individuals.

REFERENCE

Burgdorf WHC, Koester G. Multiple cutaneous tumors: what do they mean? J Cutan Pathol 1992;19:449–457

NEVOID BASAL CELL CARCINOMA SYNDROME

Synonyms

- basal cell nevus syndrome
- BCNS
- Gorlin syndrome
- Gorlin-Goltz syndrome

Skin

typically smooth, skin-colored or reddish brown papules (Figs. 7–1 and 7–2); may resemble melanocytic nevi or skin tags but are basal cell

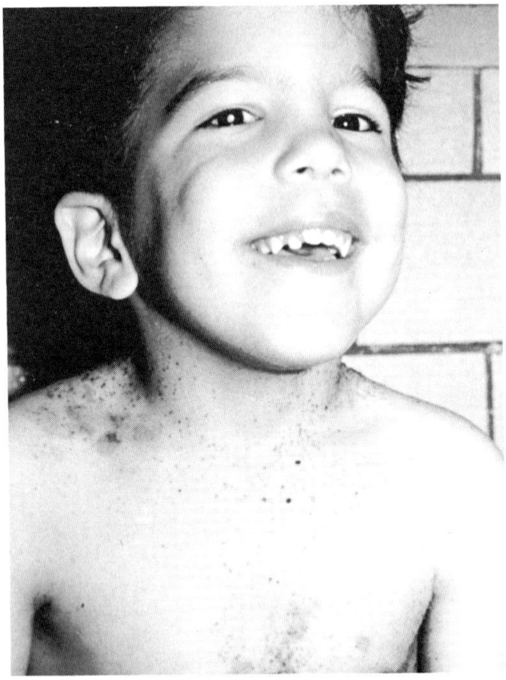

FIGURE 7–1
Nevoid basal cell carcinoma syndrome. A young child has some frontal bossing, but the striking findings are the hundreds of tiny brown papules on the neck and chest. They look like skin tags, but all are basal cell carcinomas.

carcinomas histologically; most frequently occur on face, neck, and upper trunk but may occur on virtually any cutaneous site; lesions grow and may evolve into more typical telangiectatic or ulcerated tumors

tumors appear most often in second to fourth decades but may occur much earlier or later

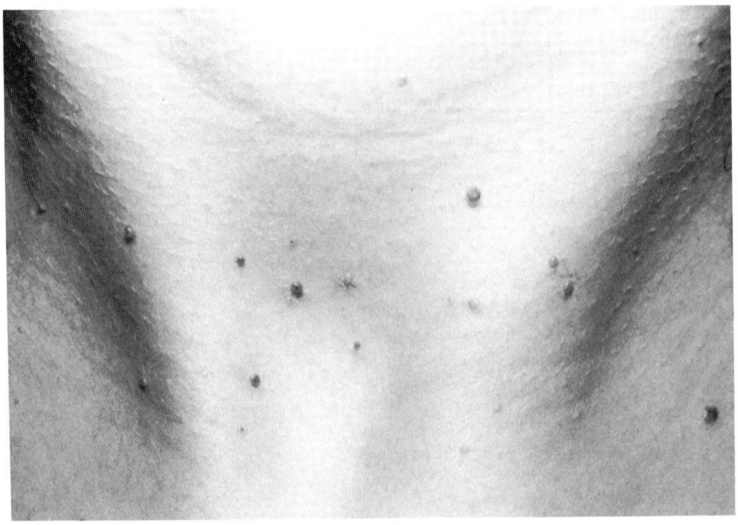

FIGURE 7–2
Multiple skin-colored and hyperpigmented papules on the neck of a child with nevoid basal cell carcinoma syndrome.

basal cell carcinomas may be present at birth or not until middle age; typically increase in number at puberty and become more invasive but only rarely metastasize

destructiveness and invasiveness of the carcinomas are variable, but they have a predilection for the eyelids and periorbital areas; severe complications include direct central nervous system invasion (e.g., facial nerve)

palmar and plantar pits in over half of patients (Fig. 7–3)

milia on face and epidermoid cysts on trunk and extremities common; acral (especially digital) epidermoid cysts characteristic (Fig. 7–4)

occasional café-au-lait macules

Non-Skin

early signs including medulloblastoma, congenital cataracts, congenital hydrocephalus, and maxillary and mandibular cysts may occur before cutaneous findings

odontogenic keratocysts of jaw in 65% to 75% of patients; more likely to be mandibular and bilateral than maxillary or unilateral

these cysts often occur in first decade of life, frequently before skin tumors appear; often are symptomatic (e.g., displacing teeth); recurrences following removal are common

ovarian (75%) and uterine fibromas, as well as other anomalies of the male and female reproductive system, including hypogonadism in males and calcified ovarian cysts in females

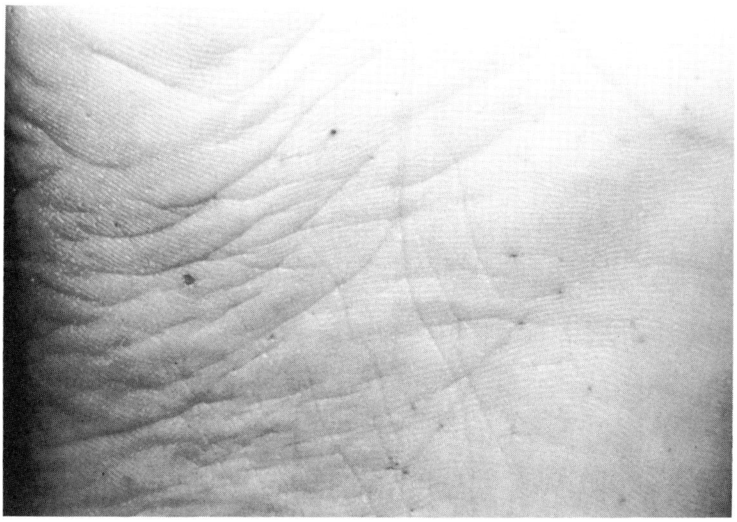

FIGURE 7–3
Multiple plantar pits on the sole of a child with nevoid basal cell carcinoma syndrome.

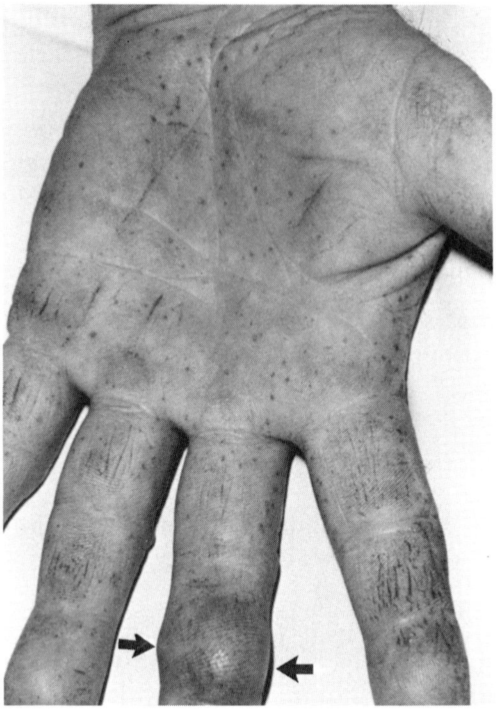

FIGURE 7–4
This palm of an adult with nevoid basal cell carcinoma syndrome shows characteristic acral or digital epidermoid cysts *(arrows)* and pitting. Sporadic epidermoid cysts are hardly ever found in the fingers. (Courtesy of Gary Peck, MD, Silver Springs, Maryland)

cerebellar medulloblastoma has been the first manifestation in some patients; if radiation is used to treat this tumor, large numbers of basal cell carcinomas develop in irradiation ports (Fig. 7–5)

other central nervous system abnormalities include congenital hydrocephalus, meningiomas, and calcification of falx cerebri, tentorium cerebelli, and diaphragma sellae

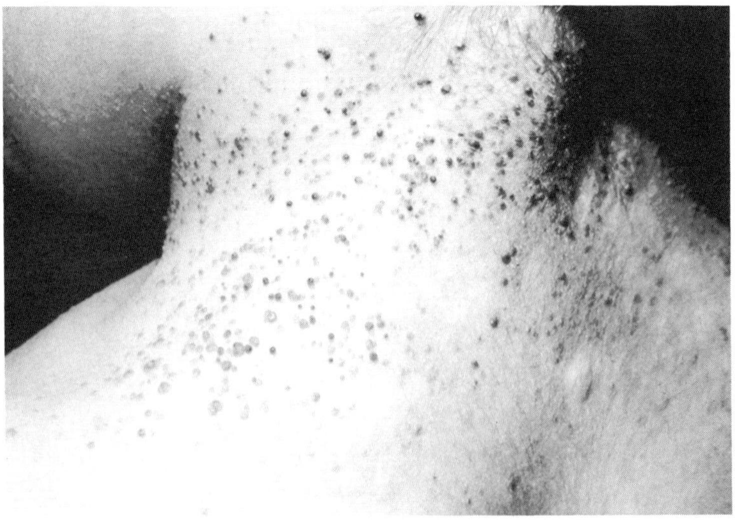

FIGURE 7–5
Myriads of hyperpigmented papules scattered over the neck and shoulders of a boy with nevoid basal cell carcinoma syndrome. This child had a medulloblastoma and received radiation therapy, after which these tumors developed.

ocular abnormalities include strabismus and, less commonly, congenital cataracts, glaucoma, and colobomas of the iris or optic tract

craniofacial abnormalities include enlarged occipitofrontal circumference, cleft lip and/or palate, and ocular hypertelorism

musculoskeletal abnormalities, most of them congenital, include rib anomalies (e.g., bifid or splayed), spina bifida occulta of cervical or thoracic vertebrae, kyphoscoliosis, pectus excavatum or carinatum, pseudocystic lesions of bones, and brachymetacarpalism

occasional musculoskeletal findings include marfanoid habitus, postaxial polydactyly, and scapular abnormalities (Sprengle's deformity); many of these findings are congenital

other less commonly reported findings include lymphomesenteric cysts of the gastrointestinal tract, maxillary fibrosarcomas, myocardial fibromas, agenesis of the corpus callosum, and fetal rhabdomyoma

Genetics

AD

whites affected more than blacks

mutation in nevoid basal cell carcinoma syndrome localized to the long arm of chromosome 9

Pathophysiology

clinical (in vivo) cutaneous hypersensitivity to x-ray irradiation

tumors not affected by sunlight, but possible increased sensitivity to ultraviolet light has been demonstrated in vitro

Laboratory Data

histopathology: basal cell carcinomas may have a unique pattern described as infundibulocystic by Walsh and Ackerman (1990); they are also more likely to be calcified or ossified as compared with sporadic basal cell carcinomas

abnormalities evident on radiography include jaw cysts, bone pseudocysts, skeletal defects, calcification of falx cerebri and tentorium cerebelli, and sella turcica bridging

Prognosis

x-ray therapy for skin lesions is contraindicated; radiation therapy is often required for the central nervous system tumors and usually induces numerous basal cell carcinomas in the radiation portals

keratocysts are often removed because of concern about fibrosarcomatous degeneration, but, ironically, preoperative radiographs may cause half of jaw fibrosarcomas

Discussion

at least 10% of patients have internal signs or other stigmata but no basal cell carcinomas

- *linear unilateral basal cell nevus with comedones:*

  linear unilateral basal cell carcinomas

  comedones and epidermoid cysts

  striae-like atrophy

  onset usually at birth

  not associated with other findings of nevoid basal cell carcinoma syndrome (which very rarely is unilateral)

  sporadic; may represent a postzygotic somatic mutation

REFERENCES

McK 109400

Barr RJ, Headley JL, Jensen JL, et al. Cutaneous keratocysts of nevoid basal cell carcinoma syndrome. J Am Acad Dermatol 1986;14:572–576

Camisa C. Unilateral nevoid basal cell carcinoma syndrome. J Am Acad Dermatol 1987;16:1270–1271

Frentz G, Munch-Petersen B, Wulf HC, et al. The nevoid basal cell carcinoma syndrome: sensitivity to ultraviolet and x-ray irradiation. J Am Acad Dermatol 1987;17:637–643

Gorlin RJ. Nevoid basal-cell carcinoma syndrome. Medicine 1987;66:98–113

Gutierrez MM, Mora RG. Nevoid basal cell carcinoma syndrome: a review and case report of a patient with unilateral basal cell nevus syndrome. [Review]. J Am Acad Dermatol 1986;15:1023–1030

Johnson AD, Hebert AA, Esterly NB. Nevoid basal cell carcinoma syndrome: bilateral ovarian fibromas in a 3½ year-old girl. J Am Acad Dermatol 1986;14:371–374

Maddox WD, Winkelmann RK, Harrison EGJ, et al. Multiple nevoid basal cell epitheliomas, jaw cysts, and skeletal defects: a clinical syndrome. JAMA 1964;188:106–111

Peck GL. Long-term retinoid therapy is needed for maintenance of cancer chemopreventive effect. Dermatologica 1987;1:138–144

Pratt MD, Jackson R. Nevoid basal cell carcinoma syndrome: a 15-year follow-up of cases in Ottawa and the Ottawa Valley. J Am Acad Dermatol 1987;16:964–970

Reis A, Kuster W, Linss G, et al. Localisation of gene for the naevoid basal cell carcinoma syndrome. [Letter]. Lancet 1992; 339:617

Southwick GJ, Schwartz RA. The basal cell nevus syndrome: disasters occurring among a series of 36 patients. Cancer 1979; 44:2294–2305

Walsh N, Ackerman AB. Infundibulocystic basal cell carcinoma: a newly described variant. Mod Pathol 1990;3:599–608

BASAL CELL CARCINOMAS, COARSE SPARSE HAIR, AND MILIA

a kindred with basal cell carcinomas, sparse scalp and body hair, eyebrows, and eyelashes, and widespread milia reported

patients lacked features of nevoid basal cell carcinoma syndrome, including palmar or plantar pits, keratocysts of the jaw, rib or vertebral abnormalities, or abnormal calcification on skull radiography

AD

McK 109390
Oley CA, Sharpe H, Chenevix-Trench G. Basal cell carcinomas, coarse sparse hair, and milia. Am J Med Genet 1992;43:799–804

BAZEX SYNDROME

Synonyms

- follicular atrophoderma and basal cell carcinomas

Skin

at birth or in early infancy, follicular "atrophoderma" (i.e., patulous follicles or "pits") most commonly on the dorsa of hands, lower back, and extensor surface of elbows; occasional involvement of face and dorsa of feet

follicular pits resemble "ice pick marks" or "exaggerated follicular funnels"

clinically, basal cell carcinomas are light brown papules that may resemble melanocytic nevi; develop most commonly on central face or eyelids in second or third decade, rarely in first decade

other reported findings include keratosis pilaris of popliteal and buttock areas, milia-like papules on face, upper trunk, and flexural areas

generalized or localized (limited to head and face) hypohidrosis or anhidrosis

hypotrichosis, with pili torti on microscopic examination

Genetics

AD or X-linked dominant

Laboratory Data

some tumors show histopathologic features of trichoepitheliomas

Discussion

kindred reported with no basal cell carcinomas

the nevoid basal cell carcinoma syndrome (see main entry) also has basal cell carcinomas resembling melanocytic nevi and may have follicular atrophoderma-like lesions

Bazex syndrome also refers to paraneoplastic acrokeratosis, a totally unrelated acquired disorder

REFERENCES

McK 109520

Bazex A, Dupre A, Christol B. Atrophodermic folliculaire, proliferations baso-cellulaires et hypotrichose. Ann Dermatol Syphilol 1966;93:251–254

Curth HO. The genetics of follicular atrophoderma. Arch Dermatol 1978;114:1479–1483

Gould DJ, Barker DJ. Follicular atrophoderma with multiple basal cell carcinomas (Bazex). Br J Dermatol 1978;99:431–435

Mehta VR, Potdar R. Bazex syndrome: follicular atrophoderma and basal cell epitheliomas. Int J Dermatol 1985;24:444–446

Plosila M, Kiistala R, Niemi KM: The Bazex syndrome: follicular atrophoderma with multiple basal cell carcinomas, hypotrichosis and hypohidrosis. Clin Exp Dermatol 1981;6:31–41

Tuzun Y, Mat MC, Serdaroglu S, et al. Follicular atrophoderma with scrotal tongue. Pediatr Dermatol 1987;4:328–331

ROMBO SYNDROME

vasodilation with cyanosis of lips, hands, and feet in first decade

yellowish papules and follicular atrophy of face (atrophoderma vermiculatum)

facial milia and telangiectases

sparse body and facial hair and eyelashes and eyebrows in adulthood

basal cell carcinomas and rarely trichoepitheliomas develop in adulthood

AD

McK 180730

Ashinoff R, Jacobson M, Belsito DV. Rombo syndrome: A second case report and review. J Am Acad Dermatol 1993;28:1011–1014

Michaelsson G, Olsson E, Westermark P. The Rombo syndrome: a familial disorder with vermiculate atrophoderma, milia, hypotrichosis, trichoepitheliomas, basal cell carcinomas and peripheral vasodilation with cyanosis. Acta Derm Venereol 1981; 61:497–503

GARDNER SYNDROME

Synonym

- intestinal polyposis type III

Skin

epidermoid cysts measuring up to greater than 15 cm in size in 65% of patients (Fig. 7–6); they arise during childhood or adolescence and usually precede onset of polyposis by 10 to 15 years; face and neck are predominant sites

desmoid tumors, which are deep, poorly defined fibrous tissue tumors, arise at sites of trauma, surgical scars or de novo; most commonly on anterior abdominal wall; 75% occur in women, often following obstetric or gynecologic surgery

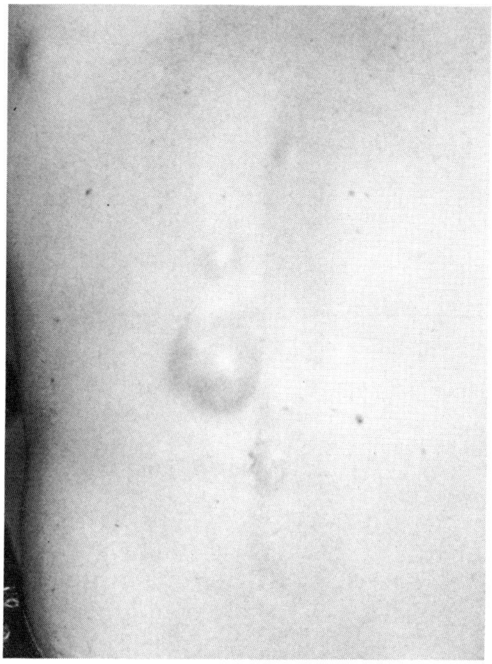

FIGURE 7–6
Gardner syndrome. This patient has multiple epidermoid cysts.

poorly circumscribed subcutaneous fibromas; occasional lipomas, leiomyomas, fibrosarcomas, neurofibromas, and oral fibromas

dental abnormalities include rudimentary, supernumerary, and unerupted teeth; odontomas; and dentigerous cysts

Non-Skin

hundreds of gastrointestinal polyps may be present, which are more likely to involve the colon and rectum than the small intestine or stomach; frequently detected during early adulthood but may be detected earlier

diagnosis is usually made based on signs and symptoms of polyposis, which include abdominal pain and bleeding; usually, however, these do not occur until malignant degeneration has ensued

adenocarcinoma of the colon occurs in 50% of cases by fourth decade; incidence eventually approaches 100%

osteomas of the skull (mostly facial bones) and mandible usually present by late childhood or adolescence; they occur in membranous bone in over 75% of cases, and precede onset of polyposis by 10 to 15 years

osteomas and epidermoid cysts increase in number and size with age, but eventually stabilize

multiple pigmented bilateral ocular fundus lesions in majority of patients are an early, specific and sensitive marker of the disease

other associated neoplasms include hepatoblastoma and carcinoid tumors as well as ovarian, adrenal, and thyroid carcinomas; these may precede or follow detection of colonic polyposis

Genetics

AD

Laboratory Data

histopathology: epidermoid cysts may occasionally have features of pilomatricomas

Prognosis

early detection of disease may allow earlier prophylactic colectomy before malignant transformation of polyps

genetic counseling is crucial; diagnosis often not established until well into reproductive age

relatives of patients with newly diagnosed Gardner syndrome should also be carefully examined; ophthalmologic and gastrointestinal examinations and dental radiographs (which detect the jaw osteomas commonly seen as an early finding) should be obtained in all suspected cases of Gardner syndrome and in family members at risk

fibrous tumors may compress crucial organs, causing surgical emergency; mesenteric, retroperitoneal, or abdominal wall fibromatosis frequently occurs 1 to 2 years after intestinal tract surgery

Discussion

cutaneous findings may be very subtle (e.g., only a few epidermoid cysts may be present)

Oldfield syndrome (premalignant polyposis and epidermoid cysts) is the same as Gardner syndrome

familial polyposis of the colon (intestinal polyposis type I) may be allelic with Gardner syndrome, but no soft tissue tumors or osteomas are seen; massive numbers of polyps in the colon with carcinomatous degeneration in nearly every patient

REFERENCES

McK 175100

Cooper PH, Fechner RE. Pilomatricoma-like changes in the epidermal cysts of Gardner's syndrome. J Am Acad Dermatol 1983;8:639–644

Gardner EJ, Richards RC. Multiple cutaneous and subcutaneous lesions occurring simultaneously with hereditary polyposis and osteomatosis. Am J Hum Genet 1953; 5:139–147

Gardner EJ, Stephens FE. Cancer of the lower digestive tract in one family group. Am J Hum Genet 1950;2:41–48

Kratzer GL, Kasumi A, Krush AJ. Gardner syndrome: study and follow-up of a family. Am J Med Genet 1991;41:393–397

Leppard BJ, Bussey HJR. Gardner's syndrome with epidermoid cysts showing features of pilomatrixomas. Clin Exp Dermatol 1976; 1:75–82

Naylor EW, Gardner EJ, Richards RC. Desmoid tumors and mesenteric fibromatosis in Gardner's syndrome. Arch Surg 1979; 114:1181–1185

Oldfield MC. The association of familial polyposis of the colon with multiple sebaceous cysts. Br J Surg 1954;41:534–541

Traboulsi EI, Krush AJ, Gardner EJ, et al.

Prevalence and importance of pigmented ocular fundus lesions in Gardner's syndrome. N Engl J Med 1987;316:661–667
Traboulsi EI, Murphy SF, de la Cruz ZC, et al. A clinicopathologic study of the eyes in familial adenomatous polyposis with extracolonic manifestations (Gardner's syndrome). Am J Ophthalmol 1990;110:550–561

TURCOT SYNDROME

occasional café-au-lait macules

colonic polyposis

malignant tumors of the central nervous system include glioblastomas, medulloblastomas, and astrocytomas

very rare and heterogeneous; some autosomal dominant cases clearly related to Gardner syndrome; other cases are clearly not representative of Gardner syndrome and some may be AR

McK 276300
Baughman FA Jr, List CF, Williams JR, et al. The glioma-polyposis syndrome. N Engl J Med 1969;281:1345–1346
Lewis JH, Ginsberg AL, Toomey KE. Turcot's syndrome: evidence for autosomal dominant inheritance. Cancer 1983;51:524–528
Michels VV, Stevens JC. Basal cell carcinoma in a patient with intestinal polyposis. Clin Genet 1982;22:80–82
Tops CMJ, Vasen HFA, van Berge Henegouwen G, et al. Genetic evidence that Turcot syndrome is not allelic to familial adenomatous polyposis. Am J Med Genet 1992; 43:888–893
Yaffee HS. Gastric polyposis and soft tissue tumors: a variant of Gardner's syndrome. Arch Dermatol 1964;89:806–808

TORRE SYNDROME

Synonym

- Muir-Torre syndrome

Skin

multiple yellowish, flesh-colored or translucent papules and nodules are most commonly located on the trunk and face (Fig. 7–7); these are usually sebaceous tumors

some lesions are crateriform with a hyperkeratotic plug, typical for a keratoacanthoma

it is difficult, especially on the face, to distinguish between sebaceous tumors and keratoacanthomas

Non-Skin

multiple primary low-grade visceral malignancies, most commonly carcinomas of the gastrointestinal tract, but also of other sites, including lung and genitourinary systems

occasional colonic polyps

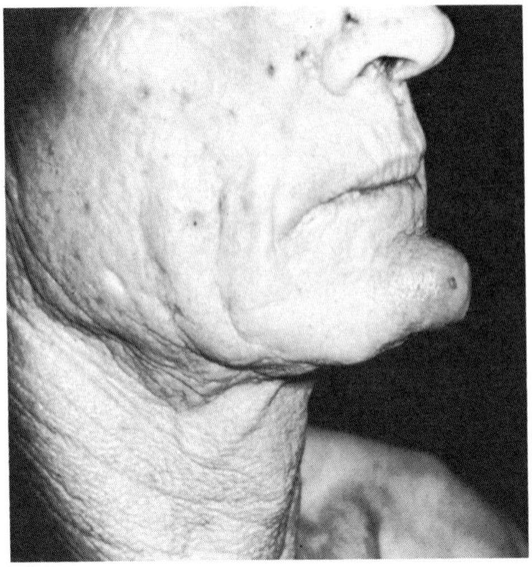

FIGURE 7–7
Torre syndrome. The protuberant chin represents a sebaceous carcinoma that metastasized to the jaw. Around the nasolabial folds and across the cheeks are numerous hyperkeratotic papules and ulcerated lesions, which are sebaceous neoplasms and keratoacanthomas.

Genetics

AD in patients who are part of the "cancer family syndrome"; most cases are sporadic

Laboratory Data

wide and unusual histopathologic spectrum of sebaceous neoplasia that does not conform to the usual descriptions for these entities; commonly termed *sebaceous adenomas, sebaceous hyperplasia, sebaceous epitheliomas,* and *sebaceous carcinomas*

a single lesion may show histologic features of both a keratoacanthoma and a sebaceous neoplasm

Prognosis

in 50%, visceral malignancies occur before the development of sebaceous tumors

visceral malignancies are low grade; early recognition of sebaceous neoplasms may improve survival

Discussion

Torre syndrome is one of the phenotypic expressions of the larger set termed the *cancer family syndrome* (McK 11440)

some patients described as having multiple keratoacanthomas and visceral malignancies may actually have Torre syndrome with few or no sebaceous lesions

REFERENCES

McK 158320

Banse-Kupin L, Morales A, Barlow M. Torre's syndrome: report of two cases and review of the literature. J Am Acad Dermatol 1984;10:803–817

Burgdorf WH, Pitha J, Fahmy A. Muir-Torre

syndrome: histologic spectrum of sebaceous proliferations. Am J Dermatopathol 1986;8:202–208

Fahmy A, Burgdorf WH, Schosser RH, et al. Muir-Torre syndrome: report of a case and reevaluation of the dermatopathologic features. Cancer 1982;49:1898–1903

Finan MC, Connolly SM. Sebaceous gland tumors and systemic disease: a clinicopathologic analysis. Medicine 1984;63:232–242

Housholder MS, Zeligman I. Sebaceous neoplasms associated with visceral carcinomas. Arch Dermatol 1980;116:61–64

Lynch HT, Fusaro RM, Roberts L, et al. Muir-Torre syndrome in several members of a family with a variant of the cancer family syndrome. Br J Dermatol 1985;113:295–301

Lynch HT, Lynch PM, Pester J, et al. The cancer family syndrome: rare cutaneous phenotypic linkage of Torre's syndrome. Arch Intern Med 1981;141:607–611

Muir EG, Yates-Bell AJ, Barlow KA. Multiple primary carcinomata of the colon, duodenum and larynx associated with keratoacanthomata of the face. Br J Surg 1967;54:191–195

Spielvogel RL, DeVillez RL, Roberts LC. Oral isotretinoin therapy for familial Muir-Torre syndrome. J Am Acad Dermatol 1985;12:475–480

Stone MS, Duncan WC, McGavran MH. Torre's syndrome: exacerbation of cutaneous manifestations with immunosuppression. J Am Acad Dermatol 1986;15:1101–1103

Torre D. Multiple sebaceous tumors. Arch Dermatol 1968;98:549–551

MULTIPLE KERATOACANTHOMAS, FERGUSON-SMITH TYPE

Synonyms

- multiple self-healing epithelioma
- familial primary self-healing squamous epithelioma of the skin

Skin

skin-colored to reddish nodules with central crust overlying a keratin-filled crater that closely resemble solitary keratoacanthomas but with a greater tendency to ulcerate (Fig. 7–8)

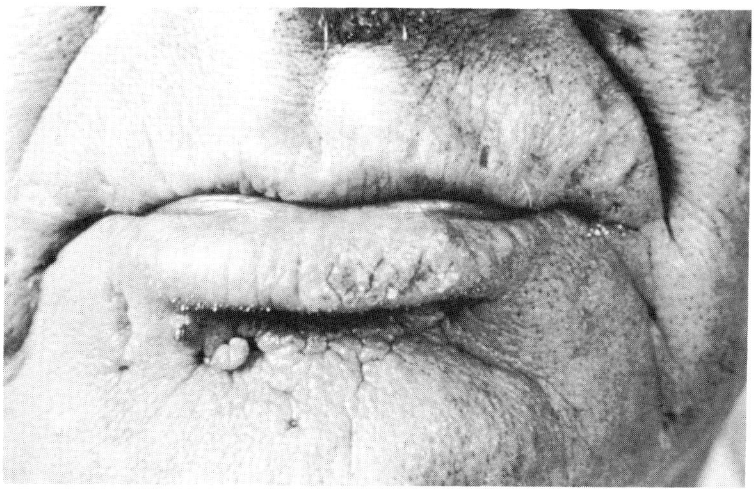

FIGURE 7–8
Multiple keratoacanthomas, Ferguson-Smith type. There are numerous hyperkeratotic papules about the mouth as well as some crateriform scars. (Courtesy of Dr. John A. Hunter, Edinburgh, Scotland)

predominantly occur in exposed areas of face, ears, neck, hands, and extensor extremities; rarely other sites are involved, including the trunk or oral mucous membranes

usually begin in adolescence or early adult life

lesions appear on scalp in majority of cases, unlike solitary keratoacanthomas, which rarely affect the scalp

lesions number from a few to hundreds and occur singly or in crops

typically enlarge over 2 to 4 weeks and begin to regress 1 to 2 months later, frequently leaving a scar

Genetics

AD

gene responsible for this syndrome localized to chromosome 9q

Laboratory Data

histopathology: typical features of solitary keratoacanthomas, occasionally with deeper or more perineural involvement, hence the term *self-healing squamous epithelioma*

Discussion

in Torre syndrome (see main entry), some patients have only multiple keratoacanthomas and internal malignancy, but most also have multiple sebaceous neoplasms

Ferguson-Smith syndrome is rare and limited to several Scottish pedigrees

- *eruptive keratoacanthomas (keratoacanthomas, multiple, Grzybowski type):*

  lesions are numerous, small, but persistent, most commonly affecting the face, trunk, and proximal extremities; usually do not appear until adulthood

  may affect oral or laryngeal mucosae, but palms and soles are spared

  pruritus may be prominent

  acquired

REFERENCES

McK 132800

Elewski BE, Gilgor RS. Eruptive lesions and malignancy. Int J Dermatol 1985;24:617–629

Ferguson Smith MA, Wallace DC, James ZH, et al. Multiple self-healing squamous epithelioma. Birth Defects 1971;7(8):157–163

Mackie RM. Epidermal skin tumours. In: Champion RH, Burton JL, Ebling FJG, eds. Textbook of Dermatology. Oxford, Blackwell Scientific Publications, 1992: 1472–1473

Winkelmann RK, Brown J. Generalized eruptive keratoacanthoma: report of cases. Arch Dermatol 1968;97:615–623

Young SK, Larsen PE, Markowitz NR. Generalized eruptive keratoacanthoma. Oral Surg 1986;62:422–426

COWDEN SYNDROME

Synonym

- multiple hamartoma syndrome

Skin

association of facial papules, acral keratoses, and mucosal lesions

flesh-colored papules 1 to 5 mm in size with either a flat-topped or verrucous appearance are found most reliably on the face in a periorificial and perinasal distribution (Fig. 7–9); onset is usually in adolescence

individual papules also appear elsewhere on face, nose, ears, and on dorsa of hands or wrists; they may resemble flat warts or lesions of acrokeratosis verruciformis; rarely, lesions are located more proximally on the trunk

palmoplantar keratoses are present in approximately 40% of cases

mucosal papules 1 to 3 mm in size are found on the gingival, labial, and palatal surfaces (Fig. 7–10); sometimes papillomatous lesions are found on the buccal, faucial, and oropharyngeal surfaces

confluent mucosal lesions may have a "cobblestone" appearance

if the tongue is involved, a "scrotal" or fissured appearance may result (Fig. 7–11)

multiple lipomas, hemangiomas, neuromas, and acanthosis nigricans reported

Non-Skin

craniomegaly with a prominent forehead noted early in life

there is a high incidence of fibrocystic disease of breast, thyroid adenomas, and gastrointestinal tract polyposis

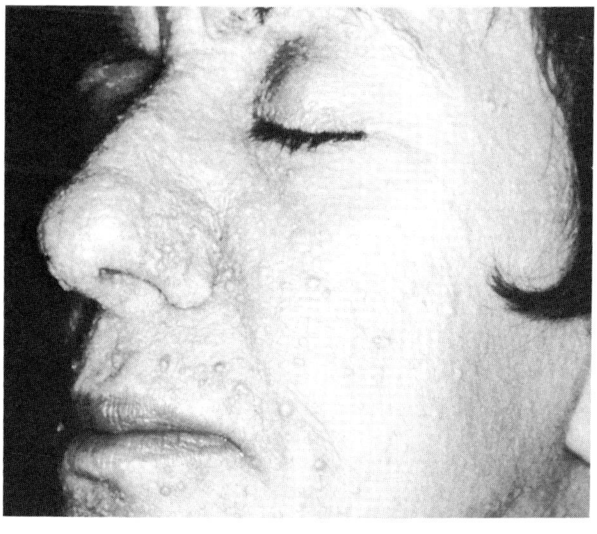

FIGURE 7–9
Cowden syndrome. Multiple flesh-colored papules distributed over the face with accentuation in the perinasal and perioral areas. (Courtesy of Benjamin K. Fisher, MD, Toronto, Ontario)

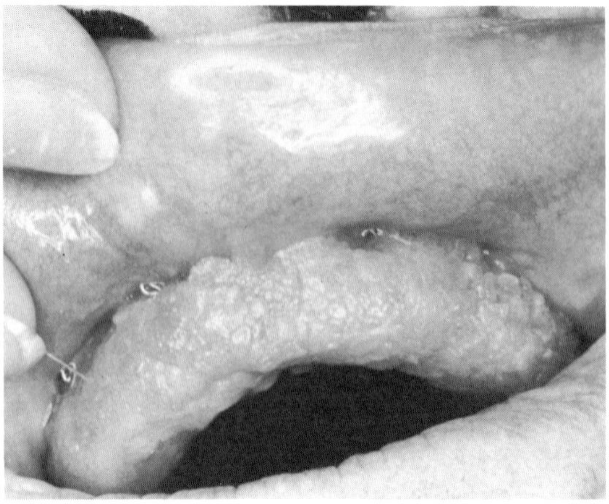

FIGURE 7–10
Cowden syndrome. Confluent mucosal papules giving the gingiva a cobblestone appearance. (Courtesy of Benjamin K. Fisher, MD, Toronto, Ontario)

multiple facial, oral, and acral papules often precede development of breast and thyroid disease

nearly all women develop fibrocystic disease of the breasts; at least 25% develop carcinoma

thyroid disease in two thirds of patients, including goiters, adenomas, and follicular adenocarcinomas; the latter occurs in 3% to 5% of men and women

Genetics

AD

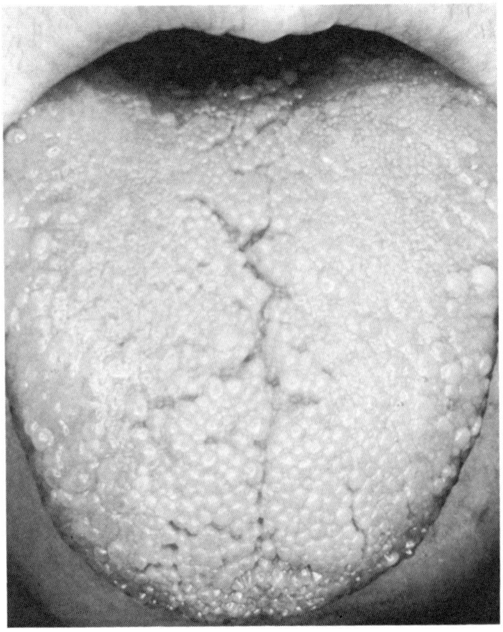

FIGURE 7–11
Cowden syndrome. Fissured tongue studded with papules resulting in a cobblestone appearance. (Courtesy of Benjamin K. Fisher, MD, Toronto, Ontario)

Laboratory Data

histopathology of facial lesions show features of trichilemmoma in most cases, but individual lesions may not show these findings; some mimic verrucae

histopathologic findings of the oral and acral lesions include broad bundles of hypocellular collagen in plate-like or whorled configuration with occasional giant cells; have been described as sclerotic fibroma

Prognosis

some recommend prophylactic mastectomies because of 25% incidence of breast carcinoma

Discussion

Lhermitte-Duclos syndrome of cerebellar hamartomas is identical to Cowden syndrome

REFERENCES

McK 158350

Albrecht S, Haber RM, Goodman JC, Duvic M. Cowden syndrome and Lhermitte-Duclos disease. Cancer 1992;70:869–876

Barax CN, Lebwohl M, Phelps RG. Multiple hamartoma syndrome. J Am Acad Dermatol 1987;17:342–346

Elston DM, James WD, Rodman OG, et al. Multiple hamartoma syndrome (Cowden's disease) associated with non-Hodgkin's lymphoma. Arch Dermatol 1986;122:572–575

Graham RM, Emmerson RW. Multiple hamartoma and neoplasia syndrome. Clin Exp Dermatol 1985;10:262–268

Salem OS, Steck WD. Cowden's disease (multiple hamartoma and neoplasia syndrome): a case report and review of the English literature. J Am Acad Dermatol 1983; 8:686–696

Starink TM, van der Veen JP, Arwert F, et al. The Cowden syndrome: a clinical and genetic study in 21 patients. Clin Genet 1986;29:222–233

Starink TM. Cowden's disease: analysis of fourteen new cases. J Am Acad Dermatol 1984;11:1127–1141

Swart JG, Lekkas C, Allard RH. Oral manifestations in Cowden's syndrome: report of four cases. Oral Surg 1985;59:264–268

Williard W, Borgen P, Bol R, et al. Cowden's disease: a case report with analyses at the molecular level. Cancer 1992;69:2969–2974

MULTIPLE MUCOSAL NEUROMA SYNDROME

Synonym

- multiple endocrine neoplasia syndrome type 2B

Skin

multiple mucosal nodules, some pedunculated, in nearly every patient (Fig. 7–12); onset usually in the first decade, before endocrine neoplasia in most

enlarged, blubbery lips and nodules and eversion of eyelids are the most visible findings; neuromas usually affect labial, lingual, buccal, and

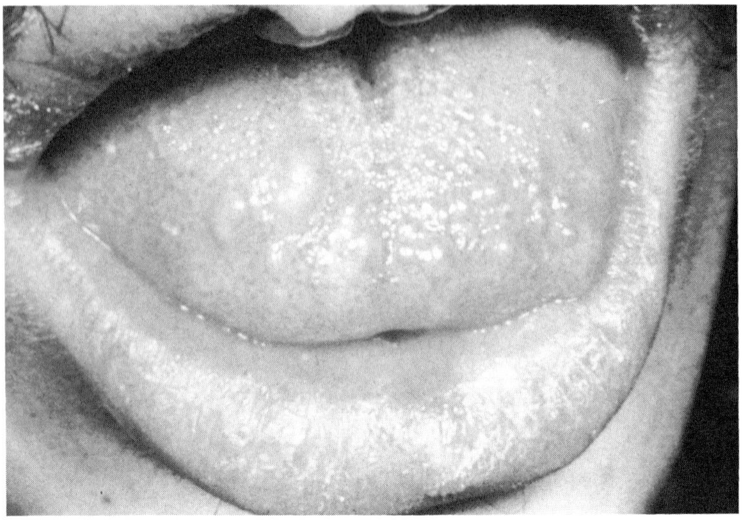

FIGURE 7–12
Multiple mucosal neuroma syndrome. There are nodules on both the tongue and lips. (Courtesy of Robert J. Gorlin, DDS, MS, Minneapolis, Minnesota)

conjunctival mucosae but also may affect the larynx and nasal mucosae

eversion of eyelids may occur spontaneously (Fig. 7–13)

rare cutaneous neuromas

occasional café-au-lait macules and/or lentigines

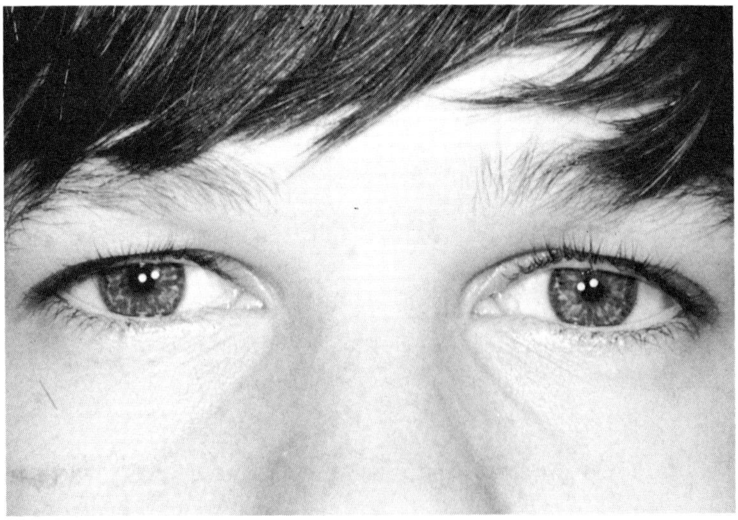

FIGURE 7–13
Multiple mucosal neuroma syndrome. The upper eyelids are everted or folded up, as is often done during an examination searching for a foreign object. However, this occurs spontaneously in these patients and is almost pathognomonic for this disorder. (Courtesy of Robert J. Gorlin, DDS, MS, Minneapolis, Minnesota)

Non-Skin

medullary carcinoma of the thyroid in nearly every patient, usually presenting after the first decade of life but may appear in infancy as presenting sign

pheochromocytomas in half, most frequently appearing in the second or third decades; usually multiple, often bilateral

marfanoid habitus common (Fig. 7–14); other skeletal abnormalities include high-arched palate and pectus excavatum

corneal nerve hypertrophy may be detected on ophthalmologic examination

disabling, intractable diarrhea may result from chemical mediators released by thyroid carcinoma

Genetics

AD

Prognosis

prompt referral to an endocrinologist is recommended for serial basal and pentagastrin-stimulated calcitonin levels and carcinoembryonic antigen levels to detect medullary thyroid carcinoma while it is still in the occult stage, as well as meta-iodobenzylguanidine (MIBG) scintigraphy to detect pheochromocytomas

50% of those with thyroid carcinoma already have metastatic disease at time of diagnosis

prophylactic thyroidectomy and replacement therapy recommended

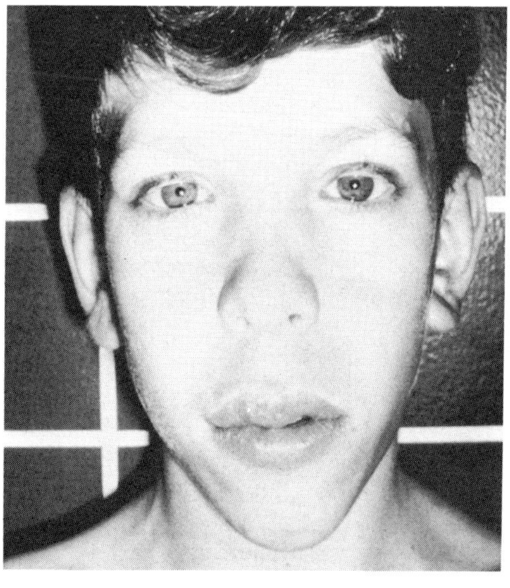

FIGURE 7–14
Multiple mucosal neuroma syndrome. The young patient has a marfanoid facies with prominent lips. (Courtesy of Robert J. Gorlin, DDS, MS, Minneapolis, Minnesota)

Discussion

the numerical designation of the multiple endocrine neoplasia syndromes has changed so often that terms such as multiple mucosal neuroma syndrome may be less confusing

REFERENCES

McK 162300

Cunliffe WJ, Hudgson P, Fulthorpe JJ, et al. A calcitonin-secreting medullary thyroid carcinoma associated with mucosal neuromas, marfanoid features, myopathy and pigmentation. Am J Med 1970;48:120–126

Dyck PJ, Carney JA, Sizemore GW, et al. Multiple endocrine neoplasia, type 2b: Phenotype recognition, neurological features and their pathological basis. Ann Neurol 1979;6:302–314

Gorlin RJ, Cohen MM Jr, Levin LS. Syndromes of the Head and Neck. 3rd ed. New York, Oxford University Press, 1990:385–392

Gorlin RJ, Sedano HO, Vickers RA, et al. Multiple mucosal neuromas, pheochromocytoma and medullary carcinoma of the thyroid—a syndrome. Cancer 1968;22: 293–299

Kirk JF, Flowers FP, Ramos-Caro FA, Browder JF. Multiple endocrine neoplasia type III: case report and review. Pediatr Dermatol 1991;8:124–128

Vasen HFA, van der Feltz M, Raue F, et al. The natural course of multiple endocrine neoplasia type IIb: a study of 18 cases. Arch Intern Med 1992;152:1250–1252

White MP, Goel KM, Connor JM, Coutts NA. Mucosal neuroma syndrome—a phenotype for malignancy. Arch Dis Child 1985; 60:876–877

SIPPLE SYNDROME (MULTIPLE ENDOCRINE NEOPLASIA SYNDROME TYPE 2)

parathyroid hyperplasia, pheochromocytoma and medullary carcinoma of the thyroid

cutaneous amyloidosis reported in some kindreds

AD

McK 171400

Donovan DT, Levy ML, Furst EJ, et al. Familial cutaneous lichen amyloidosis in association with multiple endocrine neoplasia type 2A: a new variant. Henry Ford Hosp Med J 1989;37:147–150

Gagel RF, Levy ML, Donovan DT, et al. Multiple endocrine neoplasia type 2a associated with cutaneous lichen amyloidosis. Ann Intern Med 1989;111:802–806

EPIDERMODYSPLASIA VERRUCIFORMIS

Synonym

- Lewandowsky-Lutz disease

Skin

papules that resemble flat warts on the face and neck

scaly plaques similar to those seen in tinea versicolor on the trunk and extremities lesions may be flesh-colored, erythematous, hyperpigmented, or hypopigmented; commonly coalesce into large plaques

onset in early childhood; lesions do not regress

a range of 25% to 80% of patients are reported to develop squamous cell carcinoma in warty lesions, especially in sun-exposed sites, usually beginning in adulthood

Genetics

mostly sporadic, but AR in 25% of patients

XLR also reported (McK 305350)

Pathophysiology

due to human papillomavirus (HPV) infection; inherited inability to resist infection with selected strains of HPV

many HPV strains are found predominantly or exclusively in patients with epidermodysplasia verruciformis

certain strains (e.g., HPV 5) are associated with malignant degeneration of skin lesions

defects in cell-mediated immunity reported and believed by some to be essential in the pathogenesis of the disease

Laboratory Data

paradoxically, increased natural killer cell activity reported

Prognosis

etretinate therapy has been useful in some cases

Discussion

widespread HPV infections resembling epidermodysplasia verruciformis may occur in transplant recipients and patients with acquired immunodeficiency syndrome; these lesions have a high rate of malignant degeneration, especially in sun-exposed skin

REFERENCES

McK 226400

McK 305350 (XLR form)

Androphy EJ, Dvoretzky I, Lowy DR. X-linked inheritance of epidermodysplasia verruciformis: Genetic and virologic studies of a kindred. Arch Dermatol 1985;121:864–868

Androphy EJ. Human papillomavirus: current concepts. [Review]. Arch Dermatol 1989;125:683–685

Bahru J, Loo DSC, Tay CH, et al. Epidermodysplasia verruciformis of Lewandowsky and Lutz. Arch Dermatol 1972;105:73–78

Jablonska S, Orth G, Jarzabek-Chorzelska M, et al. Twenty-one years of follow-up studies of familial epidermodysplasia verruciformis. Dermatologica 1979;158:309–327

Kaminski M, Pawinska M, Jablonska S, et al. Increased natural killer cell activity in patients with epidermodysplasia verruciformis. Arch Dermatol 1985;121:84–86

Majewski S, Malejczyk J, Jablonska S, et al. Natural cell-mediated cytotoxicity against various target cells in patients with epidermodysplasia verruciformis. J Am Acad Dermatol 1990;22:423–427

Majewski S, Skopinska-Rozewska E, Jablonska S, et al. Partial defects of cell-mediated immunity in patients with epidermodysplasia verruciformis. J Am Acad Dermatol 1986;15:966–973

Orth G, Jablonska S, Jarzabek-Chorzelska M, et al. Characteristics of the lesions and risk of malignant conversion associated with the type of human papillomavirus involved in epidermodysplasia verruciformis. Cancer Res 1979;39:1074–1082

FAMILIAL ATYPICAL MOLE–MELANOMA SYNDROME

Synonyms

- familial atypical multiple mole–melanoma syndrome
- FAMMM syndrome
- familial dysplastic nevus syndrome
- B-K mole syndrome

Skin

large numbers of atypical-appearing melanocytic nevi (so-called dysplastic nevi), typically on upper trunk and limbs, tending to spare the face

clinically, these lesions are papules or plaques characterized by variegated topography; asymmetry; polycyclic, notched, or blurred borders; and variable coloring, sometimes a haphazard mixture of pink, red, brown, or black

nevi can arise in childhood and continue to develop during adolescence and adulthood

some have an increased number of nevi that appear during puberty or pregnancy

increased incidence of malignant melanomas occurring at younger age as compared with general population; also, some report a better prognosis than sporadic melanoma

Non-Skin

increased risk for development of intraocular malignant melanoma

Genetics

AD

the gene for this syndrome has been mapped to chromosome 1p

Prognosis

whether these nevi are premalignant, a marker of an increased melanoma risk, or neither is controversial

Discussion

some kindred members with melanoma may not manifest "atypical nevi"

the dysplastic nevus syndrome has been classified into types A, B, C, D-1, and D-2 based on personal and family history of melanoma and dysplastic nevi, with the risk of melanoma increasing from A to D-2; we confine our comments to the familial forms and not sporadic dysplastic nevi, whose significance, if different from other melanocytic nevi, is unclear

some dispute the concept of "dysplastic nevi" being distinct from other types of melanocytic nevi in their biologic behavior; furthermore, they state that these lesions have not been shown to be either premalignant or a marker of increased melanoma risk

some report an increased incidence of gastrointestinal and breast carcinoma, sarcoma, and lymphoreticular malignancies, but others have not found such a predilection

REFERENCES

McK 155600

Bale SJ, Dracopoli NC, Tucker MA, et al. Mapping the gene for hereditary cutaneous malignant melanoma–dysplastic nevus to chromosome 1p. N Engl J Med 1989; 320:1367–1372

Clark WH Jr, Reimer RR, Greene M, et al. Origin of familial malignant melanomas from heritable melanocytic lesions: the B-K mole syndrome. Arch Dermatol 1978; 114:732–738

Greene MH, Clark WH Jr, Tucker MA, et al. Acquired precursors of cutaneous malignant melanoma: the familial dysplastic nevus syndrome. N Engl J Med 1985;312:91–97

Greene MH, Tucker MA, Clark WH Jr, et al. Hereditary melanoma and the dysplastic nevus syndrome: the risk of cancers other than melanoma. J Am Acad Dermatol 1987;16:792–797

Lynch HT, Frichot BC III, Lynch JF. Familial atypical multiple mole-melanoma syndrome. J Med Genet 1978;15:352–356

Lynch HT, Fusaro RM, Danes BS, et al. A review of hereditary malignant melanoma including biomarkers in familial atypical multiple mole melanoma syndrome. Cancer Genet Cytogenet 1983;8:325–358

National Institutes of Health consensus conference. Diagnosis and treatment of early melanoma. JAMA 1992;9:1314–1319

NEUROCUTANEOUS MELANOSIS SYNDROME

giant (> 20 cm in adult) congenital melanocytic nevi of the skin almost invariably involving posterior midline or multiple (≥ 3) congenital cutaneous melanocytic nevi

melanocytic proliferations involving pia-arachnoid membranes

usually neurologic manifestations within first 2 years; less frequently as late as second or third decades; signs of increased intracranial pressure, ataxia, cranial nerve palsies, bowel/bladder dysfunction, seizures, and mental retardation resulting in early death

hydrocephalus common

increased risk for central nervous system melanoma (40% to 60% of patients) sporadic, but may be due to a lethal AD gene surviving in a mosaic state by somatic mutation

McK 249400

Happle R. Lethal genes surviving by mosaicism: a possible explanation for sporadic birth defects involving the skin. J Am Acad Dermatol 1987;16:899–906

Kadonaga JN, Barkovich AJ, Edwards MSB, Frieden IJ. Neurocutaneous melanosis in association with Dandy-Walker complex. Pediatr Dermatol 1992;9:37–43

Kadonaga JN, Frieden IJ. Neurocutaneous melanosis: definition and review of the literature. J Am Acad Dermatol 1991; 24:747–755

Zuniga S, Las Heras J, Benveniste S. Neurocutaneous melanosis with extensive intracerebral and spinal cord involvement; report of two cases. J Neurosurg 1984; 61:782–785

Multiple Adnexal Tumors

For almost every type of adnexal tumor there is an autosomal dominant syndrome in which multiple lesions are seen. Some of the inherited syndromes are listed below. In general, the incidence of the acquired tumors is much higher than the dominantly inherited multiple lesions.

REFERENCES

Brownstein MH. The genodermatopathology of adnexal tumors. J Cutan Pathol 1984;11:457–465

Burgdorf WHC, Koester G. Multiple appendageal tumors. J Cutan Pathol 1992;19:449–457

Jelinek JE. Aspects of heredity, syndromic associations, and course of conditions in which cutaneous lesions occur solitarily or in multiplicity. J Am Acad Dermatol 1982;7:526–540

MULTIPLE CYLINDROMAS

Synonyms

- Ancell-Spiegler syndrome
- Spiegler tumor
- turban tumors

Skin

multiple pink to red nodules and tumors, most frequently on scalp ("turban" distribution when extensive) and forehead (Fig. 7–15)

less frequently on face and trunk

onset usually in adult life, occasionally earlier

malignant degeneration reported

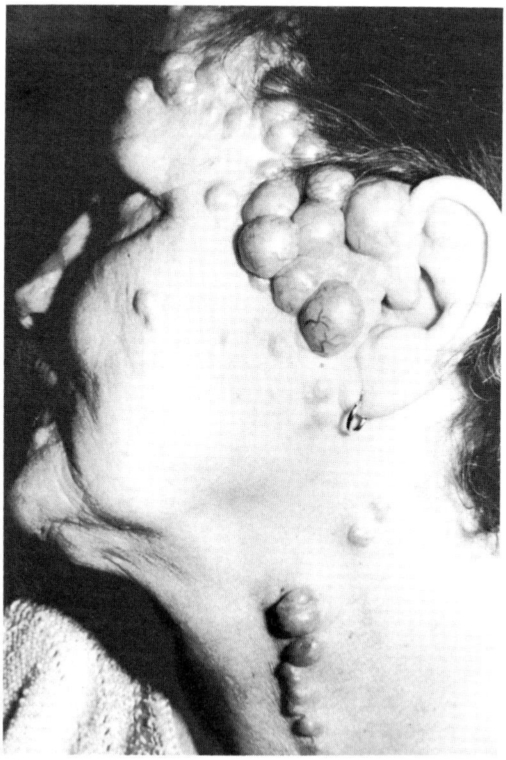

FIGURE 7–15
Multiple cylindromas. Pink nodules with surface telangiectases grouped at the temple, in the preauricular area, and in a linear distribution on the neck. (Courtesy of Benjamin K. Fisher, MD, Toronto, Ontario)

Genetics

AD

female preponderance has led to speculation of XLD inheritance

Discussion

there is much overlap among the multiple adnexal tumor syndromes; many closely related tumors may be found in the same patient or pedigree

REFERENCES

McK 123850

Crain RC, Helwig EB. Dermal cylindroma (dermal eccrine cylindroma). Am J Clin Pathol 1961;35:504–515

Rockerbie N, Solomon AR, Woo TY, et al. Malignant dermal cylindroma in a patient with multiple dermal cylindromas, trichoepitheliomas, and bilateral dermal analogue tumors of the parotid gland. Am J Dermatopathol 1989;11:353–359

Welch JP, Wells RS, Kerr CB. Ancell-Spiegler cylindromas (turban tumours) and Brooke-Fordyce trichoepitheliomas: evidence for a single genetic entity. J Med Genet 1968;5:29–35

TRICHOEPITHELIOMAS, MULTIPLE

Synonyms

- Brooke tumors
- epithelioma adenoides cysticum

Skin

multiple papules measuring a few to several millimeters are seen mostly on the central face (nasolabial fold, nose, forehead and upper lip), but also on the scalp, neck, and upper trunk (Fig. 7–16)

most lesions arise in second decade of life, before or during adolescence

Genetics

AD

females affected more than males

Discussion

- *familial multiple desmoplastic trichoepitheliomas:*

  separate kindreds with exclusively solitary or multiple lesions reported

  however, sporadic cases with solitary or multiple lesions are much more common

  AD

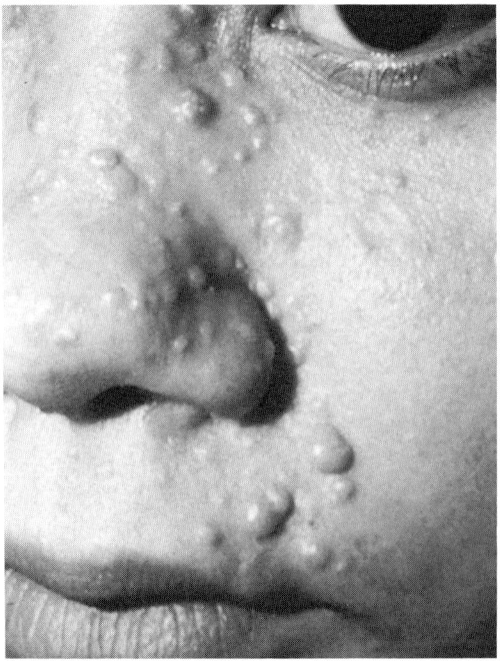

FIGURE 7–16
Multiple trichoepitheliomas. Variably sized skin-colored nodules scattered over the nose, upper lip, and chin.

REFERENCES

McK 132700
Anderson DE, Howell JB. Epithelioma adenoides cysticum: genetic update. Br J Dermatol 1976;95:225–232
Dervan PA, O'Hegarty M, O'Loughlin S, et al. Solitary familial desmoplastic trichoepithelioma: a study by conventional and electron microscopy. Am J Dermatopathol 1985;7:277–282
Pariser RJ. Multiple hereditary trichoepitheliomas and basal cell carcinomas. J Cutan Pathol 1986;13:111–117
Ziprkowski L, Schewach-Millet M. Multiple trichoepithelioma in a mother and two children. Dermatologica 1966;132:248–256

BROOKE-FORDYCE SYNDROME

multiple cylindromas associated with multiple trichoepitheliomas

AD, but more common in females

multiple cylindromas (Ancell-Spiegler syndrome) and multiple trichoepitheliomas (Brooke tumors) may overlap

McK 313100
Welch JP, Wells RS, Kerr CB. Ancell-Spiegler cylindromas (turban tumours) and Brooke-Fordyce trichoepitheliomas: evidence for a single genetic entity. J Med Genet 1968;5:29–35

MULTIPLE FIBROFOLLICULOMAS, TRICHODISCOMAS, AND ACROCHORDONS

Synonyms

- Birt-Hogg-Dubé syndrome
- Hornstein-Knickenberg syndrome

Skin

numerous skin-colored papules (fibrofolliculomas, perifollicular fibromas, and trichodiscomas) appearing on the scalp, forehead, face, neck, and upper trunk, in association with acrochordons (Figs. 7–17 and 7–18)

papules appear in adolescence or in young adulthood

Non-Skin

most patients do not have internal malignancy, but there are reports of increased incidence of thyroid carcinoma or gastrointestinal malignancies

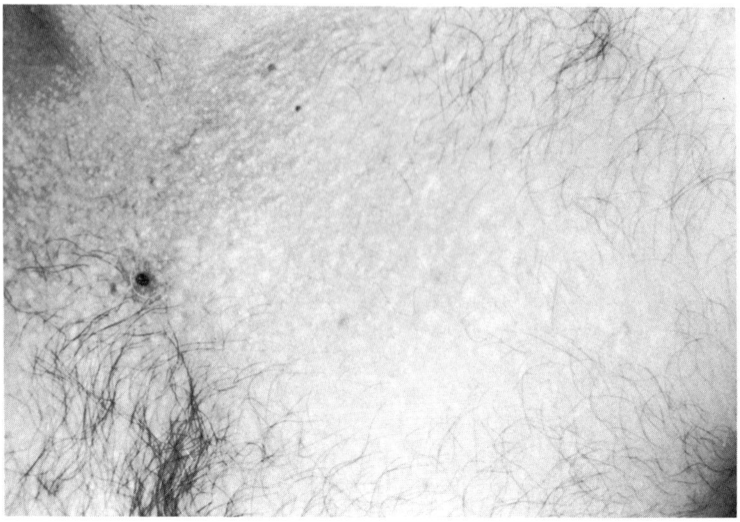

FIGURE 7–17
Multiple fibrofolliculomas, trichodiscomas, and acrochordons. There are hundreds of tiny papules on the chest. About 10 of these were biopsied; half revealed fibrofolliculomas, the others were trichodiscomas. The patient died several years later of metastatic carcinoma of the colon.

Genetics

AD

Laboratory Data

the trichodiscomas are actually fibrous tumors, probably closely related to the other follicular-oriented proliferations

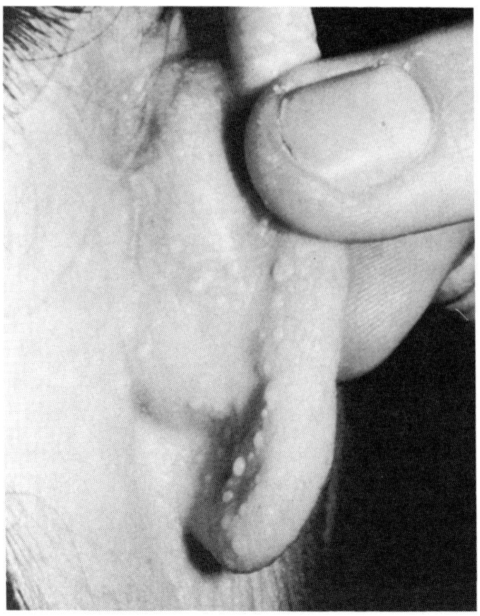

FIGURE 7–18
This patient and several family members had numerous warty papules around the ears but lacked other evidence of the syndrome of multiple fibrofolliculomas, trichodiscomas, and acrochordons. (Courtesy of Elliot Foucar, MD, Albuquerque, New Mexico; reprinted with permission from Foucar K, Rosen T, Foucar E, Cochran RJ. Fibrofolliculoma: a clinicopathologic study. Cutis 1981;28:429–432)

Discussion

the original report postulated an association with an increased incidence of hereditary medullary carcinoma of the thyroid in family members whether they had skin lesions or not

familial multiple trichodiscomas (Mck 190340) and multiple fibrofolliculomas are seen without systemic disease in different pedigrees

REFERENCES

McK 135150

Balus L, Crovato F, Breathnach AS. Familial multiple trichodiscomas. J Am Acad Dermatol 1986;15:603–607

Birt AR, Hogg GR, Dubé WJ. Hereditary multiple fibrofolliculomas with trichodiscomas and acrochordons. Arch Dermatol 1977; 113:1674–1677

Camarasa JG, Calderon P, Moreno A. Familial multiple trichodiscomas. Acta Derm Venereol 1988;68:163–165

Fujita WH, Barr RJ, Headley JL. Multiple fibrofolliculomas with trichodiscomas and acrochordons. Arch Dermatol 1981;117:32–35

Rongioletti F, Hazini R, Gianotti G, Rebora A. Fibrofolliculomas, tricodiscomas and acrochordons (Birt-Hogg-Dubé) associated with intestinal polyposis. Clin Exp Dermatol 1989;14:72–74

Starink TM, Brownstein MH. Fibrofolliculoma: solitary and multiple types. J Am Acad Dermatol 1987;17:493–496

Starink TM, Kisch LS, Meijer CJ. Familial multiple trichodiscomas: a clinicopathologic study. Arch Dermatol 1985;121:888–891

Ubogy-Rainey Z, James WD, Lupton GP, et al. Fibrofolliculomas, trichodiscomas, and acrochordons: the Birt-Hogg-Dubé syndrome. J Am Acad Dermatol 1987;16:452–457

HEREDITARY PILAR CYSTS

Synonyms

- hereditary trichilemmal cysts
- wens

Skin

multiple cysts on scalp; rarely on face, neck, trunk, or scrotum; usually appear during third decade, but may first present at birth or as late as eighth decade

leukonychia totalis in some families

Genetics

AD

Laboratory Data

histopathology: 2% of "epidermoid cysts" show features of proliferating trichilemmal cysts (pilar tumors)

Discussion

no association with polyposis coli (which may be associated with multiple epidermoid cysts in Gardner syndrome)

REFERENCES

Leppard BJ, Sanderson KV, Wells RS. Hereditary trichilemmal cysts: hereditary pilar cysts. Clin Exp Dermatol 1977;2:23–32

Leppard BJ, Sanderson KV. The natural history of trichilemmal cysts. Br J Dermatol 1976;94:379–390

MULTIPLE PILOMATRICOMAS (MULTIPLE BENIGN CALCIFYING EPITHELIOMAS OF MALHERBE)

firm, stony hard nodules, usually of head and neck; onset from childhood to adulthood

association with myotonic dystrophy reported in some families

AD

McK 132600

Cantwell AR, Reed WB. Myotonia atrophica and multiple calcifying epithelioma of Malherbe. Acta Derm Venereol 1965;45:387–390

Chiaramonti A, Gilgor RS. Pilomatricomas associated with myotonic dystrophy. Arch Dermatol 1978;114:1363–1365

Harper PS. Calcifying epithelioma of Malherbe. Arch Dermatol 1972;106:41–45

Hills RJ, Ive FA. Familial multiple pilomatrixomas. Br J Dermatol 1992;127:194–195

STEATOCYSTOMA MULTIPLEX

Synonyms

- sebocystomatosis
- hereditary epidermal polycystic disease

Skin

multiple (commonly hundreds) rounded cystic nodules on trunk, especially over sternum, and proximal extremities (Fig. 7–19); other areas including buttocks, thighs, axillae, and scrotum may be involved

onset is usually at puberty; patients with earlier onset may note increase in number of lesions at puberty, after which disease becomes stationary

lesions may be localized (e.g., to the axilla or scrotum); usually symmetrically distributed

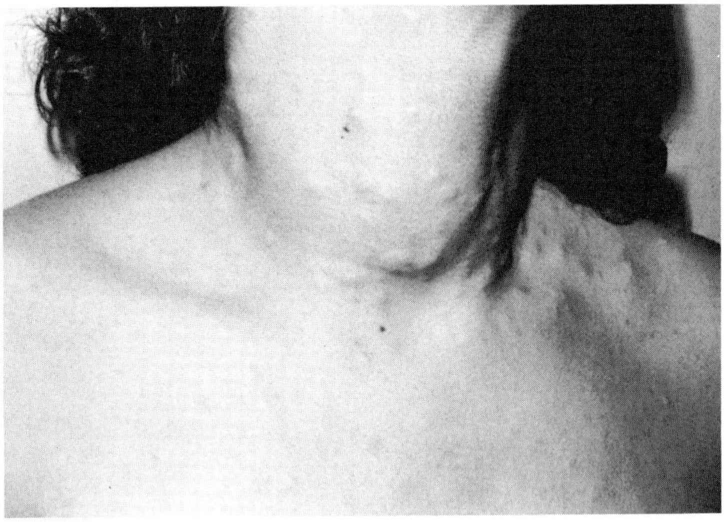

FIGURE 7–19
Steatocystoma multiplex. Multiple, cystic, skin-colored nodules distributed over the anterior neck, shoulders, and chest. (Courtesy of Benjamin K. Fisher, MD, Toronto, Ontario)

characteristically, an "oily" material may be extruded when lesions are incised; rarely, lesions are calcified

association with natal teeth and/or hidradenitis suppurativa reported

Genetics

AD

Discussion

may overlap with multiple eruptive vellus hair cysts

REFERENCES

McK 184500

Barone JG, Brown AS, Gisser SD, et al. Steatocystoma multiplex with bilateral preauricular sinuses in four generations. Ann Plast Surg 1988;21:55–57

McDonald RM, Reed WB. Natal teeth and steatocystoma multiplex complicated by hidradenitis suppurativa. Arch Dermatol 1976;112:1132–1134

Nishimura M, Kohda H, Urabe A. Steatocystoma multiplex: a facial papular variant. Arch Dermatol 1986;122:205–207

Noojin RO, Reynolds JP. Familial steatocystoma multiplex: twelve cases in three generations. Arch Dermatol 1948;57:1013–1018

Plewig G, Wolff HH, O B-F. Steatocystoma multiplex: anatomic reevaluation, electron microscopy, and autoradiography. Arch Dermatol Res 1982;272:363–380

ERUPTIVE VELLUS HAIR CYSTS

multiple 1- to 4-mm slightly red-brown to bluish papules most frequently found on chest and flexural limbs but may be found anywhere (Fig. 7–20)

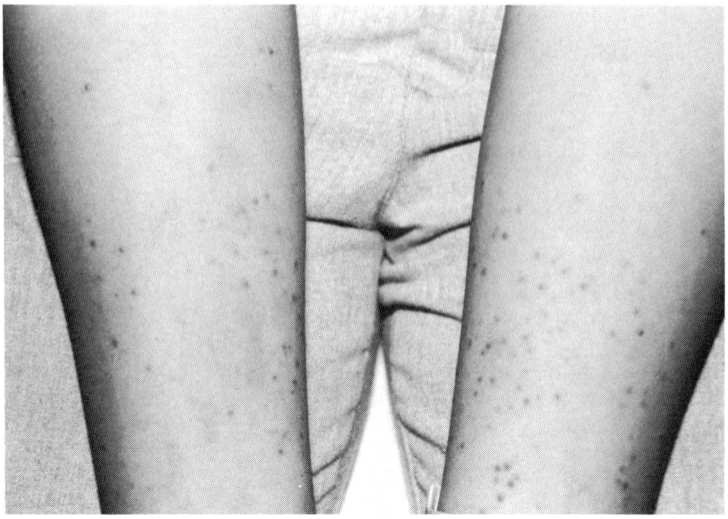

FIGURE 7–20
Eruptive vellus hair cysts. Multiple, tiny, hyperpigmented papules distributed on the flexural surfaces of the forearms in a child.

usually appear in first or second decade but may be present at birth or occur in adulthood

AD and sporadic cases reported

Esterly NB, Fretzin DF, Pinkus H. Eruptive vellus hair cysts. Arch Dermatol 1977;113:500–503

Grimalt R, Gelmetti C. Eruptive vellus hair cysts: case report and review of the literature. Pediatr Dermatol 1992;9:98–102

Mayron R, Grimwood RE. Familial occurrence of eruptive vellus hair cysts. Pediatr Dermatol 1988;5:94–96

Ohtake N, Kubota Y, Takayama O, et al. Relationship between steatocystoma multiplex and eruptive vellus hair cysts. J Am Acad Dermatol 1992;26:876–878

Sanchez-Yus E, Aguilar-Martinez A, Cristobal-Gil MC, et al. Eruptive vellus hair cyst and steatocystoma multiplex: two related conditions? J Cutan Pathol 1987;15:40–42

Stiefler RE, Bergfeld WF. Eruptive vellus hair cysts—an inherited disorder. J Am Acad Dermatol 1980;3:425–429

FAMILIAL SYRINGOMAS

multiple skin-colored to yellowish papules usually localized to anterior trunk and extremities, rarely facial (Fig. 7–21)

onset usually appearing in childhood

AD

most instances of multiple syringomas are nonfamilial

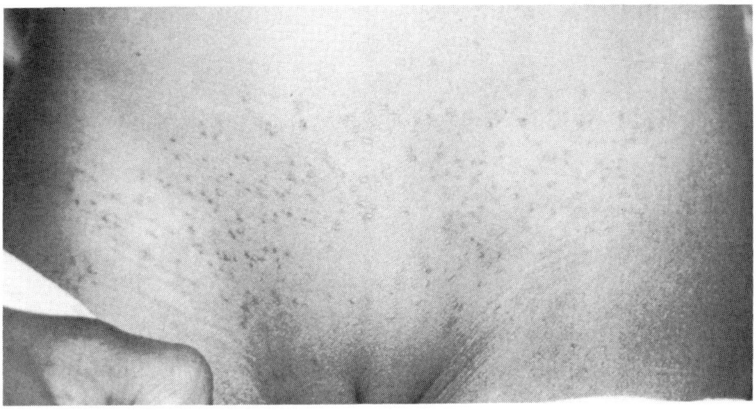

FIGURE 7–21
Multiple syringomas. Numerous small, skin-colored papules scattered over the lower abdomen and groin of an 8-year-old girl. Her mother had involvement of the torso.

McK 186600

Hashimoto K, Blum D, Fukaya T, et al. Familial syringoma: case history and application of monoclonal anti-eccrine gland antibodies. Arch Dermatol 1985;121:756–760

Ribera M, Servitje O, Peyri J, et al. Familial syringoma clinically suggesting milia. [Letter]. J Am Acad Dermatol 1989; 20:702–703

Yesudian P, Thambiah A. Familial syringoma. Dermatologica 1975;150:32–35

NICOLAU-BALUS SYNDROME

vermiculate atrophoderma on cheeks from early infancy

eruptive syringomas and milia on trunk and extremities

AD

Dupré A, Carrère S, Bonafé J, et al. Syringomes éruptifs géneralisés, grains de milium et atrophodermie vermiculée. Dermatologica 1981;162:281–286

Nicolau SG, Balus L. Sur un cas de génodermatose polydysplasique. Ann Dermatol Venereol 1961;88:385–396

BUSCHKE-OLLENDORFF SYNDROME

Synonym

- dermatofibrosis lenticularis disseminata

Skin

yellowish papules, plaques, and nodules distributed symmetrically over back, buttocks, arms, and thighs

may be confluent, forming cobblestone plaques or streaks, especially in antecubital or popliteal fossae; rarely, lesions are solitary

onset in early childhood to postpubertal period; rarely, present at birth

Non-Skin

osteopoikilosis of epiphyses and metaphyses, usually of long bones; no associated symptoms; may be present at birth, and no further changes occur after puberty

rare supernumerary ribs and vertebrae

precocious puberty reported

Genetics

AD

Laboratory Data

radiographs disclose osteopoikilosis (round densities in long bones)

cutaneous lesions are best classified as connective tissue nevi with thickened, branching dermal elastic fibers histopathologically

Discussion

within a family, skin lesions may occur without osteopoikilosis, and vice versa

REFERENCES

McK 166700

Atherton DJ, Wells RS. Juvenile elastoma and osteopoikilosis (the Buschke-Ollendorff syndrome). Clin Exp Dermatol 1982; 7:109–113

Cole GW, Barr RJ. An elastic tissue defect in dermatofibrosis lenticularis disseminata: Buschke-Ollendorff syndrome. Arch Dermatol 1982;118:44–46

Schorr WF, Opitz JM, Reyes CN. The connective tissue nevus–osteopoikilosis syndrome. Arch Dermatol 1972;106:208–214

Trattner A, David M, Rothem A, et al. Buschke-Ollendorff syndrome of the scalp: histologic and ultrastructural findings. J Am Acad Dermatol 1991;24:822–824

Uitto J, Santa Cruz DJ, Starcher BC, et al. Biochemical and ultrastructural demonstration of elastin accumulation in the skin lesions of the Buschke-Ollendorff syndrome. J Invest Dermatol 1981;76:284–287

FAMILIAL CUTANEOUS COLLAGENOMA

Synonyms

- familial connective tissue nevi
- cardiomyopathy-hypogonadism-collagenoma syndrome

Skin

asymptomatic but potentially disfiguring collagenous nodules (from a few millimeters to several centimeters in size) symmetrically distributed on trunk and upper arms, mostly on upper two thirds of the back

onset in adolescence

may have marked increase in number of nodules during pregnancy

Non-Skin

cardiac abnormalities including cardiomyopathy

other abnormalities include hypogonadism, testicular failure, and deafness

Genetics

AD

Laboratory Data

histopathology: accumulations of dense, coarse, hypocellular collagen bundles in dermis

Discussion

these lesions can be thought of as multiple connective tissue nevi of the collagen type; absence of osteopoikilosis allows separation from Buschke-Ollendorff syndrome

REFERENCES

McK 115250

Henderson RR, Wheeler CE Jr, Abele DC. Familial cutaneous collagenoma: report of cases. Arch Dermatol 1968;98:23–27

Sacks HN, Crawley IS, Ward JA, et al. Familial cardiomyopathy, hypogonadism, and collagenoma. Ann Intern Med 1980;93:813–817

Smith LR, Bernstein BD. Eruptive collagenoma. Arch Dermatol 1978;114:1710–1711

Uitto J, Santa Cruz DJ, Eisen AZ. Familial cutaneous collagenoma: genetic studies on a family. Br J Dermatol 1979;101:185–195

JUVENILE HYALINE FIBROMATOSIS

Synonym

- mesenchymal dysplasia

Skin

multiple cutaneous papules, nodules, and tumors, several millimeters to 5 cm in size; usually noted between 2 and 5 years of age, rarely before 2 months of age

involvement of head, back, and extremities, with special predilection for nose, ear, scalp, and knees

new lesions may continue to appear into adulthood, although most form in childhood; lesions do not spontaneously resolve

gingival thickening in most

slow, painless progression

Non-Skin

flexion contractures, which usually appear before skin lesions, are prominent in almost all patients

poorly developed musculature and muscle weakness

punched-out osteolytic lesions of bone in half of patients, especially long bones and phalanges

intelligence normal in most

Genetics

AR; clear documentation of inheritance lacking in many reports; many sporadic cases

Pathophysiology

exact biochemical nature of the amorphous deposits undetermined

Laboratory Data

characteristic histopathologic features of spindle cells embedded in a homogeneous eosinophilic matrix (lacks well-formed collagen fibers); resembles cartilage

Prognosis

a very disfiguring disease with physical disabilities due to deformities and contractures

effective treatment lacking; radiation therapy is not helpful, and surgical removal of fibrous lesions is difficult because of adherence to tendons

REFERENCES

McK 228600
Camarasa JG, Moreno A. Juvenile hyaline fibromatosis. J Am Acad Dermatol 1987;16:881–883
Fayad MN, Yacoub A, Salman S, et al. Juvenile hyaline fibromatosis: two new patients and review of the literature. Am J Med Genet 1987;26:123–131
Kan AE, Rogers M. Juvenile hyaline fibromatosis: an expanded clinicopathologic spectrum. Pediatr Dermatol 1989;6:68–75
Puretic S, Puretic B, Fiser-Herman M, Adamcic M. A unique form of mesenchymal dysplasia. Br J Dermatol 1962;74:8–19
Quintal D, Jackson R. Juvenile hyaline fibromatosis: a 15-year follow-up. Arch Dermatol 1985;121:1062–1063
Remberger K, Krieg T, Kunze D, et al. Fibromatosis hyalinica multiplex (juvenile hyalin fibromatosis): light microscopic, electron microscopic, immunohistochemical, and biochemical findings. Cancer 1985; 56:614–624

INFANTILE SYSTEMIC HYALINOSIS

diffusely thickened, inflexible skin in infancy

papules on face, trunk, and perianal skin

hyperpigmentation over metacarpophalangeal joints of hands and malleoli

gingival hyperplasia

frequent severe infections

persistent diarrhea and failure to thrive

painful joint contractures

AR

widespread deposition of hyaline material in skin and internal organs

death in infancy or early childhood

some consider this a severe form of juvenile hyaline fibromatosis

McK 236490
Bedford CD, Sills JA, Sommelet-Olive D, et al. Juvenile hyaline fibromatosis: a report of two severe cases. J Pediatr 1991;119:404–410
Glover MT, Lake BD, Atherton DJ. Clinical, histologic and ultrastructural findings in two cases of infantile systemic hyalinosis. Pediatr Dermatol 1992;9:255–258
Glover MT, Lake BD, Atherton DJ. Infantile systemic hyalinosis: newly recognized disorder of collagen? Pediatrics 1991;87:228–234
Landing BH, Nadorra R. Infantile systemic hyalinosis. Pediatr Pathol 1986;6:55–97

DERMOCHONDROCORNEAL DYSTROPHY (FRANÇOIS SYNDROME)

cutaneous nodules of hands and face with variable onset in first decade; gingival involvement reported osteochondrodystrophy of bones of hands and feet; limitation of joint mobility

bilateral corneal opacities

AR

histopathology: increased collagen, decreased elastic tissue, and vacuolized histiocytic cells in dermis

McK 221800

Caputo R, Sambvani N, Monti M, et al. Dermochondrocorneal dystrophy (François' syndrome): report of a case. Arch Dermatol 1988;124:424–428

François J. Distrophie dermo-chondro-cornéenne familiale. Ann Oculist 1949; 182:409–441

INFANTILE MYOFIBROMATOSIS (CONGENITAL GENERALIZED FIBROMATOSIS; CONGENITAL MULTIPLE FIBROMATOSIS; SOLITARY CONGENITAL FIBROMATOSIS)

nodules in skin (Fig. 7–22), subcutis, muscle, bone, and internal organs, which are usually solitary but sometimes multiple

onset usually at birth or in first few weeks of life

most sporadic; some AR and AD cases reported

lesions caused by proliferation of myofibroblasts

patients with lesions confined to soft tissue and bone usually have a good prognosis; spontaneous remission may occur or lesions can be excised; patients with multiple visceral lesions have poor prognosis

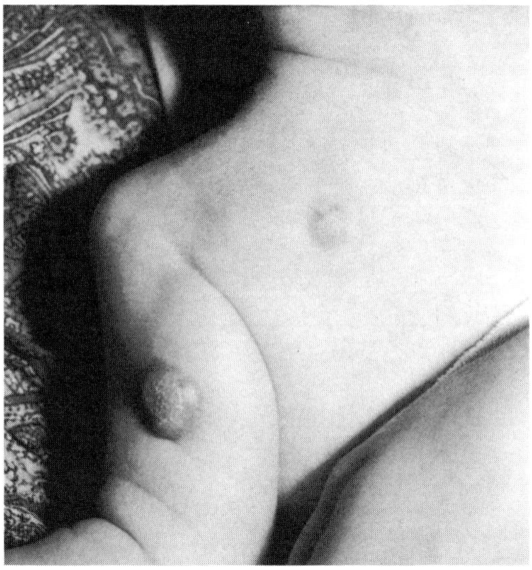

FIGURE 7–22

Two nodules on the arm and back in an infant with infantile myofibromatosis. Note the resemblance to hemangiomas.

McK 228550
Chung EB, Enzinger FM. Infantile myofibromatosis. Cancer 1981;48:1807–1818
Venencie PY, Bigel P, Desgruelles C, et al. Infantile myofibromatosis: report of two cases in one family. Br J Dermatol 1987;117:255–259
Wiswell TE, Davis J, Cunningham BE, et al. Infantile myofibromatosis: the most common fibrous tumor of infancy. J Pediatr 1988;23:314–318
Wiswell TE, Sakas EL, Stephenson SR, et al. Infantile myofibromatosis. Pediatrics 1985; 76:981–984

FAMILIAL HISTIOCYTIC DERMATOARTHRITIS

multiple erythematous nodules of face and limbs with onset in first or second decade

destructive symmetrical arthritis, predominantly of hands and wrists

ocular findings include glaucoma, uveitis, and cataracts

possible AD

McK 142730
Valente M, Parenti A, Cipriani R, Peserico A. Familial histiocytic dermatoarthritis: histologic and ultrastructural findings in two cases. Am J Dermatopathol 1987;9:491–496
Zayid I, Farraj S. Familial histiocytic dermatoarthritis: a new syndrome. Am J Med 1973;54:793–800

GRANULOMATOUS SYNOVITIS, UVEITIS, AND CRANIAL NEUROPATHIES (JABS SYNDROME; FAMILIAL GRANULOMATOUS ARTHRITIS, IRITIS, AND RASH)

widespread papular eruption

joint, eye, and nerve involvement

AD

histopathology: noncaseating granulomas in biopsy specimens of cutaneous and noncutaneous lesions

may be confused with sarcoidosis

McK 186580
Blau EB. Familial granulomatous arthritis, iritis, and rash. J Pediatr 1985,107:689–693
Jabs DA, Houk JL, Bias WB, Arnett FC. Familial granulomatous synovitis, uveitis, and cranial neuropathies. Am J Med 1985,78:801–804
Pastores GM, Michels VV, Stickler GB, et al. Autosomal dominant granulomatous arthritis, uveitis, skin rash, and synovial cysts. J Pediatr 1990;117:403–408

HEREDITARY PROGRESSIVE MUCINOUS HISTIOCYTOSIS

slowly progressive eruption of multiple pea-sized nodules on face, trunk, and extremities appearing in late childhood

bleeding into nodules after minor trauma is excessive

probable AD

increased acid mucopolysaccharide deposition in lesions; resembles focal mucinosis histopathologically in older lesions

a non–Langerhans cell histiocytosis

McK 142630

Bork K, Hoede N. Hereditary progressive mucinous histiocytosis in women: report of three members in a family. Arch Dermatol 1988;124:1225–1229

MULTIPLE CUTANEOUS LEIOMYOMATA

Skin

multiple (few to several hundred) 2- to 12-mm nodules in an arciform or linear arrangement, most commonly on the extensor surfaces of the extremities, as well as the trunk, face, and neck (Fig. 7–23)

lesions may appear from infancy to seventh decade and increase in size and number with age

one third of cases are unilateral

paroxysms of pain may occur later in course

rare malignant transformation reported

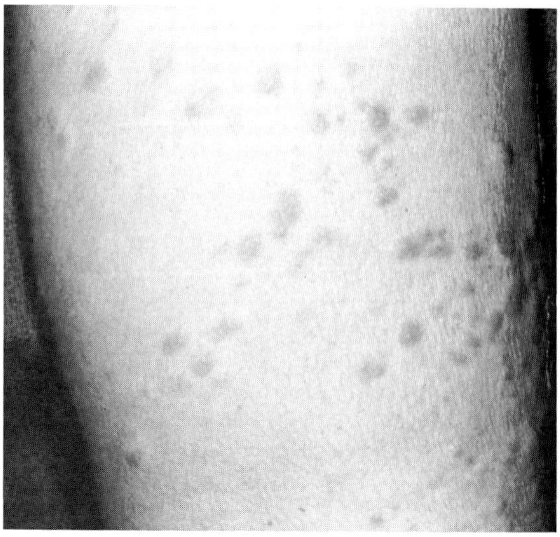

FIGURE 7–23
Multiple cutaneous leiomyomas. Numerous red papulonodules scattered over the forearm, some in linear array.

Non-Skin

occasional multiple uterine leiomyomata

Genetics

AD

Pathophysiology

lesions arise from arrectores pilorum muscle

Prognosis

surgically excised lesions may recur

pain relief with nitroglycerin and nifedipine reported

Discussion

solitary or multiple leiomyomata that arise from arrectores pilorum muscle are tender and sometimes painful, whereas leiomyomata arising from dartoic muscles are rarely painful

REFERENCES

McK 150800

Fisher WC, Helwig EB. Leiomyomas of the skin. Arch Dermatol 1963;88:510–520

Reed WB, Walker R, Horowitz R. Cutaneous leiomyomata with uterine leiomyomata. Acta Derm Venereol 1973;53:409–416

FAMILIAL URTICARIA PIGMENTOSA

Skin

usually symmetrical, orange-brown papulonodules most frequently found on trunk and extremities but may be found elsewhere; may be single or multiple

lesions may have onset in infancy, childhood, or adulthood

when lesions are stroked, urticaria develops in lesions (Darier sign)

occasional flushing episodes

Genetics

AD and AR cases reported

Discussion

most cases of urticaria pigmentosa are nonfamilial

REFERENCES

McK 154800
Anstey A, Lowe DG, Kirby JD, Horton MA. Familial mastocytosis: a clinical, immunophenotypic, light and electron microscopic study. Br J Dermatol 1991;125:583–587
Fowler JF Jr, Parsley WM, Cotter PG. Familial urticaria pigmentosa. Arch Dermatol 1986;122:80–81
James MP, Eady RA. Familial urticaria pigmentosa with giant mast cell granules: a clinical, light, and electron microscopic study. Arch Dermatol 1981;117:713–718
Shaw JM. Genetic aspects of urticaria pigmentosa. Arch Dermatol 1968;97:137–138

FAMILIAL MULTIPLE LIPOMATOSIS

Synonym

- hereditary lipomatosis

Skin

multiple discrete, encapsulated lipomas, several millimeters to 6 cm in size (occasionally larger) symmetrically distributed on trunk, arms, forearms (most frequent location), and thighs but sparing the neck and shoulders; may occur elsewhere, even in mouth and gastrointestinal tract

lesions are usually noted in third decade but can develop up to the fifth decade and initially grow rapidly, then stabilize

pain is rare but may be noted in early growth phase

rare malignant degeneration

Genetics

AD

male to female ratio: 2:1

REFERENCES

McK 151900
Dolph JL, Demuth RJ, Miller SH. Familial multiple lipomatosis. Plast Reconstr Surg 1980;66:620–622
Leffell DJ, Braverman IM. Familial multiple lipomatosis: report of a case and a review of the literature. J Am Acad Dermatol 1986;15:275–279
Mohar N. Familial multiple lipomatosis. Acta Derm Venereol 1980;60:509–513
Rabbiosi G, Borroni G, Scuderi N. Familial multiple lipomatosis. Acta Derm Venereol 1977;57:265–267

MULTIPLE SYMMETRICAL LIPOMATOSIS

Synonyms

- benign symmetrical lipomatosis

- Madelung disease
- Launois-Bensaude syndrome

Skin

symmetrical fat deposits with two different patterns

type 1 has a predominantly circumscribed "horse-collar" distribution (neck and shoulder girdle) with reduction or atrophy of univolved adipose tissue (Fig. 7–24)

type 2 manifests a more diffuse pattern of lipomatosis while sparing the distal extremities, hands, and feet; the latter finding helps to distinguish patients with type 2 from those with simple obesity

onset in adulthood, usually later than in familial multiple lipomatosis

Non-Skin

most patients have peripheral motor, sensory, and autonomic neuropathies

Genetics

mostly sporadic but familial cases reported

male to female ratio: 4:1 to 15:1

Pathophysiology

may be related to a localized defect in catecholamine-induced lipolysis associated with alcoholism or other factors

Discussion

later onset, different sites of involvement, and lack of encapsulation help distinguish these tumors from familial multiple lipomatosis

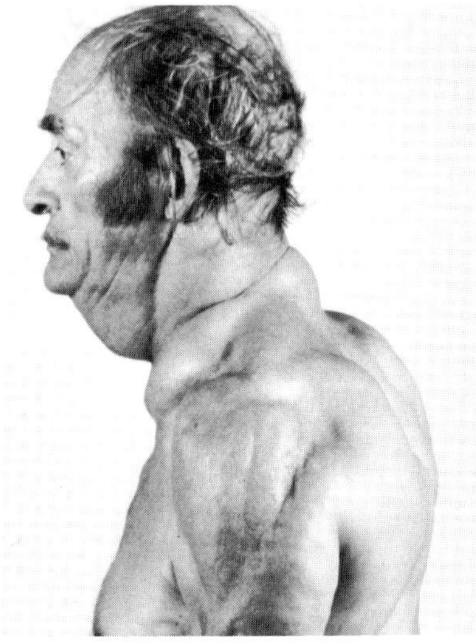

FIGURE 7–24
Benign symmetrical lipomatosis. Extensive fatty deposits about the neck and shoulder girdle.

REFERENCES

McK 151800

Enzi G. Multiple symmetric lipomatosis: an updated clinical report. Medicine 1984;63:56–64

Findlay GH, Duvenage M. Acquired symmetrical lipomatosis of the hands—a distal form of the Madelung-Launois-Bensaude syndrome. Clin Exp Dermatol 1989;14:58–59

Ruzicka T, Vieluf D, Landthaler M, et al. Benign symmetric lipomatosis Launois-Bensaude: report of ten cases and review of the literature. [Review]. J Am Acad Dermatol 1987;17:663–674

DERCUM DISEASE (ADIPOSIS DOLOROSA)

tender fatty tumors involve the trunk and limbs, sparing the face and hands

onset in adulthood, mostly in obese postmenopausal women

mostly sporadic but some familial cases reported

pain may be relieved for weeks to months by a single infusion of intravenous lidocaine

McK 103200

Bonatus TJ, Alexander AH. Dercum's disease (adiposis dolorosa): a case report and review of the literature. Clin Orthop 1986;1205:251–253

Petersen P, Kastrup J. Dercum's disease (adiposis dolorosa): treatment of the severe pain with intravenous lidocaine. Pain 1987;28:77–80

MICHELIN-TIRE BABY (FOLDED SKIN WITH LIPOMATOUS NEVUS)

generalized increased folding of skin with increased underlying fatty tissue is usually present at birth (Fig. 7–25)

possible spontaneous improvement

mostly sporadic, but AD cases reported

cases without underlying lipomatous nevi reported

probably represents many entities; has been associated with underlying lipomatosis, smooth muscle hamartomas and idiopathic scarring; when isolated, has been called multiple benign annular creases

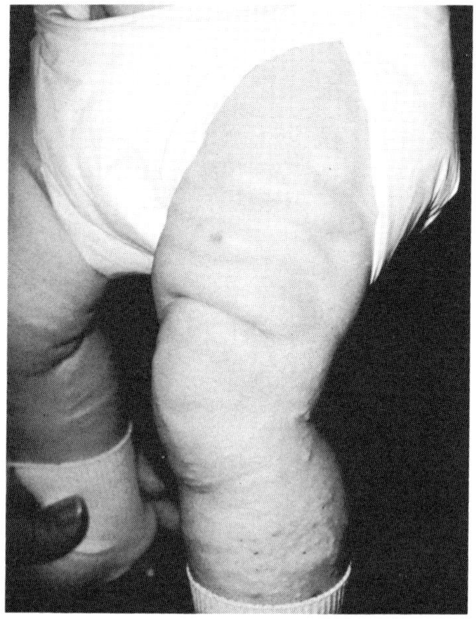

FIGURE 7–25
Michelin-tire baby. Numerous folds of fat are seen on the legs.

McK 156610
Burgdorf WHC, Doran CK, Worret WI. Folded skin with scarring: Michelin tire baby syndrome? J Am Acad Dermatol 1982;7:90–93
Glover MT, Malone M, Atherton DJ. Michelin-tire baby syndrome resulting from diffuse smooth muscle hamartoma. [Review]. Pediatr Dermatol 1989;6:329–331
Kunze J. The "Michelin tire baby syndrome": an autosomal dominant trait. [Letter]. Am J Med Genet 1986;25:169–171
Niikawa N, Ishikiriyama S, Shikimani T. The "Michelin tire baby" syndrome—an autosomal dominant trait. [Letter]. Am J Med Genet 1985;22:637–638
Ross CM. Generalized folded skin with an underlying lipomatous nevus: "the Michelin tire baby." Arch Dermatol 1969;100:320–323

MULTIPLE ANGIOLIPOMAS

subcutaneous tumors of extremities and trunk often appearing shortly after puberty

frequently painful

usually sporadic but AR cases reported

patients with familial multiple lipomatosis may also have multiple angiolipomas

McK 206550
Belcher RW, Czarnetzki BM, Carney JF, et al. Multiple (subcutaneous) angiolipomas: clinical, pathologic, and pharmacologic studies. Arch Dermatol 1974;110:583–585
Hapnes SA, Boman H, Skeie SO. Familial angiolipomatosis. Clin Genet 1980;17:202–208
Heymann WR, Fiorillo A, Simons J. Eruptive familial angiolipomas occurring during pregnancy. Cutis 1988;42:525–526

Tumors and Proliferative Disorders—Abbreviated Entries

JUVENILE COLLOID MILIUM

translucent yellowish brown papules on nose, upper lip, and upper cheeks; posterior neck and dorsa of hands may be involved

onset before puberty

probable AR

pathogenesis unknown; far more common acquired type of colloid milium, associated with prolonged sun exposure; occurs in adulthood

Handfield-Jones SE, Atherton D, Black MM. Juvenile colloid milium. Br J Dermatol 1991;125(suppl 38):80–81

Handfield-Jones SE, Atherton DJ, Black MM, Hashimoto K, McKee PH. Juvenile colloid milium: clinical, histological and ultrastructural features. J Cutan Pathol 1992;19:434–438

Hashimoto K, Nakayama H, Chimenti S, et al. Juvenile colloid milium: immunohistochemical and ultrastructural studies. J Cutan Pathol 1989;16:164–174

CUTANEOUS NODULES WITH URINARY TRACT ABNORMALITIES

0.5- to 2-cm nodules on lower extremities

hydronephrosis and urinary tract abnormalities

AD

histopathology: epidermal hyperkeratosis and acanthosis overlying spindle cell proliferation and increased collagen in dermis

McK 163850

Gelfarb M, Hyman AB. Multiple noduli cutanei. Arch Dermatol 1962;85:89–94

Selmanowitz VJ, Lerer WN, Orentreich N. Multiple noduli cutanei and urinary tract abnormalities: a possible significant association. Cancer 1970;26:1256–1260

CHAPTER

8

Dysplasias and Malformations

A wide spectrum of disorders have been classified in this chapter under the rubric of dysplasias and malformation syndromes. The etiologies of these disorders are unknown in most instances, and their nosology is controversial. We have, therefore, for practical purposes, divided these complicated entities into two groups: (1) those with abnormalities of structure originating primarily from ectoderm and (2) those with malformations of structures derived from more than one of the three germ layers.

Ectodermal Dysplasias

Ectodermal dysplasias are a heterogeneous group of conditions that are difficult to classify and whose etiologies are poorly understood. Various schemata have been used to classify ectodermal dysplasias, such as the "1–2–3–4" system of Freire-Maia and Pinhiero. In this system, the ectodermal dysplasias are classified by the clinical findings of

1. hair abnormalities
2. dental defects
3. nail abnormalities
4. sweating abnormalities

Although this schema is not perfect, categorization does allow cases to be compared more readily.

The most common hereditary ectodermal dysplasia syndromes are listed in fuller detail and presented first. Less common hereditary ectodermal dysplasias follow and are grouped by their "1–2–3–4" classification. We have not included nonhereditary ectodermal dysplasias or the large number of syndromes in which dental defects are the only ectodermal manifestation.

REFERENCES

Freire-Maia N, Pinhiero M. Ectodermal Dysplasia: A Clinical and Genetic Study. New York, Alan R. Liss, 1984

Salinas CF, Opitz JM, Paul NW, eds. Recent advances in ectodermal dysplasias. Birth Defects 1988;24(2)

HYPOHIDROTIC ECTODERMAL DYSPLASIA

Synonyms

- Christ-Siemens-Touraine syndrome
- anhidrotic ectodermal dysplasia

Skin

manifestations present from birth

sparse, fine, fair scalp hair (hypotrichosis); sparse eyebrows and eyelashes, especially laterally; mustache and beard hair usually normal in distribution and texture

diffuse scaling of skin in newborn (appears "post mature"); may be an early clue to diagnosis

wrinkling and darkening of periorbital skin (Fig. 8–1)

sweat and mucous glands are absent or greatly reduced in number; decreased number of sweat pores on epidermal ridges

atopy and xerosis common

nails are usually normal

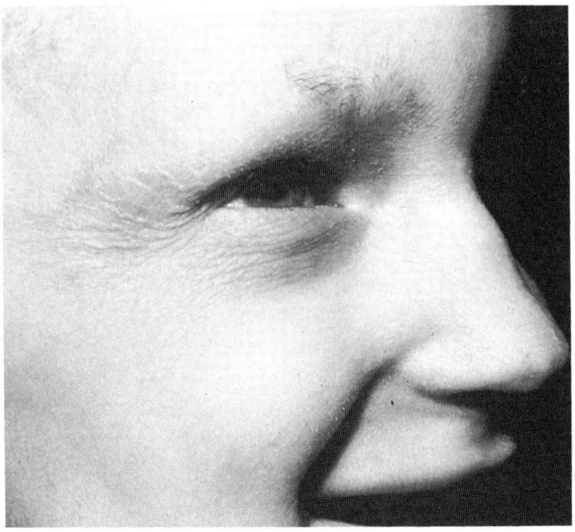

FIGURE 8–1
Fine wrinkling and hyperpigmentation around the eyes of a boy with hypohidrotic ectodermal dysplasia.

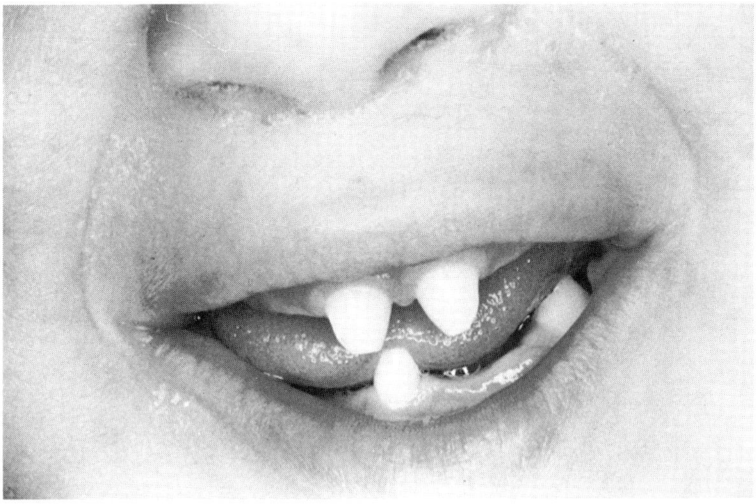

FIGURE 8–2
Partial anodontia with abnormally shaped teeth in a child with hypohidrotic ectodermal dysplasia.

both deciduous and permanent teeth are reduced in number and malformed, typically being cone-shaped or peg-shaped; occasional delayed eruption (Fig. 8–2)

Non-Skin

initial sign may be intermittent fever in first weeks of life owing to impaired heat regulation; hyperpyrexia may result in seizures

distinctive facies recognizable by as early as 1 year of age; features include prominent frontal bossing and supraorbital ridges, protruding ears, eyes with a mongolian slant, depressed nasal bridge, hypoplasia of midface, large nostrils, pseudorhagades, and prominent lips with lack of lip support because of hypodontia or anodontia (Fig. 8–3)

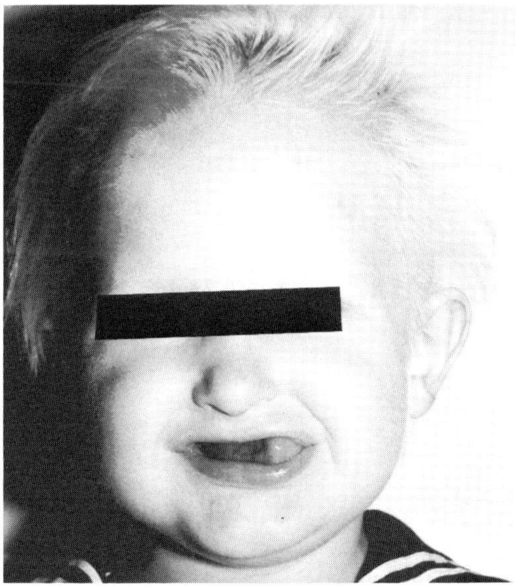

FIGURE 8–3
Typical facies of a boy wtih hypohidrotic ectodermal dysplasia showing the depressed nasal bridge and prominent forehead, chin, and ears. Note light-colored, fly-away hair and absence of teeth.

normal intelligence

occasional hypoplastic or absent areolae and nipples

short stature is common; may be result of failure to thrive

absence of mucous glands may lead to otitis, pharyngitis, hoarseness, rhinitis and nasal crusting (which may cause feeding difficulties in infants), destruction of the nasal septum, decreased senses of taste and smell, increased incidence of respiratory infections, and chronic obstructive airway disease

eye abnormalities include decreased tearing and photophobia

Genetics

XLR

rare AD and AR (McKusick 224900) forms reported, but their validity has been challenged

purported examples of AR hypohidrotic ectodermal dysplasia possibly explained by marked lyonization

Laboratory Data

jaw radiographs in infants with fever of unknown origin suspected of this diagnosis may be useful, since dental abnormalities (e.g., absent tooth buds) may be detected

decreased sweat secretion (including in carriers) determined by starch-iodine or iontophoretic methods

identification of gene defect (localized to chromosome Xq) makes carrier detection and prenatal diagnosis feasible

Prognosis

up to 30% mortality in infancy or early childhood due to severe illnesses including hyperpyrexia, sepsis, respiratory infections, and failure to thrive

following early childhood, growth and development proceed more normally and mortality and morbidity are greatly reduced

early diagnosis may help prevent heat intolerance and allow for favorable influence on ultimate height obtained

patients should avoid smoking because of already increased risk for chronic obstructive airway disease

Discussion

about 70% of heterozygote females have clinical manifestations including hypohidrosis (e.g., patchy areas of decreased sweating), hypotrichosis, hypodontia or conical teeth, and breast abnormalities; manifestations are usually minor, but severe cases have been reported with findings including respiratory infections, failure to thrive in infancy, and heat intolerance; dental abnormalities are the most helpful indicators of the carrier state

REFERENCES

McK 305100

Berg D, Weingold DH, Abson KG, Olsen EA. Sweating in ectodermal dysplasia syndromes. Arch Dermatol 1990;126;1075–1079

Clarke A, Burn J. Sweat testing to identify carriers of X linked hypohidrotic ectodermal dysplasia. J Med Genet 1991;28:330–333

Clarke A, Phillips DI, Brown R, et al. Clinical aspects of X-linked hypohidrotic ectodermal dysplasia. Arch Dis Child 1987; 62:989–996

Clarke A. Hypohidrotic ectodermal dysplasia. J Med Genet 1987;24:659–663

Crawford PJM, Aldred MJ, Clarke A. Clinical and radiographic dental findings in X-linked hypohidrotic ectodermal dysplasia. J Med Genet 1991;28:181–185

Executive and Scientific Advisory Boards, National Foundation for Ectodermal Dysplasias. Scaling skin in the neonate: a clue to the early diagnosis of X-linked hypohidrotic ectodermal dysplasia (Christ-Siemens-Touraine syndrome). J Pediatr 1989;114:600–602

Gilgenkrantz S, Blanchet-Bardon C, Nazzaro V, et al. Hypohidrotic ectodermal dysplasia: clinical study of a family of 30 over three generations. Hum Genet 1989;81: 120–122

Passarge E, Fries E. X chromosome inactivation in X-linked hypohidrotic ectodermal dysplasia. Nature 1973;245:58–59

Settineri WM, Salzano FM, De Melo E, Freitas MJ. X-linked anhidrotic ectodermal dysplasia with some unusual features. J Med Genet 1976;13:212–216

Sybert VP. Hypohidrotic ectodermal dysplasia: argument against an autosomal recessive form clinically indistinguishable from X-linked hypohidrotic ectodermal dysplasia (Christ-Siemens-Touraine syndrome). Pediatr Dermatol 1989;6:76–81

Viljoen DL, Winship WS. A new form of hypohidrotic ectodermal dysplasia. Am J Med Genet 1988;31:25–32

Wright JT, Finley WH. X-linked recessive hypohidrotic ectodermal dysplasia: manifestations and management. Ala J Med Sci 1986;23:84–87

Zonana J, Clarke A, Sarfarazi M, et al. X-linked hypohidrotic ectodermal dysplasia: localization within the region Xq11-21.1 by linkage analysis and implications for carrier detection and prenatal diagnosis. Am J Hum Genet 1988;43:75–85

RAPP-HODGKIN HYPOHIDROTIC ECTODERMAL DYSPLASIA

Skin

sparse, fair scalp and eyebrow hair with a "steel wool" texture; eyelashes and body hair also sparse

occasional pili torti or pili canaliculi

recalcitrant, crusted, inflammatory scalp dermatitis in some (Fig. 8–4); may cause scarring alopecia

hypohidrosis; may cause heat intolerance

hypoplastic dermatoglyphics

narrow, dystrophic nails

teeth decreased in number and often conical; prone to caries

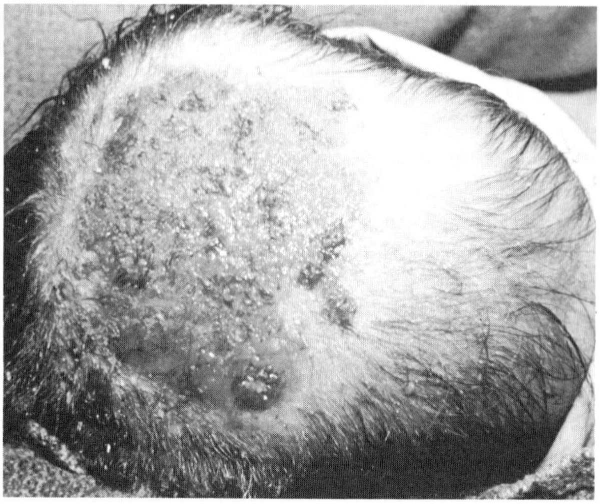

FIGURE 8–4
Rapp-Hodgkin hypohidrotic ectodermal dysplasia. Chronic exudative inflammatory dermatitis of the scalp with alopecia.

Non-Skin

abnormal craniofacies including cleft lip and palate, prominent forehead, abnormal ears (e.g., cup-shaped), hypoplastic maxilla, narrow nose, foreshortened and widened columella, thin upper lip, small mouth, and hypoplastic uvula (Fig. 8–5)

occasional minor syndactyly of toes

frequent recurrent otitis media (may be related to abnormal craniofacies)

occasional deafness

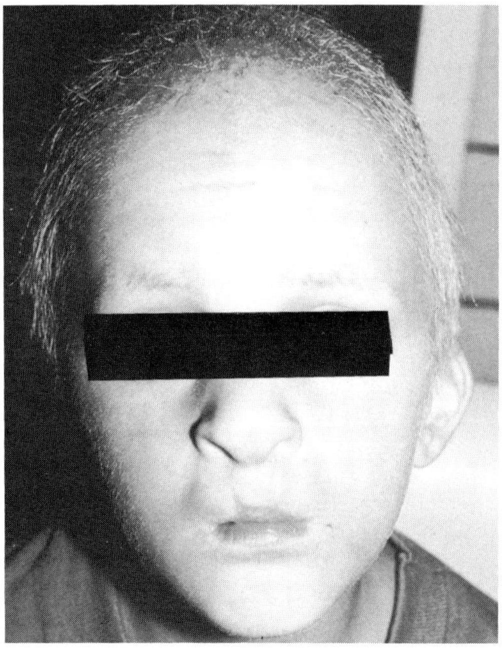

FIGURE 8–5
Characteristic facies of a patient with Rapp-Hodgkin hypohidrotic ectodermal dysplasia: sparse scalp hair and eyebrows, repaired bilateral cleft lip, prominent forehead, and cup-shaped ears.

eye abnormalities including conjunctivitis, epiphora, and absence of lacrimal puncta

occasional hypospadias

Genetics

probable AD

Laboratory Data

scanning electron microscopy of hair shafts: longitudinal twisting and canal-like depressions

REFERENCES

McK 129400

Crawford PJ, Aldred MJ, Clarke A, et al. Rapp-Hodgkin syndrome: an ectodermal dysplasia involving the teeth, hair, nails, and palate: report of a case and review of the literature. Oral Surg 1989;67:50–62

Felding IB, Björklund LJ. Rapp-Hodgkin ectodermal dysplasia. Pediatr Dermatol 1990;7:126–131

O'Donnell BP, James WD. Rapp-Hodgkin ectodermal dysplasia. J Am Acad Dermatol 1992;27:323–326

Rodini EOS, Freitas JAS, Richieri-Costa A. Rapp-Hodgkin syndrome: report of a Brazilian family. Am J Med Genet 1990; 36:463–466

Salinas CF, Montes GM. Rapp-Hodgkin syndrome: observations on ten cases and characteristic hair changes (pili canaliculi). Birth Defects 1988;24:149–168

Schroeder HWJ, Sybert VP. Rapp-Hodgkin ectodermal dysplasia. J Pediatr 1987; 110:72–75

Silengo MC, Davi GF, Bianco R, et al. Distinctive hair changes (pili torti) in Rapp-Hodgkin ectodermal dysplasia syndrome. Clin Genet 1982;21:297–300

Walpole IR, Goldblatt J. Rapp-Hodgkin hypohidrotic ectodermal dysplasia syndrome. Clin Genet 1991;39:114–120

HIDROTIC ECTODERMAL DYSPLASIA

Synonyms

- Clouston syndrome
- French Canadian ectodermal dysplasia

Skin

scalp hypotrichosis ranges from mild to complete alopecia and is usually present from birth; hair, when present, is thin and fragile; eyebrows, eyelashes, and body hair may be sparse or absent

palmoplantar keratoderma

knuckles, elbows, and nipples may be markedly hyperpigmented

squamous cell carcinoma of nail beds or palmar skin reported

white plaques on oral mucosa

nail dystrophy ranges from slight thickening and discoloration to marked scarring and anonychia (Fig. 8–6)

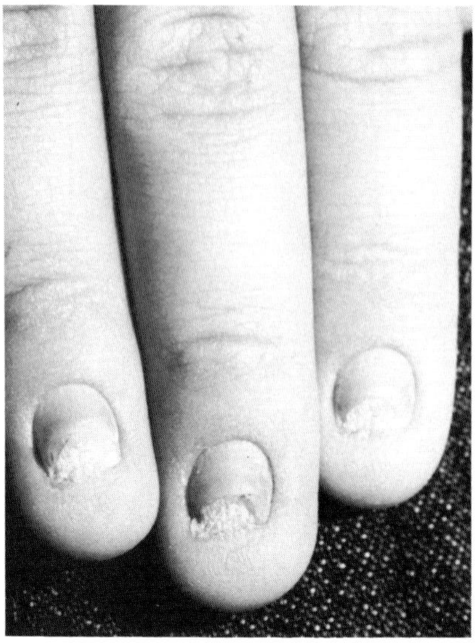

FIGURE 8–6
Thickened foreshortened dystrophic nails of a patient with hidrotic ectodermal dysplasia.

Non-Skin

frequent neurologic defects include mental retardation and stammering

eye abnormalities are common and include pterygium formation and congenital cataracts

Genetics

AD

in North America, increased incidence among French Canadians

Prognosis

hair abnormalities stable, but nail and skin changes may worsen

REFERENCES

McK 129500

Clouston HR. A hereditary ectodermal dystrophy. Can Med Assoc J 1929;21:18–31

George DI Jr, Escobar VH. Oral findings of Clouston's syndrome (hidrotic ectodermal dysplasia). Oral Surg 1984;57:258–262

Gold RJM, Scriver CR. The characterization of hereditary abnormalities of keratin: Clouston's ectodermal dysplasia. Birth Defects 1971;7:91–95

Hazen PG, Zamora I, Bruner WE, Muir WA. Premature cataracts in a family with hidrotic ectodermal dysplasia. Arch Dermatol 1980;116:1385–1387

Rajagopalan K, Tay CH. Hidrotic ectodermal dysplasia: study of a large Chinese pedigree. Arch Dermatol 1977;113:481–484

Wilkinson RD, Schopflocher P, Rozenfeld M. Hidrotic ectodermal dysplasia with diffuse eccrine poromatosis. Arch Dermatol 1977; 113:472–476

Williams M, Fraser FC. Hydrotic ectodermal dysplasia: Clouston's family revisited. Can Med Assoc J 1967;96:36–38

ECTRODACTYLY, ECTODERMAL DYSPLASIA, AND CLEFT LIP AND PALATE SYNDROME

Synonym

- EEC syndrome

Skin

sparse, fair scalp hair, eyebrows, and eyelashes (Fig. 8–7); absence of pubic and axillary hair reported

occasional xerostomia and fissured tongue

occasional hypohidrosis, diminished sebaceous glands with xerosis, and pigment dilution of skin and hair

nail abnormalities include pitting, ridging, brittleness, and thinning

dental abnormalities include microdontia, enamel hypoplasia, and increased caries

Non-Skin

cleft lip and/or palate

ectrodactyly (unilateral or bilateral aplasia of the middle ray) results in characteristic "lobster claw" deformity of hands and feet (Fig. 8–8)

lacrimal duct abnormalities (e.g., absent lacrimal puncta) are associated with tearing, blepharitis, dacryocystitis, keratoconjunctivitis, and photophobia; occasional corneal ulcers and scarring

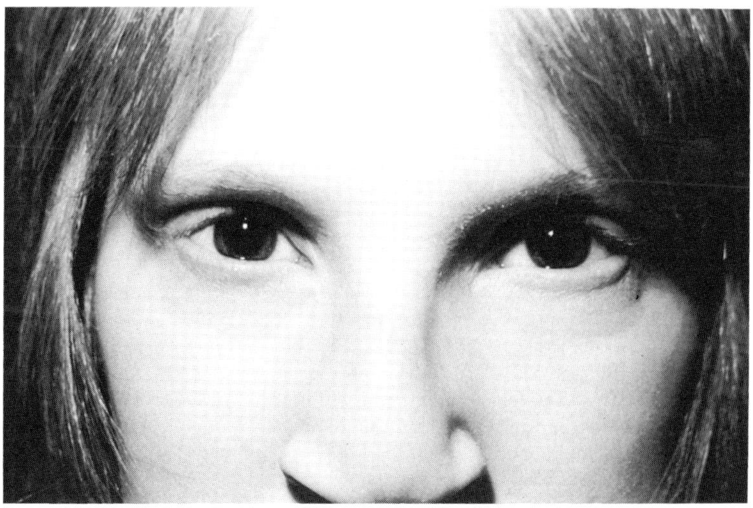

FIGURE 8–7
Sparse brows and lashes, thickening of the lower lids, and blepharitis in a patient with ectrodactyly, ectodermal dysplasia, and cleft lip and palate syndrome. Characteristic nasal contour for cleft lip and palate may be seen.

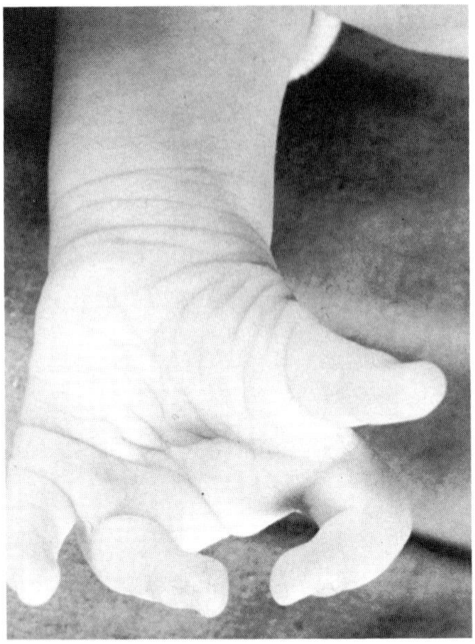

FIGURE 8–8
Characteristic lobster-claw deformity of the hand in a young child with ectrodactyly, ectodermal dysplasia, and cleft lip and palate syndrome. (Courtesy of Lester Weiss, MD, Detroit, Michigan)

occasional deafness, nipple hypoplasia, and renal and genitourinary tract anomalies

Genetics

AD and possible AR cases reported; many sporadic cases

Prognosis

regular ophthalmologic care may prevent chronic dacryocystitis and corneal scarring

Discussion

expressivity is quite variable and no single feature is obligatory (e.g., cleft lip or palate alone or ectrodactyly alone may be the only manifestation)

REFERENCES

McK 129900

McK 129810

Anneren G, Andersson T, Lindgren PG, Kjartansson S. Ectrodactyly-ectodermal dysplasia-clefting syndrome (EEC): the clinical variation and prenatal diagnosis. Clin Genet 1991;40:257–262

Majewski F, Kuster W. EEC syndrome sine sine? Report of a family with oligosymptomatic EEC syndrome. Clin Genet 1988; 33:69–72

Nardi AC, Ferreira U, Netto NR, et al. Urinary tract involvement in EEC syndrome: a clinical study in 25 Brazilian patients. Am J Med Genet 1992;44:803–806

Rodini ES, Richieri-Costa A. EEC syndrome: report on 20 new patients, clinical and genetic considerations. Am J Med Genet 1990;37:42–53

Rosenmann A, Shapira T, Cohen MM. Ectrodactyly, ectodermal dysplasia and cleft palate (EEC syndrome): report of a family and review of the literature. Clin Genet 1976;9:347–353

Wallis CE. Ectrodactyly (split-hand/split-foot) and ectodermal dysplasia with normal lip and palate in a four-generation kindred. Clin Genet 1988;34:252–257

AEC SYNDROME

Synonyms

- ankyloblepharon, ectodermal dysplasia, and cleft lip and palate syndrome
- Hay-Wells syndrome

Skin

ankyloblepharon filiforme adnatum (congenital adhesion of the margins of the upper and lower eyelids by fibrous bands); rudimentary eyelashes

coarse, sparse, wiry scalp hair; eyebrows also affected

recalcitrant, crusted inflammatory scalp dermatitis in some (Fig. 8–9); may cause scarring alopecia

hypohidrosis

occasional palmoplantar keratoderma

absent or dystrophic nails (Fig. 8–10)

hypodontia, anodontia, or pointed and widely spaced teeth; may erode or be lost

facial and nail changes at birth; other findings develop later in infancy

Non-Skin

craniofacial abnormalities include broad nasal bridge and sunken, hypoplastic maxilla

cleft palate and rarely cleft lip

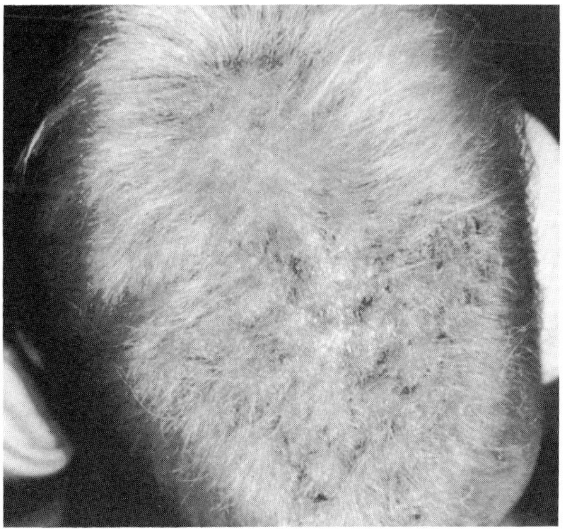

FIGURE 8–9
Chronic inflammatory dermatitis of the scalp associated with alopecia in a patient with ankyloblepharon, ectodermal dysplasia, and cleft lip and palate syndrome. (Courtesy of Tor Shwayder, MD, Detroit, Michigan)

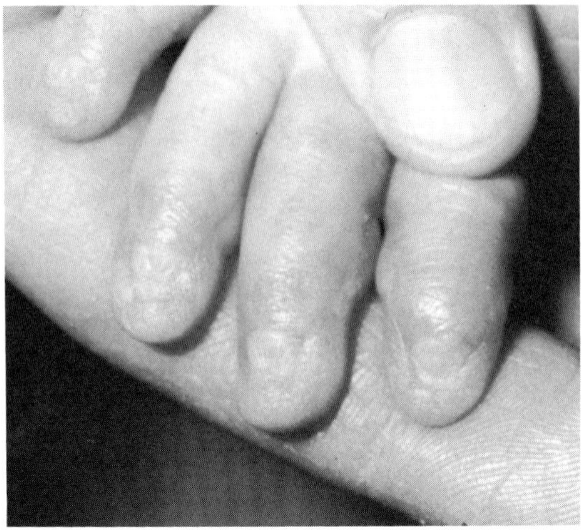

FIGURE 8–10
Ankyloblepharon, ectodermal dysplasia, and cleft lip and palate syndrome. Same infant as in Figure 8–9. The nails are hypoplastic and dystrophic. (Courtesy of Tor Shwayder, MD, Detroit, Michigan)

Genetics

AD

Laboratory Data

electron microscopy of hair shaft: longitudinal fluting and focal defects of cuticle

REFERENCES

McK 106260

Greene SL, Michels VV, Doyle JA. Variable expression in ankyloblepharon–ectodermal defects–cleft lip and palate syndrome. Am J Med Genet 1987;27:207–212

Hay RJ, Wells RS. The syndrome of ankyloblepharon, ectodermal defects and cleft lip and palate: an autosomal dominant condition. Br J Dermatol 1976;94:277–289

Shwayder TA, Lane AT, Miller ME. Hay-Wells syndrome. Pediatr Dermatol 1986;3:399–402

Spiegel J, Colton A. AEC syndrome: ankyloblepharon, ectodermal defects, and cleft lip and palate: report of two cases. J Am Acad Dermatol 1985;12:810–815

Ectodermal Dysplasias—Abbreviated Entries

GROUP 1–2 (HAIR–TEETH)

Gorlin-Chaudry-Moss syndrome (craniofacial dysostosis with hypertrichosis and hypodontia)

trichodental syndrome

acrorenal–ectodermal dysplasia–lipoatrophic diabetes syndrome (AREDYLD syndrome) alopecia-anosmia-deafness-hypogonadism syndrome (Johnson neuroectodermal syndrome)

oculo-osteocutaneous syndrome

taurodontia, absent teeth, sparse hair

Walbaum-Dehaene-Schlemmer syndrome

Mikaelian syndrome (ectodermal dysplasia and neurosensory deafness)

pilodental dysplasia with refractive errors

ectodermal dysplasia, ectrodactyly, and macular dystrophy

ectodermal dysplasia with blindness in sibs on the Island of Rodrigues

GROUP 1–2–3 (HAIR–TEETH–NAILS)

trichodento-osseous syndrome

hair, tooth, and nail syndromes

Witkop tooth-nail syndrome (hypodontia and nail dysgenesis; Witkop syndrome)

tooth and nail syndrome of Fried

odontotrichomelic syndrome (tetramelic ectodermal dysplasia)

odonto-onychodysplasia with alopecia

dento-oculocutaneous syndrome

dermo-odontodysplasia

oculotrichodysplasia

cranioectodermal dysplasia (Sensenbrenner syndrome)

GAPO syndrome (growth retardation, alopecia, pseudoanodontia, progressive optic atrophy syndrome)

lacrimo-auriculo-dento-digital syndrome (LADD syndrome; Levy-Hollister syndrome)

ectodermal dysplasia, Margarita type

ectodermal dysplasia with corkscrew hairs

GROUP 1–2–3–4 (HAIR–TEETH–NAILS–SWEATING)

Rosselli-Gulienetti ectodermal dysplasia

hypohidrotic ectodermal dysplasia with papillomas and acanthosis nigricans

odonto-onycho-hypohidrotic dysplasia with midline scalp defect

Jorgenson syndrome (Basan syndrome)

Zanier-Roubicek syndrome

XTE syndrome (xeroderma, talipes, and enamel defect syndrome; XTE syndrome of Moynahan)

Salamon syndrome

GROUP 1–2–4 (HAIR–TEETH–SWEATING)

melanoleucoderma (Berlin syndrome)

GROUP 1–3 (HAIR–NAILS)

CHANDS (curly hair, ankyloblepharon, and nail dysplasia syndrome; Baughman syndrome)

Coats' reaction retinal angiomas, hair and nail defects, and intracranial calcification

cataracts, alopecia, and sclerodactyly

GROUP 1–3–4 (HAIR–TEETH–SWEATING)

hypohidrotic ectodermal dysplasia with hypothyroidism syndrome (HEDH syndrome; ANOTHER syndrome)

hypohidrotic ectodermal dysplasia, primary hypothyroidism, and agenesis of the corpus callosum

GROUP 1–4 (HAIR–SWEATING)

Kirghizian dermato-osteolysis

Group 2–3–4 (TEETH–NAILS–SWEATING)

amelo-onychohypohidrotic dysplasia

GROUP 2–3 (TEETH–NAILS)

nail dystrophy–deafness syndrome

sensorineural hearing loss, enamel hypoplasia, and nail abnormalities

GROUP 2–4 (TEETH–SWEATING)

amelocerebrohypohidrosis syndrome (epilepsy and yellow teeth)

GROUP 3–4 (NAILS–SWEATING)

absence of dermal ridge patterns, onychodystrophy, and palmoplantar anhidrosis

MISCELLANEOUS ECTODERMAL DYSPLASIAS

hypohidrosis with neurolabyrinthitis

simple anhidrosis

familial generalized anhidrosis

triphalangeal thumbs-onychodystrophy-deafness syndrome (deafness, onychodystrophy, and digital anomalies; deafness–onycho-osteodystrophy–mental retardation [DOOR syndrome])

GROUP 1–2 (HAIR–TEETH)

GORLIN-CHAUDHRY-MOSS SYNDROME (CRANIOFACIAL DYSOSTOSIS WITH HYPERTRICHOSIS AND HYPODONTIA)

hypertrichosis of scalp, arms, legs, and back

dental abnormalities include hypodontia and microdontia

short stature

craniofacial abnormalities include craniosynostosis and midface hypoplasia, downward slanting palpebral fissures, and high-arched palate

ocular abnormalities include eyelid colobomas, inability to completely open or close eyes, and microphthalmia

bilateral hearing loss

hypoplasia of the distal phalanges of fingers and toes

radiographs show premature synostosis of the coronal suture, brachycephaly, and maxillary underdevelopment

McK 233500

Gorlin RJ, Chaudhry AP, Moss ML. Craniofacial dysostosis, patent ductus arteriosus, hypertrichosis, hypoplasia of labia majora, dental and eye anomalies—a new syndrome? J Pediatr 1960;56:778–785

Ippel PF, Gorlin RJ, Lenz W, et al. Craniofacial dysostosis, hypertrichosis, genital hypoplasia, ocular, dental and digital defects: Confirmation of the Gorlin-Chaudry-Moss syndrome. Am J Med Genet 1992;44:518–522

TRICHODENTAL SYNDROME

short, fine, lusterless scalp hair; lateral eyebrows may be absent

hypodontia

AD

electron microscopy of hair shaft: cuticular abnormalities

shortness of hair may be due to shortened anagen phase

Kersey PJ. Tricho-dental syndrome: a disorder with a short hair cycle. Br J Dermatol 1987;116:259–263
Salinas CF, Spector M. Tricho-dental syndrome. In: Brown AC, Crounse RG, eds. Hair, Trace Elements, and Human Illness. New York, Praeger, 1980:240–256

ACRORENAL-ECTODERMAL DYSPLASIA–LIPOATROPHIC DIABETES SYNDROME (AREDYLD SYNDROME)

sparse, fine, slow-growing scalp hair; scant axillary and pubic hair

hypoplastic and hypopigmented areolae and hypoplastic labia minora

dental abnormalities include natal teeth, enamel dysplasia, and premature loss

lipoatrophic diabetes

musculoskeletal abnormalities including short stature

craniofacial abnormalities

renal abnormalities

AR

McK 207780
Breslau-Siderius EJ, Toonstra J, Baart JA, et al. Ectodermal dysplasia: Lipoatrophy, diabetes mellitus, and amastia: A second case of the AREDYLD syndrome. Am J Med Genet 1992;44:374–377
Pinheiro M, Freire-Maia N, Chautard-Freire-Maia EA, et al. AREDYLD: a syndrome combining an acrorenal field defect, ectodermal dysplasia, lipoatrophic diabetes, and other manifestations. Am J Med Genet 1983;16:29–33

ALOPECIA-ANOSMIA-DEAFNESS-HYPOGONADISM SYNDROME (JOHNSON NEUROECTODERMAL SYNDROME)

AD

McK 147770
Johnson VP, McMillin JM, Aceto TJ, et al. A newly recognized neuroectodermal syndrome of familial alopecia, anosmia, deafness, and hypogonadism. Am J Med Genet 1983;15:497–506

OCULO-OSTEOCUTANEOUS SYNDROME

fair skin

sparse, fair hair

palmoplantar keratoderma

limb and digit abnormalities

hypoplastic nipples

abnormal genitalia

possible AR

McK 211370
Tuomaala P, Haapanen E. Three siblings with similar anomalies in the eyes, bones and skin. Acta Ophthalmol 1968;46:365–372

TAURODONTIA, ABSENT TEETH, SPARSE HAIR

possible AR

McK 272980
Gorlin RJ. A selected miscellany: oligodontia, taurondontia, and sparse hair growth. Birth Defects 1975;11:39–50
Stenvik A, Zachrisson BU, Svatun B. Taurodontism and concomitant hypodontia in siblings. Oral Surg 1972;33:841–845
Stoy PJ. Taurodontism associated with other dental anomalies. Dent Pract 1960;10:202–205

WALBAUM-DEHAENE-SCHLEMMER SYNDROME

sparse, blond scalp hair in early childhood followed by alopecia; sparse body hair

dental abnormalities

abnormal dermatoglyphics

short stature

flat nasal bridge and enlarged nasal tip

possible AR

Walbaum R, Dehaene P, Schlemmer H. Dysplasie ectodermique: une forme autosomique recessive? Arch Fr Pediatr 1971;28:435–442

MIKAELIAN SYNDROME (ECTODERMAL DYSPLASIA AND NEUROSENSORY DEAFNESS)

sparse brittle scalp hair

increased dental caries

sensorineural deafness

coarse facial features

arachnodactyly

probable AR

McK 224800
Mikaelian DO, Der Kaloustian VM, Shahin NA, Barsoumian VM. Congenital ectodermal dysplasia with hearing loss. Arch Otolaryngol 1970;92:85–89

PILODENTAL DYSPLASIA WITH REFRACTIVE ERRORS

sparse, thin, brittle, scalp hair; pili annulati demonstrated on microscopic examination

dental abnormalities

ocular abnormalities include hyperopia

possible AR

McK 262020
Kopysc Z, Barczyk K, Krol E. A new syndrome in the group of euhidrotic ectodermal dysplasia: pilodental dysplasia with refractive errors. Hum Genet 1985;70:376–378

ECTODERMAL DYSPLASIA, ECTRODACTYLY, AND MACULAR DYSTROPHY (EEM SYNDROME)

probable AR

McK 225280
Ohdo S, Hirayama K, Terawaki T. Association of ectodermal dysplasia, ectrodactyly, and macular dystrophy: the EEM syndrome. J Med Genet 1983;20:52–57

ECTODERMAL DYSPLASIA WITH BLINDNESS IN SIBS ON THE ISLAND OF RODRIGUES

fine, sparse scalp hair

malaligned teeth

ocular abnormalities include microphthalmos, microcornea, and sclerocornea; results in blindness

short stature

abnormal craniofacies

probable AR

McK 268320

Wallis CE, Beighton P. Ectodermal dysplasia with blindness in sibs on the island of Rodrigues. J Med Genet 1992;29:323–325

GROUP 1–2–3 (HAIR–TEETH–NAILS)

TRICHODENTO-OSSEOUS SYNDROME (TDO I SYNDROME)

tightly curled hair at birth, which frequently straightens by second or third decade; long eyelashes

small, pitted, widely spaced teeth with defective enamel that may subsequently erode and become discolored; sequelae include early caries, gingival abscesses, and eventual total loss of teeth by the third decade

nails are brittle and show white transverse banding in childhood

craniofacial abnormalities include dolichocephaly, frontal bossing, and square jaw

increased bone density, most evident in skull but also in long bones

physical development normal

AD

hair shafts are normal microscopically

TDO II syndrome also has curly hair and same dental changes as in TDO I syndrome but no discoloration of the enamel; long bones do not appear to have increased density but macrocephaly is present; whether these two forms represent true heterogeneity is not known

McK 190320

Jorgenson RJ, Warson RW. Dental abnormalities in the tricho-dento-osseous syndrome. Oral Surg 1973;36:693–700

Lichtenstein JR, Warson RW, Jorgenson RJ, McKusick VA. The tricho-dento-osseous syndrome. Am J Hum Genet 1972;24:569–582

Lichtenstein JR, Warson RW. Syndrome of dental anomalies, curly hair and sclerotic bones. Birth Defects 1971;7(7):308–311

Quattromani F, Shapiro SD, Young RS, et al.

Clinical heterogeneity in the tricho-dento-osseous syndrome. Hum Genet 1983; 64:116–121
Robinson GC, Miller JR, Worth HM. Hereditary enamel hypoplasia, its association with characteristic hair structure. Pediatrics 1966;37:498–502
Shapiro SD, Quattromani FL, Jorgenson RJ, Young RS. Tricho-dento-osseous syndrome: heterogeneity or clinical variability? Am J Med Genet 1983;16:225–236

HAIR, TOOTH, AND NAIL SYNDROMES

Various ectodermal dysplasias with hair, dental, and nail abnormalities have been described with designations using permutations of the roots "tricho-" and "onycho-." We use the term *hair, tooth, and nail syndromes* as a generic descriptor for this group of diseases. We list the diseases using the nomenclature from the published descriptions but wish to point out that the terminology overlaps and is confusing.

- *tricho-odonto-onychial dysplasia*

a single family with hypotrichosis, hypodontia, and additional findings of linear atrophy of nose, hyperpigmentation, mild hearing loss, and hypoplastic breasts and nipples

AD

McK 129510
Tsakalakos N, Jordaan FH, Taljaard JJ, et al. A previously undescribed ectodermal dysplasia of the tricho-odonto-onychial subgroup in a family. Arch Dermatol 1986; 122:1047–1053

- *tricho-onychodental (TOD) syndrome*

sparse, curly scalp hair; easily plucked

decreased facial, axillary, and pubic hair

nail dystrophy

hypohidrosis

dental anomalies include taurodontic molars and abnormalities of dentin and enamel

AD

Koshiba H, Kimura O, Nakata M, Witkop CJ Jr. Clinical, genetic, and histologic features of the tricho-onychodental (TOD) syndrome. Oral Surg 1978;46:376–385

- *tricho-odonto-onychodermal syndrome*

scalp hypotrichosis

aplasia cutis of scalp

palmar keratoderma

onychodysplasia

dental abnormalities

absent nipples

sporadic occurrence

Pinheiro, M, Pereira LC, Freire MN. A previously undescribed condition: tricho-odonto-onychodermal syndrome: a review of the tricho-odonto-onychial subgroup of ectodermal dysplasias. Br J Dermatol 1981; 105:371–382

■ *odonto-onychodermal dysplasia*

normal to sparse scalp hair and eyebrows

palmoplantar hyperhidrosis and hyperkeratosis

atrophy, telangiectasia, and scaling of facial skin

hypodontia with coniform or hypoplastic teeth

short, thickened toenails; fingernails normal

AR

McK 257980

Fadhil M, Ghabra TA, Deeb M, Der Kaloustian VM. Odonto-onychodermal dysplasia: a previously apparently undescribed ectodermal dysplasia. Am J Med Genet 1983;14:335–346

■ *tricho-odonto-onychial dysplasia*

scalp hair is dry and brittle in general and sparse over the crown

enamel hypoplasia

nail dystrophy

palmoplantar keratoderma

supernumerary nipples

AR

McK 275450

Pinheiro M, Freire-Maia N, Roth AJ. Tricho-odonto-onychial dysplasia: a new mesoectodermal dysplasia. Am J Med Genet 1983;15:67–70

WITKOP TOOTH-NAIL SYNDROME (HYPODONTIA AND NAIL DYSGENESIS; WITKOP SYNDROME)

scalp hair is fine, fair, and sparse in some; eyebrows and eyelashes may be affected

hypoplasia and occasionally koilonychia of nails, especially on toes

permanent teeth and occasionally deciduous teeth are absent or cone-shaped

eclabium

prominent ears

AD

although skin may have dry appearance, sweat tests are normal, allowing this syndrome to be distinguished from various hypohidrotic ectodermal dysplasias

McK 189500

Giansanti JS, Long SM, Rankin JL. The tooth and nail type of autosomal dominant ectodermal dysplasia. Oral Surg 1974;37:576–582

Hudson CD, Witkop CJ Jr. Autosomal dominant hypodontia with nail dysgenesis: report of twenty-nine cases in six families. Oral Surg 1975;39:409–423

TOOTH AND NAIL SYNDROME OF FRIED

fine, short hair

nails thin, small, and concave

teeth decreased in number and peg-shaped

normal sweating

AR

normal sweating, dental findings, and autosomal inheritance distinguish it from hypohidrotic ectodermal dysplasia

Fried K. Autosomal recessive hidrotic ectodermal dysplasia. J Med Genet 1977;14:137–139

ODONTOTRICHOMELIC SYNDROME (TETRAMELIC ECTODERMAL DYSPLASIA)

hypotrichosis, hypoplastic nails, and hypodontia

hypoplastic nipples and areolae

severe limb abnormalities include absence deformities and ectrodactyly

abnormal craniofacies including deformed auricles, large nose, and protruding lips

AR

McK 273400
Pavone L, Rizzo R, Tine A, et al. A case of the Freire-Maia odontotrichomelic syndrome: nosology with EEC syndrome. Am J Med Genet 1989;33:190–193

ODONTO-ONYCHODYSPLASIA WITH ALOPECIA

alopecia of scalp, eyebrows and eyelashes, pubes, and axillae

brittle nails

dental abnormalities include enamel hypoplasia, hypodontia, and microdontia

other abnormalities include palmoplantar hyperkeratosis, supernumerary nipples, myopia, and simian creases

probable AR

Pinheiro M, Freire MN, Gollop TR: Odonto-onychodysplasia with alopecia: a new pure ectodermal dysplasia with probable autosomal recessive inheritance. Am J Med Genet 1985;20:197–202

DENTO-OCULOCUTANEOUS SYNDROME

nail abnormalities including horizontal ridging and onychoschizia

hyperpigmented and thickened skin over finger interphalangeal joints

dental abnormalities including taurodontia

juvenile glaucoma

facial abnormalities including ectropion and absence of the cupid's bow of upper lip

syndactyly and clinodactyly

possible AD with complete syndrome expressed only in the homozygous state

McK 200970
Ackerman JL, Ackerman AL, Ackerman AB. A new dental, ocular and cutaneous syndrome. Int J Dermatol 1973;12:285–289

DERMO-ODONTODYSPLASIA

dry, slowly growing scalp and facial hair; sparse axillary and pubic hair

palmoplantar hyperkeratosis; dry, thin skin elsewhere in some

occasional brittle and dystrophic nails

dental abnormalities include microdontia, hypodontia, and persistence of deciduous teeth

AD

McK 125640
Pinheiro M, Freire-Maia N. Dermo-odontodysplasia: an eleven-member, four generation pedigree with an apparently hitherto undescribed pure ectodermal dysplasia. Clin Genet 1983;24:58–68
Pinheiro M, Gomes-de-Sa-Filho FP, Freire-Maia N. New cases of dermo-odontodysplasia? Am J Med Genet 1990;36:161–166

OCULOTRICHODYSPLASIA

generalized hypotrichosis; sparse distal two thirds of eyebrows and eyelashes

brittle nails

xeroderma

dental abnormalities

retinitis pigmentosa

probable AR

McK 257960
Cecatto-De-Lima L, Pinheiro M, Freire-Maia N. Oculotrichodysplasia (OTD): a new probably autosomal recessive condition. J Med Genet 1988;25:430–432

CRANIOECTODERMAL DYSPLASIA (SENSENBRENNER SYNDROME)

sparse, fine, slow-growing scalp hair

nails short and broad

dental abnormalities include hypodontia and small, widely spaced teeth with enamel dysplasia

craniofacial abnormalities include dolichocephaly (with sagittal suture synostosis in some), frontal bossing, epicanthal folds, anteverted nares, eclabium, and antimongoloid palpebral fissures

musculoskeletal abnormalities include short limbs, short and narrow thorax, and brachydactyly

probable AR

McK 218330
Levin LS, Perrin JC, Ose L, et al. A heritable syndrome of craniosynostosis, short thin hair, dental abnormalities, and short limbs: cranioectodermal dysplasia. J Pediatr 1977;90:55–61
Young ID. Cranioectodermal dysplasia (Sensenbrenner's syndrome). J Med Genet 1989;26:393–396

GAPO SYNDROME (GROWTH RETARDATION, ALOPECIA, PSEUDOANODONTIA, PROGRESSIVE OPTIC ATROPHY SYNDROME)

alopecia of scalp and eyebrows with onset in early childhood

pseudoanodontia

growth retardation

progressive optic atrophy in some

craniofacial abnormalities include frontal bossing and midfacial hypoplasia

progeroid appearance emphasized by some authors

AR

McK 230740
Gagliardi AR, Gonzalez CH, Pratesi R. GAPO syndrome: report of three affected brothers. Am J Med Genet 1984;19:217–223
Manouvrier-Hanu S, Largilliere C, Benalioua M, et al. The GAPO syndrome. Am J Med Genet 1987;26:683–688
Tipton RE, Gorlin RJ. Growth retardation, alopecia, pseudo-anodontia, and optic atrophy—the GAPO syndrome: report of a patient and review of the literature. Am J Med Genet 1984;19:209–216
Wajntal A, Koiffmann CP, Mendonca BB, et al. GAPO syndrome (McKusick 23074)—a connective tissue disorder: report on two affected sibs and on the pathologic findings in the older. Am J Med Genet 1990;37:213–223

LACRIMO-AURICULO-DENTO-DIGITAL (LADD) SYNDROME (LEVY-HOLLISTER SYNDROME)

frequent xerostomia

nail dysplasia

dental abnormalities include hypodontia, small peg-shaped lateral maxillary incisors, and enamel hypoplasia

variable digital anomalies include syndactyly and triphalangeal thumbs

cup-shaped pinnae with mixed conductive/sensorineural hearing deficit

hypoplasia or aplasia of components of the lacrimal system with sequelae including chronic dacryocystitis and conjunctivitis

AD

McK 149730

Bamforth JS, Kaurah P. Lacrimo-auriculo-dento-digital syndrome: evidence for lower limb involvement and severe congenital renal anomalies. Am J Med Genet 1992;43:932–937

Roodhooft AM. Lacrimo-auriculo-dento-digital (LADD) syndrome with renal and foot anomalies. Clin Genet 1990;38:228–232

Thompson E, Pembrey M, Graham JM. Phenotypic variation in LADD syndrome. J Med Genet 1985;22:382–385

Wiedemann HR, Drescher J. LADD syndrome: report of new cases and review of the clinical spectrum. Eur J Pediatr 1986; 144:579–582

ECTODERMAL DYSPLASIA, MARGARITA TYPE

cleft lip and palate

syndactyly

sparse short scalp hair and sparse eyebrows and eyelashes

onychodysplasia

dental abnormalities include hypodontia

probable AR

McK 225060

Bustos T, Simosa V, Pinto-Cisternas J, et al. Autosomal recessive ectodermal dysplasia: I. An undescribed dysplasia/malformation syndrome. Am J Med Genet 1991;41:398–404

ECTODERMAL DYSPLASIA WITH CORKSCREW HAIRS

light-colored, lusterless hair at birth

progressive universal hair loss beginning in childhood; complete alopecia by sixth decade; follicular plugging of scalp

hairs described as corkscrew, an exaggeration of pili torti

palmoplantar keratoderma

other cutaneous abnormalities include occipital keloids, xerosis, widespread dermatitis, and extensive keratosis pilaris

onychodysplasia

dental abnormalities

abnormal craniofacies including malar hypoplasia, broad nose, anteverted pinnae, and cleft lip or palate

syndactyly

hair shaft microscopy: repeated, up to 360° twists along longitudinal axis of hair shaft and flattening; cuticle disorganized and focally clumped

Abramovits-Ackerman W, Bustos T, Simosa-Leon V, et al. Cutaneous findings in a new syndrome of autosomal recessive ectodermal dysplasia with corkscrew hairs. J Am Acad Dermatol 1992;27:917–921

Whiting DA, Jenkins T, Whitcomb MJ. Corkscrew hair: a unique type of congenital alopecia in pili torti. In: Brown AC, Crounse RG, eds. Hair, Trace Elements, and Human Illness. New York, Praeger, 1980:228–239

GROUP 1–2–3–4 (HAIR–TEETH–NAILS–SWEATING)

ROSSELLI-GULIENETTI ECTODERMAL DYSPLASIA

sparse, fine, woolly scalp hair

possible mild hypohidrosis

toenail hypoplasia

dental abnormalities include hypodontia and oligodontia

frontal bossing and depression of nasal bridge

cleft lip and palate

popliteal and perineal pterygia and syndactyly

external genitalia abnormalities

probable AR

may be forme fruste of EEC syndrome

some of the case reports cited here are considered by some to represent separate syndromes

McK 225000
Bowen P, Armstrong HB. Ectodermal dysplasia, mental retardation, cleft lip–palate and other anomalies in three sibs. Clin Genet 1976;9:35–42
Ogur G, Yuksel M. Association of syndactyly, ectodermal dysplasia, and cleft lip and palate: report of two sibs from Turkey. J Med Genet 1988;25:37–40
Rodini ESO, Richieri-Costa A. Autosomal recessive ectodermal dysplasia, cleft lip/palate, mental retardation, and syndactyly: the Zlotogora-Ogur syndrome. Am J Med Genet 1990;36:473–476
Rosselli D, Gulienetti R. Ectodermal dysplasia. Br J Plast Surg 1961;14:190–204
Zlotogora J, Zilberman Y, Tenebaum A, Wexler MR. Cleft lip and palate, pili torti, malformed ears, partial syndactyly of fingers and toes, and mental retardation: a new syndrome? J Med Genet 1987;24:291–293

HYPOHIDROTIC ECTODERMAL DYSPLASIA WITH PAPILLOMAS AND ACANTHOSIS NIGRICANS

generalized sparse, slow-growing hair

acanthosis nigricans in flexures of neck, axillae, and groin

hypohidrosis

papillomas

palmoplantar hyperkeratosis

short and dystrophic nails

dental abnormalities include hypoplastic or absent teeth

Freire-Maia N, Pinheiro M. Ectodermal Dysplasias: A Clinical and Genetic Study. New York, Alan R. Liss, 1984:57–58

ODONTO-ONYCHOHYPOHIDROTIC DYSPLASIA WITH MIDLINE SCALP DEFECT

congenital absence of skin on scalp

hypohidrosis

dental abnormalities include delayed eruption

fingernail dystrophy

hypoplastic breasts, areolae, and nipples

adrenocortical cyst, renal abscess, and hypertension

possible AD

McK 129550
Tuffli GA, Laxova R. New, autosomal dominant form of ectodermal dysplasia. Am J Med Genet 1983;14:381–384

JORGENSON SYNDROME (BASAN SYNDROME)

sparse, coarse scalp hair with marked loss during adolescence

hypohidrosis, nail dystrophy, and dermatoglyphic abnormalities

dental abnormalities including brown discoloration

AD inheritance probable but XLD cannot be excluded

McKusick appears to equate this condition with Basan syndrome; others consider them separate entities

McK 129200
Basan M. Ektodermale Dysplasie, fehlendes Papillarmuster, Nagelveraenderungen und Vierfingerfurche. Arch Klin Exp Dermatol 1965;222:546–557
Jorgenson RJ. Ectodermal dysplasia with hypotrichosis, hypohidrosis, defective teeth and unusual dermatoglyphics (Basan syndrome?). Birth Defects 1974:10(4):323–325
Reed T, Schreiner RL. Absence of dermal ridge patterns: genetic heterogeneity. Am J Med Genet 1983;16:81–88

ZANIER-ROUBICEK SYNDROME

scalp hypotrichosis, brittle nails, hypohidrosis, and dental abnormalities including cone-shaped teeth and yellow transverse streaks in enamel

AD

some distinguish this entity from hypohidrotic ectodermal dysplasia on the basis of normal eyebrows and eyelashes, transverse streaks in dental enamel, and presence of palmoplantar sweating

McK 129490
Jorgenson RJ, Dowben JS, Dowben SL. Autosomal dominant ectodermal dysplasia. J Craniofac Genet Dev Biol 1987;7:403–412
Zanier JM, Roubicek MM. Hidrotic ectodermal dysplasia with autosomal dominant transmission. Proceedings of the Fifth International Congress on Human Genetics, Mexico City, 1976: communication 273

XTE SYNDROME (XERODERMA, TALIPES, AND ENAMEL DEFECT SYNDROME; XTE SYNDROME OF MOYNAHAN)

generalized dry, red, scaly skin; bullae on exposed areas during warm weather

sparse, coarse scalp hair; absent lower lid eyelashes

dystrophic nails

dental abnormalities include defective tooth enamel and yellowish discoloration; enamel defects noted in heterozygotes

talipes

small lacrimal puncta

sweat glands decreased in number and size on skin biopsy

Moynahan EJ. XTE (xeroderma, talipes and enamel defect): a new heredofamilial syndrome. Two cases: homozygous inheritance of a dominant gene. Proc R Soc Med 1970;63:447–448

SALAMON SYNDROME

sparse, brittle scalp hair and hair shaft abnormalities including pili torti and trichorrhexis nodosa

hypohidrosis

nail dystrophy

dental abnormalities include tooth hypoplasia

bird-like facies

ocular abnormalities include blepharoconjunctivitis, keratitis, and retinal atrophy

probable AR

Salamon T, Cubela V, Bogdanovic B, et al. Uber ein Geschwisterpaar mit einer eigenartigen ektodermalen Dysplasie. Arch Klin Exp Dermatol 1967;230:60–68

Salamon T, Mahrle G, Beighton E. The hairs in the syndrome of Netherton and in a peculiar form of ectodermal dysplasia. Derm Monatschr 1974;160:362–372

Salamon T, Milicevic M. Uber eine besondere Form der ektodermalen Dysplasie mit Hypohidrosis, Hypotrichosis, Hornhautveranderungen, Nagel- und Anderen anomalien bei einem Geschwisterpaar. Arch Klin Exp Dermatol 1964;220:564–575

GROUP 1–2–4 (HAIR–TEETH–SWEATING)

MELANOLEUCODERMA (BERLIN SYNDROME)

hypotrichosis, hypodontia (but no conical teeth), hypohidrosis, generalized mottled pigmentation, anetopoikilodermatous lesions over joints, and prominent palmoplantar hyperkeratosis

depressed nasal bridge, furrows around eyes and mouth, prominent mental and physical retardation

AR

McK 246500
Berlin C. Congenital generalized melanoleucoderma associated with hypodontia, hypotrichosis, stunted growth, and mental retardation occurring in two brothers and two sisters. Dermatologica 1961;123:227–243

GROUP 1–3 (HAIR–NAILS)

CHANDS (CURLY HAIR, ANKYLOBLEPHARON, AND NAIL DYSPLASIA SYNDROME; BAUGHMAN SYNDROME)

curly hair, congenital ankyloblepharon filiformis (congenital adhesion of the margins of the upper and lower eyelids by fibrous bands), and hypoplastic nails

normal sweating

ataxia

AR

McK 214350
Baughman FA Jr. CHANDS: the curly hair–ankyloblepharon–nail dysplasia syndrome. Birth Defects 1971;7:100–102
Toriello HV, Lindstrom JA, Waterman DF, et al. Re-evaluation of CHANDS. J Med Genet 1979;16:316–317

TRICHO-ONYCHODYSPLASIA WITH XERODERMA

absence of all hair from birth

generalized scaling and xeroderma

nail dystrophy

possible AR

Freire-Maia N, Pinheiro M. Ectodermal Dysplasias: A Clinical and Genetic Study. New York, Alan R. Liss, 1984:159–160.

COATS' REACTION RETINAL ANGIOMAS, HAIR AND NAIL DEFECTS, AND INTRACRANIAL CALCIFICATION

sparse, fair-colored, wiry scalp hair

nail dysplasia

ocular abnormalities include bilateral retinal abnormalities (Coats disease) and strabismus

possible AR

cranial calcification

Tolmie JL, Browne BH, McGettrick PM, Stephenson BP. A familial syndrome with Coats' reaction retinal angiomas, hair and nail defects and intracranial calcification. Eye 1988;2:297–303

CATARACTS, ALOPECIA, AND SCLERODACTYLY

congenital alopecia universalis

palmoplantar hyperkeratosis

nail dystrophy

sclerodactyly

pseudoainhum, deforming bands and nodules on hands and feet

joint contractures of distal extremities

bilateral congenital cataracts

McK 212360
Wallis C, Ip FSL, Beighton P. Cataracts, alopecia, and sclerodactyly: a previously apparently undescribed ectodermal dysplasia syndrome on the Island of Rodrigues. Am J Med Genet 1989;32:500–503

GROUP 1–3–4 (HAIR–TEETH–SWEATING)

HYPOHIDROTIC ECTODERMAL DYSPLASIA WITH HYPOTHYROIDISM (HEDH) SYNDROME (ANOTHER SYNDROME)

possibly distinct hypohidrotic ectodermal dysplasia with hypothyroidism

findings include those designated by the acronym ANOTHER:

Alopecia

Nail dystrophy

Ophthalmic complications (bilateral conjunctivitis and tearing)

Thyroid dysfunction

Hypohidrosis

Ephelides and enteropathy

Respiratory infections due to ciliary dyskinesia

AR, or possibly X-linked

McK 225050

Pike MG, Baraitser M, Dinwiddie R, Atherton DJ. A distinctive type of hypohidrotic ectodermal dysplasia featuring hypothyroidism. J Pediatr 1986;108:109–111

Pinheiro M, Penna FJ, Freire-Maia N. Two other cases of ANOTHER syndrome? Family report and update. Clin Genet 1989;35:237–242

HYPOHIDROTIC ECTODERMAL DYSPLASIA, PRIMARY HYPOTHYROIDISM, AND AGENESIS OF THE CORPUS CALLOSUM

this and hypohidrotic ectodermal dysplasia with hypothyroidism may be X-linked and part of a contiguous gene syndrome

---

McK 225040

Fryns JP, Chrzanowska K, van den Berghe H. Hypohidrotic ectodermal dysplasia, primary hypothyroidism, and agenesis of the corpus callosum. J Med Genet 1989;26:520–521

GROUP 1–4 (HAIR–SWEATING)

KIRGHIZIAN DERMATO-OSTEOLYSIS

widespread cutaneous ulcerations

nail dystrophy

arthro-osteolysis

keratitis

possible AR

McK 221810
Kozlova SI, Altshuler BA, Kravchenko VL. Self-limited autosomal recessive syndrome of skin ulceration, arthroosteolysis with pseudoacromegaly, keratitis and oligodontia in a Kirghizian family. Am J Med Genet 1983;15:205–210

GROUP 2–3–4 (TEETH–NAILS–SWEATING)

AMELO-ONYCHOHYPOHIDROTIC DYSPLASIA

scaling and crusting of scalp

generalized xerosis and keratosis pilaris of buttocks and extensor extremities

onycholysis and subungual hyperkeratosis

facial hypohidrosis

enamel defect and unerupted teeth that undergo resorption within the alveolar bone of the jaws

AD

McK 104570
Witkop CJ Jr, Brearley LJ, Gentry WC. Hypoplastic enamel, onycholysis, and hypohidrosis inherited as autosomal dominant trait: a review of ectodermal dysplasia syndromes. Oral Surg 1975;39:71–86

GROUP 2–3 (TEETH–NAILS)

NAIL DYSTROPHY–DEAFNESS SYNDROME

dysplastic nails, sensorineural deafness, dental abnormalities, syndactyly, and polydactyly

AD

McKusick considers this the AD form of triphalangeal thumbs–onycho-dystrophy–deafness (DOOR) syndrome

---

McK 124480

Robinson GC, Miller JR, Bensimon JR. Familial ectodermal dysplasia with sensorineural deafness and other anomalies. Pediatrics 1962;30:797–802

SENSORINEURAL HEARING LOSS, ENAMEL HYPOPLASIA, AND NAIL ABNORMALITIES

nail dystrophy including leukonychia

enamel hypoplasia of permanent teeth

severe bilateral sensorineural hearing loss

possible AR

McK 234580

Heimler A, Fox JE, Hershey JE, Crespi P. Sensorineural hearing loss, enamel hypoplasia, and nail abnormalities in sibs. Am J Med Genet 1991;39:192–195

GROUP 2–4 (TEETH–SWEATING)

AMELOCEREBROHYPOHIDROSIS SYNDROME (EPILEPSY AND YELLOW TEETH)

hypohidrosis

enamel hypoplasia causing yellow discoloration of teeth

seizures in infancy or early childhood

muscular spasticity

progressive central nervous system degeneration

possible X-linked inheritance; AR kindred reported

death in first or second decade

McK 226750

Christodoulou J, Hall RK, Menahem S, et al. A syndrome of epilepsy, dementia and amelogenesis imperfecta: genetic and clinical features. J Med Genet 1988;25:827–830.

Kohlschutter A, Chappuis D, Meier C, et al. Familial epilepsy and yellow teeth—a disease of the CNS associated with enamel hypoplasia. Helv Paediat Acta 1974; 29:283–294

GROUP 3–4 (NAILS–SWEATING)

ABSENCE OF DERMAL RIDGE PATTERNS, ONYCHODYSTROPHY, AND PALMOPLANTAR ANHIDROSIS

AD

Freire-Maia N, Pinheiro M. Ectodermal Dysplasias: A Clinical and Genetic Study. New York, Alan R. Liss, 1984:181
Reed T, Schreiner RL. Absence of dermal ridge patterns: genetic heterogeneity. Am J Med Genet 1983;16:81–88

MISCELLANEOUS ECTODERMAL DYSPLASIAS

HYPOHIDROSIS WITH NEUROLABYRINTHITIS

AD

McK 125050
Helweg-Larsen HF, Ludvigsen K. Congenital familial anhidrosis and neurolabyrinthitis. Acta Derm Venereol 1946;26:489–505

SIMPLE ANHIDROSIS

complete isolated absence of eccrine sweat glands

AR; very rare

McK 206600
Frydman M, Cohen HA, Kauschansky A, Matoth Y. Familial simple hypohidrosis with abnormal palmar dermal ridges. Am J Med Genet 1988;31:591–596
Juhlin L. Absence of eccrine sweat glands without other ectodermal defects. Acta Derm Venereol 1980;60:73
Mahloudji M, Livingston KE. Familial and congenital simple anhidrosis. Am J Dis Child 1967;113:477–479

FAMILIAL GENERALIZED ANHIDROSIS

generalized anhidrosis and heat intolerance

inheritance unclear; AD versus XLR

on biopsy, sweat glands morphologically intact

McK 106190
Dann EJ, Epstein Y, Sohar E. Familial generalized anhidrosis. Isr J Med Sci 1990; 26:451–453
Ingber A. Familial generalized anhidrosis. Isr J Med Sci 1990;26:457–458

TRIPHALANGEAL THUMBS–ONYCHODYSTROPHY–DEAFNESS SYNDROME (DEAFNESS, ONYCHODYSTROPHY, AND DIGITAL ANOMALIES; DEAFNESS-ONYCHO-OSTEODYSTROPHY-MENTAL RETARDATION [DOOR SYNDROME])

absent or hypoplastic fingernails and toenails

abnormal dermatoglyphics

sensorineural deafness

triphalangeal ("finger-like") thumbs and great toes

mental retardation and/or epilepsy (recessive form only)

AR mostly, but AD cases also reported (see nail dystrophy–deafness syndrome)

increased 2-oxoglutarate in plasma and urine reported

McK 220500
Feinmesser M, Zelig S. Congenital deafness associated with onychodystrophy. Arch Ophthalmol 1961;74:507–508
Nevin NC, Thomas PS, Calvert J, et al. Deafness, onycho-osteodystrophy, mental retardation (DOOR) syndrome. Am J Med Genet 1982;13:325–332
Patton MA, Krywawych S, Winter RM, et al. DOOR syndrome (deafness, onycho-osteodystrophy, and mental retardation): elevated plasma and urinary 2-oxoglutarate in three unrelated patients. Am J Med Genet 1987;26:207–215

Other Dysplasias or Malformation Syndromes

EHLERS-DANLOS SYNDROME

Ehlers-Danlos syndrome (EDS) refers to a group of disorders with the chief findings of extensible skin and/or hypermobile joints. Presently, all types are defined on the basis of specific and different defects in collagen metabolism. The salient features of the Ehlers-Danlos subtypes are listed in Table 8–1.

TABLE 8–1
EHLERS-DANLOS SYNDROME

Type; Synonym (McKusick Number)	Inheritance	Skin	Joints	Other	Biochemical Defect
I; gravis (McK 130000)	AD	Marked hyperextensibility and fragility; poor wound healing (atrophic scars); prominent bruising; molluscoid pseudotumors, subcutaneous calcified spherules; varicose veins	Marked large and small joint hypermobility	Herniae; premature delivery	Not known; possible abnormal processing of procollagen
II; mitis (McK 130010)	AD	Moderate hyperextensibility and fragility; moderate bruisability; mild scarring	Mild hypermobility	Herniae (fewer than type 1)	Not known
III; benign hypermobile (McK 130020)	AD	Mild skin hyperextensibility and fragility	Marked large and small joint hypermobility; common joint dislocation		Not known
IV; arterial ecchymotic (McK 225350; McK 130050)	AR or AD	Thin, translucent and fragile; recurrent ecchymoses; no hyperextensibility	Normal mobility except small hand joints	Prematurity, low birth weight and failure to thrive; frequent arterial, bowel (especially colon), or uterine rupture often causes death	Diminished or abnormal type III collagen
V; X-linked (McK 305200)	XLR	Similar to type II, except bruising may be more extensive	Mild to moderative hypermobility	Short stature; herniae; mitral and tricuspid valve prolapse	Lysyl oxidase deficiency reported
VI; ocular (McK 225400)	AR	Soft; moderate hyperextensibility, fragility and scarring	Marked hypermobility; kyphoscoliosis	Ocular fragility (corneal tears, intraocular hemorrhage, eyeball rupture); keratoconus; blue sclerae	Lysyl hydroxylase deficiency
VII; arthrochalasis multiplex congenita (McK 225410)	AR or AD	Moderate skin fragility, hyperextensibility, and bruising; slight scarring	Marked hypermobility; hip dislocations	Scoliosis; short stature	Procollagen aminoprotease deficiency (AR form); probable structural mutation of pro alpha-2 (AD form)
VIII; periodontal (McK 130080)	AD	Marked fragility; atrophic pigmented scars; minimal hyperextensibility	Moderate joint laxity	Periodontitis and tooth loss	Decreased type III collagen
IX; "X-linked cutis laxa type" (McK 304150)	XLR	Soft; slight hyperextensibility	Mild joint hypermobility	Occipital horns; carpal bone fusion; broad short clavicles; bladder diverticula; herniae; rhizomelic limb shortening	Abnormal copper metabolism; lysyl oxidase deficiency
X; fibronectin-deficient (McK 225310)	AR	Soft; mild hyperextensibility; striae	Mild hypermobility		Abnormal fibronectin

Modified from Pinnell SR, McKusick VA. Heritable disorders of connective tissue with skin changes. In: Fitzpatrick TB, Eisen AZ, Wolff K, et al., eds. Dermatology in General Medicine. New York, McGraw-Hill, 1987:1780–1783.

EHLERS-DANLOS SYNDROME TYPE I

Synonyms

- Ehlers-Danlos syndrome, gravis type
- cutis hyperelastica

Skin

markedly extensible skin with hyperelasticity; after stretching, skin returns to normal shape without rugae or wrinkles; also known as India rubber skin (Fig. 8–11)

skin is soft, smooth, and thin

bony prominences more noticeable due to reduced subcutaneous fat

increased skin fragility; minor trauma results in gaping, "fish mouth" wounds (Fig. 8–12); surgical sutures frequently tear through skin

scars resulting from injury are "papyraceous" (i.e., thin, wrinkled, and atrophic); typical sites include elbows, knees, shins, and forehead

hematomas are easily induced by trauma because of increased fragility of blood vessels; some subcutaneous hematomas resolve into bulging, patulous scars ("molluscoid" pseudotumors)

diezogenic papules common

occasional elastosis perforans serpiginosa

Non-Skin

craniofacial abnormalities include frontal bossing, hypertelorism, epicanthal folds, and broad nasal bridge

ears project outward and downward ("lop ears")

hyperextensible and more easily dislocated, lax joints; occasional congenital dislocation of the hip

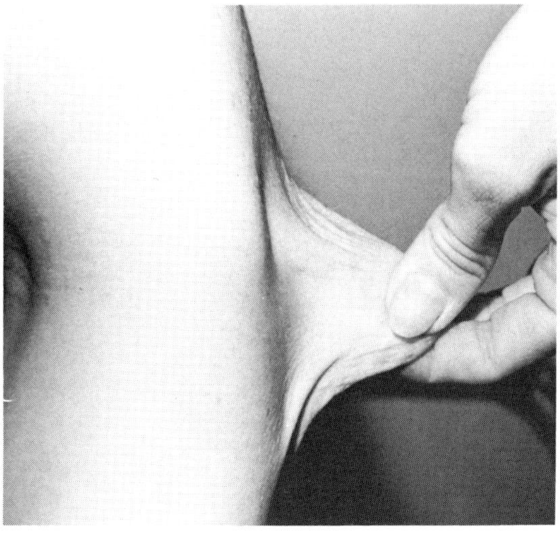

FIGURE 8–11
Hyperextensible skin in a patient with Ehlers-Danlos syndrome type I.

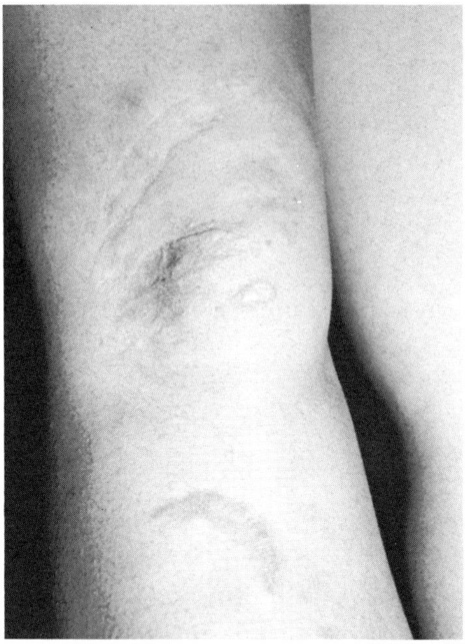

FIGURE 8–12
Multiple "fish mouth" scars over the knee and pretibial area in a patient with Ehlers-Danlos syndrome, type I.

other skeletal abnormalities include pes planus in about half of patients and scoliosis

premature birth of affected individuals due to early rupture of fetal membranes

cardiovascular abnormalities are common and include tetrology of Fallot, aortic aneurysms, atrioseptal defects, pulmonary artery stenosis, and spontaneous large vessel rupture

gastrointestinal abnormalities include melena, hematemesis, multiple herniae (related to muscular hypotonicity; umbilical, hiatal), diverticula, and rectal prolapse

eye abnormalities include strabismus, myopia, easily everted eyelids, and blue sclerae; less commonly, keratoconus, ectopia lentis, ocular hemorrhages, angioid streaks, and retinal detachment

normal general physical and mental development

Genetics

AD

Pathophysiology

pathogenesis and biochemical defect(s) unknown

Laboratory Data

skin biopsy unhelpful

Rumpel-Leede sign may be positive

Prognosis

prolonged bleeding after tooth extraction or with epistaxis

complications that may shorten life expectancy include cardiac defects, arterial rupture, and intestinal perforation

Discussion

EDS type I has the most severe skin findings

individuals of a given family may have a wide range of disease severity

some individuals may have localized forms

cutis laxa has lax but wrinkled and rugated skin as opposed to smooth skin in EDS

prematurity is a major criterion for separating EDS types I and II

REFERENCES

McK 130000

Barabas AP. Ehlers-Danlos syndrome associated with prematurity and premature rupture of foetal membranes. Br Med J 1966;2:682–684

Beighton P, Price A, Lord J, Dickson E. Variants of the Ehlers-Danlos syndrome: clinical, biochemical, haematological, and chromosomal features of 100 patients. Ann Rheum Dis 1969;28:228–245

Byers PH, Holbrook KA. Molecular basis of clinical heterogeneity in the Ehlers-Danlos syndrome. Ann NY Acad Sci 1985;460: 198–310

Danlos H. Un cas de cutis laxa avec tumeurs par contusion chronique des coudes et des genoux. Bull Soc Fr Dermatol Syph 1908;19:70–72

Ehlers E. Cutis laxa, Neigung zu Hemorrhagien in der Haut, Lockerung mehrerer Artikulationen. Dermatol Z 1901;8:173–174

McKusick VA. Heritable Disorders of Connective Tissue. 4th ed. St. Louis, CV Mosby, 1972

Owen SM, Durst RD. Ehlers-Danlos syndrome simulating child abuse. Arch Dermatol 1984;120:97–101

Pierard GE, Pierard-Franchimont C, Lapiere CM. Histopathological aid at the diagnosis of the Ehlers-Danlos syndrome, gravis and mitis types. Int J Dermatol 1983;22:300–304

Pinnell SR. The skin in Ehlers-Danlos syndrome. [Letter]. J Am Acad Dermatol 1987;16:399–400

Pope FM, Nicholls AC. Molecular abnormalities of collagen in human disease. Arch Dis Child 1987;62:523–528

Prockop DJ, Kivirikko KI. Heritable diseases of collagen. N Engl J Med 1984;311:376–386

Sulica VI, Cooper PH, Pope M, et al. Cutaneous histologic features in Ehlers-Danlos syndrome. Arch Dermatol 1979;115:40–42

EHLERS-DANLOS SYNDROME TYPE II (EHLERS-DANLOS SYNDROME, MITIS TYPE)

joint hypermobility is limited to digits

AD

pathogenesis and biochemical defect undetermined, but abnormalities in fibrillogenesis demonstrated

mild clinical features

prematurity (not a feature of EDS type II) is a major criterion for separating EDS types I and II

McK 130010
Beighton P. The Ehlers-Danlos Syndrome. London, William Heinemann, 1970
Rizzo R, Contri MB, Micali G, et al. Familial Ehlers-Danlos syndrome type II: abnormal fibrillogenesis of dermal collagen. Pediatr Dermatol 1987;4:197–204

EHLERS-DANLOS SYNDROME TYPE III (EHLERS-DANLOS SYNDROME, BENIGN HYPERMOBILE TYPE)

mild skin findings

marked large joint hypermobility (Fig. 8–13)

AD

biochemical defect unknown

do not confuse with familial generalized articular hypermobility, which lacks skin, cardiac, and other findings of Ehlers-Danlos syndrome

McK 130020
Beighton P, Price A, Lord J, Dickson E. Variants of the Ehlers-Danlos syndrome: clinical, biochemical, haematological, and chromosomal features of 100 patients. Ann Rheum Dis 1969;28:228–245
Beighton P. The Ehlers-Danlos Syndrome. London, William Heinemann, 1970
Jessee EF, Owen DS Jr, Sagar KB. The benign hypermobile joint syndrome. Arthritis Rheum 1980;23:1053–1056
Viljoen D, Goldblatt J, Thompson D, Beighton P. Ehlers-Danlos syndrome: yet another type? Clin Genet 1987;32:196–201

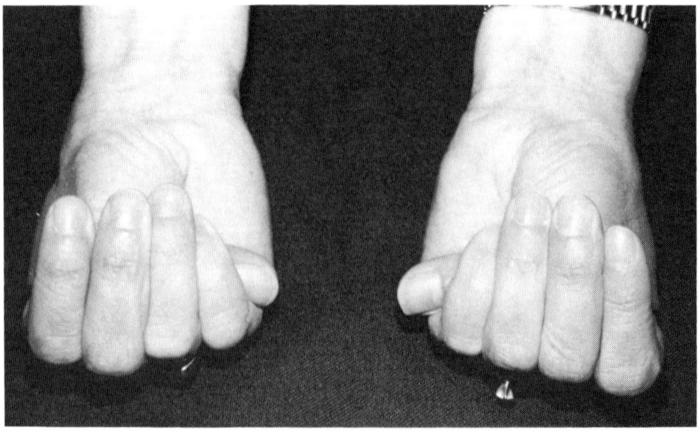

FIGURE 8–13
Hyperextensibility of the joints in Ehlers-Danlos syndrome, type III.

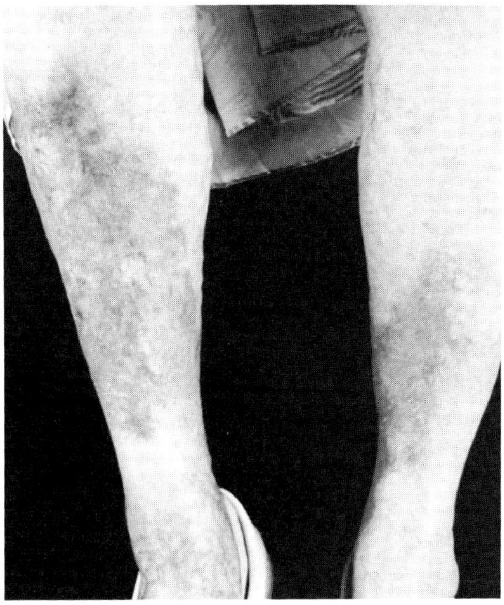

FIGURE 8–14
Ehlers-Danlos syndrome, type IV. Atrophic symmetrical reddish plaques over the tibia are common, probably caused by repeated trauma. This patient was 70 years old and had survived numerous cardiac complications of this syndrome.

EHLERS-DANLOS SYNDROME TYPE IV (EHLERS-DANLOS SYNDROME, ECCHYMOTIC TYPE; EHLERS-DANLOS SYNDROME, ARTERIAL TYPE)

marked bruisability

skin thin, translucent, and fragile; extremities are more severely affected than trunk, giving an "acrogeric" appearance (Fig. 8–14)

increased incidence of arterial rupture

increased incidence of visceral perforation, especially of colon and the gravid uterus

AR; AD in some families (McK 130050); very rare

abnormalities in type III collagen synthesis

decreased life span; patients rarely survive into the fifth decade

type IV has the greatest mortality of all types of Ehlers-Danlos syndrome

compared with other types of Ehlers-Danlos syndrome, skin hyperextensibility and joint hypermobility are mild or absent

- *Ehlers-Danlos syndrome type IV-D:*

  has clinical features of EDS type IV, but cultured fibroblasts synthesize and secrete normal amounts of type III collagen

McK 225350
McK 130050
Barabas AP. Heterogeneity of the Ehlers-Danlos syndrome: description of three clinical types and a hypothesis to explain the basic defects. Br Med J 1967;2:612–613
Byers PH, Holbrook KA, Barsh GS, et al. Altered secretion of type III procollagen in a form of type IV Ehlers-Danlos syndrome. Lab Invest 1981;44:336–341
Byers PH, Holbrook KA, McGillivray B, et al. Clinical and ultrastructural heterogeneity

of type IV Ehlers-Danlos syndrome. Hum Genet 1979;47:141–150
Gertsch P, Loup PW, Lochman A, Anani P. Changing patterns in the vascular form of Ehlers-Danlos syndrome. Arch Surg 1986;121:1061–1064
Pope FM, Martin GR, Lichtenstein JR, et al. Patients with Ehlers-Danlos syndrome type IV lack type III collagen. Proc Natl Acad Sci USA 1975;72:1314–1316
Pope FM, Narcisi P, Nicholls AC, et al. Clinical presentations of Ehlers Danlos syndrome type IV. Arch Dis Child 1988;63:1016–1025
Sulh HMB, Steinmann B, Rao VH, et al. Ehlers-Danlos syndrome type IV D: an autosomal recessive disorder. Clin Genet 1984;25:278–287

EHLERS-DANLOS SYNDROME TYPE V (EHLERS-DANLOS SYNDROME, "X-LINKED TYPE")

short stature, herniae, mitral and tricuspid valve prolapse, and moderate joint hypermobility

XLR

lysyl oxidase deficiency

McK 305200
Beighton P. X-linked recessive inheritance in the Ehlers-Danlos syndrome. Br Med J 1968;2:409–411
Beighton P, Curtis D. X-linked Ehlers-Danlos syndrome type V: the next generation. Clin Genet 1985;27:472–478

EHLERS-DANLOS SYNDROME TYPE VI (EHLERS-DANLOS SYNDROME, HYDROXYLYSINE-DEFICIENT TYPE; EHLERS-DANLOS SYNDROME, OCULAR TYPE)

hyperextensible and moderately fragile skin

marked joint hypermobility and kyphoscoliosis

ocular fragility; blindness from retinal detachment or ocular rupture may occur

AR

lysyl hydroxylase deficiency (caused by mutation of gene encoding lysyl hydroxylase or chromosome 1p)

McK 225400
Elsas LJ II, Miller RL, Pinnell SR. Inherited human collagen lysyl hydroxylase deficiency: ascorbic acid response. J Pediatr 1978;92:378–384
Krieg T, Feldmann U, Kessler W, Muller PK. Biochemical characteristics of Ehlers-Danlos syndrome type VI in a family with one affected infant. Hum Genet 1979;46:41–49
Pinnell SR, Krane SM, Kenzora JE, Glimcher MJ. Heritable disorder with hydroxylysine-deficient collagen. Hydroxylysine-deficient collagen disease. N Engl J Med 1972;286:1013–1020
Wenstrup RJ, Murad S, Pinnell SR. Ehlers-Danlos syndrome type VI: clinical manifestations of collagen lysyl hydroxylase deficiency. J Pediatr 1989;115:405–409

EHLERS-DANLOS SYNDROME TYPE VII (EHLERS-DANLOS SYNDROME, ARTHROCHALASIS MULTIPLEX CONGENITA TYPE)

moderate skin hyperextensibility

moderate joint hypermobility and hip dislocations

short stature

AR; AD cases also reported

procollagen amino protease deficiency (formerly called procollagen peptidase deficiency)

variant reported having dominant inheritance with marked joint hypermobility and hip dislocations, due to probable structural mutation of pro-alpha-2 (I) collagen (McK 130060)

McK 225410
McK 130060
Cole WG, Evans R, Sillence DO. The clinical features of Ehlers-Danlos syndrome type VII due to a deletion of 24 amino acids from the pro-alpha-1(I) chain of type I procollagen. J Med Genet 1987;24:698–701
Lichtenstein JR, Martin GR, Kohn LD, et al. Defect in conversion of procollagen to collagen in a form of Ehlers-Danlos syndrome. Science 1973;182:298–299

EHLERS-DANLOS SYNDROME TYPE VIII (EHLERS-DANLOS SYNDROME, PERIODONTOSIS TYPE)

marked skin fragility, especially over shins

severe generalized periodontitis (loss of deciduous and adult teeth)

AD

decreased type III collagen

McK 130080
Lapiere CM, Nusgens BV. Ehlers-Danlos type VIII skin has a reduced proportion of type III collagen. J Invest Dermatol 1981;76:422
Nelson DL, King RA. Ehlers-Danlos syndrome type VIII. J Am Acad Dermatol 1981; 5:297–303
Stewart RE, Hollister DW, Rimoin DL. A new variant of Ehlers-Danlos syndrome: an autosomal dominant disorder of fragile skin, abnormal scarring, and generalized periodontosis. Birth Defects 1983;13:85–93

EHLERS-DANLOS SYNDROME TYPE IX (EHLERS-DANLOS SYNDROME, X-LINKED CUTIS LAXA TYPE; OCCIPITAL HORN SYNDROME)

hyperextensible skin

bony occipital horns

herniae

XLR

may be allelic to Menkes syndrome

abnormal copper metabolism

lysyl oxidase deficiency

cases formerly classified as X-linked cutis laxa are now classified as Ehlers-Danlos syndrome type IX

McK 304150

Byers PH, Siegel RC, Holbrook KA, et al. X-linked cutis laxa: defective cross-linked formation in collagen due to decreased lysyl oxidase activity. N Engl J Med 1980;303:61–65

Tsukahara M, Shinkai H, Asagami C, et al. A disease with features of cutis laxa and Ehlers-Danlos syndrome: report of a mother and daughter. Hum Genet 1988;78:9–12

EHLERS-DANLOS SYNDROME TYPE X (EHLERS-DANLOS SYNDROME, FIBRONECTIN-DEFICIENT TYPE)

easy bruisability

hyperextensible skin

hyperextensible joints

AR

abnormal fibronectin

platelet aggregation defect corrected by human fibronectin

McK 225310

Arneson MA, Hammerschmidt DE, Furcht LT, King RA. A new form of Ehlers-Danlos syndrome: fibronectin corrects defective platelet function. JAMA 1980;244:144–147

Hammerschmidt DE, Arneson MA, Larson SL, et al. Maternal Ehlers-Danlos syndrome type X: successful management of pregnancy and parturition. JAMA 1982; 248:2487–2488

COFFIN-LOWRY SYNDROME

loose, easily stretched skin

frequent varicose veins and acrocyanosis

dental abnormalities

dermatoglyphic abnormalities include transverse hypothenar crease

abnormal craniofacies include microcephaly, hypoplastic mandible, hypoplastic zygoma, ocular hypertelorism, antimongoloid slant of palpebral fissures, frontal bossing, large low-set ears, broad nose with thick alae nasi, long philtrum, thin upper lip, and thick lower lip

skeletal abnormalities include pectus carinatum, kyphoscoliosis, severe joint laxity, and characteristic broad, thick, hyperextensible fingers that taper distally

muscle hypotonia

mental retardation

inheritance unclear, possibly XLD or AR

milder manifestations in female relatives

McK 303600

Gorlin RJ. Lapsus—caveat emptor: Coffin-Lowry syndrome vs Coffin-Siris syndrome—an example of confusion compounded. [Letter]. Am J Med Genet 1981;10:103–104

Gorlin RJ, Cohen MM Jr, Levin LS. Syndromes of the Head and Neck. 3rd ed. New York, Oxford University Press, 1990:827–829

Hunter AGW, Partington MW, Evans JA. The Coffin-Lowry syndrome: experience from four centres. Clin Genet 1982;21:321–335

Lowry RB, Miller JR, Fraser FC. A new dominant gene mental retardation syndrome: associated with small stature, tapering fingers, characteristic facies and possible hydrocephalus. Am J Dis Child 1971; 121:496–500

Temtany SA, Miller DJ, Hussels-Maumenee I. The Coffin-Lowry syndrome: an inherited faciodigital mental retardation syndrome. J Pediatr 1975;86:724–731

PSEUDOXANTHOMA ELASTICUM

Synonyms

- Grönblad-Strandberg syndrome
- systematized elastorrhexis

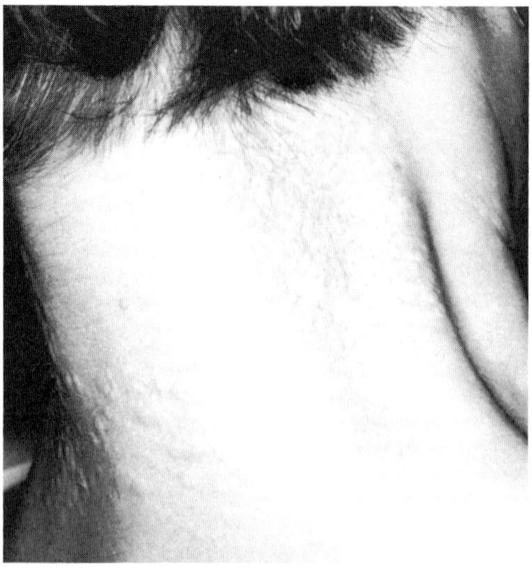

FIGURE 8–15
Yellowish, waxy papules of pseudoxanthoma elasticum in a reticulated pattern on the posterior neck. (Courtesy of Benjamin K. Fisher, MD, Toronto, Ontario)

Skin

waxy yellowish papules in a linear or reticulated pattern paralleling lines of skin cleavage (Figs. 8–15 and 8–16); tend to become confluent, forming plaques; surrounding skin may be livid or telangiectatic

lesions arise insidiously in childhood, adolescence, or early adulthood but may arise as late as eighth decade

in severe cases, skin becomes wrinkled and redundant, hanging in folds

lesions are symmetrically distributed and have a predilection for skin folds; affected areas of neck or axillae appear like "chicken skin"; sparing of scalp, palms, and soles

follicular openings become patulous and plugged

occasional striae distensae on abdominal skin

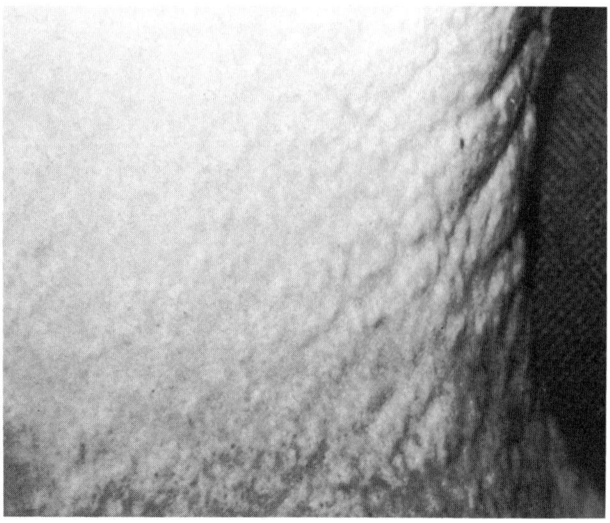

FIGURE 8–16
Closer view of pseudoxanthoma elasticum shows typical "chicken skin" appearance with whitish bumps laced by furrows. (Courtesy of Kenneth Neldner, MD, Lubbock, Texas)

occasional elastosis perforans serpiginosa

rare involvement of oral mucosa, most commonly the gingivolabial groove

Non-Skin

angioid streaks of ocular fundi in most, usually appearing in third or fourth decade, but may develop at any age; caused by rupture of elastic tissue in Bruch's membrane

ocular hemorrhages, unrelated to angioid streaks, are major cause of visual loss

other retinal changes include disciform macular degeneration, drusen, retinal pigmentation, and subretinal neovascularization

occasional blue sclerae

increased incidence of hypertension, aortic aneurysms, diminished peripheral pulses, and angina pectoris; thought to be due to elastic tissue degeneration with calcification of arterial media

Genetics

AR; less commonly AD; see Discussion re Pope classification *below*

Laboratory Data

histopathology: swollen and irregularly clumped elastic fibers, frequently calcified and easily visible, in mid and lower dermis

if more typical lesions are not available, biopsy specimens may be best obtained from scars (e.g., previous biopsy sites)

calcifications may be noted in radiographs

Prognosis

prognosis poor due to arterial rupture (e.g., cerebral or gastrointestinal hemorrhage)

cutaneous, ocular, or vascular abnormalities may follow separate courses (e.g., angioid streaks may be only sign of disease for many years)

early ophthalmologic intervention and avoidance of contact sports and refraining from smoking may decrease morbidity and mortality

Discussion

Pope classified patients with pseudoxanthoma elasticum into four clinical types (two AR forms: McK 264800 and 264810 and two AD forms: McK 177850 and 177860) to allow for better prognostication; however, some dispute the accuracy of the Pope classification and its purported usefulness in predicting prognosis. A new classification of PXE was described at a consensus conference.

widespread lesions of PXE may resemble cutis laxa

- *perforating calcific elastosis (perforating calcific elastosis of the umbilicus)*

  considered to be a localized form of pseudoxanthoma elasticum

  usually in black females

  acquired

REFERENCES

McK 264800
McK 177860
McK 264810
McK 177850
Lebwohl M, Neldner K, Pope M, et al. Classification of pseudoxanthoma elasticum: Report of a consensus conference. J Am Acad Dermatol 1994;30:103–107
Lebwohl M, Phelps RG, Yannuzzi L, et al. Diagnosis of pseudoxanthoma elasticum by scar biopsy in patients without characteristic skin lesions. N Engl J Med 1987;317:347–350
Mallette LE, Mechanick JI. Heritable syndrome of pseudoxanthoma elasticum with abnormal phosphorus and vitamin D metabolism. Am J Med 1987;83:1157–1162
Neldner KH. Pseudoxanthoma elasticum. Clin Dermatol 1988;6:1–59
Pope FM. Autosomal dominant pseudoxanthoma elasticum. J Med Genet 1974; 11:152–157
Pope FM. Historical evidence for the genetic heterogeneity of pseudoxanthoma elasticum. Br J Dermatol 1975;92:493–509
Pope FM. Two types of autosomal recessive pseudoxanthoma elasticum. Arch Dermatol 1974;110:209–212
Rongioletti F, Bertamino R, Rebora A. Generalized pseudoxanthoma elasticum with deficiency of vitamin K–dependent clotting factors. J Am Acad Dermatol 1989; 21:1150–1152
Somasundaram V, Premalatha S, Rao NR, et al. Periumbilical perforating pseudoxanthoma elasticum. Int J Dermatol 1987; 26:536–537
Viljoen D. Pseudoxanthoma elasticum (Grönblad-Strandberg syndrome). J Med Genet 1988;25:488–490
Viljoen DL, Pope FM, Beighton P. Heterogeneity of pseudoxanthoma elasticum: delineation of a new form? Clin Genet 1987; 32:100–105

FOCAL DERMAL HYPOPLASIA

Synonyms

- Goltz syndrome
- Goltz-Gorlin syndrome

Skin

variable spectrum of ectodermal and mesodermal defects present at birth; may affect any body area (Figs. 8–17 through 8–20)

cutaneous depressions with atrophy, scarring, hyperpigmentation, hypopigmentation ("marble streaks"), and/or telangiectases; lesions highly variable, including cribriform, linear, oval, or round patterns

most frequently involves trunk and extremities and, to lesser extent, scalp, cheek, neck, and ears

widely distributed, soft, reddish yellow nodules, most commonly on extremities in linear or reticular pattern

single or multiple localized congenital absence(s) of skin

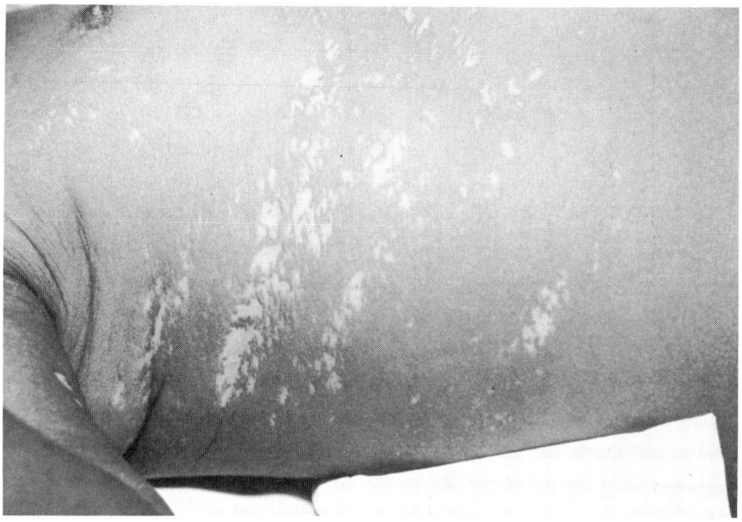

FIGURE 8–17
Patterned hypopigmented atrophic lesions on the torso of an infant with focal dermal hypoplasia.

papillomatous growths on various mucosae, periorificial areas or skin folds, especially lips; may involve oral cavity, esophagus, perineum (may be mistaken for perianal verrucae), and inguinal or axillary areas (Fig. 8–21)

occasional sparse, brittle scalp hair or areas of complete alopecia

nails may be normal, dystrophic, or absent

dental abnormalities include hypodontia, oligodontia, and enamel defects

Non-Skin

musculoskeletal defects include short stature and abnormalities of the hands and feet such as syndactyly, polydactyly, and hypoplasia or absence of digits

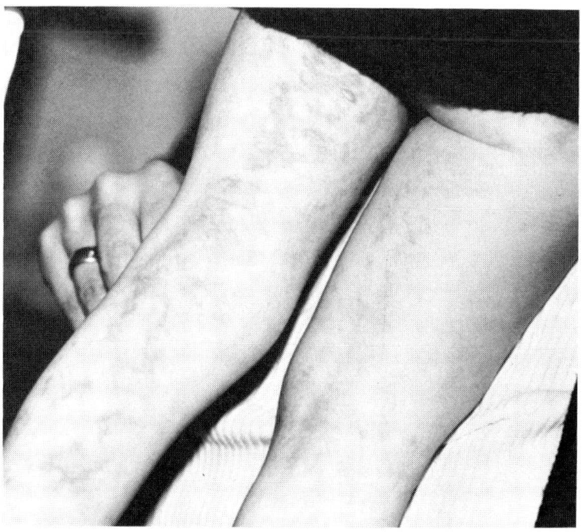

FIGURE 8–18
Focal dermal hypoplasia. Erythematous atrophic and herniated patches are arranged in a linear fashion.

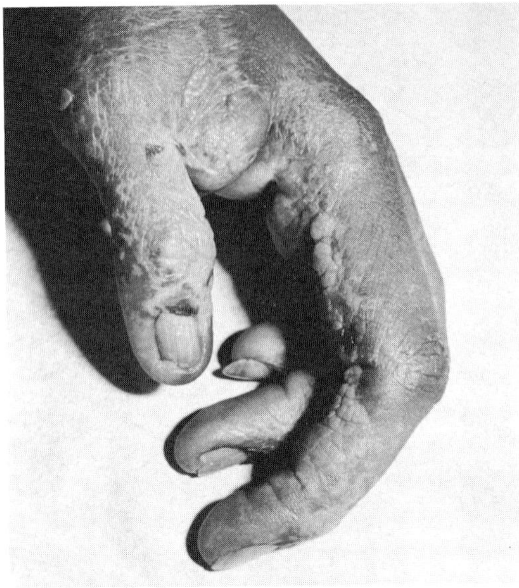

FIGURE 8–19
Multiple soft reddish nodules, atrophy, and pigmentary change on the hand of a young woman with focal dermal hypoplasia. Note absence of a digit (congenital).

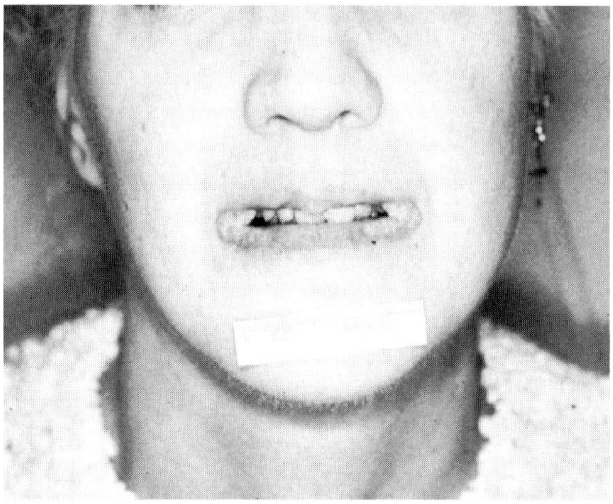

FIGURE 8–20
Focal dermal hypoplasia. Numerous papillomas are present around the mouth. The patient also had abnormal hands and feet but no other signs of dermal hypoplasia. (Courtesy of Herman Solomon, MD, Wichita, Kansas)

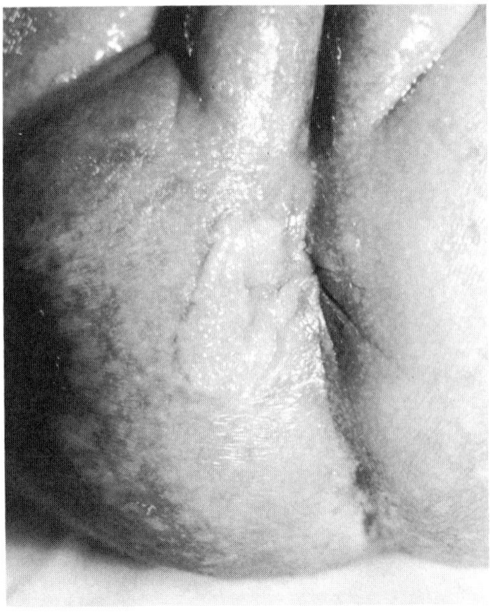

FIGURE 8–21
Perianal papillomas in an infant with focal dermal hypoplasia.

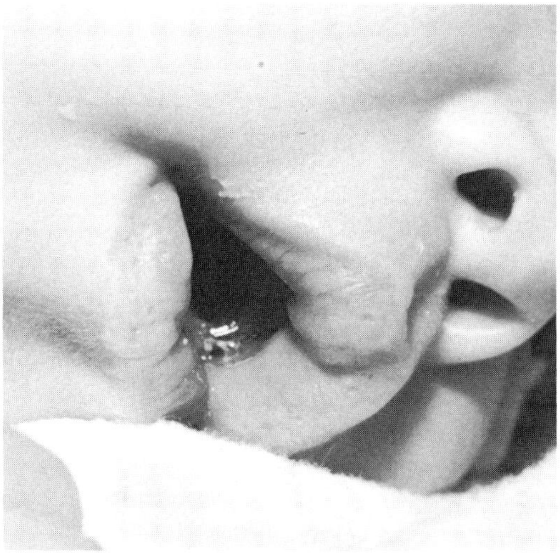

FIGURE 8–22
Multiple pits on the lips of a newborn with focal dermal hypoplasia.

craniofacial abnormalities include facial and ear asymmetry, lip pits, gingival hyperplasia, double frenulum, hemihypoplasia of tongue, and cleft lip, palate, and tongue (Fig. 8–22)

eye abnormalities include strabismus, cataracts, hypertelorism, and colobomata of iris, retina, choroid, or optic nerve (Color Fig. 8–1)

otic abnormalities may result in neurosensory or conductive hearing loss

mental retardation common

Genetics

most cases sporadic, but possible XLD reported; XLD suggested by female proponderance; cases in males represent new mutations or possibly autosomal inheritance with high male lethality; father to daughter transmission reported

male to female ratio: 1:11

Laboratory Data

see Figure 8–23

radiographs reveal osteopathia striata (radiopaque longitudinal streaks in long bones) in virtually every patient; improves or resolves with age

histopathology: thinning of dermis with subcutaneous tissue close to the epidermis; these "herniations" may be due to heterotopic fat

Prognosis

cutaneous changes gradually worsen

the only increased mortality risks are due to rare cardiac or renal defects

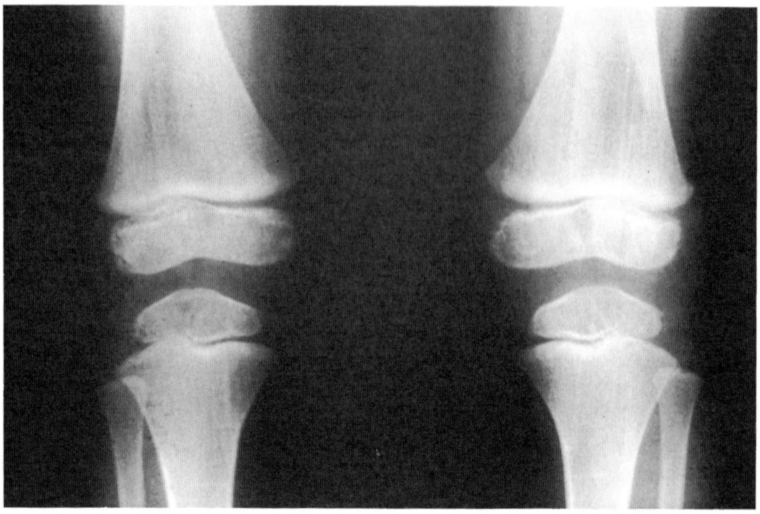

FIGURE 8–23
This radiograph shows osteopathia striata, which is a pathognomonic finding in focal dermal hypoplasia. It is best seen in the epiphyses of long bones and may resolve as the patient grows older.

Discussion

variability of expression may be due to early embryologic random inactivation of the X chromosome carrying the mutant gene

- *linear skin defects and congenital microphthalmia*

  linear erythematous erosions on face and neck at birth

  eye abnormalities include microphthalmia, corneal opacities, and orbital cysts

  XLD with deletion on short arm of X chromosome

  McK 309801

REFERENCES

McK 305600

al Gazali LI, Mueller RF, Caine A, et al. Two 46,XX,t(X;Y) females with linear skin defects and congenital microphthalmia: a new syndrome at Xp22.3. J Med Genet 1990;27:59–63

Allanson J, Richter S. Linear skin defects and congenital microphthalmia: a new syndrome at Xp22.2. J Med Genet 1991;28:143–144

Brinson RR, Schuman BM, Mills LR, et al. Multiple squamous papillomas of the esophagus associated with Goltz syndrome. Am J Gastroenterol 1987;82:1177–1179

Burgdorf WHB, Dick GF, Sonderberg HD. Focal dermal hypoplasia in a father and daughter. J Am Acad Dermatol 1981; 4:273–277

Howell JB, Freeman RG. Cutaneous defects of focal dermal hypoplasia: an ectomesodermal dysplasia syndrome. J Cutan Pathol 1989;16:237–258

Mahe A, Couturier J, Mathe C, et al. Minimal focal dermal hypoplasia in a man: a case of father-to-daughter transmission. J Am Acad Dermatol 1991;25:879–881

Moore DJ, Mallory SB. Goltz syndrome. Pediatr Dermatol 1989;6:251–253

Wechsler MA, Papa CM, Haberman F, et al. Variable expression in focal dermal hypoplasia: an example of differential X-chromosome inactivation. Am J Dis Child 1988;142:297–300

Wilson Jones E, Marks R, Pongsehirun D. Naevus superficialis lipomatosus. Br J Dermatol 1975;93:121–133

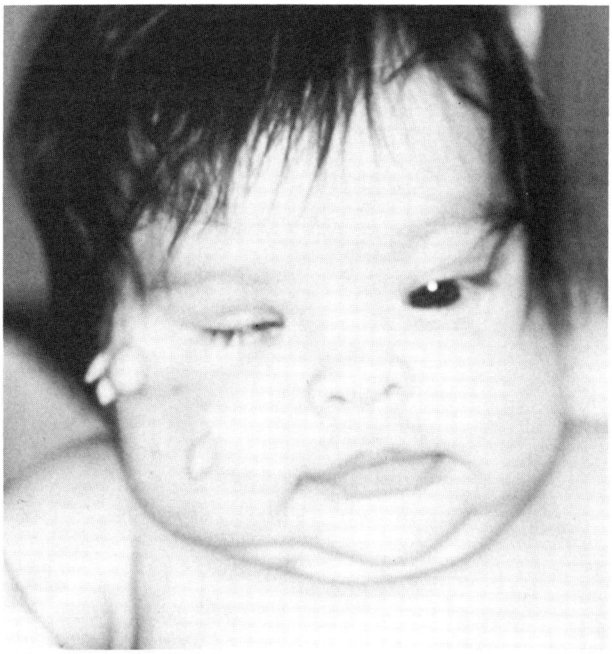

FIGURE 8–24
Oculocerebrocutaneous syndrome. Multiple skin tags are seen over the face of this infant. (Courtesy of Carol Clericuzio, MD, Albuquerque, New Mexico)

OCULOCEREBROCUTANEOUS SYNDROME (DELLEMAN-OORTHUYS SYNDROME)

focal, "punched-out" skin defects, mostly on alae nasi

orbital cysts and periorbital "skin tags" (Fig. 8–24)

cerebral malformations include porencephaly

sporadic occurrence; may be due to lethal AD gene with survival in mosaic state

report of infant with skin tags containing striated muscle; some skin tags showed spontaneous and independent movement

McK 164180

Happle R. Lethal genes surviving by mosaicism: a possible explanation for sporadic birth defects involving the skin. J Am Acad Dermatol 1987;16:899–906

Happle R, Steijlen PM. Enzephalokraniokutane lipomatose. Hautarzt 1993;44:19–22

Loggers HE, Oosterwijk JC, Overweg-Plandsoen WC, et al. Encephalocraniocutaneous lipomatosis and oculocerebrocutaneous syndrome. Ophthalmol Pediatr Genet 1992;13:171–177

Sahn EE, Garen PD, Shashidhar P, Levkoff AH, et al. Multiple rhabdomyomatous mesenchymal hamartomas of skin. Am J Dermatopathol 1990;12:485–491

Wilson RD, Traverse L, Hall JG. Oculocerebrocutaneous syndrome. Am J Ophthalmol 1985;99:142–148

FOCAL FACIAL DERMAL DYSPLASIA

Synonyms

- familial focal dermal dysplasia
- bitemporal aplasia cutis congenita
- Brauer syndrome
- bitemporal forceps marks syndrome
- Setleis syndrome

Skin

scar-like depressions on temples with or without forehead and chin (median scar-like ridge) involvement; bilateral in 90% (Fig. 8–25); present at birth

occasional leonine facies

some patients have complete absence of upper and lower lid eyelashes or multiple rows of eyelashes on upper lids and absence of lashes on lower lid; eyebrows may be slanted sharply upward and laterally

Genetics

AD and AR cases reported; perceived AR transmission may be due to observer error or low expressivity of a dominant gene

Discussion

probably unrelated to aplasia cutis congenita (see main entry), but this is controversial; in focal facial dermal dysplasia, the lack of ulcerated lesions at birth and the presence of scar tissue on biopsy argue against a relationship

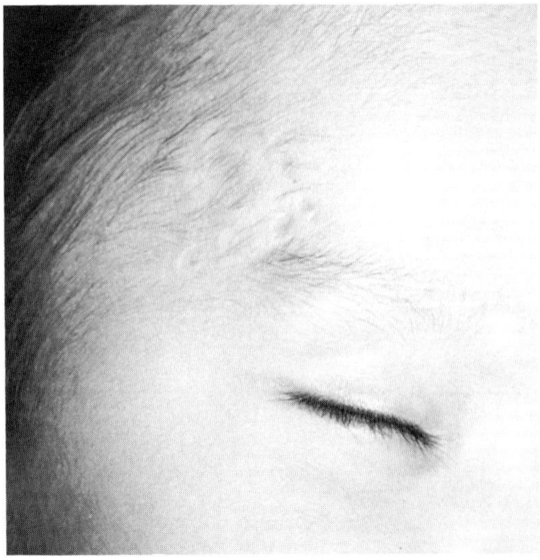

FIGURE 8–25
Focal facial dermal dysplasia. Grouped, atrophic, annular lesions on the temple. This child had bilateral lesions noted at birth.

Kowalski and Fenske suggested the following classification of focal facial dermal dysplasia (FFDD), which separates affected patients into three categories:

- *type I (autosomal dominant FFDD)*

  typical scar-like facial lesions without significant other facial anomalies

  AD

- *type II (autosomal recessive FFDD)*

  typical scar-like facial lesions without significant other facial anomalies

  AR

- *type III (FFDD with other facial features; Setleis syndrome)*

  bitemporal scar-like depressions

  periorbital puffiness

  eyebrows may be slanted sharply upward and laterally; sparse laterally

  eyelash abnormalities

  abnormalities of nose include flattening of nasal bridge, bulbous nasal tip, and nasal septum that extends below alae nasi

  abnormal facies

  mostly AR; possibly AD or XLD

REFERENCES

McK 136500

McK 227260

Brauer A. Hereditaerer symmetrischer Naevus aplasticus bei 38 Personen. Dermatol Wochenschr 1929;89:1163–1168

Di Lernia V, Neri I, Patrizi A. Focal facial dermal dysplasia: two familial cases. J Am Acad Dermatol 1991;25:389–391

Kowalski DC, Fenske NA. The focal facial dermal dysplasias: report of a kindred and a proposed new classification. J Am Acad Dermatol 1992;27:575–582

Magid ML, Prendiville JS, Esterly NB. Focal facial dermal dysplasia: bitemporal lesions resembling aplasia cutis congenita. J Am Acad Dermatol 1988;18:1203–1207

Marion RW, Chitayat D, Hutcheon G, Goldberg R, Shprintzen RJ, Cohen MM Jr. Autosomal recessive inheritance in the Setleis bitemporal "forceps marks" syndrome. Am J Dis Child 1987;141:895–897

McGeoch AH, Reed WB. Familial focal facial dermal dysplasia. Arch Dermatol 1973; 107:591–595

Rudolph RI, Schwartz W, Leyden JJ. Bitemporal aplasia cutis congenita: occurrence with other cutaneous abnormalities. Arch Dermatol 1974;110:615–618

Rudolph RI, Schwartz W, Leyden JJ. Emendation to "bitemporal aplasia cutis congenita." Arch Dermatol 1974;110:636

Setleis H, Kramer B, Valcarcel M, et al. Congenital ectodermal dysplasia of the face. Pediatrics 1963;32:540–548

CUTIS LAXA

Synonyms

- dermatochalasis
- generalized elastolysis

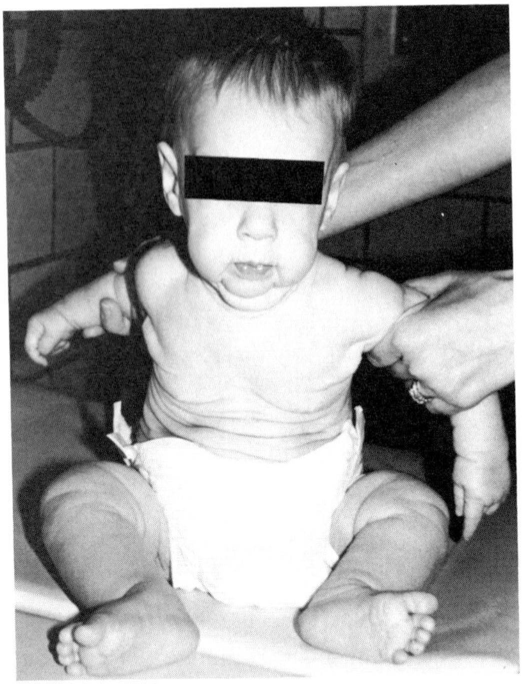

FIGURE 8–26
Generalized laxity of the skin in an infant with cutis laxa. Note the double chin and sagging cheeks.

Skin

generalized loose, wrinkled skin gives a "bloodhound" or prematurely aged appearance (Figs. 8–26 through 8–28); present at birth but may be inconspicuous in some

overhanging, pendulous skin folds, especially at wrists, knees, and ankles

skin may feel coarse; follicular openings often patulous

after stretching, skin is slow to return to normal shape

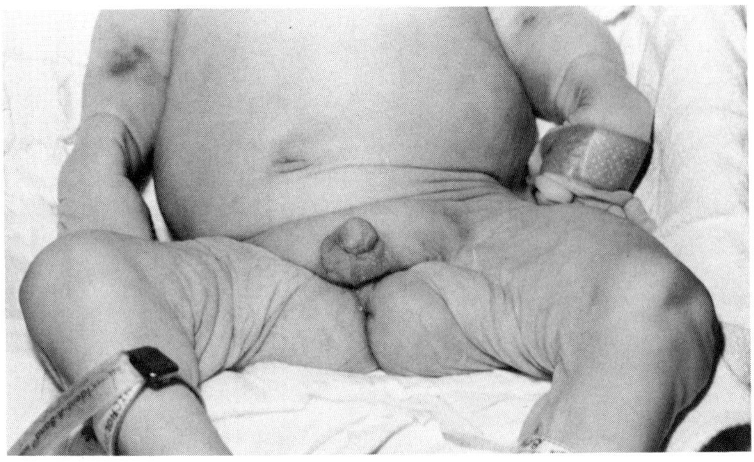

FIGURE 8–27
Marked laxity of the skin over the lower torso and limbs of an infant with severe cutis laxa and multiple joint dislocations.

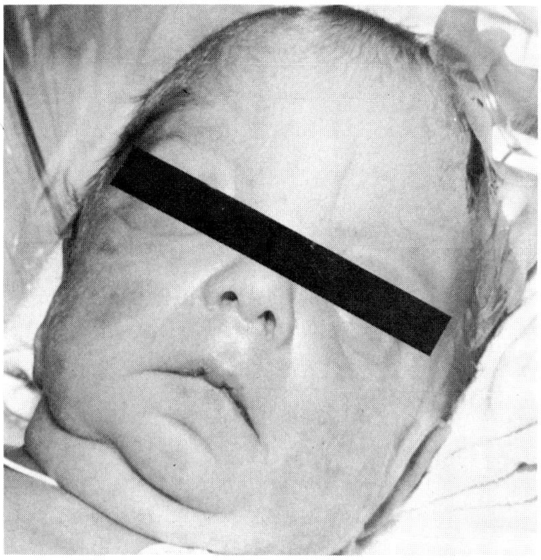

FIGURE 8–28
This newborn with cutis laxa already has a droopy face.

wide range in severity; skin folds may be markedly pendulous

no increase in bruisability (cf. Ehlers-Danlos syndrome)

Non-Skin

pulmonary emphysema is the most common systemic manifestation and may develop in infancy or later

cardiovascular complications including arterial aneurysms in some

laxity of vocal cords results in deepening of voice

hooked nose, everted nostrils, and long upper lip are typical and are not seen in acquired cutis laxa

males commonly have impotence, infantile genitalia, and scant body hair

inguinal, ventral, and diaphragmatic herniae; occasional pectus excavatum, ligament laxity, and congenital hip dislocation

bladder or gastrointestinal diverticula and prolapse of uterus or rectum

Genetics

AR; less commonly, AD

Laboratory Data

histopathology: dermal elastic fibers are decreased in numbers, fragmented, and granular; ends of fibers tapered while middle portions thickened; eventually, all elastic fibers are lost but collagen bundles remain normal

Prognosis

condition generally worsens with age but may stabilize

cor pulmonale and congestive heart failure secondary to emphysema may develop

life expectancy may be shortened by pulmonary and cardiovascular complications, which are most frequent in AR forms; AD forms have better prognosis

Discussion

AD form generally does not have serious internal manifestations, and cutaneous findings usually do not become evident until adolescence or adulthood

in acquired cases of "cutis laxa," changes tend to be localized and occur after puberty; often preceded by inflammatory disease (e.g., erythema multiforme, contact dermatitis, drug eruptions [especially penicillamine], and acute febrile neutrophilic dermatosis); systemic manifestations may occur; postinflammatory elastolysis and cutis laxa is probably a variant

- *granulomatous slack skin*

  cutaneous T-cell lymphoma in which pendulous redundant skin produces cutis laxa–like appearance; acquired

- *elastoderma*

  acquired condition causing laxity of skin but with an increase rather than decrease in elastic tissue or elastin

REFERENCES

McK 219100

McK 123700 (AD form)

Damkier A, Brandrup F, Starklint H. Cutis laxa: autosomal dominant inheritance in five generations. Clin Genet 1991;39:321–329

Fisher BK, Page E, Hanna W. Acral localized acquired cutis laxa. J Am Acad Dermatol 1989;21:33–40

Fitzsimmons JS, Fitzsimmons EM, Guibert PR, et al. Variable clinical presentation of cutis laxa. Clin Genet 1985;28:284–295

Gardner LI, Sanders-Fay K, Bifano EM. Congenital cutis laxa syndrome: relation of joint dislocations to oligohydramnios. Arch Dermatol 1986;122:1241–1243

Goltz RW, Hult AM, Goldfarb M, Gorlin RJ. Cutis laxa: a manifestation of generalized elastolysis. Arch Dermatol 1965;92:373–387

Greenbaum SS, Krull EA, Rubin MG, et al. Localized acquired cutis laxa in one of identical twins. Int J Dermatol 1989; 28:402–406

Kornberg RL, Hendler SS, Oikarinen AI, et al. Elastoderma: disease of elastin accumulation within the skin. N Engl J Med 1985;312:771–774

Lewis PG, Hood AF, Barnett NK, Holbrook KA. Postinflammatory elastolysis and cutis laxa: a case report. J Am Acad Dermatol 1990;22:40–48

Muster AJ, Bharati S, Herman JJ, et al. Fatal cardiovascular disease and cutis laxa following acute febrile neutrophilic dermatosis. J Pediatr 1983;102:243–248

AMBIGUOUS GENITALIA ASSOCIATED WITH SKELETAL ABNORMALITIES, CUTIS LAXA, CRANIOSTENOSIS, PSYCHOMOTOR RETARDATION, AND FACIAL ABNORMALITIES (SCARF SYNDROME)

possible XLR

McK 312830
Koppe R, Kaplan P, Hunter A, et al. Ambiguous genitalia associated with skeletal abnormalities, cutis laxa, craniostenosis, psychomotor retardation, and facial abnormalities (SCARF syndrome). Am J Med Genet 1989;34:305–312

CUTIS LAXA WITH BONE DYSTROPHY

ligamentous laxity and retarded physical and motor development also seen

AR; lethal in males

McK 219200
Allanson J, Austin W, Hecht F. Congenital cutis laxa with retardation of growth and motor development: a recessive disorder of connective tissue with male lethality. Clin Genet 1986;29:133–136
Debré R, Marie J, Seringe P. Cutis laxa avec dystrophies osseuses. Bull Mem Soc Med Hosp Paris 1037;53:1038–1039
Fitzsimmons JS, Fitzsimmons EM, Guibert PR, et al. Variable clinical presentation of cutis laxa. Clin Genet 1985;28:284–295

CUTIS LAXA, CORNEAL CLOUDING, MENTAL RETARDATION (DeBARSY SYNDROME)

probable AR

McK 219150
Karnes PS, Shamban AT, Olsen DR, et al. De Barsy syndrome: report of a case, literature review, and elastin gene expression studies of the skin. Am J Med Genet 1992;42:29–34
Kunze J, Majewski F, Montgomery P, et al. De Barsy syndrome—an autosomal recessive, progeroid syndrome. Eur J Pediatr 1985;144:348–354

HEMOLYTIC ANEMIA, CONGENITAL, WITH EMPHYSEMA AND CUTIS LAXA

possible AR

McK 235360
Anderson CE, Finklestein JZ, Nussbaum E, et al. Association of hemolytic anemia and early-onset pulmonary emphysema in three siblings. J Pediatr 1984;105:247–251

MENTAL DEFICIENCY, MACROCRANIUM, PECULIAR FACIES, AND CARDIAC AND SKELETAL ANOMALIES (CANTU SYNDROME)

lax skin

possible AD vs. XLD

McK 114620
Cantu JM, Sanchez-Corona J, Hernandes A, et al. Individualization of a syndrome with mental deficiency, macrocranium, peculiar facies, and cardiac and skeletal anomalies. Clin Genet 1982;22:172–179

LENZ-MAJEWSKI HYPEROSTOTIC DWARFISM

possible AD

McK 151050
Kaye CI, Fischer DE, Esterly NB. Cutis laxa, skeletal anomalies and ambiguous genitalia. Am J Dis Child 1974;127:115–117
Lenz WD, Majewski F. A generalized disorder of the connective tissues with progeria, choanal atresia, symphalangism, hypoplasia of dentine and craniodiaphyseal hyperostosis. Birth Defects 1974;10:133–136

BLEPHAROCHALASIS (DERMATOLYSIS PALPEBRARUM)

insidious progressive relaxation and dark discoloration of skin of upper eyelids; lids droop over eyes by adulthood

AD

possibly due to localized elastic tissue defect

McK 110000
Custer PL, Tenzel RR, Kowalczyk AP. Blepharochalasis syndrome. Am J Ophthalmol 1985;99:424–428

ASCHER SYNDROME

blepharochalasis, mostly of upper lids

enlargement of upper lip ("double" lip); onset in infancy

variable nontoxic thyroid enlargement

AD

McK 109900
Gorlin RJ, Cohen MM Jr, Levin LS. Syndromes of the Head and Neck. 3rd ed. New York, Oxford University Press, 1990:420–422
Navas J, Rodriguez-Pichardo A, Camacho F. Ascher syndrome: a case study. Pediatr Dermatol 1991;8:122–123

WRINKLY SKIN SYNDROME

Skin

wrinkled skin involving dorsa of hands and feet at birth; may also involve abdomen

palmoplantar creases increased in number

skin is dry and less extensible ("hypoelastic")

prominent cutaneous vascular pattern on chest

Non-Skin

hypotonia and low birth weight

musculoskeletal abnormalities include winged scapulae and congenital hip dysplasia

mild to moderate psychomotor retardation

microcephaly and midface hypoplasia in one third of patients

Genetics

AR

Laboratory Data

histopathology: decreased number and length of dermal elastic fibers

REFERENCES

McK 278250

Casamassima AC, Wesson SK, Conlon CJ, et al. Wrinkly skin syndrome: phenotype and additional manifestations. Am J Med Genet 1987;27:885–893

Goodman RM, Duksin D, Legum C, et al. The wrinkly skin syndrome and cartilage-hair hypoplasia (a new variant?) in sibs of the same family. Prog Clin Biol Res 1982;104:205–214

Hurvitz SA, Baumgarten A, Goodman RM. The wrinkly skin syndrome: a report of a case and review of the literature. Clin Genet 1990;38:307–313

RESTRICTIVE DERMOPATHY

Skin

see Figure 8–29

skin is thickened, scaly, and nonpliant; irregular shiny erythematous thinned patches are seen

sparse eyebrows and eyelashes; scalp hair occasionally sparse

occasional nail hypoplasia

Non-Skin

intrauterine growth retardation

short umbilical cord

abnormal craniofacies including microcephaly or macrocephaly, widened sutures of skull, micrognathia, small pinched nose, ectropion, and immobile mouth with everted lips

pulmonary hypoplasia

defective bone formation; widespread contractures

Genetics

AR

Pathophysiology

disorder of skin growth and differentiation

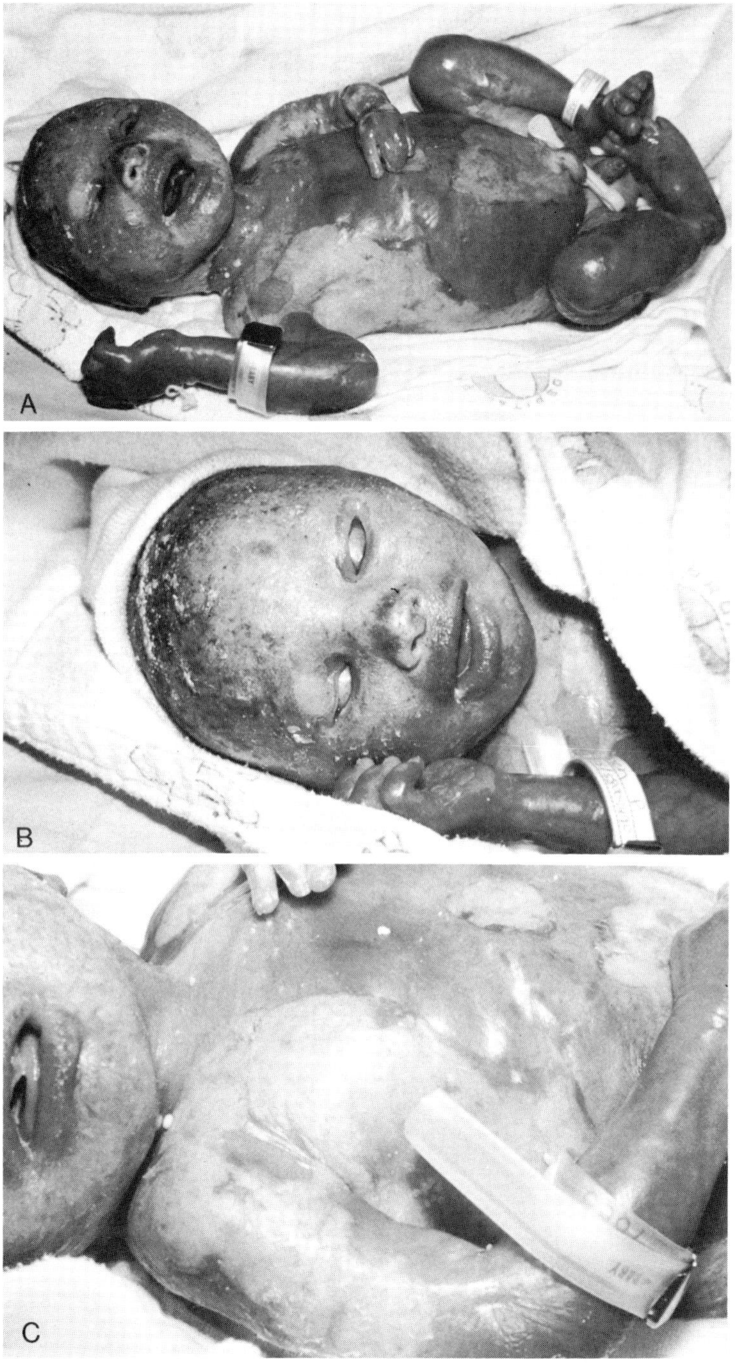

FIGURE 8–29

Restrictive dermopathy. *A,* Large areas of thinned, atrophic, membranous skin alternating with areas of thickened skin. The limbs are held in flexion. *B,* Facies similar to those in "collodion babies." Note the sparse hair, ectropion, and fixed open mouth. *C,* Close-up of the skin showing both the thickened and atrophic areas. Note the hypoplastic nails.

Laboratory Data

histopathology: hyperkeratosis, acanthosis, and absent rete ridge pattern; thin dermis with collagen bundles oriented parallel to the epidermis and absence of elastic tissue fibers; decreased number and size of dermal adnexal structures

poor fibroblast growth in vitro and ultrastructurally; degenerating fibroblasts reported

Prognosis

lethal in newborn period

REFERENCES

McK 275210

Happle R, Stekhoven JH, Hamel BCJ, et al. Restrictive dermopathy in two brothers. Arch Dermatol 1992;128:232–235

Holbrook KA, Dale BA, Witt DR, et al. Arrested epidermal morphogenesis in three newborn infants with a fatal genetic disorder (restrictive dermopathy). J Invest Dermatol 1987;88:330–339

Lowry RB, Machin GA, Morgan K, et al. Congenital contractures, edema, hyperkeratosis, and intrauterine growth retardation: a fatal syndrome in Hutterite and Mennonite kindreds. Am J Med Genet 1985;22:531–543

Mok Q, Curley R, Tolmie JL, et al. Restrictive dermopathy: a report of 3 cases. J Med Genet 1990;27:315–319

Paige DG, Lake BD, Bailey AJ, Ramani P, Harper JI. Restrictive dermopathy: a disorder of fibroblasts. Br J Dermatol 1992;127:630–634

Toriello HV. Invited editorial comment on "restrictive" dermopathy and report of another case. Birth Defects 1988;24(2);103–108

Verloes A, Mulliez N, Gonzales M, et al. Restrictive dermopathy, a lethal form of arthrogryposis multiplex with skin and bone dysplasias: three new cases and review of the literature. Am J Med Genet 1992;43:539–547

Welsh KM, Smoller BR, Holbrook KA, Johnston K. Restrictive dermopathy: report of two affected siblings and a review of the literature. Arch Dermatol 1992;128:228–231

Witt DR, Hayden MR, Holbrook KA, et al. Restrictive dermopathy: a newly recognized autosomal recessive skin dysplasia. Am J Med Genet 1986;24:631–648

NEU-LAXOVA SYNDROME

Skin

widespread ichthyosiform scaling

increased subcutaneous fat and atrophic musculature

generalized edema

nails may be absent

Non-Skin

severe intrauterine growth retardation

abnormal craniofacies including microcephaly, sloping forehead, protuberant eyes and hypoplasia of eyelids, flat nose, large and deformed ears, everted lips, and micrognathia; occasional bilateral cleft palate short neck

musculoskeletal abnormalities include osteopenia, short limbs and joint contractures, hypoplastic digits, rockerbottom feet, and syndactyly

variable central nervous system abnormalities

microphthalmia and cataracts reported

Genetics

AR

Laboratory Data

prenatal diagnosis possible by ultrasonography

Prognosis

most affected infants are stillborn or die within hours or days after birth

Discussion

features similar to those of restrictive dermopathy

REFERENCES

Manjunath NC, Sreenivas V. New manifestations of Neu-Laxova syndrome. Am J Med Genet 1990;35:55–59

Meguid NA, Temtamy SA. Neu-Laxova syndrome in two Egyptian families. Am J Med Genet 1991;41:30–31

Neu RL, Kajii T, Gardener L, et al. A lethal syndrome of microcephaly with multiple congenital anomalies in three siblings. Pediatrics 1971;47:610–612

Ostrovskaya T, Lazjuk G. Cerebral abnormalities in the Neu-Laxova syndrome. Am J Med Genet 1988;30:747–756

Tolmie JL, Mortimer G, Doyle D, et al. The Neu-Laxova syndrome in female sibs: clinical and pathological features with prenatal diagnosis in the second sib. Am J Med Genet 1987;27:175–182

WINCHESTER SYNDROME

Skin

diffuse thickening, hyperpigmentation, and hypertrichosis of skin (Fig. 8–30)

hypertrophy of gums and lips

Non-Skin

musculoskeletal abnormalities with onset usually in first year of life include dwarfism, joint contractures, osteoporosis, and acro-osteolysis of elbows and carpal and tarsal bones

coarse facial features in some

corneal opacities in early childhood

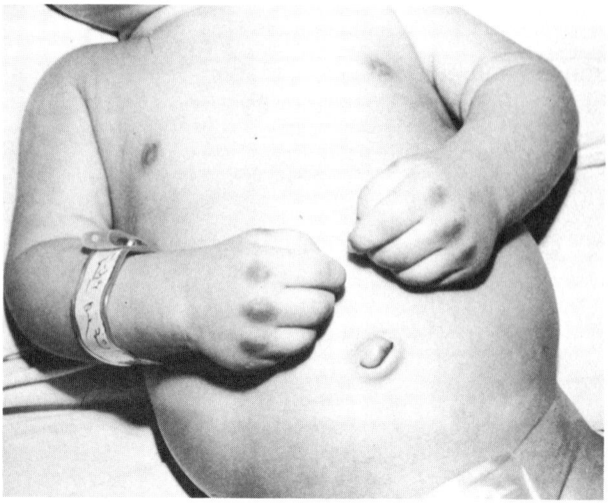

FIGURE 8–30
Winchester syndrome. Diffuse thickening of the skin of the hands with hyperpigmentation over the knuckles. (Courtesy of Amir H. Mehregan, MD, Monroe, Michigan)

Genetics

AR

Laboratory Data

characteristic osteoporosis and osteolysis detected radiographically (Fig. 8–31)

Prognosis

joint stiffness and contractures are progressive, leading to clawing of hands and flexion deformities of limbs with difficulty walking

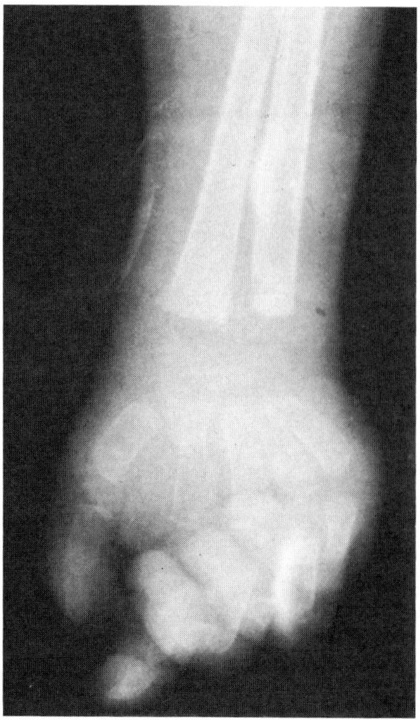

FIGURE 8–31
Winchester syndrome. Radiograph of the lower arms and hands showing osteolysis and osteoporosis. (Courtesy of Amir H. Mehregan, MD, Monroe, Michigan)

REFERENCES

McK 277950
Cohen AH, Hollister DW, Reed WB. The skin in the Winchester syndrome. Arch Dermatol 1975;111:230–236
Hollister SW. The Winchester syndrome: a non-lysosomal connective tissue disease. J Pediatr 1974;84:701–709
Nabai H, Mehregan AH, Mortezai A, et al. Winchester syndrome: report of a case from Iran. J Cutan Pathol 1977;4:281–285
Winchester P, Grossman H, Lim WN, Danes BS. A new acid mucopolysaccharidosis with skeletal deformities simulating rheumatoid arthritis. AJR 1969;106:121–128
Winter RM. Winchester's syndrome. J Med Genet 1989;26:772–775

STIFF SKIN SYNDROME

Synonym

- congenital fascial dystrophy

Skin

localized areas of stony-hard skin, firmly bound to underlying tissues; involves buttocks and upper thighs most severely

onset at birth or in early childhood; nonprogressive

mild generalized hypertrichosis

Non-Skin

limited joint mobility

Genetics

AD and possible AR cases reported

Pathophysiology

similar findings seen in the tight-skin mouse

Laboratory Data

histopathology: abnormal amounts of acid mucopolysaccharides in dermis

fascial thickening up to four times normal

amianthoid-like fibrils and collagen abnormalities are detectable by electron microscopy

large, metachromatically staining cells in dermis and fibroblast culture

normal urine mucopolysaccharide excretion

REFERENCES

McK 184900
McK 228020
Esterly NB, McKusick VA. Stiff skin syndrome. Pediatrics 1971;47:360–369

Jablonska S, Groniowski J, Krieg T, et al. Congenital fascial dystrophy—a noninflammatory disease of fascia: the stiff skin syndrome. Pediatr Dermatol 1984;2:87–97

Jablonska S, Schubert H, Kikuchi I. Congenital fascial dystrophy: stiff skin syndrome—a human counterpart of the tight-skin mouse. J Am Acad Dermatol 1989;21:943–950

Kikuchi I, Inoue S, Hamada K, et al. Stiff skin syndrome. Pediatr Dermatol 1985;3:48–53

PARANA HARD-SKIN SYNDROME

gradual, generalized hardening of skin and subcutaneous tissue beginning at 2 to 3 months of age; spares eyelids, neck, and ears; eventually the patient becomes encased in immovable "cast"

generalized hyperpigmentation

widespread hypertrichosis

growth retardation

joint contractures and immobilization

parotid gland enlargement

pulmonary insufficiency, which has caused death in some

probable AR

McK 260530

Cat I, Rodrigues-Magdalena NI, Parolin-Marinoni L, et al. Parana hard-skin syndrome: study of seven families. Lancet 1974; 1:215–216

APLASIA CUTIS CONGENITA

Synonym

- congenital absence of the skin

Skin

2 to 3 cm in diameter (range 0.5 to over 10 cm) erosion, ulceration, or scarred bald area on scalp, usually at or close to parietal hair whorl (Fig. 8–32); shape is variable, being round, oval, linear, rhomboidal, or stellate

scalp defect may have associated hypertrichosis of adjacent skin

hypertrophic scarring may result with healing

defects occasionally extend into muscle and bone, especially with larger lesions; may also extend to dura and meninges and be associated with hemorrhage, sagittal sinus thrombosis, or meningitis

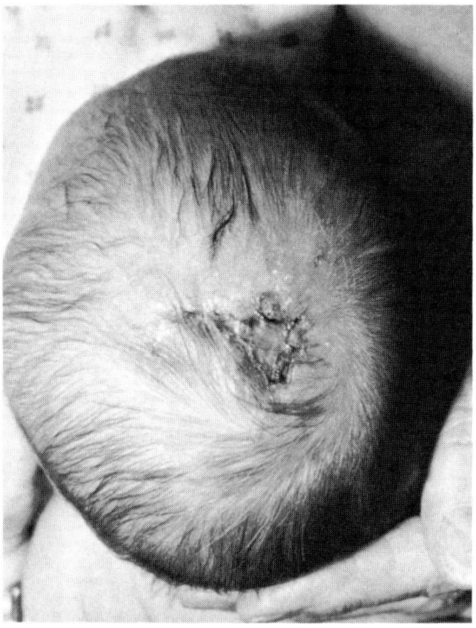

FIGURE 8–32
Aplasia cutis congenita. Large, stellate, crusted erosion on the vertex of a newborn.

less commonly, lesions are multiple, and rarely widespread (Figs. 8–33 and 8–34); uncommonly appear on trunk and extremities; rarely on face

Non-Skin

a heterogeneous group of disorders, some with major associated anomalies; see Discussion and Table 8–2

prematurity of birth common

Genetics

a heterogeneous group of disorders; see Discussion and Table 8–2

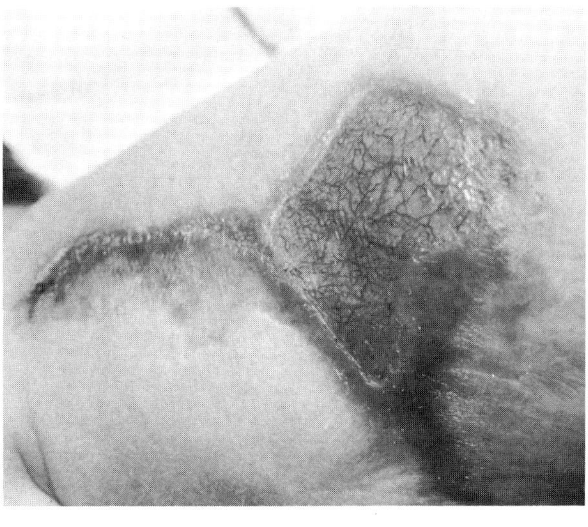

FIGURE 8–33
Aplasia cutis congenita. This infant had symmetrically placed membranous patches on the lateral torso.

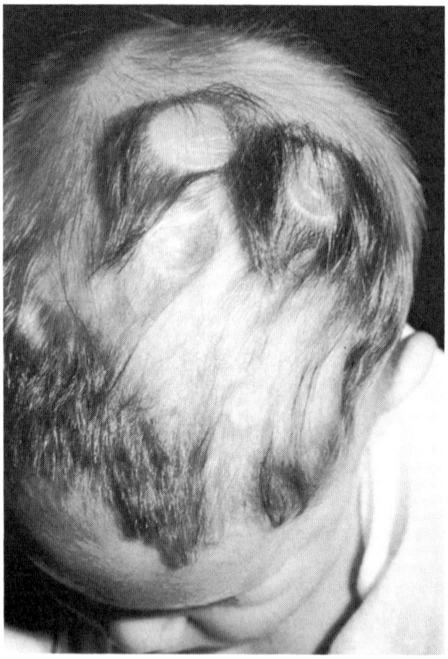

FIGURE 8–34
Multiple areas of aplasia cutis congenita on the scalp in association with hypertrichosis.

Pathophysiology

a variety of etiologies exist; see Discussion and Table 8–2

cases affecting both infants or just one infant in births of monozygotic twins reported

Laboratory Data

histopathology: healed lesions show atrophic epidermis overlying areas of fibrosis in the dermis and complete absence of adnexal structures

up to 30% of cases with scalp defects have radiolucent areas of the calvarium that spontaneously improve

Prognosis

lesions usually heal uneventfully with scarring within a few months, sometimes have already healed in utero

grafts may be indicated in large scalp defects that are more likely to extend to meninges and be associated with hemorrhage, venous thromboses, and meningitis

increased incidence of stillbirth and neonatal death reported in siblings

Discussion

The term *aplasia cutis congenita* (ACC) incorporates a heterogeneous group of disorders in which congenital localized absence of skin (CLAS) is seen, sometimes alone or in association with a wide variety of anomalies. Some authors contend that the term CLAS is preferable to ACC since ACC implies a failure

TABLE 8–2
CLASSIFICATION OF APLASIA CUTIS CONGENITA (ACC)

ACC Grouping	Inheritance	Area Affected by ACC	Selected Other Findings
Group 1 Scalp ACC without multiple anomalies	AD and sporadic	Scalp, usually vertex; single lesion in about two thirds	
Group 2 Scalp ACC with associated limb abnormalities	AD	Midline scalp close to scalp hair whorl; solitary or multiple	Limb reduction abnormalities; lower limbs more severely affected than upper limbs Association with postaxial polydactyly may represent a separate genetic entity (McK 181250)
Group 3 Scalp ACC with associated epidermal and organoid nevi	Sporadic	Scalp; may be asymmetrical	Some cases associated with ophthalmologic and neurologic abnormalities
Group 4 ACC overlying embryologic malformations	Varies; depends on underlying condition	Abdomen, lumbar skin, scalp, and elsewhere	Meningomyelocele Spinal dysraphia Cranial stenosis Congenital midline porencephaly Leptomeningeal angiomatosis Omphalocele Gastroschisis Ectopia of ear
Group 5 ACC with associated fetus papyraceus or placental infarcts	Sporadic	Scalp, trunk, axillae and extremities; involvement is multiple and mostly symmetrical; lesions may have linear or stellate configuration	Fibrous constriction bands on limbs
Group 6a ACC with epidermolysis bullosa (EB) usually localized, without multiple congenital anomalies	AD or AR, depending on EB subtype (see chapter on epidermolysis bullosa)	Extremities	
Group 6b ACC with gastrointestinal atresia (McK 207730)	AR	Large areas on extremities and torso	Many associated abnormalities reported, including pyloric or duodenal atresia, abnormal craniofacies, and nail dystrophy
Group 7 ACC localized to extremities without blistering	AD and AR	Pretibial areas; dorsal aspects of hands and feet; extensor wrists	
Group 8 ACC caused by specific teratogens		Scalp (due to methimazole); any area (due to varicella or herpes simplex infection)	Imperforate anus (methimazole) Other sequelae of varicella and herpes simplex infection
Group 9 ACC associated with malformation syndromes	Varies; depends on associated syndrome	Scalp; any location	Malformation syndromes include: Trisomy 13 4p⁻ syndrome Oculocerebrocutaneous syndrome (Delleman-Orthuys syndrome) Focal facial dermal dysplasia Johanson-Blizzard syndrome Focal dermal hypoplasia Amniotic band disruption complex XY gonadal dysgenesis

Table continued on following page

TABLE 8–2
CLASSIFICATION OF APLASIA CUTIS CONGENITA (ACC) *Continued*

ACC Grouping	Inheritance	Area Affected by ACC	Selected Other Findings
Adams-Oliver syndrome (McK 100300)	AD; AR and sporadic cases also reported	Scalp	Included in group 2 Skull and limb defects Cutis marmorata telangiectatica congenita reported

References:
Frieden IJ. Aplasia cutis congenita: a clinical review and proposal for classification. J Am Acad Dermatol 1986;14:646–660
Sybert VP. Aplasia cutis congenita: a report of 12 new families and review of the literature. Pediatr Dermatol 1985:3:1–14
Bork K, Pfeifle J. Multifocal aplasia cutis congenita, distal limb hemimelia, and cutis marmorata telangiectatica in a patient with Adams-Oliver syndrome. Br J Dermatol 1992;127:160–163
Atherton DJ. Naevi and other developmental defects. In: Champion RH, Burton JL, Ebling FJG, eds. Textbook of Dermatology. Oxford, Blackwell Scientific Publications, 1992:518–524.
Buttiens M, Fryns JP, Jonckheere P, et al. Scalp defect associated with postaxial polydactyly: confirmation of a distinct entity with autosomal dominant inheritance. Hum Genet 1985;71:86–88
Carmi R, Sofer S, Karplus M, et al. Aplasia cutis congenita in two sibs discordant for pyloric atresia. Am J Med Genet 1982;11:319–328
Toriello HV, Higgins JV, Waterman DF. Autosomal-recessive aplasia cutis congenita—report of two affected sibs. [Letter]. Am J Med Genet 1983;15:153–156

of development whereas in many instances the findings are believed to be related to trauma.

There have been many case reports associating ACC with a wide variety of diseases and anomalies. For this reason, various classifications of ACC have been proposed. Frieden (1986) classified ACC into nine groups; Table 8–2 follows this schema. Sybert (1985) suggested another classification, as follows:

type I: lesions limited to scalp

type II: body lesions with or without scalp lesions

type IIA: body lesions with or without limb defects

type III: scalp lesions with or without limb defects

type IV: cases with lesions of epidermolysis bullosa

type IVA: Bart syndrome (see main entry)

Because of heterogeneity of ACC and because the term has been used rather loosely in the literature with reference to a wide variety of diseases and findings, case reports and series using this term should be interpreted with care. This is especially true since partial-thickness skin loss (e.g., skin erosion or denudation) is not uncommon in neonatal period and almost never represents ACC.

Besides the entities listed in Table 8–2, there are other entities in which ACC is seen or in which ACC is considered in the differential diagnosis. These include

- *scalp-ear-nipple syndrome*

  midline posterior scalp nodules with histologic findings of ACC, multiple external ear deformities, and rudimentary or absent nipples

  AD

  McK 181270

- *ACC with intestinal lymphangiectasia*

  ACC of vertex of scalp and lymphedema of limbs at birth

  possible AR

  McK 207731

- *ACC, ear malformations, facial paresis, and dermal sinuses*

  AD

  McK 134100

- *congenital vertex alopecia (aplastic nevus)*

  may be a minor variant of aplasia cutis congenita but skin is normal in appearance apart from absence of adnexae; sporadic occurrence

- *injury due to obstetric forceps or scalp electrode*

REFERENCES

McK 107600

Anderson CE, Hollister D, Szalay GC. Autosomal dominantly inherited cutis aplasia congenita, ear malformations, right-sided facial paresis, and dermal sinuses. Birth Defects 1979;15(5B):265–270

Bronspiegel N, Zelnick N, Rabinowitz, et al. Aplasia cutis congenita and intestinal lymphangiectasia: an unusual association. Am J Dis Child 1985;139:509–513

Butler DF, Berger TG, James WD, et al. Bart's syndrome: microscopic, ultrastructural, and immunofluorescent mapping features. Pediatr Dermatol 1986;3:113–118

Finlay AY, Markes R. An hereditary syndrome of lumpy scalp, odd ears and rudimentary nipples. Br J Dermatol 1978;99:423–430

Frieden IJ. Aplasia cutis congenita: a clinical review and proposal for classification. J Am Acad Dermatol 1986;14:646–660

Fryns JP, de Cock P, van den Berghe H. Occipital scalp defect associated with valvular pulmonary stenosis. A new entity? Clin Genet 1992;42:97–99

Jones EM, Hersh JH, Yusk JW. Aplasia cutis congenita, cleft palate, epidermolysis bullosa, and ectrodactyly: a new syndrome? Pediatr Dermatol 1992;9:293–297

Lestringant G, al Towairky A. Three siblings with extensive aplasia cutis congenita of the scalp and underlying bone defect: autosomal recessive inheritance. [Letter]. Int J Dermatol 1989;28:278–279

Leung RCS, Beer WE, Mehta HK. Aplasia cutis congenita presenting as a familial triad of atrophic alopecia, ocular defects, and a peculiar scarring tendency of the skin. Br J Dermatol 1988;118:715–720

Levin DL, Nolan KS, Esterly NB. Congenital absence of skin. J Am Acad Dermatol 1980;2:203–206

McMurray BR, Martin LW, St. John Dignan P, Fogelson MH. Hereditary aplasia cutis congenita and associated defects: three instances in one family and a survey of reported cases. Clin Pediatr 1977;16:610–614

Sanchez Pedreño GP, Rodriguez Pichardo A, Camacho Martinez F, et al. Aplasia cutis congenita. J Am Acad Dermatol 1985; 13:429–433

Santos H, Cordeiro I, Menezes I. Aplasia cutis congenita associated with congenital heart defect, not a coincidence? [Letter]. Am J Med Genet 1989;34:614–615

Steinberg RD, Ethington J, Esterly NB. Lumpy scalp syndrome. Int J Dermatol 1990; 29:657–658

Sybert VP. Aplasia cutis congenita: a report of 12 new families and review of the literature. Pediatr Dermatol 1985;3:1–14

Yagupsky P, Reuveni H, Karplus M, et al. Aplasia cutis congenita in one of monozygotic twins. Pediatr Dermatol 1986;3:403–405

JOHANSON-BLIZZARD SYNDROME

aplasia cutis of scalp and sparse hair

absence or hypoplasia of the alae nasi and pancreatic insufficiency with failure to thrive are characteristic

other common ectodermal and mesodermal abnormalities include short stature, mental retardation, dental anomalies, deafness, and anorectal anomalies

AR

McK 243800

Day DW, Israel JN. Johanson-Blizzard syndrome. Birth Defects 1978;14:275–287

Gould NS, Paton JB, Bennett AR. Johanson-Blizzard syndrome: clinical and pathological findings in 2 sibs. Am J Med Genet 1989;33:194–199

Hurst JA, Baraitser M. Johanson-Blizzard syndrome. J Med Genet 1989;26:45–48

PROTEUS SYNDROME

Skin

large variety of hyperplasias, neoplasms, and malformations, many forming soft tissue masses, including

- distinctive cerebriform masses of the soles and, less commonly, the palms (Fig. 8–35); masses composed of fibrous and fatty tissue
- vascular tumors and malformations, many subcutanous, produce characteristic soft masses; vascular and related tumors include lymphan-

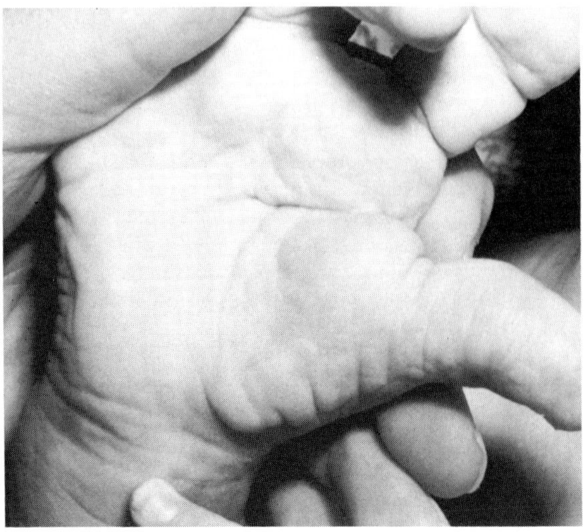

FIGURE 8–35
Early cerebriform change on the palm of an infant with Proteus syndrome. Note the thickened areas on the thenar eminence.

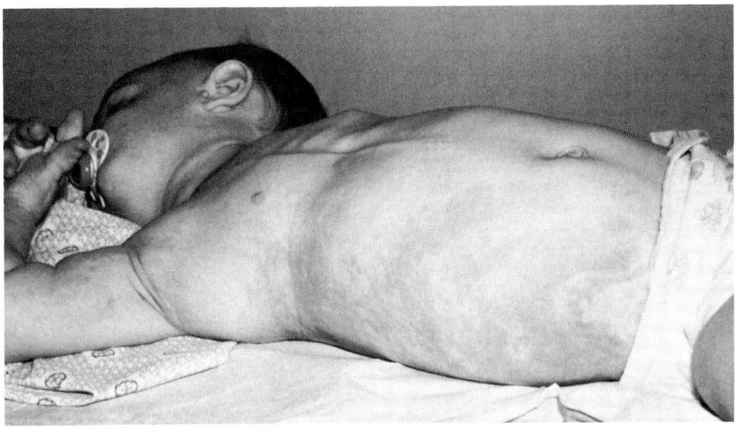

FIGURE 8–36
Patterned epidermal nevi on the torso of the child with Proteus syndrome shown in Figure 8–35. A lipoma was also present in the axillary area.

giomas, hemolymphangiomas, and lipohemangiomas; vascular malformations include port wine stains

- lipomas, especially of abdomen
- epidermal nevi in linear and whorled patterns, which may follow lines of Blaschko, on trunk, neck, and extremities; same areas may have hypopigmented and/or hyperpigmented streaks (Fig. 8–36)

cutaneous findings frequently present at birth but may develop in infancy

occasional dental abnormalities

Non-Skin

birth weight may be high

increased growth rate in infancy and early childhood causes asymmetrical hypertrophy of virtually any body part, including total or segmental hemihypertrophy, asymmetrical macrocephaly, and gigantism of fingers and toes (Figs. 8–37 through 8–39); macrodactyly is considered characteristic but is not invariably present

other musculoskeletal abnormalities include kyphoscoliosis, cranial exostoses, and hip dislocation

neurologic abnormalities include epilepsy; mental function usually normal, but mental retardation reported

eye abnormalities include strabismus, epibulbar tumor, and enlarged globe

Genetics

mostly sporadic

may be due to a lethal AD gene surviving in a mosaic state by somatic mutation

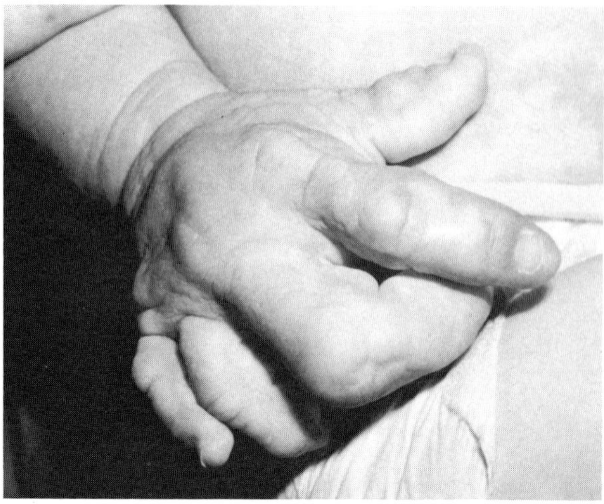

FIGURE 8–37
Proteus syndrome. Same infant as in Figures 8–35 and 8–36. Note macrodactyly.

one case with partial expression revealed mosaic duplication of a portion of chromosome 1

Laboratory Data

histopathology: cerebriform masses of palms and soles show increased collagen or fat

Prognosis

more severe and more rapidly progressive cases usually have earlier age at onset

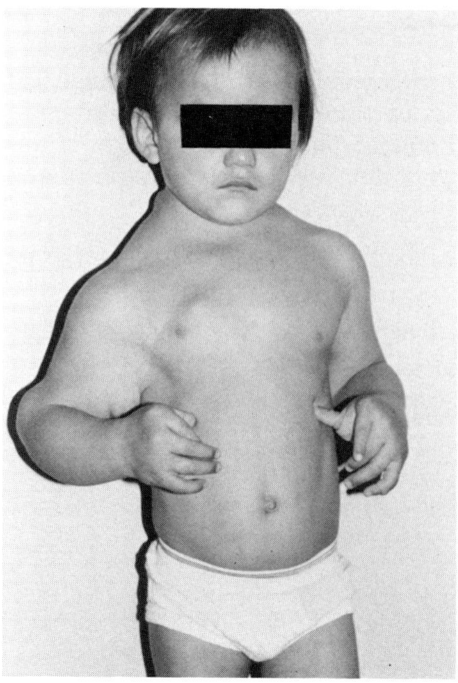

FIGURE 8–38
Proteus syndrome. The child has marked asymmetrical limb overgrowth. (Courtesy of Jon Aase, MD, Albuquerque, New Mexico)

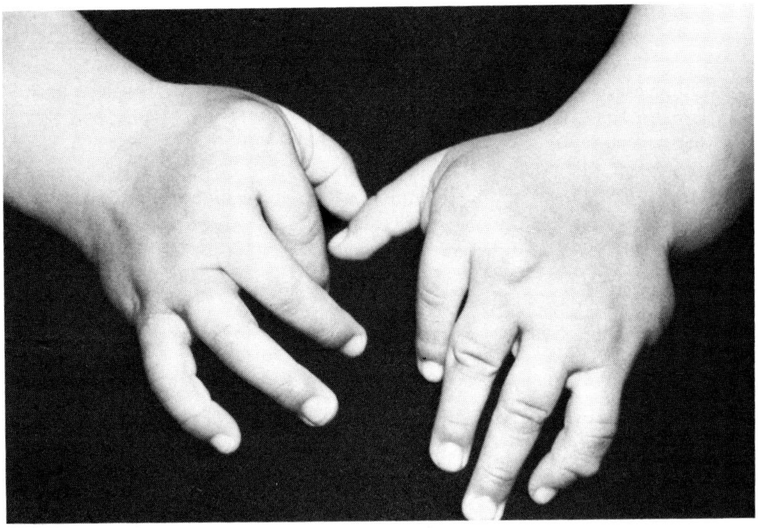

FIGURE 8–39
Proteus syndrome. The hands are large and show ulnar deviation. (Courtesy of Jon Aase, MD, Albuquerque, New Mexico)

Discussion

the "Elephant Man," Joseph Merrick, is believed to have suffered from this disease rather than from neurofibromatosis

Klippel-Trenaunay-Weber syndrome and neurofibromatosis are two principal entities that must be ruled out before a diagnosis of Proteus syndrome can be made

- *encephalocraniocutaneous lipomatosis*

  nosology controversial; some consider it a distinct entity from Proteus syndrome characterized by severe mental retardation, seizures, unilateral frontotemporal lipomatosis, ipsilateral leptomeningeal and cerebral lipomatosis, cerebral malformations and calcification, and lipomas of the skull, eye, and heart; others believe it represents a circumscribed form of Proteus syndrome; sporadic occurrence

REFERENCES

McK 176920

Bialer MG, Riedy MJ, Wilson WG. Proteus syndrome versus Bannayan-Zonana syndrome: a problem in differential diagnosis. Eur J Pediatr 1988;148:122–125

Clark RD, Donnai D, Rogers J, et al. Proteus syndrome: an expanded phenotype. Am J Med Genet 1987;27:99–117

Cohen MM Jr. Understanding Proteus syndrome, unmasking the elephant man, and stemming elephant fever. Neurofibromatosis 1988;1:260–280

Costa T, Krafchik BR. Proteus syndrome. Pediatr Dermatol 1989;6:344–345

Goodship J, Redfearn A, Milligan D, Gardner-Medwin D, Burn J. Transmission of Proteus syndrome from father to son? J Med Genet 1991;28:781–785

Happle R, Steijlen PM. Enzephalokraniokutane lipomatose. Hautarzt 1993;44:19–22

Loggers HE, Dosterwijk JC, Overweg-Plandsoen WC, et al. Encephalocraniocutaneous lipomatosis and oculocerebrocutaneous syndrome. Ophthalmol Pediatr Genet 1992;13:171–177

Mayatepek E, Kurczynski TW, Ruppert ES, et al. Expanding the phenotype of the Proteus syndrome: a severely affected patient

with new findings. Am J Med Genet 1989;32:402–406
McCall S, Ramzy MI, Cure JK, Pai GS. Encephalocraniocutaneous lipomatosis and the Proteus syndrome: distinct entities with overlapping manifestations. Am J Med Genet 1992;43:662–668
Nazzaro V, Cambiaghi S, Montagnani A, et al. Proteus syndrome: ultrastructural study of linear verrucous and depigmented nevi. J Am Acad Dermatol 1991;25:377–383
Samlaska CP, Levin SW, James WD, et al. Proteus syndrome. Arch Dermatol 1989; 125:1109–1114
Tibbles JA, Cohen MM Jr. The Proteus syndrome: the Elephant Man diagnosed. Br Med J [Clin Res] 1986;293:683–685
Vaughn RY, Selinger AD, Howell CG, et al. Proteus syndrome: diagnosis and surgical management. J Pediatr Surg 1993;28:5–10
Wiedemann HR, Burgio GR. Encephalocraniocutaneous lipomatosis and Proteus syndrome. Am J Med Genet 1986;25:403–404

BANNAYAN-RILEY-RUVALCABA SYNDROME (BANNAYAN-ZONANA SYNDROME; RILEY-SMITH SYNDROME; RUVALCABA-MYHRE-SMITH SYNDROME)

multiple cutaneous tumors consisting of combinations of lipomatous, angiomatous, and lymphangiomatous tissue; usually develop in mid childhood

occasional lymphedema of lower limbs

may have pigmented macules on genitalia

macrocephaly at birth

pseudopapilledema in some

hamartomas in viscera, serosal cavities, and bones

increased birth size; postnatal growth deficiency

mental retardation

ileal and colonic polyps

Hashimoto thyroiditis

AD

Bannayan-Zonana syndrome and Riley-Smith syndrome are the same; some distinguish Ruvalcaba-Myhre-Smith syndrome from this group, whose major features are genital pigmented macules and intestinal polyps

differs from Proteus syndrome by lack of features including skull exostoses, epidermal nevi, and palmoplantar masses

McK 153480
Cohen MM Jr. Bannayan-Riley-Ruvalcaba syndrome: renaming three formerly recognized syndromes as one etiologic entity. [Letter]. Am J Med Genet 1990;35:291
DiLiberti JH, Weleber RG, Budden S. Ruvalcaba-Myhre-Smith syndrome: a case with probable autosomal-dominant inheritance and additional manifestations. Am J Med Genet 1983;15:491–495
DiLiberti JH. Comments on Dr. Cohen's letter. [Letter]. Am J Med Genet 1990;35:292
Dvir M, Beer S, Aladjem M. Heredofamilial syndrome of mesodermal hamartomas, macrocephaly, and pseudopapilledema. Pediatrics 1988;81:287–290

Gorlin RJ, Cohen MM, Condon LM, Burke BA. Bannayan-Riley-Ruvalcaba syndrome. Am J Med Genet 1992;44:307–314
Gretzula JC, Hevia O, Schachner LS, et al. Ruvalcaba-Myhre-Smith syndrome. Pediatr Dermatol 1988;5:28–32
Higginbottom MC, Schultz P. The Bannayan syndrome: an autosomal dominant disorder consisting of macrocephaly, lipomas, hemangiomas, and risk for intracranial tumors. Pediatrics 1982;69:632–634
Klein JA, Barr RJ. Bannayan-Zonana syndrome associated with lymphangiomyomatous lesions. Pediatr Dermatol 1990;7:48–53
Miles JH, Zonana J, McFarlane J, et al. Macrocephaly with hamartomas: Bannayan-Zonana syndrome. Am J Med Genet 1984;19:225–234
Riley HD Jr, Smith WR. Macrocephaly, pseudopapilledema and multiple hemangiomata: a previously undescribed heredofamilial syndrome. Pediatrics 1960;26:293–300

PACHYDERMOPERIOSTOSIS

Synonyms

- idiopathic hypertrophic osteoarthropathy
- Touraine-Solente-Galé syndrome

Skin

furrowing and thickening of skin of face, scalp, legs, forearms, hands, and feet resulting in coarsening of the facial features and cutis verticis gyrata (Fig. 8–40)

onset is usually after puberty, but rarely in infancy

thickening of the eyelids causes prominent pseudoptosis and an “angry,” “worried,” or prematurely aged appearance

thickened skin may be hyperhidrotic, particularly that of the hands and feet

increased seborrhea and acne, especially of face and forehead

clubbing and increased convexity of the nails results in a “watch-glass” appearance

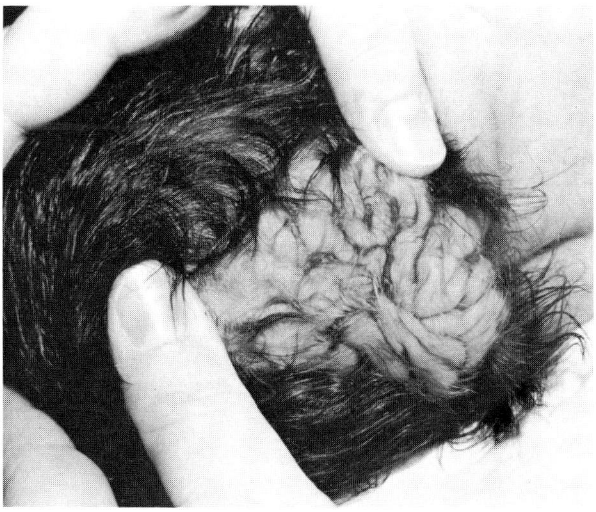

FIGURE 8–40
Cutis verticis gyrata on the posterior scalp of a newborn. This infant had multiple congenital anomalies.

Non-Skin

periosteal proliferation and soft tissue hyperplasia, causing thickening of fingers and toes, clubbing of terminal phalanges and "spade-like" enlargement of hands and feet, cylindrical thickening of legs and forearms; these joints may be painful

other joints may be hyperextensible, due to thickened but lax ligaments, with occasional effusions; eventually, however, ankylosis of joints may occur

Genetics

usually sporadic; AD cases reported

male to female ratio: 9:1

females have less severe disease than males

Laboratory Data

histopathology: increased collagen and mucin deposition; trapping of cutaneous adnexa, which are also increased in number

radiographs show prominent periosteal proliferation (especially of tibiae and fibulae) and soft tissue thickening

Prognosis

condition progressive for several years, then stable

Discussion

a secondary, nonfamilial form is associated with a primary neoplasm, usually carcinoma of lung (hypertrophic pulmonary osteoarthropathy)

abortive forms may exist with variable clinical features (e.g., isolated cutis verticis gyrata or simple hereditary clubbing)

association with severe anemia and gastric hypertrophy reported

- *cutis vertis gyrata*

  cutis verticis gyrata is a descriptive term and may be seen in many acquired and congenital diseases including acromegaly, inflammatory diseases (e.g., dermatitis and psoriasis), neoplasms (e.g., large melanocytic nevi and neurofibromas), systemic diseases (e.g., myxedema), and following trauma

  some cases inherited (mostly AR) in association with neurologic abnormalities, especially mental retardation

  McK 219300

  McK 304200

- *acromegaly*

also may show cutis verticis gyrata and "spade-like" hands; acromegaly differentiated by enlargement of tongue, mandible, nose, and supraorbital ridges; caused by a pituitary adenoma

REFERENCES

McK 167100
Akesson HO. Cutis verticis gyrata and mental deficiency in Sweden: I. Epidemiologic and clinical aspects. Acta Med Scand 1964;175:115–127
Akesson HO. Cutis verticis gyrata and mental deficiency in Sweden: II. Genetic aspects. Acta Med Scand 1964;177:459–464
Curth HO, Firschein IL, Alpert M. Familial clubbed fingers. Arch Dermatol 1961; 83:828–836
Hambrick GW, Carter DM. Pachydermoperiostosis. Arch Dermatol 1966;94:594–608
Herman MA, Massaro D, Katz S, Sachs M. Pachydermoperiostosis: clinical spectrum. Arch Intern Med 1965;116:918–923
Lindmaier A, Raff M, Seidl G, Jurecka W. Pachydermoperiostose. Hautarzt 1989;40: 752–757
Martinez-Lavin M, Pineda C, Valdez T, et al. Primary hypertrophic osteoarthropathy. Semin Arthritis Rheum 1988;17:156–162
Venencie PY, Boffa GA, Delmas PD, et al. Pachydermoperiostosis with gastric hypertrophy, anemia, and increased serum bone Gla-protein levels. Arch Dermatol 1988; 124:1831–1834

CARTILAGE-HAIR HYPOPLASIA SYNDROME

Synonym

- metaphyseal chondrodysplasia, McKusick type

Skin

short, silky, sparse, and light-colored scalp hair; occasional complete alopecia

eyebrows, eyelashes, body hair, and beard may be sparse

skin is baggy around large joints

nails short and broad

Non-Skin

metaphyseal dysostosis due to cartilage hypoplasia results in dwarfism with disproportionately short limbs and pudgy hands

occasional chest deformities and posterior projection of the heel

joints of fingers, wrists, and feet are lax and hyperextensible; in contrast, elbows are hypoextensible

head size and intelligence normal

increased infections (e.g., respiratory)

occasional defects in intestinal absorption or megacolon and resultant diarrhea

Genetics

AR

most kindreds reported in Old Order Amish, Finland, and England

Pathophysiology

impaired T-cell–mediated immunity reported

Laboratory Data

tensile strength of hair and diameter reduced; hair shafts are elliptical in cross section

radiographic findings include irregularly scalloped metaphyses with sclerotic margins, cystic radiolucencies in bony metaphyses, and flattened epiphyses; findings can be mild or absent by adulthood

lymphopenia common

Prognosis

increased susceptibility to some viral infections (e.g., varicella), which may be fatal

life expectancy decreased

Discussion

the actor who played the character of "E.T." in the movie by that name suffered from cartilage-hair hypoplasia syndrome

REFERENCES

McK 250250

Brennan TE, Pearson RW. Abnormal elastic tissue in cartilage-hair hypoplasia. Arch Dermatol 1988;124:1411–1414

Coupe RL, Lowry RB. Abnormality of the hair in cartilage-hair hypoplasia. Dermatologica 1970;141:329–334

Gorlin RJ. Cartilage-hair-hypoplasia and Hodgkin disease. Am J Med Genet 1992;44:539

Makitie O. Cartilage-hair hypoplasia in Finland: epidemiological and genetic aspects of 107 patients. J Med Genet 1992;29:652–655

McKusick VA, Eldridge R, Hostetler JA, et al. Dwarfism in the Amish: II. Cartilage-hair hypoplasia. Bull Johns Hopkins Hosp 1965;116:285–326

van der Burgt I, Haraldsson A, Oosterwijk JC, et al. Cartilage hair hypoplasia, metaphyseal chondrodysplasia type McKusick: description of seven patients and review of the literature. Am J Med Genet 1991; 41:371–380

IMMUNODEFICIENCY WITH SHORT-LIMBED DWARFISM

redundant skin folds around neck and large joints

generalized scaling and erythema

hair light in color, reduced in diameter, and sparse

head normal, but extremities are short and hands are pudgy

may have the hematologic and associated findings of severe combined immunodeficiency

AR

Feigin RD, Middlekamp JN, Kissane JM, Warren RJ. Agammaglobulinemia and thymic dysplasia associated with ectodermal dysplasia. Pediatrics 1971;47:143–147

Gatti RA, Platt N, Pomerance HH, et al. Hereditary lymphopenic agammaglobulinemia associated with a distinctive form of short-limbed dwarfism and ectodermal dysplasia. J Pediatr 1969;75:675–684

Gotoff SP, Esterly NB, Gottbrath E, et al. Granulomatous reaction in an infant with combined immunodeficiency disease and short-limbed dwarfism. J Pediatr 1972; 80:1010–1017

van der Burgt I, Haraldsson A, Oosterwijk JC, et al. Cartilage-hair hypoplasia, metaphyseal chondrodysplasia type McKusick: description of seven patients and review of the literature. Am J Med Genet 1991;41:371–380

CHONDROECTODERMAL DYSPLASIA

Synonym

- Ellis–van Creveld syndrome

Skin

hair normal in most patients but is fine, sparse, and brittle in some

nail abnormalities include brittleness, furrowing, and hypoplasia or absence

dental anomalies frequent and include neonatal teeth, partial anodontia, hypodontia, and/or delayed eruption

sulcus between upper lip and gum often absent

Non-Skin

acromesomelic dwarfism (greater shortening of distal extremities compared with proximal)

other skeletal abnormalities include small thorax, syncarpalism, synmetacarpalism, bilateral ulnar polydactyly, and rarely extra toes

mental retardation in some

congenital heart defects in about half

genital anomalies in about one third including cryptorchidism and hypospadias

Genetics

AR

many cases among the Pennsylvania Amish

Laboratory Data

radiographs: cone-shaped epiphyses of hands are pathognomonic

Prognosis

around half of patients die in first 6 months of life due to congenital heart disease

Discussion

some family members may have limited stigmata

REFERENCES

McK 225500

Blackburn MG, Belliveau RE. Ellis-van Creveld syndrome: a report of previously undescribed anomalies in two siblings. Am J Dis Child 1971;122:267–270

Douglas WF, Schonholtz GJ, Geppert LJ. Chondroectodermal dysplasia (Ellis-van Creveld syndrome). Am J Dis Child 1959;97:473–478

Ellis RWB, van Crevald S. A syndrome characterized by ectodermal dysplasia, polydactyly, chondrodysplasia and congenital morbus cordis. Arch Dis Child 1940;15:65–84

Rosemberg S, Carneiro PC, Zerbini MC, Gonzalez CH. Brief clinical report: chondroectodermal dysplasia (Ellis-van Creveld) with anomalies of CNS and urinary tract. Am J Med Genet 1983;1:291–295

Walls WL, Altman DH, Winslow OP. Chondroectodermal dysplasia (Ellis-van Creveld syndrome). Am J Dis Child 1959;89:118–124

COFFIN-SIRIS SYNDROME

Synonym

- fifth digit syndrome

Skin

sparse scalp hair

hypertrichosis of eyelashes and eyebrows; occasional synophrys

bilateral hypoplastic or absent nails, predominantly involving fifth fingers or toes

Non-Skin

abnormal craniofacies including microcephaly, coarsening of features, flat and broad nasal bridge, broad and upturned nasal tip, wide mouth, and prominent lips

low birth weight; feeding problems in infancy

constant but variable mental and physical retardation

musculoskeletal abnormalities include bilateral hypoplasia or aplasia of terminal phalanges of fifth fingers and toes, joint laxity, and muscle hypotonia

recurrent respiratory infections

Genetics

AR

Discussion

because of abnormalities including digital hypoplasia, some cases of fetal hydantoin syndrome have been misdiagnosed as Coffin-Siris syndrome

REFERENCES

McK 135900

Carey JC, Hall BD. The Coffin-Siris syndrome: five new cases including two siblings. Am J Dis Child 1978;132:667–671

D'Souza SW, Robertson IG, Donnai D, Mawer G. Fetal phenytoin exposure, hypoplastic nails and jitteriness. Arch Dis Child 1990;65:320–324

Feingold M. The Coffin-Siris syndrome. Am J Dis Child 1978;132:660–661

Gorlin RJ. Lapsus—caveat emptor: Coffin-Lowry syndrome vs Coffin-Siris syndrome—an example of confusion compounded. [Letter]. Am J Med Genet 1981;10:103–104

Haspeslagh M, Fryns JP, van den Berghe, H. The Coffin-Siris syndrome: report of a family and further delineation. Clin Genet 1984;26:374–378

Levy P, Baraitser M. Coffin-Siris syndrome. J Med Genet 1991;28:338–341

Tunnessen WWJ, McMillan JA, Levin MB. The Coffin-Siris syndrome. Am J Dis Child 1978;132:393–395

ACROFACIAL DYSOSTOSIS (WEYERS SYNDROME; CURRY-HALL SYNDROME)

hypoplastic or dysplastic nails

dental abnormalities include conical teeth

skeletal abnormalities include short stature, anomalies of mandible, and postaxial polydactyly

AD

McK 193530

Roubicek M, Spranger J. Syndrome of polydactyly, conical teeth and nail dysplasia. Am J Med Genet 1985;20:205–206

Shapiro SD, Jorgenson RJ, Salinas CF. Brief clinical report: Curry-Hall syndrome. Am J Med Genet 1984;17:579–583

EPIDERMAL NEVUS SYNDROME

Synonyms

- Solomon syndrome
- Schimmelpfennig-Feuerstein-Mims syndrome
- nevus sebaceus syndrome

Skin

single or multiple flesh-colored to brownish papules and plaques with a mamillated to verrucoid texture, located most frequently on head and neck (Fig. 8–41); trunk next most frequently involved site, but nevi may occur anywhere (Figs. 8–42 through 8–44)

nevi may be grouped in plaques, in linear distribution unilaterally (as in nevus unius lateris), or widespread (as in ichthyosis hystrix)

onset at birth or within first year of life in majority of cases

other skin findings include hypopigmentation, café-au-lait spots, and hemangiomas

Non-Skin

skeletal abnormalities, most commonly kyphosis and scoliosis, in about two thirds of patients

neurologic abnormalities in one third of patients, especially with midline or extensive epidermal nevi (especially of the head and neck); epilepsy and variable mental retardation are most common manifestations

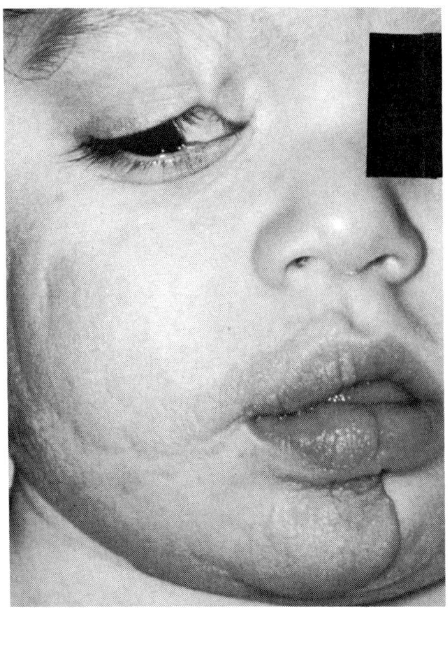

FIGURE 8–41
Multiple sebaceous nevi on the face of a child with linear nevus sebaceus syndrome. Note the midline cutoff and coloboma of the right upper eyelid. (Courtesy of Edward A. Krull, MD, Detroit, Michigan)

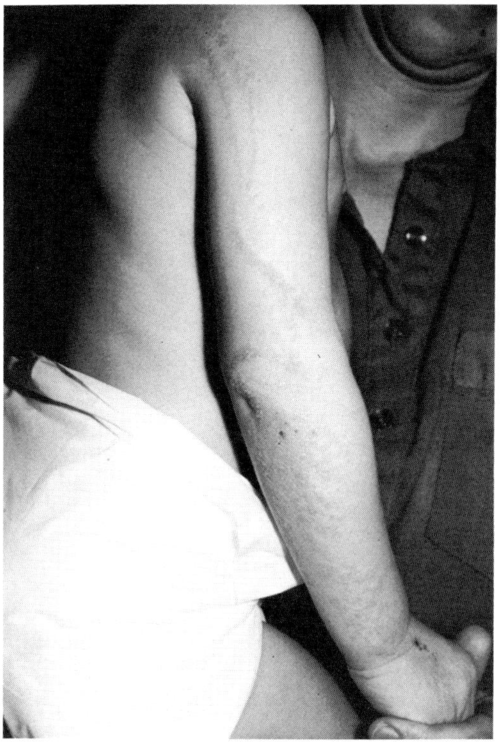

FIGURE 8–42
Linear inflammatory verrucous epidermal nevus on the arm of a toddler. This child had multiple lesions elsewhere on the body associated with intense pruritus.

ocular findings present in up to half of patients, either caused by direct extension of the nevus or present as intrinsic abnormalities

renal malformations include horseshoe, solitary, or hypoplastic kidney, ectopic ureter, and double urinary collecting system

Genetics

mostly sporadic occurrence; AD cases reported

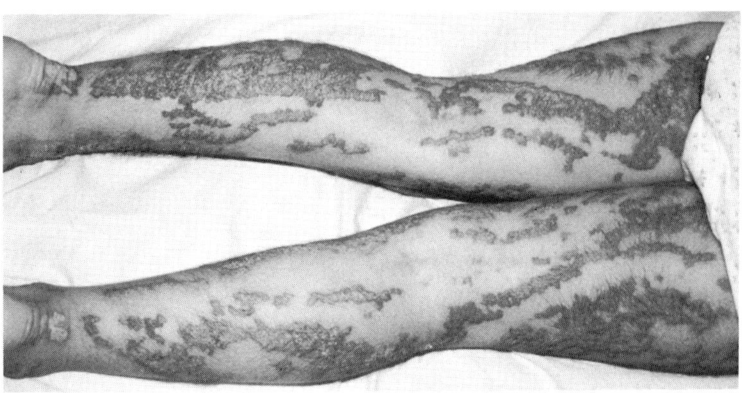

FIGURE 8–43
Multiple hyperpigmented verrucous epidermal nevi covering the thighs and legs of a young girl. Her arms, buttocks, and face were similarly affected.

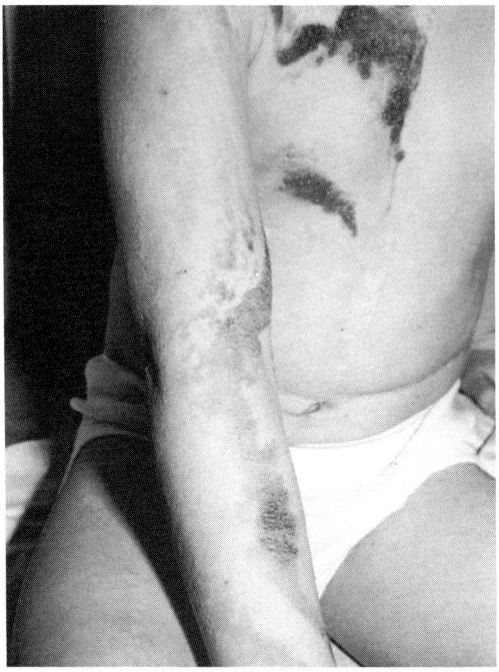

FIGURE 8–44
Multiple velvety plaques on the right torso and arm. This child had extensive cutaneous lesions and multiple other findings of epidermal nevus syndrome.

may be due to a lethal AD gene surviving in mosaic state by somatic mutation

Discussion

an individual with only a linear epidermal nevus, which on histopathology shows epidermolytic hyperkeratosis, can have a child with widespread bullous congenital ichthyosiform erythroderma

instead of subclassifying the nevoid epidermal lesions, such as "nevus sebaceus," "nevus comedonicus," and "inflammatory linear verrucous epidermal nevus (ILVEN)," as well as the various designations of epidermal nevi such as "nevus unius lateris" and "ichthyosis hystrix," some authors propose the use of the generic term *epidermal nevus,* since a single biopsy specimen may incorporate more than one histopathologic pattern

in contrast, some authors propose that there are many distinct epidermal nevus syndromes, such as epidermal nevus syndrome, Proteus syndrome (see main entry), CHILD syndrome (see main entry), and linear nevus sebaceus syndrome (see below), with each type of epidermal nevus representing the cutaneous manifestation of a different mosaic phenotype

- *linear nevus sebaceus syndrome (nevus sebaceus syndrome)*

  orange-tan, verrucous, hairless, unilateral plaque on scalp; projects linearly onto cheek, ear, nose, eyelid, or mucous membranes; some lesions extend to other body surfaces

  mental retardation

epilepsy

ocular coloboma and lipodermoid of conjunctiva

sporadic; may be due to a lethal AD gene surviving in mosaic state by somatic mutation

McK 165630

REFERENCES

McK 163200

Benedetto L, Sood U, Blumenthal N, et al. Familial nevus sebaceus. J Am Acad Dermatol 1990;23:130–132

Eichler C, Flowers FP, Ross J. Epidermal nevus syndrome: case report and review of clinical manifestations. Pediatr Dermatol 1989;6:316–320

Goldberg LH, Collins SA, Siegel DM. The epidermal nevus syndrome: case report and review. Pediatr Dermatol 1987;4:27–33

Happle R. How many epidermal nevus syndromes exist? J Am Acad Dermatol 1991;25:550–556

Happle R. Lethal genes surviving by mosaicism: a possible explanation for sporadic birth defects involving the skin. J Am Acad Dermatol 1987;16:899–906

Hodge JA, Ray MC, Flynn KJ. The epidermal nevus syndrome. Int J Dermatol 1991; 30:91–98

Rogers M, McCrossin I, Commens C. Epidermal nevi and the epidermal nevus syndrome: a review of 131 cases. J Am Acad Dermatol 1989;20:476–488

Rogers M. Epidermal nevi and the epidermal nevus syndromes: a review of 233 cases. Pediatr Dermatol 1992;4:342–344

Sahl WJ Jr. Familial nevus sebaceus of Jadassohn: occurrence in three generations. J Am Acad Dermatol 1990;22:853–854

Solomon LM, Esterly NB. Epidermal and other congenital organoid nevi. Curr Probl Pediatr 1975;6:1–56

ACANTHOSIS NIGRICANS

Skin

dark brown to black velvety plaques most commonly affecting neck, axillae, groin, and perineum, but any area of the skin or mucous membranes may be involved (Figs. 8–45 and 8–46)

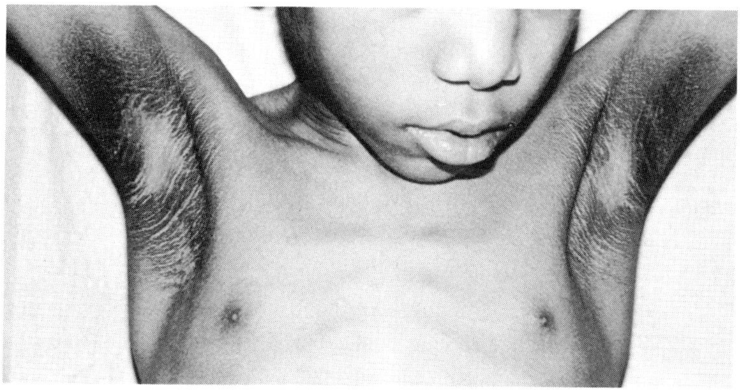

FIGURE 8–45
Acanthosis nigricans. Hyperpigmentated velvety plaques in the axillae of a boy with insulin-resistant diabetes mellitus.

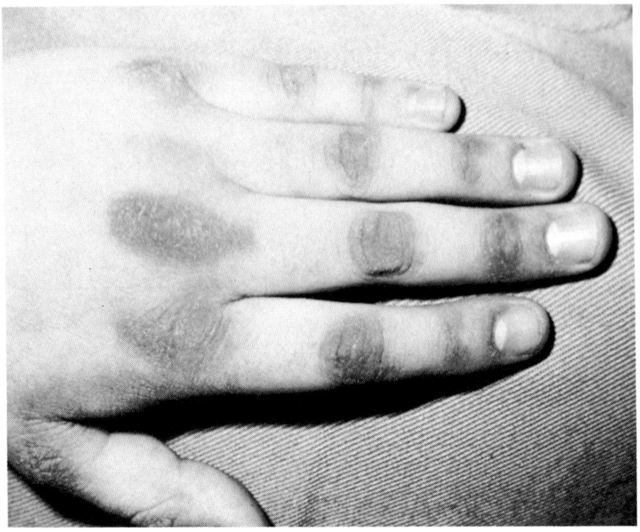

FIGURE 8–46
Brownish discoloration and hyperkeratosis over the knuckles of the hand of a young man with endocrinopathy and acanthosis nigricans.

plaques may become papillomatous or vegetating, especially in skin folds; lesions appear as white papillomatous masses when on mucosal surfaces

onset usually in early childhood, but lesions may be present at birth; usually worsens at puberty, and thereafter remains stable

Genetics

AD when inherited

Discussion

familial form of acanthosis nigricans (AN) is uncommon relative to acquired forms; these forms are traditionally described as follows:

benign AN: can be idiopathic or occur in many hereditary syndromes (e.g., Bloom syndrome, Crouzon syndrome and especially endocrine disorders with insulin resistance such as Seip syndrome and type A and B syndromes of Kahn [see later]); leprechaunism (see main entry) is another hereditary syndrome with severe insulin resistance and AN

pseudo-AN: lesions in body folds of obese individuals, more prominently in those with darker skin; lesions may improve or disappear with weight loss; since these lesions are clinically and histologically identical to those of acanthosis nigricans, the use of the term *pseudo* has been challenged

drug-induced AN: may be due, for example, to nicotinic acid, oral contraceptives, corticosteroids, pituitary extracts, and triazinate (a folic acid antagonist)

malignant AN: lesions may be extensive and appear before, simultaneous with, or after the development of an adenocarcinoma; most of these tumors are intra-abdominal, especially gastric (about two thirds of cases); malignant AN is also seen in association with lymphomas and other malignancies the nosology of acanthosis nigricans is confusing; AN may be a single disease with multiple etiologies with the common effect of increased keratinocyte proliferation by certain growth factors and/or insulin

- *insulin resistance with acanthosis nigricans, type A (type A syndrome of Kahn):*

  inherited deficiency of insulin receptors on cell surface, resulting in insulin resistance and acanthosis nigricans

  polycystic ovary disease is also seen

  possible AR

  seen mostly in females, in first 2 decades of life

- *insulin resistance with acanthosis nigricans, type B (type B syndrome of Kahn):*

  autoantibodies against cell surface insulin receptors, resulting in insulin resistance and acanthosis nigricans

  may be accompanied by other autoimmune disorders besides diabetes mellitus, including systemic lupus erythematosus, Sjögren's syndrome, vitiligo, and alopecia areata

  possible AR

  occurs mostly in females, of older age than in type A

- *insulin resistance with acanthosis nigricans, type C:*

  clinical findings similar to those in type A

  insulin resistance probably located at postreceptor levels

REFERENCES

McK 100600

Auckland G. Acanthosis nigricans heredita. Br J Dermatol 1971;84:193

Brown J, Winkelmann RK. Acanthosis nigricans: a study of 90 cases. Medicine 1968; 47:33–51

Curth HO, Aschner BM. Genetic studies on acanthosis nigricans. Arch Dermatol 1959; 79:55–66

Ellis DL, Kafka SP, Chow JC, et al. Melanoma, growth factors, acanthosis nigricans, the sign of Leser-Trélat, and multiple acrochordons: a possible role for alpha-transforming growth factor in cutaneous paraneoplastic syndromes. N Engl J Med 1987;317:1582–1587

Fukushima N, Nohara Y, Fujita H, et al. A case of insulin resistance associated with acanthosis nigricans. Tohuku J Exp Med 1984;144:129–138

Kahn CR, Flier JS, Bar RS, et al. The syndromes of insulin resistance and acanthosis nigricans: insulin receptor disorders in man. N Engl J Med 1976;294:739–745

Rendon MI, Cruz PD Jr, Sontheimer RD, Bergstresser PR. Acanthosis nigricans: a cutaneous marker of tissue resistance to insulin. J Am Acad Dermatol 1989;12:461–469

Rudiger HW, Dreyer M, Kuhnau J, Bartelheimer H. Familial insulin-resistant diabetes secondary to an affinity defect of the insulin receptor. Hum Genet 1983;64:407–411

Schwenk WF, Rizza RA, Mandarino LJ, et al. Familial insulin resistance and acanthosis nigricans: presence of a postbinding defect. Diabetes 1986;35:33–37

Tasjian D, Jarratt M. Familial acanthosis nigricans. Arch Dermatol 1984;120:1351–1354

LIPODYSTROPHIES

There is no standard nomenclature for a group of conditions variously known as lipodystrophies or lipoatrophies. Lipoatrophy refers to a loss of fat. Lipodystrophy, depending on the context, refers to either a gain or a loss of fat. Acute injury, chronic pressure, and injections (e.g., triamcinolone and insulin) are common causes of fat atrophy seen in clinical practice. Lipoatrophy may also be associated with panniculitides and connective tissue diseases. Finally, there is a highly confusing group of less well known hereditary and acquired disorders, some of which are described in this section, in which lipoatrophy may be seen in isolation or in conjunction with various systemic abnormalities.

SEIP SYNDROME

Synonyms

- Berardinelli syndrome
- lipoatrophic diabetes
- congenital generalized lipodystrophy

Skin

generalized loss of subcutaneous fat; onset at birth or within first years of life

widespread hyperpigmentation, hypertrichosis, and acanthosis nigricans develop at birth or later

Non-Skin

insulin-resistant diabetes mellitus early in life

rapid growth in first decade, when patients are tall for their age, but stature eventually average or shortened

somatic musculature and superficial veins become prominent and abdomen becomes protuberant

penis or clitoris enlarged in most children and some adults; women have no other signs of virilization

mental retardation of variable degree in about 50%

hepatosplenomegaly and cirrhosis develop in most patients

occasional renal or cardiac disease

Genetics

AR

Laboratory Data

increased triglyceride and slightly increased cholesterol levels

advanced bone age detectable radiographically

Prognosis

poor long-term prognosis mainly due to diabetes and its complications

Discussion

- *late-onset generalized lipodystrophy (Lawrence syndrome):*

  onset in adolescence or adulthood; thus, there is no childhood gigantism

  abdomen and somatic musculature less prominent than in Seip syndrome

  cutaneous features in common with Seip syndrome include hyperpigmentation, acanthosis nigricans, hypertrichosis, and a gaunt facial appearance; occasional cutaneous xanthomas

  similar internal manifestations include hepatomegaly and cirrhosis, hypertriglyceridemia, renal disease, and insulin-resistant diabetes; hepatic failure may ensue

  may occur after bacterial (e.g., pertussis) or viral infections

  acquired

REFERENCES

McK 269700
McK 200170
Aronson IK, Zeitz HJ, Variakojis D. Panniculitis in childhood. [Review]. Pediatr Dermatol 1988;5:216–230
Brubaker MM, Levan NE, Collipp PJ. Acanthosis nigricans and congenital total lipodystrophy. Arch Dermatol 1965;91:320–325
Edidin DV. Cutaneous manifestations of diabetes mellitus in children. [Review]. Pediatr Dermatol 1985;2:161–179
Flier JS, Young JB, Landsberg L. Familial insulin resistance with acanthosis nigricans, acral hypertrophy, and muscle cramps. N Engl J Med 1980;303:970–973
Janaki VR, Premalatha S, Rao NR, et al. Lawrence-Seip syndrome. Br J Dermatol 1980;103:693–696
Reed WB, Dexter R, Corley C, Fish C. Congenital lipodystrophic diabetes with acanthosis nigricans. Arch Dermatol 1965;91:326–334
Reed WB, Ragsdale W Jr, Curtis AC, Richards HJ. Acanthosis nigricans in association with various genodermatoses. Acta Derm Venereol 1968;48:465–473
Senior B, Gellis SS. The syndromes of total lipodystrophy and of partial lipodystrophy. Pediatrics 1964;33:593–611

LEPRECHAUNISM

Synonym

- Donohue syndrome

Skin

generalized decrease in subcutaneous fat

loose, wrinkled skin, especially on flexures, hands, and/or feet; orifices rugated

thickened lips and gingivae

marked hypertrichosis, especially of face

occasional acanthosis nigricans

dysplastic nails in some

Non-Skin

intrauterine growth retardation; failure to thrive

patients have a facial appearance described as "elfin" or "gnome-like," with prominent ears and a depressed nasal bridge

abdomen may be protuberant, and hands and feet are disproportionately large

decreased intelligence

nipples, breasts, clitoris, and penis may be enlarged; precocious puberty

insulin-resistant diabetes mellitus with fasting hypoglycemia

Genetics

inheritance not fully established, but familial cases reported

Pathophysiology

defective insulin binding (cellular insulin receptor defect); severe insulin resistance

Laboratory Data

general aminoaciduria

decreased serum alkaline phosphatase level

Prognosis

death occurs in infancy or early childhood

REFERENCES

McK 246200

Der Kaloustian VM, Kronfol NM, Takla R, et al. Leprechaunism: a report of two new cases. Am J Dis Child 1971;122:442–445

Donohue WL, Uchida I. Leprechaunism: a euphemism for a rare familial disorder. J Pediatr 1954;45:505–519

Frindik JP, Kemp SF, Fiser RH, et al. Phenotypic expression in Donohue syndrome (leprechaunism): a role for epidermal growth factor. J Pediatr 1985;107:428–430

Roth SI, Schedewie HK, Herzberg VK, et al. Cutaneous manifestations of leprechaunism. Arch Dermatol 1981;117:531–535

PATTERSON-DAVID SYNDROME (PATTERSON PSEUDOLEPRECHAUNISM SYNDROME)

large redundant loose folds of skin of hands and feet; present at birth

generalized "bronzed" hyperpigmentation

hypertrichosis, mostly of extremities

severe mental retardation

bony deformities and skeletal dysplasia

normal birth weight

inheritance unknown

death in childhood

McK 169170

David TJ, Webb BW, Gordon IRS. The Patterson syndrome, leprechaunism and pseudoleprechaunism. J Med Genet 1981;18:294–298

NODULAR ERYTHEMA WITH DIGITAL CHANGES (NAKAJO SYNDROME)

erythematous papules, plaques, and nodules most commonly on distal extremities, face, and forearms; condition worsens with exposure to cold

onset in infancy to early childhood

large eyes, nose, lips, and ears

disproportionately long, thick fingers with clubbing

slowly progressive growth retardation and "emaciation" due to loss of adipose tissue from upper half of body; muscles atrophic

occasional periosteal hypertrophy, mental retardation, lymphadenopathy, or cardiomegaly

AR

anemia and hypergammaglobulinemia

probably a lipodystrophy

McK 256040

Kitano Y, Matsunaga E, Morimoto T, et al. A syndrome with nodular erythema, elongated and thickened fingers, and emaciation. Arch Dermatol 1985;121:1053–1056

PARTIAL LIPODYSTROPHY

Synonyms

- partial lipoatrophy
- progressive lipodystrophy
- Barraquer-Simons disease
- Weir-Mitchell lipoatrophy

Skin

see Figures 8–47 and 8–48

in the cephalothoracic or Weir-Mitchell type there is symmetrical loss of facial fat in the first or second decade, with or without involvement of neck, arms, chest, or abdomen; lower extremities are normal

variant that spares the face described

Non-Skin

renal disease, most commonly glomerulonephritis of the membranoproliferative type, in 50%; usually follows development of lipodystrophy

Genetics

mostly sporadic; familial cases reported

male to female ratio: 1:4

Pathophysiology

C3 "nephritic factor" is IgG antibody directed against C3bBb complex and stabilizes C3bBbP from inactivation by factors H (C3b inactivator accelerator) and I (C3b inactivator)

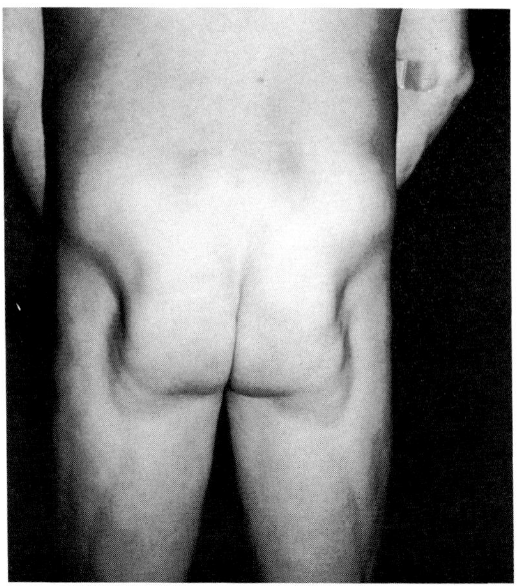

FIGURE 8–47
Absence of fat over the buttocks and thighs of a boy with partial lipodystrophy.

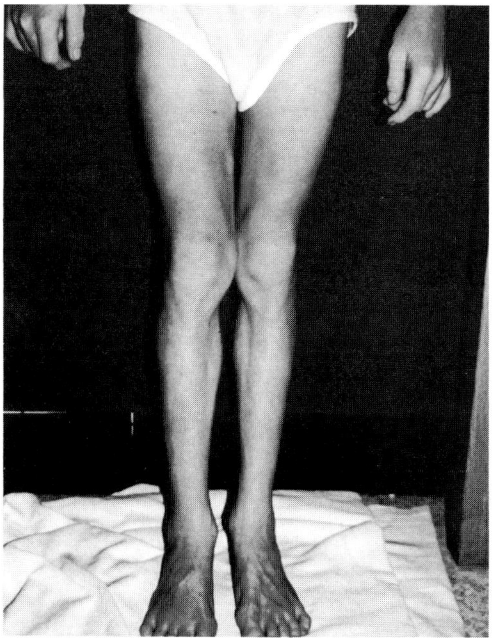

FIGURE 8–48
Absence of subcutaneous tissue on the lower extremities of a youngster with partial lipodystrophy.

glomerulonephritis may be due to the presence of serum C3-activating "nephritic factor" and accompanying C3 hypocomplementemia

Discussion

most cases acquired, often following febrile illnesses; disorders associated with partial lipodystrophy include infections (e.g., measles), insulin-resistant diabetes mellitus, central nervous system disturbances, hepatomegaly, cirrhosis, hypertriglyceridemia, myopathy, Hashimoto thyroiditis, lupus erythematosus, dermatomyositis, Raynaud syndrome, and Sjögren syndrome

in contrast to this type of partial lipodystrophy (Weir-Mitchell type), other rare forms involving the extremities and torso in different combinations have been reported with both autosomal and X-linked dominant inheritance; these forms may manifest many of the noncutaneous findings listed above for Weir-Mitchell partial lipodystrophy

localized lipodystrophies are a third clinical category of lipodystrophies and are not hereditary; they appear at birth or in the first decade most commonly and, unlike total and partial lipodystrophies, are generally not associated with systemic disease

some acquired localized lipodystrophies considered in the differential diagnosis are listed below:

- *lipoatrophia annularis, lipoatrophia semicircularis:*

  annular or semicircular depression of an extremity, ankle, or foot following tenderness and swelling of the limb

  the vast majority of cases involve women

some lesions have been attributed to trauma or wearing tight trousers

spontaneous partial or complete resolution occurs within 1 year

- *lipodystrophia centrifugalis abdominalis infantalis:*

  loss of subcutaneous fat from the abdomen with a raised, scaly, erythematous border

  occurs in infants and children

- *atrophic connective tissue panniculitis:*

  an inflammatory component precedes development of the lipoatrophy

  arthralgias

  elevated erythrocyte sedimentation rate

- *secondary lipodystrophies:*

  causes include insulin injections, lupus profundus, and factitial panniculitis

REFERENCES

McK 308980

Aronson IK, Zeitz HJ, Variakojis D. Panniculitis in childhood. [Review]. Pediatr Dermatol 1988;5:216–230

Ayala F, Lembo G, Ruggiero F, Balato N. Lipoatrophia semicircularis: report of a case. Dermatologica 1985;170:101–103

Chartier S, Buzzanga JB, Paquin F. Partial lipodystrophy associated with a type 3 form of membranoproliferative glomerulonephritis. J Am Acad Dermatol 1987; 16:201–205

Giam YC, Rajan VS, Hock OB. Lipodystrophia centrifugalis abdominalis infantilis. Br J Dermatol 1982;106:461–464

Mascaro JM, Ferrando J. Lipoatrophia semicircularis: the perils of wearing jeans? Int J Dermatol 1982;21:138–139

McLean RH, Hoefnagel D. Partial lipodystrophy and familial C3 deficiency. Hum Hered 1980;30:149–154

Rongioletti F, Rebora A. Annular and semicircular lipoatrophies: report of three cases and review of the literature. [Review]. J Am Acad Dermatol 1989;20:433–436

Roth DE, Schikler KN, Callen JP. Annular atrophic connective tissue panniculitis of the ankles. J Am Acad Dermatol 1989;21;1152–1156

Senior B, Gellis SS. The syndromes of total lipodystrophy and of partial lipodystrophy. Pediatrics 1964;33:593–612

FAMILIAL LIPODYSTROPHY OF LIMBS AND LOWER TRUNK

Synonyms

- reverse partial lipodystrophy
- Köbberling-Dunnigan syndrome

Skin

Two types have been described and their clinical findings are listed below:

- type I

  loss of subcutaneous fat on limbs; sparing of face and trunk

  prominent veins and musculature of limbs

genitalia and face appear normal

acanthosis nigricans, diabetes mellitus, hyperlipidemia, and xanthomas only in some cases

- type II

loss of subcutaneous fat on limbs and trunk but sparing face and vulva, giving appearance of rounded facies and labial hypertrophy

prominent musculature and peripheral veins

insulin-resistant diabetes mellitus and acanthosis nigricans

hyperlipoproteinemia; occasional cutaneous xanthomas

Genetics

seen almost exclusively in females; possible XLD with lethality in XY male; some cases sporadic

Discussion

the two clinical types described earlier may actually be allelic variations of a single disorder

REFERENCES

McK 151660

Burn J, Baraitser M. Partial lipoatrophy with insulin-resistant diabetes mellitus and hyperlipidemia (Dunnigan syndrome). J Med Genet 1986;23:128–130

Köbberling J, Dunnigan MG. Familial partial lipodystrophy: two types of an X-linked dominant syndrome, lethal in the hemizygous state. J Med Genet 1986;23:120–127

PINEAL HYPERPLASIA, INSULIN-RESISTANT DIABETES MELLITUS, AND SOMATIC ABNORMALITIES (MENDENHALL SYNDROME)

decreased subcutaneous fat

acanthosis nigricans

hirsutism

thickened fingernails

dental abnormalities include premature eruption

abnormal facies

abdominal protuberance and enlarged genitalia

insulin-resistant diabetes mellitus

AR

possible insulin receptor defect

pineal body hyperplasia at autopsy

McK 262190

Barnes ND, Palumbo PJ, Hayles AB, Folgar H. Insulin resistance, skin changes, and virilization: a recessively inherited syndrome possibly due to pineal gland dysfunction. Diabetologia 1974;10:285–289

Moncada VY, Hedo JA, Serrano-Rios M, Taylor SI. Insulin-receptor biosynthesis in cultured lymphocytes from an insulin-resistant patient (Rabson-Mendenhall syndrome): evidence for defect before insertion of receptor into plasma membrane. Diabetes 1986;35:802–807

Rabson SM, Mendenhall EN. Familial hypertrophy of pineal body, hyperplasia of adrenal cortex and diabetes mellitus. Am J Clin Pathol 1956;26:283–290

West RJ, Leonard JV. Familial insulin resistance with pineal hyperplasia: metabolic studies and effect of hypophysectomy. Arch Dis Child 1980;55:619–621

SHORT SYNDROME

an acronym for short stature, hyperextensibility of joints, hernia, ocular depression, Rieger anomaly, and teething delay

lipoatrophy of face and upper extremities

probable AR

Aarskog described a family with similar findings (McK 151680) that he suggested represented a separate entity based on features including less extensive lipoatrophy, lack of joint laxity, and AD inheritance

McK 269880

McK 151680

Aarskog D, Ose L, Pande H, Eide N. Autosomal dominant partial lipodystrophy associated with Rieger anomaly, short stature, and insulinopenic diabetes. Am J Med Genet 1983;15:29–38

Gorlin RJ. A selected miscellany. Birth Defects 1975;11(2):46–48

Sensenbrenner JA, Hussels IE, Levin LS. A low birthweight syndrome, ?Rieger syndrome. Birth Defects 1975;11(2):423–426

Toriello HV, Wakefield S, Komar K, et al. Report of a case and further delineation of the SHORT syndrome. Am J Med Genet 1985;22:311–314

MARFAN SYNDROME

Skin

symmetrical extensive striae of the trunk, breasts, deltoid area, hips, buttocks, and thighs in about 25% of patients

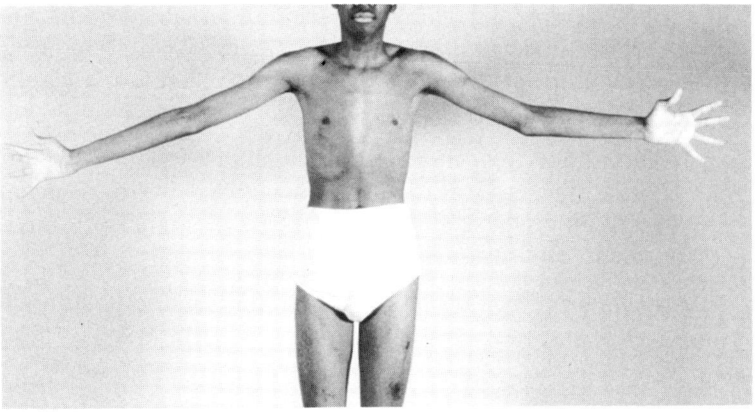

FIGURE 8–49
Note increased arm span and arachnodactyly in this young man with Marfan syndrome. (Courtesy of Lester Weiss, MD, Detroit, Michigan)

scant subcutaneous fat

occasional elastosis perforans serpiginosa

Non-Skin

musculoskeletal abnormalities include tall stature (limb length increased compared with trunk; arm span often greater than height) (Fig. 8–49), arachnodactyly, lax joints, recurrent joint dislocations, pectus carinatum or excavatum, kyphoscoliosis (which may be severe), and pes planus (Fig. 8–50)

craniofacial abnormalities include dolichocephaly, frontal bossing, and high-arched palate

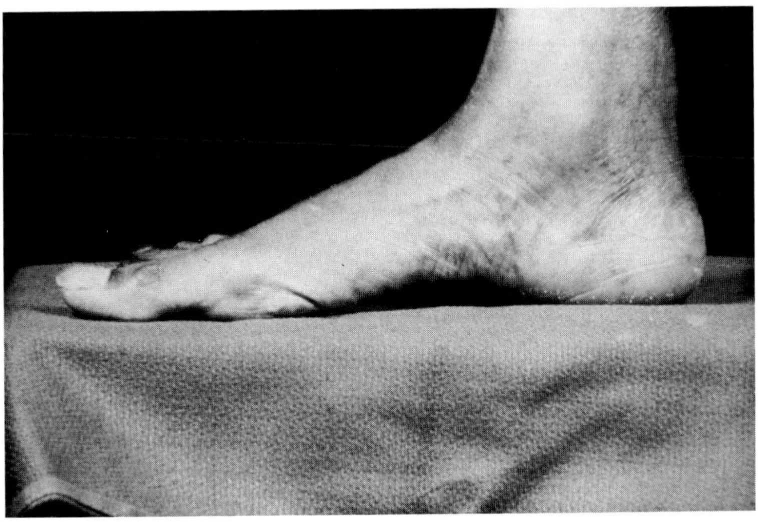

FIGURE 8–50
Marfan syndrome. Pes planus is a very common finding. It is a reflection of the joint laxity. (Courtesy of Philip Cohen, MD, Houston, Texas; reprinted with permission from Cohen PR, Schneiderman P. Clinical manifestations of the Marfan syndrome. Int J Dermatol 1989; 28:291–299)

cardiovascular abnormalities, in most or all patients, include dilatation (with associated aortic insufficiency), aneurysm or rupture of the ascending aorta, and valvular heart disease (including mitral valve prolapse and regurgitation)

eye abnormalities, in over half, include ectopia lentis (usually bilateral and symmetrical; dislocation upward in 75%), myopia, iridodonesis (tremulousness of iris due to lack of support of lens), retinal detachment, and blue sclerae

occasional pulmonary blebs, which may lead to pneumothorax

Genetics

AD; about 15% of cases due to new mutations

genetic defect responsible for Marfan syndrome mapped to chromosome 15; defective gene for fibrillin

Pathophysiology

abnormalities of the microfibrillar-fiber system

abnormal deposition of mucopolysaccharides with secondary destruction of elastic fibers in heart and blood vessels

Prognosis

cardiovascular complications are greatest cause of early mortality, and prophylactic aortic repair should be considered; death may rarely occur in infancy

Discussion

variability in expression is a hallmark; two of the three characteristic organ systems (skeletal, ocular, or cardiovascular) need to be involved to make the diagnosis; although several characteristic musculoskeletal, cardiovascular, and ocular abnormalities may be present at birth or develop anywhere from infancy to adulthood, a high index of suspicion is required to make the diagnosis

- *marfanoid hypermobility syndrome*

  features of Marfan syndrome allegedly without cardiovascular findings or ectopia lentis, but cardiovascular and possible lens abnormalities found on re-examination

REFERENCES

McK 154700

Anonymous. Fibrillin and Marfan's syndrome: a real clue? Lancet 1990;336:973–974

Burgio RG, Martini A, Cetta G, et al. Asymmetric Marfan syndrome. Am J Med Genet 1988;30:905–909

Cohen PR, Schneiderman P. Clinical manifestations of the Marfan syndrome. Int J Dermatol 1989;28:291–299

Gott VL, Pyeritz RE, Magovern GJ Jr, et al. Surgical treatment of aneurysms of the ascending aorta in the Marfan syndrome. N Engl J Med 1986;314:1070–1074

Gross DM, Robinson LK, Smith LT, et al. Se-

vere perinatal Marfan syndrome. Pediatrics 1989;84:83–89
Hollister DW, Godfrey M, Sakai LY, Pyeritz RE. Immunohistologic abnormalities of the microfibrillar-fiber system in the Marfan syndrome. N Engl J Med 1990;323:152–159
Kainulainen K, Pulkkinen L, Savolainen A, et al. Location on chromosome 15 of the gene defect causing Marfan syndrome. N Engl J Med 1990;323:935–939
Marfan syndrome: a mystery solved. J Med Genet 1992;29:73–74
Morse RP, Rockenmacher S, Pyeritz RE, et al. Diagnosis and management of infantile Marfan syndrome. Pediatrics 1990;86:888–895
Pope FM, Nicholls AC, Lewkonia RM, et al. Clinical and genetic heterogeneity of the Marfan syndrome. Curr Probl Dermatol 1987;17:95–110
Pyeritz RE. Marfan syndrome. N Engl J Med 1990;323:987–989
Sarfarazi M, Tsipouras P, Del Mastro R, et al. A linkage map of 10 loci flanking the Marfan syndrome locus on 15q: results of an international consortium study. J Med Genet 1992;29:75–80
Viljoen D, Beighton P. Marfan syndrome: a diagnostic dilemma. Clin Genet 1990;37:417–422
Walker BA, Beighton PH, Murdoch JL. The marfanoid hypermobility syndrome. Ann Intern Med 1969;71:349–352

HALLERMANN-STREIFF SYNDROME

Synonyms

- mandibulo-oculofacial dyscephaly
- François dyscephalic syndrome

Skin

hypotrichosis, most commonly of scalp (especially over the sutures), eyebrows, and eyelashes, but may involve axillary, pubic, and facial hair as well; hair usually sparse, fine, and fair

skin atrophy and telangiectases, most typically localized to the face, especially the nose

dental anomalies are virtually constant, including absence, malformation, and enamel hypoplasia of teeth with frequent caries

Non-Skin

craniofacial abnormalities include dyscephaly (most commonly brachycephaly), frontal bossing, mandibular hypoplasia, chin grooves, and a long nose with a thin, beaked tip; these defects produce a parrot-like profile (Fig. 8–51)

proportionate dwarfism

ocular abnormalities are manifold; microphthalmia and bilateral congenital cataracts, which may rupture spontaneously and resorb, are the most unique and common features; occasional blue sclerae

Genetics

sporadic occurrence; purported examples of AR and AD challenged

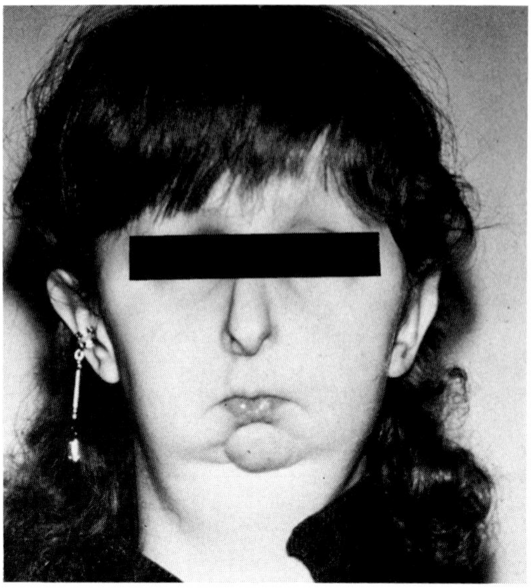

FIGURE 8–51
Hallermann-Streiff syndrome. This patient has brachycephaly with a very thin pointed nose and micrognathia. The chin grooves are a distinctive feature of this syndrome. (Courtesy of Robert J. Gorlin, DDS, MS, Minneapolis, Minnesota)

Laboratory Data

histopathology: elastic fiber fragmentation and collagen fiber abnormalities in both involved and clinically normal-appearing skin

electron microscopy of hair shaft: abnormalities of cuticle demonstrated

Prognosis

normal intelligence and life expectancy in most, but death related to feeding difficulty or respiratory infection in some

Discussion

the eponym François syndrome is more often applied to dermochondrocorneal dystrophy (see main entry)

REFERENCES

McK 234100

Cohen MM Jr. Hallermann-Streiff syndrome: a review. Am J Med Genet 1991;41:488–499

François J, Pierard J. The François dyscephalic syndrome and skin manifestations. Am J Ophthalmos 1971;71:1241–1250

François J. A new syndrome: dyscephalia with bird face and dental anomalies, nanism, hypotrichosis, cutaneous atrophy, microphthalmia, and congenital cataract. Arch Ophthalmol 1958;60:842–862

François J. François' dyscephalic syndrome. Birth Defects 1982;18:595–619

Golomb RG, Porter PS. A distinct hair shaft abnormality in the Hallermann-Streiff syndrome. Cutis 1975;16:123–129

OCULODENTOOSSEOUS SYNDROME (OCULODENTODIGITAL SYNDROME; MEYER-SCHWICKERATH SYNDROME)

sparse, dry and lusterless scalp hair in some

dental abnormalities include enamel hypoplasia

characteristic facies including small, closely set, sunken eyes, small mouth with overlapping upper lip, thin nose lacking alar flare, and small eyes with microcornea

digital abnormalities include syndactyly of fingers and dysplasia or aplasia of toe phalanges (Fig. 8–52)

unlike in Hallermann-Streiff syndrome, no micrognathia or cataracts

AD and possible AR; sporadic cases reported

McK 164200
Gorlin RJ, Cohen MM Jr, Levin LS. Syndromes of the Head and Neck. 3rd ed. New York, Oxford University Press, 1990:234–235
Judisch GF, Martin-Casals A, Hanson JW. Oculodentodigital dysplasia: four new reports and a literature review. Arch Ophthalmol 1979;97:878–884
Meyer-Schwickerath G, Gruterich E, Weyers H. Mikrophthalmussyndrome. Klin Monatsbl Augenheilkd 1957;131:18–30

KNUCKLE PADS

asymptomatic circumscribed keratotic plaques over dorsa of proximal interphalangeal joints of hands; occasionally develop over metacarpophalangeal or distal interphalangeal joints of hands (Fig. 8–53); rarely, feet involved; not all joints affected equally

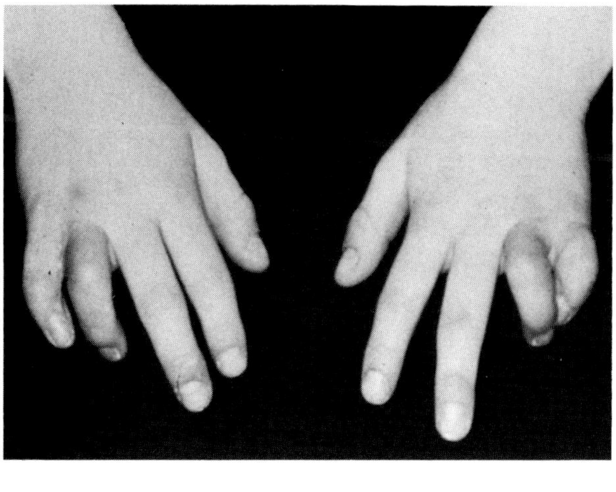

FIGURE 8–52
Oculodentoosseous syndrome. Bilaterally the fourth and fifth digits are small, and on the left they are fused. (Courtesy of Robert J. Gorlin, DDS, MS, Minneapolis, Minnesota)

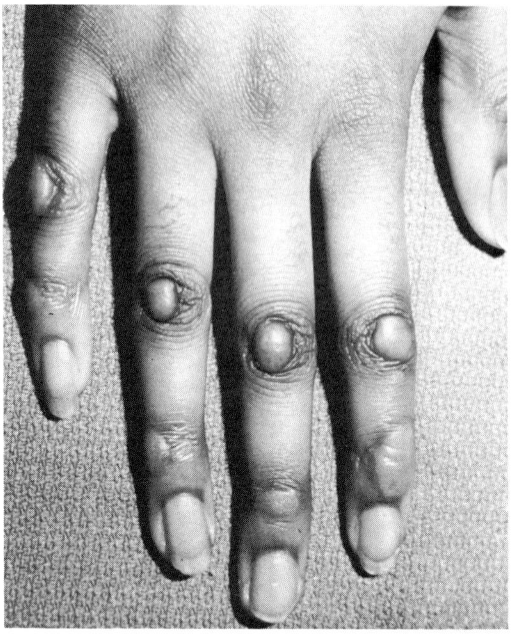

FIGURE 8–53
Knuckle pads. Circumscribed thickened plaques over the phalangeal joints of the hand. (Courtesy of Benjamin K. Fisher, MD, Toronto, Ontario)

age at onset usually in second or third decade but may develop in childhood

plaques develop slowly over months or years and persist

AD

histopathology: hyperkeratosis and acanthosis; dermal fibrosis in some lesions

acquired knuckle pads in adults are usually caused by trauma or friction, often occupational

sometimes knuckle pads are associated with Dupuytren's contracture

---

McK 149100
Paller AS, Hebert AA. Knuckle pads in children. Am J Dis Child 1986;140:915–917
Sehgal VN, Singh M, Saxena HMK. Primary knuckle pads. Clin Exp Dermatol 1979; 4:337–339

BART-PUMPHREY SYNDROME (KNUCKLE PADS, LEUKONYCHIA, AND SENSORINEURAL DEAFNESS)

knuckle pads

leukonychia totalis

occasional palmoplantar keratoderma

mixed (sensorineural and conductive) hearing loss

AD

McK 149200

Bart RS, Pumphrey RE. Knuckle pads, leukonychia and deafness: a dominantly inherited syndrome. N Engl J Med 1967; 276:202–207

Crosby EF, Vidurrizaga RH. Knuckle pads, leukonychia, deafness and keratosis palmoplantaris: report of a family. Johns Hopkins Med J 1976;139:90–92

ORAL-FACIAL-DIGITAL SYNDROME TYPE I

Synonyms

- Papillon-Léage and Psaume syndrome
- hypertrophied frenula syndrome
- orodigitofacial dysostosis

Skin

diffuse alopecia of scalp, especially the frontal area, is common (Fig. 8–54); hair may be brittle

most common oral findings are hamartomatous nodules and lobulation or clefting of tongue (Figs. 8–55 and 8–56); other findings include ankyloglossia, hypertrophied frenula, and pseudoclefting of upper lip

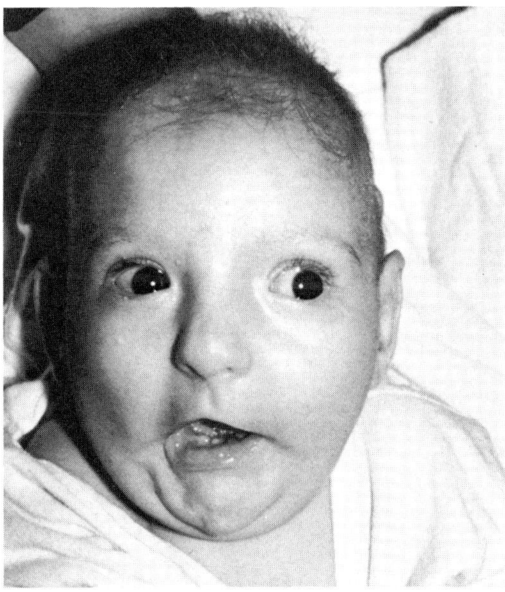

FIGURE 8–54
Characteristic appearance of an infant with oral-facial-digital syndrome. Note the sparse hair, pseudoclefting of the upper lip, and multiple milia on the face.

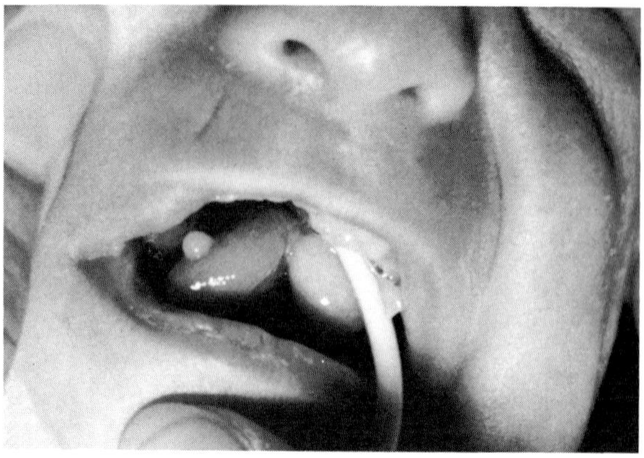

FIGURE 8–55
Oral-facial-digital syndrome. The tongue is fixed and shows the characteristic lobulation.

keratinous cysts ("milia") of skin, especially over the pinnae, face, scalp, and dorsal hands in infancy; lesions disappear spontaneously, leaving pitted scars

dental abnormalities include supernumerary canines and absence of central and lateral incisors

Non-Skin

craniofacial abnormalities include frontal bossing, micrognathia, hypoplasia of the malar bones, broad nasal root, ocular hypertelorism, dystopia canthorum (medial portion of sclerae covered by laterally displaced medial canthi), and clefting of the palate or alveolar ridge; tip of nose appears thinned due to hypoplasia of alar cartilage

digital findings include brachy-, syn-, clino-, and camptodactyly

severe mental retardation in most

Genetics

XLD

seen almost exclusively in females

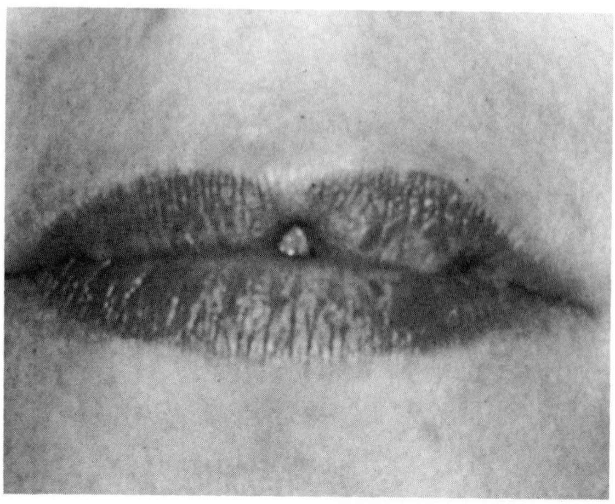

FIGURE 8–56
Oral-facial-digital syndrome. The abnormal central upper lip is easily identified. This defect has often been called the "straw drinker's hole" or "whistler's hole." (Courtesy of Robert J. Gorlin, DDS, MS, Minneapolis, Minnesota)

Laboratory Data

radiographs commonly show defects of tubular bones of the hands

Discussion

several additional subtypes of oral-facial-digital syndrome exist (types II–VII); most have AD inheritance except for type VII, which has XLD inheritance. Skin findings are uncommon. Coarse hair and preauricular skin tags are reported in type VII.

REFERENCES

McK 311200

Goodship J, Platt J, Smith R, Burn J. A male with type I orofaciodigital syndrome. J Med Genet 1991; 28:691–694

Larralde de Luna, M, Raspa ML, Ibargoyen J. Oral-facial-digital type I syndrome of Papillon-Léage and Psaume. Pediatr Dermatol 1992;9:52–56

Melnick M, Shields ED. Orofaciodigital syndrome, type I: a phenotypic and genetic analysis. Oral Surg 1975;40:599–610

Solomon LM, Fretzin DF, Pruzansky S. Pilosebaceous dysplasia in the oral-facial-digital syndrome. Arch Dermatol 1970;102:598–602

Wahrman J, Berant M, Jacobs J. The oral-facial-digital syndrome: a male-lethal condition in a boy with 47/XXY chromosomes. Pediatrics 1966;37:812–821

POPLITEAL PTERYGIUM SYNDROME

Synonym

- popliteal web syndrome

Skin

sparse, light-colored, short and brittle scalp hair and absence of eyebrows and eyelashes in some

pits or fistula of lower lip

hypodontia and enamel defects

dystrophic toenails; web over great toenail common

Non-Skin

webs, usually bilateral, extend over the popliteal area from the heel to the ischial tuberosity; occasional pterygia in other areas

craniofacial abnormalities include ankyloblepharon filiforme adnatum (filiform adhesions of the eyelids), maxillary hypoplasia, a shortened upper lip, and cleft palate and lip

genital and perineal defects include clitoromegaly, aplasia of labia majora, bifid scrotum, and cryptorchidism

musculoskeletal abnormalities include spina bifida occulta, lordosis, scoliosis, digital hypoplasia, and syndactyly of hands and feet

Genetics

AD

Discussion

there are many syndromes with pterygia; the nosology of this group of diseases is difficult

cleft lip may not be present, and other limited forms have been reported

- *ankyloblepharon filiforme adnatum and cleft palate:*

  may be a subset of the popliteal pterygium syndrome

  McK 106250

REFERENCES

McK 119500
McK 312150 (XLD cases)
Escobar V, Weaver DD. The facio-genito-popliteal syndrome. Birth Defects 1978;14:185–192
Gorlin RJ, Cohen MM Jr, Levin LS. Syndromes of the Head and Neck. 3rd ed. New York, Oxford University Press, 1990;629–631
Guillet G, Plantin P, Carsuzaa F, et al. A linear fibrous cord and ulcer of the lower limb: a limited form of a rare dysmorphic syndrome (faciogenitopopliteal syndrome). [Letter]. Arch Dermatol 1988;124:1443–1444
Hunter A. The popliteal pterygium syndrome: report of a new family and review of the literature. Am J Med Genet 1990;36:196–208
Oranje AP, Peereboom WJ, Stolz E. Hair bands in facio-genito-popliteal syndrome: a never before described hair anomaly. [Letter]. Pediatr Dermatol 1987;4:346–347

TREACHER-COLLINS SYNDROME

Synonyms

- mandibulofacial dysostosis
- Franceschetti-Klein syndrome
- Franceschetti-Zwahlen-Klein syndrome

Skin

ear tags and sinus on face between ear and angle of mouth

preauricular and temporal hairline extends anteriorly onto face; areas of circumscribed scarring alopecia reported

Non-Skin

abnormal craniofacies including hypoplastic malar bones, raised nasal bridge, hypoplastic nasal alar cartilage, cleft palate, hypoplastic mandible, and an open, "fish-like" mouth (Fig. 8–57)

ocular abnormalities include antimongoloid slant of palpebral fissures, characteristic colobomata of outer third of lower eyelid, and decreased or absent eyelashes medial to colobomata

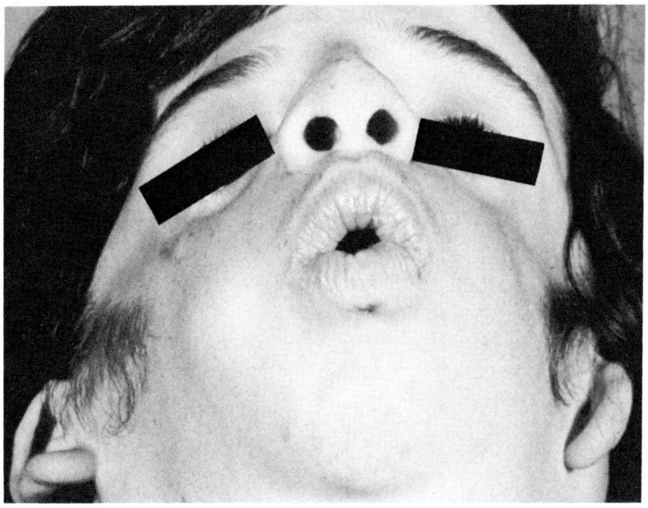

FIGURE 8–57
This patient with Treacher-Collins syndrome has hypoplasia of the malar areas, an elevated nasal bridge, a hypoplastic mandible, an open "fish-like" mouth, and malposition of the auricles. (Courtesy of Lester Weiss, MD, Detroit, Michigan)

otologic abnormalities include hearing loss (mostly conductive, due to defective ossicles), malposition of auricles, absence of external auditory canal, and microtia

Genetics

AD; mostly spontaneous mutations

Pathophysiology

primarily abnormalities of first and second branchial arch derivatives

Laboratory Data

prenatal diagnosis by fetoscopy possible in second trimester

Prognosis

prompt recognition of conductive hearing loss allows for earlier therapeutic intervention

Discussion

wide variability in expressivity

- *isotretinoin embryopathy:*

  similarities to phenotype of Treacher-Collins syndrome

  rudimentary or absent pinnae

  abnormal craniofacies including cleft palate, microstomia, and micrognathia

  cardiac defects include interrupted aortic arch, atrial septal defect, ventricular septal defect, patent ductus arteriosus, and truncus arteriosus neurologic abnormalities include cerebellar hypoplasia, microcephaly, and hydrocephalus

REFERENCES

McK 154500

Fazen LE, Elmore BA, Nadler HL. Mandibulofacial dysostosis (Treacher-Collins syndrome). Am J Dis Child 1967;113:405–410

Lammer EJ, Chen, DT, Hoar RM, et al. Retinoic acid embryopathy. N Engl J Med 1985;313:837–841

Murty PS, Hazarika P, Rajshekhar B, et al. Familial Treacher-Collins syndrome. J Laryngol Otol 1988;102:620–622

Nicolaides KH, Johansson D, Donnai D, Rodeck CH. Prenatal diagnosis of mandibulofacial dysostosis. Prenat Diagn 1984; 4:201–205

TRICHORHINOPHALANGEAL SYNDROME TYPE I

Synonym

- Giedion-Gurisch syndrome

Skin

see Figure 8–58

sparse, fair, lanugo-like scalp hair (especially frontotemporally) from birth; occasional complete alopecia; eyelash, pubic, and axillary hair may be similarly involved

eyebrows are thick medially and sparse laterally

nails thin and short; occasional koilonychia and leukonychia

Non-Skin

nose broad and pear-shaped with long ("high") philtrum

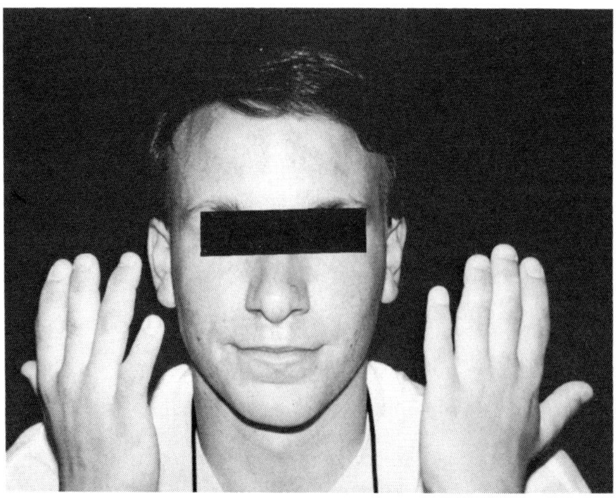

FIGURE 8–58
Trichorhinophalangeal syndrome. There are a bulbous nose and shortening of the fifth digits, particularly on the right hand. This patient's hair was relatively normal, but he had a sibling with thin hair.

deviation of the fingers and toes caused by proximal interphalangeal deformities (fusiform swelling); occasional brachymetacarpalism (usually fourth and fifth fingers)

short stature

Genetics

AD mostly; AR cases reported

chromosomal abnormalities reported

Laboratory Data

radiographs: cone-shaped epiphyses of the hands and feet

REFERENCES

McK 190350
McK 275500 (AR forms)
Besser F, Wells RS. The tricho-rhino-phalangeal syndrome (a family with three affected members). Br J Dermatol Suppl 1976;95:39–41
Buhler EM, Buhler UK, Beutler C, et al. A final word on the tricho-rhino-phalangeal syndromes. Clin Genet 1987;31:273–275
Frias JL, Felman AH, Garnica AD, et al. Variable expressivity in the trichorhinophalangeal syndrome type I. Birth Defects 1979;15:361–372
Giedion A, Burdea M, Fruchter Z, et al. Autosomal-dominant transmission of the tricho-rhino-phalangeal syndrome: report of 4 unrelated families, review of 60 cases. Helv Pediatr Acta 1973;28:249–259
McCloud DJ, Solomon LM. The tricho-rhino-phalangeal syndrome. Br J Dermatol 1977;96:403–407

TRICHORHINOPHALANGEAL SYNDROME TYPE II (LANGER-GIEDION SYNDROME)

sparse scalp hair, nail abnormalities, and loose skin

facies similar to that in type I, microcephaly, multiple cartilaginous exostoses, hypotonia associated with joint laxity, and occasional mental retardation

mostly sporadic; possible AD and AR cases reported

McK 150230
Langer LOJ, Krassikoff N, Laxova R, et al. The tricho-rhino-phalangeal syndrome with exostoses (or Langer-Giedion syndrome): four additional patients without mental retardation and review of the literature. Am J Med Genet 1984;19:81–112

APERT SYNDROME

Synonym

- acrocephalosyndactyly

Skin

acneiform eruption frequently seen around puberty; besides usual areas for acne vulgaris (face, chest, and back), lesions may extend to arms, forearms, buttocks, and thighs (Fig. 8–59)

marked seborrhea

broad, short fused nails and micronychia; may lack lunulae

association with oculocutaneous albinism reported

Non-Skin

characteristic craniofacies due to premature and irregular fusion of the coronal (and sometimes lambdoid or sagittal) sutures, resulting in oxycephaly (top of head pointed, like apex of cone)

broad, flat face with hypoplasia of nose and maxilla, giving appearance of mandibular prognathism

protuberant eyes with hypertelorism, strabismus, and downward sloping palpebral fissures

cleft palate and bifid uvula in about 25%; palate may be high arched with median furrow

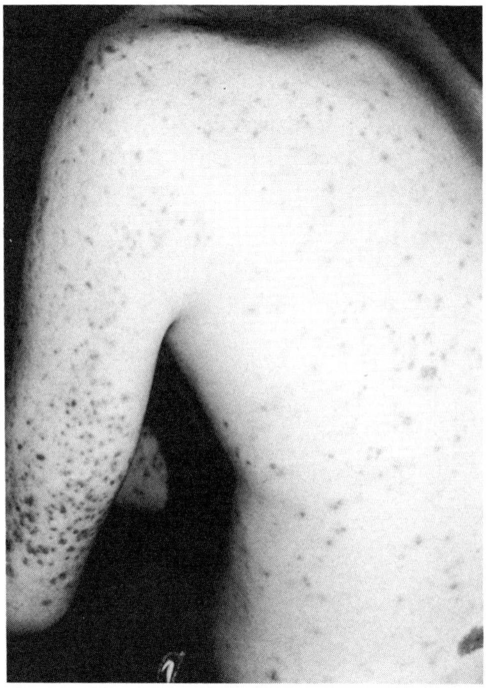

FIGURE 8–59
Apert syndrome. Extensive acne-like inflammatory papules involving the entire torso and upper extremities.

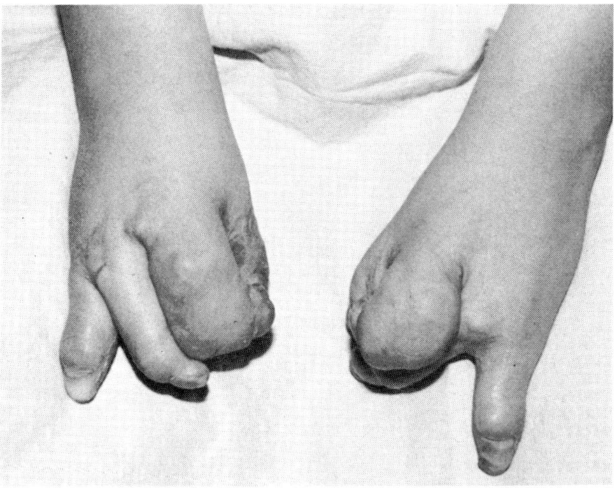

FIGURE 8–60
Mitten-like cutaneous and osseous syndactyly of the hands of a child with Apert syndrome.

progressive synostosis affecting bones other than skull including carpals, tarsals, and cervical vertebrae

variable mitten-like cutaneous and often osseous syndactyly of second to fourth digits of hands and feet, resulting in single broad nail for these digits and "flipper-like" use of thumb (Fig. 8–60)

normal to severely retarded intelligence

Genetics

mostly sporadic representing new mutations; AD transmission documented

increased paternal age associated with sporadic cases

Laboratory Data

prenatal diagnosis by fetoscopy reported

Prognosis

early craniectomy may improve intelligence

acneiform eruption may be responsive to isotretinoin

Discussion

presence of acneiform lesions on the forearms, typical of Apert syndrome, is very unusual in acne vulgaris

acneiform eruption not thought to be acne vulgaris, since the histologic findings and response to systemic antibiotics are different

variability in expression results in so-called atypical forms (e.g., some lack characteristic syndactyly and single common nail of digits 2 to 4) with exceptions of Apert and Crouzon syndromes, there are no characteristic cutaneous manifestations or associations for the many other craniosynostosis syndromes

REFERENCES

McK 101200

Erickson JD, Cohen MM Jr. A study of parental age effects on the occurrence of fresh mutations for the Apert syndrome. Ann Hum Genet 1974;38:89–96

Leonard CO, Daikoku NH, Winn K. Prenatal fetoscopic diagnosis of the Apert syndrome. Am J Med Genet 1982;11:5–9

Margolis S, Siegel IM, Choy A, Breining M. Depigmentation of hair, skin, and eyes associated with the Apert syndrome. Birth Defects 1978;14(6C):341–360

Orlow SJ. Cutaneous findings in craniofacial malformation syndromes. Arch Dermatol 1992;128:1379–1386

Parker TL, Roth JG, Esterly NB. Isotretinoin for acne in Apert syndrome. Pediatr Dermatol 1992;9:298–300

Solomon LM, Cohen MM Jr, Pruzansky S. Pilosebaceous abnormalities in Apert type acrocephalosyndactyly. Birth Defects 1971;7:193–195

Steffen C. The acneform eruption of Apert's syndrome is not acne vulgaris. Am J Dermatopathol 1984;6:213–220

CROUZON SYNDROME (CRANIOFACIAL DYSOSTOSIS)

acanthosis nigricans

increased digital dermatoglyphics

characteristic exophthalmos, hypertelorism, beaked nose, and hypoplastic maxilla (apparent mandibular prognathism)

skull brachycephalia with frontal bossing and premature closure of cranial sutures

AD

McK 123500

Breitbart AS, Eaton C, McCarthy JG. Crouzon's syndrome associated with acanthosis nigricans: ramifications for the craniofacial surgeon. Ann Plast Surg 1989;22:310–315

OTOPALATODIGITAL SYNDROME I (OPD I; TAYBI SYNDROME)

short and broad nails

generalized bone dysplasia causing multiple skeletal abnormalities including short, broad distal phalanges of thumbs and toes and, to a lesser degree, of the other digits; some authors have described "tree-frog" feet

characteristic craniofacies with cleft palate and broad nasal root mental retardation and deafness

XLR

McK 311300

Pazzaglia UE, Beluffi G. Oto-palato-digital syndrome in four generations of a large family. Clin Genet 1986;30:338–344

Salinas CF, Jorgenson RJ, Lorenzo RL. Variable expression in otopalatodigital syndrome; cleft palate in female. Birth Defects 1979;15:329–345

EAR PITS

Synonym

- auricular fistulae

Skin

unilateral or bilateral pits on ears, usually on anterior upper helix

asymptomatic or intermittent discharge of cellular debris

Genetics

AD

Discussion

may be associated with lateral cervical fistulae and branchial cleft anomalies (e.g., branchio-oto-renal syndrome, see later)

REFERENCES

McK 128700

Lipkin AF, Coker NJ, Jenkins HA. Hereditary congenital cholesteatoma: a variant of branchio-oto dysplasia. Arch Otolaryngol Head Neck Surg 1986;112:1097–1100

Takato T, Fukuda O. Hereditary occurrence of lateral cervical fistulas. Ann Plast Surg 1988;20:453–458

BRANCHIO-OTO-RENAL (BOR) SYNDROME (MELNICK-FRASER SYNDROME)

branchial arch anomalies including malformations of the external and middle ear; hearing loss; branchial cleft fistulae, sinuses, or cysts; and preauricular pits

varying degrees of renal hypoplasia

abnormal craniofacies (Potter facies) including telecanthus, epicanthal folds, lacrimal duct aplasia, flattening of the nose, and micrognathia

AD

the finding of branchial arch anomalies in a deaf child should prompt renal studies

McK 113650

Chitayat D, Hodgkinson KA, Chen M-F, et al. Branchio-oto-renal syndrome: further delineation of an underdiagnosed syndrome. Am J Med Genet 1992;43:970–975

Smith PG, Dyches TJ, Loomis RA. Clinical aspects of the branchio-oto-renal syndrome. Otolaryngol Head Neck Surg 1984;92:468–475

Other Dysplasias or Malformation Syndromes—Abbreviated Entries

RUVALCABA SYNDROME

atrophic plaques on trunk

osseous dysplasia and mental deficiency

inheritance unclear; AD and AR cases reported

McK 180870

Ruvalcaba RHA, Reichert A, Smith DW. A new familial syndrome with osseous dysplasia and mental deficiency. J Pediatr 1971; 79:450–455

Sugio Y, Kajii T. Ruvalcaba syndrome: autosomal dominant inheritance. Am J Med Genet 1984;19:741–753

SCHINZEL-GIEDION SYNDROME

generalized hypertrichosis

telangiectases over nose and cheeks

triangular, narrow, deep-set nails

delayed tooth eruption

mental and physical retardation

epilepsy, apnea, and atrioseptal and other mesodermal defects occasionally

AR

McK 269150
Schinzel A, Giedion A. A syndrome of severe midface retraction, multiple skull anomalies, clubfeet, and cardiac and renal malformations in sibs. Am J Med Genet 1978;1:361–375

DUPLICATION OF EYEBROWS, STRETCHABLE SKIN, AND SYNDACTYLY

partial double eyebrows

hypertrichosis of forehead

excessive wrinkling of periorbital skin; hyperextensible skin of face and chest

syndactyly

possible AR

McK 227210
Berkenstadt M, Zahavie H, Goodman RM. Partial duplication of the eyebrows with other congenital malformations: a new syndrome. Clin Genet 1988;33:207–210
Gross-Kieselstein E, Har-Even Y. Partial duplication of the eyebrows with other congenital malformations: a new syndrome. [Letter]. Clin Genet 1989;35:467–468

COSTELLO SYNDROME

loose skin of neck, hands, and feet; thickened palmoplantar skin

curly scalp hair

warty papules around nose and mouth and occasionally on legs and perianal skin

hypoplastic nails

mental retardation

short stature

craniofacial abnormalities

inheritance unclear

McK 218040
Costello JM. A new syndrome: mental subnormality and nasal papillomata. Aust Paediat J 1977;13:114–118

Der Kaloustian VM, Moroz B, McIntosh N, et al. Costello syndrome. Am J Med Genet 1991;41:69–73
Martin RA, Jones KL. Delineation of the Costello syndrome. Am J Med Genet 1991; 41:346–349

CHARACTERISTIC FACIAL APPEARANCE, PREAURICULAR PITS, FIFTH FINGER CLINODACTYLY, AND TETRALOGY OF FALLOT

AD

McK 187500

Jones MC, Waldman JD. An autosomal dominant syndrome of characteristic facial appearance, preauricular pits, fifth finger clinodactyly, and tetralogy of Fallot. Am J Med Genet 1985;22:135–141

DEAFNESS AND EAR PITS

preauricular ear pits that may communicate with middle ear

branchial cleft anomalies and deafness

pinnae may be deformed

AD

McK 125100

Fourman P, Fourman J. Hereditary deafness in family with ear-pits (fistula auris congenita). Br Med J 1955;2:1354–1356

NOSE PITS

present at birth

usually sporadic occurrence; AD cases reported

Halal F, Lazaro LF, Desgranges MF. Letter to the editor: dominant inheritance of nose pits. Am J Med Genet 1982;13:101–104

POLYMASTIA AND SUPERNUMERARY NIPPLES

possible association with renal anomalies in some populations

mostly sporadic occurrence; some cases possibly AD

McK 163700
Leung A. Familial supernumerary nipples. Am J Med Genet 1988;31:631–635
Leung AK, Robson WL. Polythelia. Int J Dermatol 1989;28:429–433

CONGENITAL ABSENCE OF BREAST AND NIPPLES

may result from a variety of ectodermal defects

unilateral absence associated with ipsilateral agenesis of pectoral muscles or bilateral absence associated with congenital anomalies such as cleft palate and short stature

AR, AD, or XLR, depending on associated disease

McK 113700
Kowlessar M, Orti E. Complete breast absence in siblings. Am J Dis Child 1968;115:91–92
Nelson MM, Cooper CK. Congenital defects of the breast—an autosomal dominant trait. S Afr Med J 1982;61:434–436
Trier WC. Complete breast absence: case report and review of the literature. Plast Reconstr Surg 1965;36:431–439

BENIGN BILATERAL ACROMIAL DIMPLES

AD

McK 102350
Mehes K, Meggyessy V. Autosomal dominant inheritance of benign bilateral acromial dimples. Hum Genet 1987;76:206

EXOSTOSES WITH ANETODERMIA AND BRACHYDACTYLY, TYPE E

McK 133690

Mollica F, Li Volti S, Guarneri B. New syndrome: exostoses, anetodermia, brachydactyly. Am J Med Genet 1984;19:665–667

METAPHYSEAL DYSPLASIA, ANETODERMA, AND OPTIC ATROPHY

McK 250450

Temtamy SA, El-Meligy M, Badrawy HS, et al. Metaphyseal dysplasia, anetoderma and optic atrophy: an autosomal recessive syndrome. In: Bergsma D, ed. Skeletal Dysplasias. Amsterdam, Excerpta Medica, 1974:61–71

CHAPTER

9

Hair Disorders

Disorders of hair growth and structural shaft defects can occur as isolated abnormalities or as manifestations of a syndrome. In some of these conditions, the hair defect is the outstanding and invariable feature. In others, however, the hair abnormalities may be inconstant, difficult to appreciate, or less prominent than other cutaneous findings. In addition, the abnormality in hair growth or structure may be an age-related phenomenon, demonstrable only during a particular time period.

We have included in this chapter dermatologic disorders that consist of solitary defects of hair growth and/or structure and those in which the hair abnormality is one of the major identifying features. Disorders in which the hair changes are poorly defined or nonspecific as well as those conditions in which the hair abnormality is part of a larger group of ectodermal defects (i.e., the ectodermal dysplasias) are described elsewhere in the book.

REFERENCE

Whiting DA. Structural abnormalities of the hair shaft. J Am Acad Dermatol 1987; 16:1–25

CONGENITAL HYPERTRICHOSIS LANUGINOSA

Synonyms

- familial hypertrichosis, generalized
- hypertrichosis universalis congenita

Skin

generalized, excessive, persistent growth of dark lanugo hair, usually present at birth but may not appear until late infancy or childhood (Fig. 9–1)

long eyelashes and thick eyebrows

distichiasis (extra row of eyelashes) common

hypertrichosis generally persists; at puberty, axillary and pubic hair remain downy

occasional hypodontia or anodontia

Non-Skin

mental retardation in some, but intelligence is usually normal

occasional external ear deformities

Genetics

AD

Discussion

dog-faced or *simian* are terms occasionally used to describe the hair growth in these patients

Freire-Maia distinguishes a subset of these patients under the name of hypertrichosis and dental defects

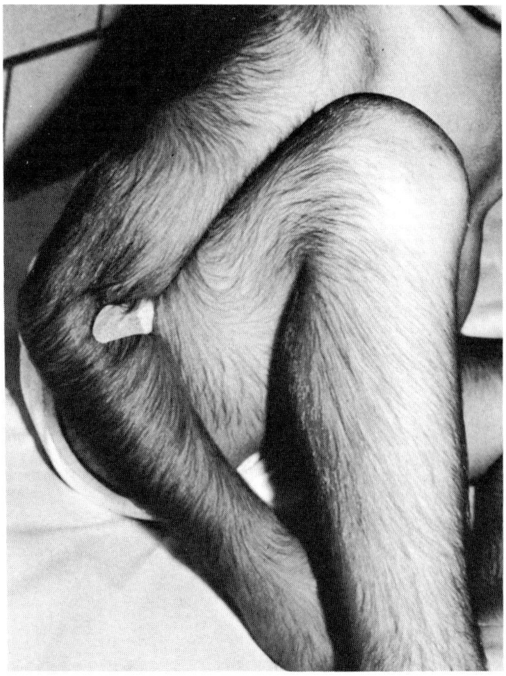

FIGURE 9–1
Long, dark lanugo hair covering the limbs of a boy with hypertrichosis lanuginosa.

- *hypertrichosis lanuginosa acquisita:*

  acquired hypertrichosis of lanugo hair may be a paraneoplastic phenomenon most often associated with lung and colon malignancies

  abrupt onset; mainly involves face and may progress to neck, shoulder, limbs, and trunk; palms and soles are spared

  in most cases, the malignancy is widely disseminated when the lanugo hair appears

  acquired

REFERENCES

McK 145700

McK 307150 (X-linked form)

Felgenhauer WR. Hypertrichosis lanuginosa universalis. J Genet Hum 1969;17:1–44

Jemec GB. Hypertrichosis lanuginosa acquisita: report of a case and review of the literature. Arch Dermatol 1986;122:805–808

Judge MR, Khaw PT, Rice NSC, et al. Congenital hypertrichosis lanuginosa and congenital glaucoma. Br J Dermatol 1991; 124:495–497

Macias-Flores MA, Garcia-Cruz D, Rivera H, et al. A new form of hypertrichosis inherited as an X-linked dominant trait. Hum Genet 1984;66:66–70

Partridge JW. Congenital hypertrichosis lanuginosa: neonatal shaving. Arch Dis Child 1987;62:623–625

Suskind R, Esterly NB. Congenital hypertrichosis universalis. Birth Defects 1971; 7:103–106

DISTICHIASIS

double row of eyelashes, usually involving all four lids

Meibomian glands absent

AD

distichiasis-lymphedema (see main entry) is a distinct syndrome

McK 126300

Fox SA. Distichiasis. Am J Ophthalmol 1962;53:14–18

Pico G. Congenital ectropion and distichiasis: etiology and hereditary factors: a report of cases and review of the literature. Am J Ophthalmol 1958;47:363–387

ALOPECIA CONGENITA

Synonyms

- familial hypotrichosis
- atrichia congenita

Skin

lanugo hair present at birth is shed, leaving almost complete alopecia; all body hair is affected, usually in proportion to alopecia of scalp

hyperkeratotic papules of scalp, face, and extremities may develop in second year; rarely, trunk becomes involved later

Genetics

AR; AD forms also reported

Pathophysiology

hair follicles are absent, attenuated, or plugged

Discussion

atrichias and hypotrichoses without other ectodermal findings are a heterogeneous group of disorders with varying degrees of severity, onset, progression, and extent; genetic mechanisms also vary—AR (as in the majority of cases of alopecia congenita) and AD (as in hereditary hypotrichosis) cases are reported, as well as sporadic cases

REFERENCES

McK 241900

Cantu JM, Sanchez-Corona J, Gonzalez-Mendoza A, et al. Autosomal recessive inheritance of atrichia congenita. Clin Genet 1980;17:209–212

Muller SA. Alopecia: syndromes of genetic significance. J Invest Dermatol 1973;60:475–492

FAMILIAL HYPOTRICHOSIS, AUTOSOMAL DOMINANT FORM (HYPOTRICHOSIS SIMPLEX)

slowly progressive, diffuse hair loss beginning between 5 and 12 years of age; few hairs remain by third decade; scalp itself appears normal

AD

McK 146520

Bentley-Phillips B, Grace HJ. Hereditary hypotrichosis: a previously undescribed syndrome. Br J Dermatol 1979;101:331–339

Kohn G, Metzker A. Hereditary hypotrichosis simplex of the scalp. Clin Genet 1987;32:120–124

Toribio J, Quinones PA. Hereditary hypotrichosis simplex of the scalp—evidence for autosomal dominant inheritance. Br J Dermatol 1974;91:687–696

FAMILIAL FOCAL ALOPECIA

noninflammatory, nonscarring patchy thinning of scalp hair of childhood onset, extensive anagen to telogen transformation and arrest

possible AD

McK 104110
Headington JT, Astle N. Familial focal alopecia: a new disorder of hair growth clinically resembling pseudopelade. Arch Dermatol 1987;123:234–237

ATRICHIA WITH PAPULAR LESIONS

normal fetal hair is shed in first months of life, followed by complete permanent alopecia and development of multiple papules, which histologically show "malformed hairs with a cystic appearance" or "epidermoid" cysts

familial occurrence documented, but inheritance is unclear, possible AR

McK 209500
Del Castillo V, Ruiz-Maldonado R, Carnevale A. Atrichia with papular lesions and mental retardation in two sisters. Int J Dermatol 1974;13:261–265
Kanzler MH, Rasmussen JE. Atrichia with papular lesions. Arch Dermatol 1986; 122:565–567
Misciali C, Tosti A, Fanti PA, Borrello P, Piraccini BM. Atrichia and papular lesions: report of a case. Dermatology 1992; 185:284–288

HEREDITARY HYPOTRICHOSIS

Synonym

- Marie-Unna hypotrichosis

Skin

at birth, hair of scalp, eyebrow, eyelashes, and body may be almost normal or may be sparse and frizzy

in early childhood, coarse and twisted terminal scalp hair develops; remainder of body hair remains sparse

around puberty, hair is progressively lost from the vertex and scalp margins; high frontal and nuchal hairlines are typical

beginning in adolescence scarring alopecia of varying extent develops; more severe in males body hair remains sparse

teeth, mucous membranes, and nails are normal

Genetics

AD

males more severely affected

Laboratory Data

hairs are uneven in caliber; irregular 90° to 180° twists of hair

electron microscopy of hair: intracellular fracturing of cuticular cells reported

Discussion

atrichias and hypotrichoses without other ectodermal findings are a heterogeneous group of disorders with varying degrees of severity, onset, progression, and extent; genetic mechanisms also vary—AR (as in the majority of cases of familial hypotrichosis) and AD (as in hereditary hypotrichosis) cases are reported, as well as sporadic cases

hypotrichosis is found in many of the ectodermal dysplasias or ectodermal dysplasia malformation syndromes; many kindreds thought to have familial hypotrichosis were eventually found to have various ectodermal dysplasias

REFERENCES

McK 146550

Bentley-Phillips B, Grace HJ. Hereditary hypotrichosis: a previously undescribed syndrome. Br J Dermatol 1979;101:331–339

Hess RO, Uno H. Hereditary hypotrichosis of the scalp. Am J Med Genet 1991;39:125–129

Marren P, Wilson C, Dawber RPR, Walshe MM. Hereditary hypotrichosis (Marie-Unna type) and juvenile macular degeneration (Stargardt's maculopathy). Clin Exp Dermatol 1992;17:189–191

Solomon LM, Esterly NB, Medenica M. Hereditary trichodysplasia: Marie-Unna's hypotrichosis. J Invest Dermatol 1971;57:389–400

Stevanovic DV. Hereditary hypotrichosis congenita: Marie-Unna type. Br J Dermatol 1970;83:331–337

MENKES KINKY HAIR SYNDROME

Synonyms

- trichopoliodystrophy
- kinky hair syndrome
- steely hair syndrome

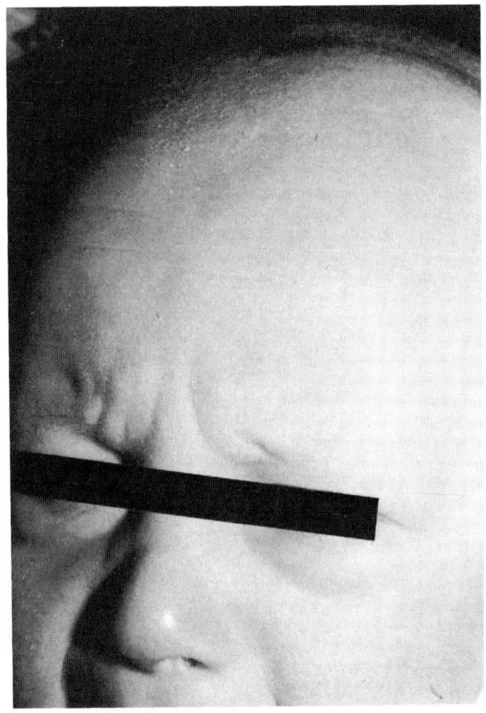

FIGURE 9–2
Sparse, lusterless, lightly pigmented hair in an infant with Menkes kinky hair syndrome. The hair is extremely short caused by breakage at defective areas in the hair shaft.

Skin

scalp hair at birth may be normal or light-colored and sparse (Fig. 9–2)

by about 3 months of age the scalp hair is sparse, coarse, kinky, and light colored but darkens as child ages

eyebrows may show same changes

skin is lax and has a peculiar doughy consistency

generalized or localized decrease in skin pigmentation in patients and female carriers reported

Non-Skin

child appears normal initially, but severe motor, mental, and physical retardation including lethargy, drowsiness, and feeding difficulties become apparent from first to third month of life onward

cerebral and cerebellar degeneration as well as focal or general epilepsy

micrognathia and high-arched palate

impaired temperature regulation (hypothermia) and increased susceptibility to infection may be apparent in early infancy

arteries grossly tortuous; intracranial hemorrhage reported; fragmentation of arterial elastic fibers microscopically

skeletal abnormalities in infancy include wormian bones of the skull and metaphyseal spurring

Genetics

XLR

Pathophysiology

some have postulated that a partial block in intestinal absorption of copper causes marked systemic copper deficiency

others note that liver copper stores are low at birth despite normal copper levels in neonatal and maternal serum and amniotic fluid; complex defect of copper metabolism including transport and cellular availability suspected

Laboratory Data

microscopically, the hair typically shows pili torti; trichorrhexis nodosa, trichoclasis, and trichoptilosis are also seen

hair analysis reveals a nine-fold increase in free sulfhydryl content

low plasma copper and ceruloplasmin levels

heterozygotes may be detected by abnormal copper metabolism in skin fibroblasts; normal serum copper levels

prenatal diagnosis is possible by detection of abnormal copper metabolism in amniotic fluid cells

Prognosis

death usually occurs by third or fourth year of life due to failure to thrive, but survival to adolescence is reported

systemic copper therapy is, at best, of minimal benefit

Discussion

the heterogeneity of hair shaft abnormalities in Menkes kinky hair syndrome is also typical of many other diseases with hair shaft abnormalities, including arginosuccinic aciduria and the trichothiodystrophies (see main entries)

monilethrix has been repeatedly reported as a finding in this disease, but it may actually be due to an optical effect resembling beading resulting from the twisting of the hair (pili torti) along its longitudinal axis

heterozygotes may have pili torti

REFERENCES

McK 309400

Danks DM, Stevens BJ, Campbell PE, et al. Menkes kinky-hair syndrome: an inherited defect in the intestinal absorption of copper with widespread effects. Birth Defects 1974;10:132–137

Garnica AD, Frias JL, Rennert OM. Menkes kinky hair syndrome: is it a treatable disorder? Clin Genet 1977;11:154–161

Gerdes AM, Tonnesen T, Horn N, et al. Clinical expression of Menkes syndrome in females. Clin Genet 1990;38:452–459

Hamer DH. Metallothionein gene regulation in Menkes' syndrome. Arch Dermatol 1987; 123:1384a–1385a

Hart DB. Menkes syndrome: an updated review. J Am Acad Dermatol 1983;9:145–152

Menkes JH, Alter M, Steigleder GK, et al. A sex-linked recessive disorder with retardation of growth, peculiar hair, and focal cerebral and cerebellar degeneration. Pediatrics 1962;29:764–779

Moore CM, Howell RR. Ectodermal manifestations in Menkes disease. Clin Genet 1985;28:532–540

Sander C, Niederhoff H, Horn N. Life-span and Menkes kinky hair syndrome: report of a 13-year course of this disease. Clin Genet 1988;33:228–233

Whiting DA. Structural abnormalities of the hair shaft. J Am Acad Dermatol 1987; 16:1–25

GIANT AXONAL NEUROPATHY

kinky, light-colored scalp hair

chronically progressive, peripheral mixed neuropathy with onset in early childhood; characteristic leg posture

probable AR

distention of axons by tightly woven neurofilaments demonstrated ultrastructurally

McK 256850

Asbury AK, Gale MK, Cox SC, et al. Giant axonal neuropathy: a unique case with segmental neurofilamentous masses. Acta Neuropathol 1972;20:237–247

Berg BO, Rosenberg SH, Asbury AK. Giant axonal neuropathy. Pediatrics 1972;49:894–899

Carpenter S, Karpati G, Andermann F, Gold R. Giant axonal neuropathy: a clinically and morphologically distinct neurological disease. Arch Neurol 1974;31:312–316

MONILETHRIX

Synonyms

- beaded hair
- spindle hair

Skin

alopecia may be present at birth

hair shaft abnormalities are not evident until 2 to 3 months later as neonatal lanugo hair is shed; rare cases of onset in childhood or early adulthood

distribution may be segmental or patchy; nape of neck and occipital scalp most commonly involved, but hair on any part of the body may be affected

affected areas are nearly bald; hair appears dry, coarse, and brittle, commonly breaking after reaching a length of 2.5 cm; often, beading is difficult to see in remaining stubble reddish follicular papules in the affected area are typical (Fig. 9–3); keratosis pilaris may be noted elsewhere including on the neck and extensor extremities

nail and dental abnormalities reported

Non-Skin

rare associated findings include cataracts and mental or motor retardation

Genetics

AD

AR inheritance also reported but not proved

Laboratory Data

see Figure 9–4

electron microscopy: constrictions show cuticle abnormalities, thinned cortex, and an absent or virtually absent medulla, while "beaded" areas are normal

constrictions occur at 0.7- to 1.0-mm intervals

beading usually affects entire shaft but may be segmental

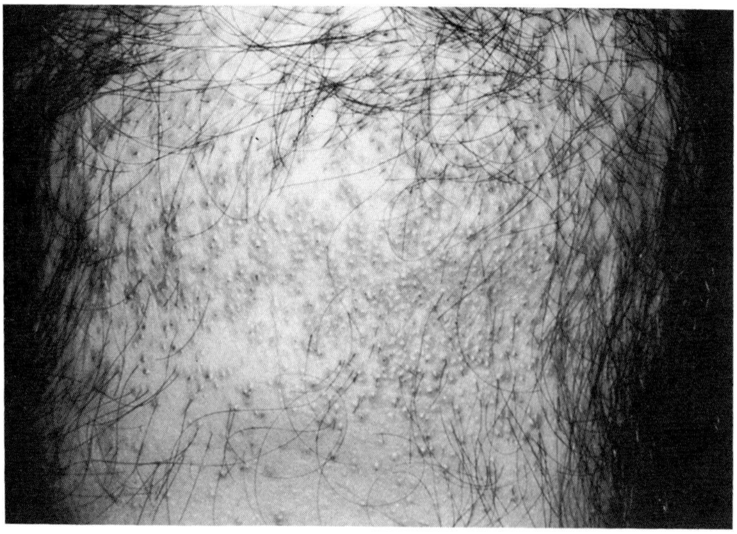

FIGURE 9–3
Posterior scalp of a patient with monilethrix showing sparse hair and hyperkeratotic papules. (Courtesy of Benjamin K. Fisher, MD, Toronto, Ontario)

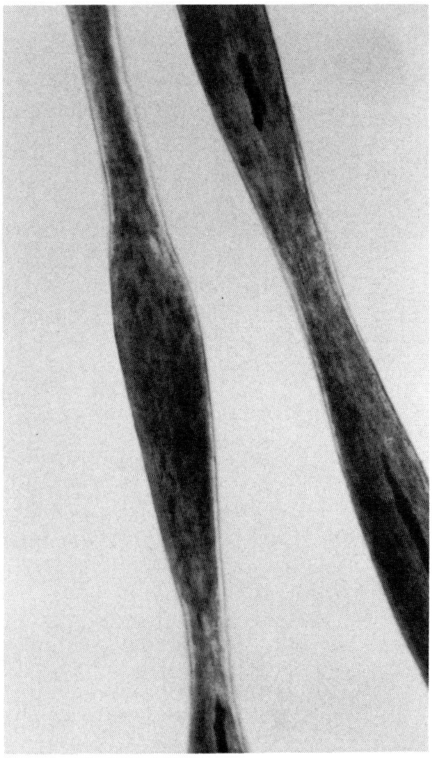

FIGURE 9–4
Beaded hair from a patient with monilethrix. The wider sections are the normal portions of the shafts.

Prognosis

general health is usually good

monilethrix and keratosis pilaris may improve with age, puberty, and pregnancy; or in summer

rare complete spontaneous remission

Discussion

in a small number of cases, the disease does not appear until puberty

individuals of affected families may show keratosis pilaris only but may pass on the gene for monilethrix; minimal expressivity manifested in this manner could account for reports of apparent recessive inheritance

trichotillomania may mimic segmental distribution of monilethrix

REFERENCES

McK 158000
McK 252200
Baker H. An investigation of monilethrix. Br J Dermatol 1962;74:24–30
Schaap T, Even PZ, Hodes ME, et al. The genetic analysis of monilethrix in a large inbred kindred. Am J Med Genet 1982; 11:469–474
Summerly R, Donaldson EM. Monilethrix: a family study. Br J Dermatol 1962;74:387–391
Wennersten G. Monilethrix. Acta Derm Venereol 1971;51:232
Whiting DA. Structural abnormalities of the hair shaft. J Am Acad Dermatol 1987; 16:1–25

PSEUDOMONILETHRIX

thinning or unruliness of scalp hair appearing in prepubertal children due to hair breakage, often following trauma to hair including brushing and combing

AD

reported in peoples of Dutch, German, British, and Indian origin

variable sized nodes ("beading"), irregularly spaced along hair shaft, consisting of indentations

irregular twisting at 25° to 200° without flattening of shafts

breaks in apparently normal shafts with brush-like ends

reducing trauma to hair may improve condition greatly

some cases, if not all, can be attributed to hair trauma alone and are considered artifactual

McK 177750

Bentley-Phillips B, Baylis MAH. A previously undescribed hereditary hair anomaly (pseudo-monilethrix). Br J Dermatol 1973; 89:159–167

Whiting DA. Structural abnormalities of the hair shaft. J Am Acad Dermatol 1987; 16:1–25

Zitelli JA. Pseudomonilethrix: an artifact. Arch Dermatol 1986;122:688–690

PILI ANNULATI

Synonym

- ringed hair

Skin

hair of normal diameter having alternating segments of light and dark color; involves entire hair shaft or may be limited to a segment; may be fragile

involves scalp hair, usually diffusely, but may be limited to certain areas; may involve axillary or mustache hair

noted at birth or in early or late childhood

decreased rate of growth

some persons report hair shaft fragility while others do not

Genetics

AD; AR also reported; up to 50% of cases sporadic

Laboratory Data

caliber of hair shaft is normal

in reflected light, abnormal segments are light-colored

in transmitted light (e.g., light microscopy), abnormal segments are dark

electron microscopy: abnormal segments have pockets of air in the cortex

cystine content of hair may be low, but sulfur content is normal

Prognosis

frequently, patients find hair cosmetically acceptable or even attractive

Discussion

- *pseudo-pili annulati*

  unusual variant of hair with bright bands at intervals along the hair shaft

  caused by twisting or curling of hair shaft and conspicuous only in blonde hair

  acquired

  no treatment required; considered attractive

- *bubble hair*

  hair is straight and stiff with a "singed" appearance

  probably acquired

  localized areas of brittleness and alternating light and dark bands

REFERENCES

McK 180600

Ashley LM, Jacques RS. Four generations of ringed hair. J Hered 1950;41:82–84

Brown VM, Crounse RG, Abele DC. An unusual new hair shaft abnormality: "bubble hair." J Am Acad Dermatol 1986;15:1113–1117

Dini G, Casigliani R, Rindi L, et al. Pili annulati: optical and scanning electron microscopic studies. Int J Dermatol 1988;27:256–257

Price VH, Thomas RS, Jones FT. Pseudopili annulati: an unusual variant of normal hair. Arch Dermatol 1970;102:354–358

Snell GD, Foley F. Inheritance of ringed hair. J Hered 1932;23:155–157

Whiting DA. Structural abnormalities of the hair shaft. J Am Acad Dermatol 1987;16:1–25

LOOSE ANAGEN SYNDROME

Skin

hair in anagen phase is slow-growing and easily and painlessly pulled out; intermittent bald patches usually trauma related

occurs mainly in blond girls 2 to 5 years of age; in time, there is spontaneous improvement in growth but the "looseness" of the hair remains

hair may be matted over occiput

no increase in fragility or breakage

Genetics

AD

Laboratory Data

anagen to telogen ratio is normal, but the inner root sheath is swollen and prematurely keratinized, ultrastructurally; proximal cuticle is coiled and likened to a "rumpled sock appearance"

Prognosis

rarely need haircut; no treatment available

REFERENCES

Baden HP, Kvedar JC, Magro CM. Loose anagen hair as a cause of hereditary hair loss in children. Arch Dermatol 1992;128:1349–1353

Hamm W, Traupe H. Loose anagen hair of childhood: the phenomenon of easily pluckable hair. J Am Acad Dermatol 1989; 20:242–248

Price VH, Gummer CL. Loose anagen syndrome. J Am Acad Dermatol 1989;20:249–256

PILI TORTI

Synonym

- twisted hair

Skin

hair usually normal at birth; gradual onset of brittle, frizzy, or bushy scalp hair with variable alopecia (Fig. 9–5); usual onset between 1 and 2 years of age, but ranges from birth to adulthood

findings vary, ranging from subtle hair loss to stubbly hair to complete alopecia; variable fragility of hair causes different clinical appearances

occasional involvement of eyebrows and other body hair

hair abnormalities improve in childhood and are often absent after puberty; however, in some persons the condition is lifelong

keratosis pilaris in some individuals

dental abnormalities include enamel hypoplasia

Genetics

AD; AR and sporadic cases reported

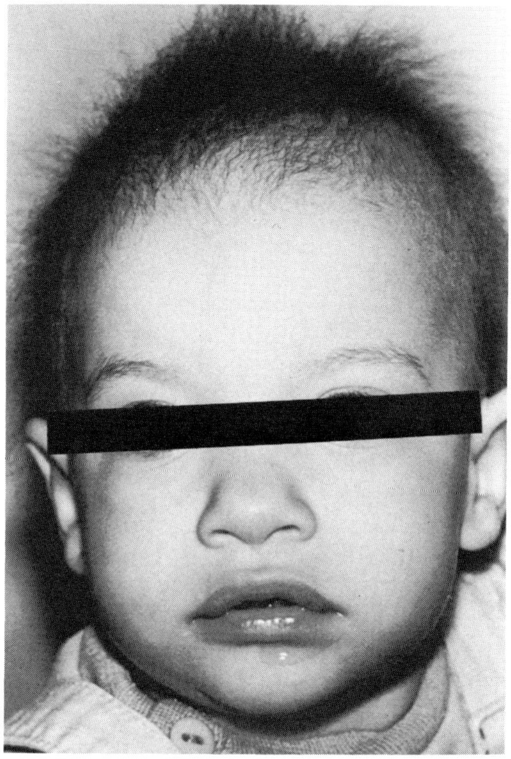

FIGURE 9–5
Unruly hair of variable length in an infant with pili torti.

male to female ratio is 1:2

Laboratory Data

see Figure 9–6

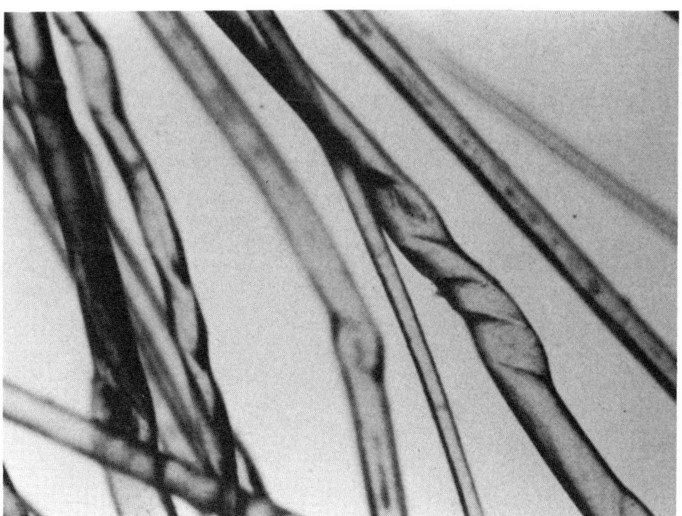

FIGURE 9–6
Pili torti. On microscopic examination, multiple twists are seen along the shafts of several hairs.

hair appears spangled in reflected light

microscopically, hair shafts flattened and, at irregular intervals, twisted 180° around the long axis

Discussion

isolated pili torti is uncommon and is usually seen in association with other defects (see below)

twisted hairs similar to those found in pili torti may be seen in association with other hair shaft abnormalities, including trichorrhexis nodosa (e.g., in arginosuccinic aciduria), monilethrix, and trichorrhexis invaginata (Netherton syndrome)

pili torti appearing after puberty is due to a second, genetically distinct form that is AD

REFERENCES

McK 261900

Appel B, Messina SJ. Pili torti hereditaria. N Engl J Med 1942;226:912–915

Nichamin SJ. Twisted hairs (pili torti). Am J Dis Child 1958;95:612–615

Patel HP, Unis ME. Pili torti in association with citrullinemia. J Am Acad Dermatol 1985;12:203–206

Whiting DA. Structural abnormalities of the hair shaft. J Am Acad Dermatol 1987; 16:1–25

BJÖRNSTAD SYNDROME

sparse, curly scalp hair; occasional thinning of lateral eyebrows

pili torti on microscopic examination

sensorineural deafness

AR

McK 262000

Cremers CW, Geerts SJ. Sensorineural hearing loss and pili torti. Ann Otol Rhinol Laryngol 1979;88:100–104

Petit A, Dontenwille MM, Blanchet-Bardon C, Civatte J. Pili torti with congenital deafness. (Björnstad's syndrome): report of three cases in one family, suggesting autosomal dominant transmission. Clin Exp Dermatol 1993;18:94–95

Scott MJ Jr, Bronson DM, Esterly NB. Björnstad syndrome and pili torti. Pediatr Dermatol 1983;1:45–50

Whiting DA. Structural abnormalities of the hair shaft. J Am Acad Dermatol 1987; 16:1–25

CRANDALL SYNDROME

sparse scalp hair and eyelashes; absent eyebrows and body hair

pili torti on microscopic examination

deafness

hypogonadism

probable AR

McK 262000
Crandall BF, Samec L, Sparkes RS, Wright SW. A familial syndrome of deafness, alopecia, and hypogonadism. J Pediatr 1973;82:461–465

PILI TORTI AND ONYCHODYSPLASIA (PILI TORTI, BEARE TYPE)

a subgroup of pili torti with onset in childhood of sparse scalp, axillary, and pubic hair

short, brittle nails

mental retardation

AD

Beare JM. Congenital pilar defect showing features of pili torti. Br J Dermatol 1952; 64:366–372

TRICHOTHIODYSTROPHY

The term *trichothiodystrophy* connotes the findings of short, brittle, sulfur-deficient hair. Trichothiodystrophy appears in association with many syndromes having neuroectodermal defects (see main entries for Tay, Marinesco-Sjögren, Sabinas brittle hair, and onychotrichodysplasia and neutropenia syndromes and Discussion); they may represent variations of a single syndrome or many syndromes with the common feature of trichothiodystrophy

Skin

dry, coarse, brittle hair at birth (Fig. 9–7)

persistent alopecia of scalp, eyebrows, and eyelashes may result from hair breakage and is aggravated by mechanical trauma

secondary sexual hair as well as body hair may be similarly affected

may have ichthyosiform skin changes and/or photosensitivity depending on the particular disorder

nail abnormalities include dystrophic changes and koilonychia

dental abnormalities reported

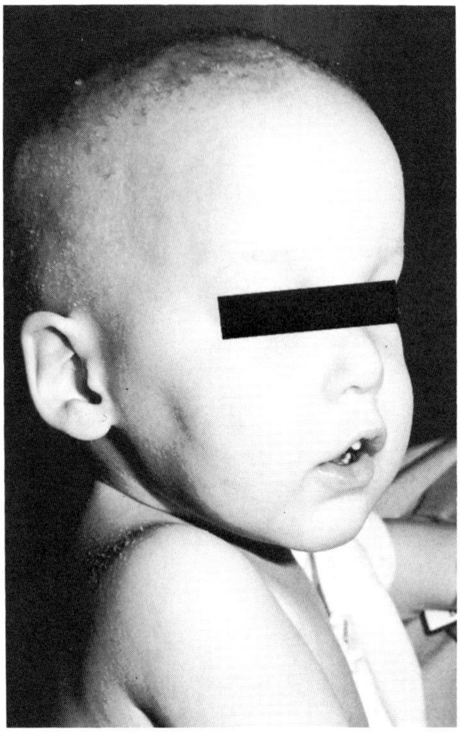

FIGURE 9–7
Short, sparse hair (trichothiodystrophy) and ichthyosiform scales over the entire skin surface in a patient with Tay syndrome.

Non-Skin

a variety of extracutaneous findings have been reported, the most salient of which are

- growth retardation
- mental retardation
- abnormal craniofacies, including microcephaly, micrognathia, and protruding ears
- cataracts
- recurrent infections

Genetics

AR; XLR also reported

Laboratory Data

see Figure 9–8

the diagnosis of trichothiodystrophy requires sulfur-deficient hair and one of the following three findings: (1) trichoschisis, (2) absent or defective cuticle on microscopic examination, or (3) characteristic light and dark banding (tiger tail pattern) on polaroscopy

hair sample shows 50% decrease in cystine/cysteine and sulfur content

evaluation for photosensitivity and DNA repair defects may be indicated in patients with suspected trichothiodystrophy (see PIBI[D]S syndrome)

Discussion

Syndromes with trichothiodystrophy not described elsewhere (except Tay syndrome) follow:

- *BIDS syndrome (Amish brittle hair syndrome)*

  an acronym for Brittle, cystine-deficient hair, Intellectual impairment, Decreased fertility, and Short stature

  AR

  McK 234050

- *IBIDS syndrome (Ichthyosis, Brittle hair, Impaired intelligence, Decreased fertility, and Short stature; Tay syndrome)*

  see main entry for Tay syndrome

  an acronym for lamellar Ichthyosis plus BIDS; present at birth

  IBIDS is same as Tay syndrome

  AR

  McK 242170

  McK 275550

- *PIBI[D]S syndrome*

  an acronym for Photosensitivity plus IBIDS; the [D] indicates that decreased fertility has not been established

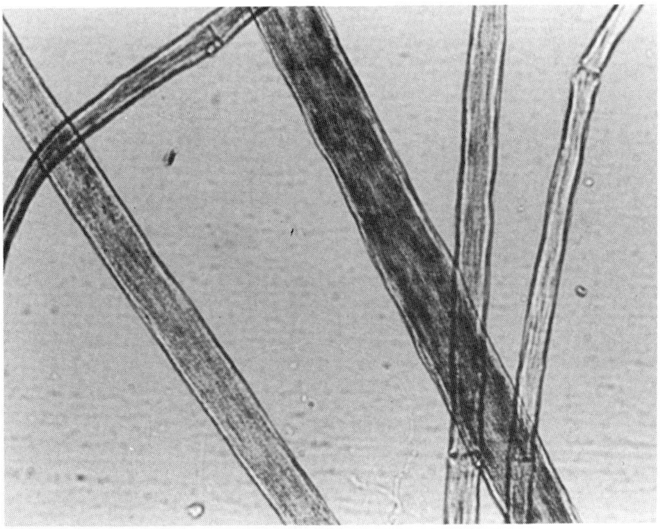

FIGURE 9–8
Several hair shafts show the clean breaks (trichoschisis) characteristic of hairs from patients with trichothiodystrophy.

some believe that PIBI[D]S syndrome is an entity distinct from BIDS and IBIDS syndromes and in some cases represents xeroderma pigmentosum complementation group D (XP-D); in addition, some patients with trichothiodystrophy and photosensitivity may have the same repair abnormalities as patients with xeroderma pigmentosum complementation group D but do not develop the skin cancers (see Xeroderma Pigmentosum, Complementation Group D)

in addition, some authors state that features distinguishing PIBI[D]S from IBIDS or Tay syndrome include skin changes most closely resembling ichthyosis vulgaris, absence of hypogonadism, and inappropriately sociable behavior (cf. IBIDS, with lamellar-like congenital ichthyosis and usually hypogonadism)

AR

McK 278730

- *SIBIDS:*

  IBIDS plus osteosclerosis

REFERENCES

McK 234050

Brown AC, Belser RB, Crounse RG, et al. A congenital hair defect: trichoschisis with alternating birefringence and low sulfur content. J Invest Dermatol 1970;54:496–509

Chapman S. The trichothiodystrophy syndrome of Pollitt. Pediatr Radiol 1988; 18:154–156

Hersh JH, Klein LR, Joyce MR, et al. Trichothiodystrophy and associated anomalies: a variant of SIBIDS or new symptom complex? Pediatr Dermatol, 1993;10:117–122

Hordinsky MK, Briden B, Berry SA. Friable hair, urea cycle dysfunction, and trichothiodystrophy: a new X-linked genodermatosis. Curr Probl Dermatol 1987;17:52–60

Itin PH, Pittelkow MR. Trichothiodystrophy: review of sulfur-deficient brittle hair syndromes and association with the ectodermal dysplasias. [Review]. J Am Acad Dermatol 1990;22:705–717

Jackson CE, Weiss L, Watson JHL. "Brittle" hair with short stature, intellectual impairment and decreased fertility: an autosomal recessive syndrome in an Amish kindred. Pediatrics 1974;54:201–207

Jorizzo JL, Atherton DJ, Crounse RG, et al. Ichthyosis, brittle hair, impaired intelligence, decreased fertility and short stature (IBIDS syndrome). Br J Dermatol 1982; 106:705–710

Lehmann AR, Arlett CF, Broughton BC, et al. Trichothiodystrophy, a human DNA repair disorder with heterogeneity in the cellular response to ultraviolet light. Cancer Res 1988;48:6090–6096

Pollitt RJ, Jenner FA, Davies M. Sibs with mental and physical retardation and trichorrhexis nodosa with abnormal amino acid composition of the hair. Arch Dis Child 1968;43:211–216

Price VH, Odom RB, Ward WH, Jones FT. Trichothiodystrophy: sulfur-deficient brittle hair as a marker for a neuroectodermal symptom complex. Arch Dermatol 1980; 116:1375–1384

Przedborski S, Ferster A, Goldman S, et al. Trichothiodystrophy, mental retardation, short stature, ataxia and gonadal dysfunction in three Moroccan siblings. Am J Med Genet 1990;35:566–573

Rebora A, Crovato F. PIBI(D)S syndrome—trichothiodystrophy with xeroderma pigmentosum (group D) mutation. J Am Acad Dermatol 1987;16:940–947

Tay CH. Ichthyosiform erythroderma, hair shaft abnormalities, and mental and growth retardation. Arch Dermatol 1971; 104:4–13

Van Neste D, Caulier B, Thomas P, et al. PIBIDS: Tay's syndrome and xeroderma pigmentosum [letter]. J Am Acad Dermatol 1985;12:372–373

MARINESCO-SJÖGREN SYNDROME

Skin

fair, short, thin, sparse scalp hair from birth

brittle nails

dental abnormalities include malformed teeth and absent lateral incisors

Non-Skin

bilateral cataracts at birth or in infancy

cerebellar ataxia usually apparent when the child is learning to walk, but adult onset also described

dysarthria

nystagmus

psychomotor retardation

muscular hypotonia, weakness, and atrophy

hypergonadotrophic hypogonadism

short stature

Genetics

AR

Laboratory Data

histopathology: internal root sheath fails to keratinize completely

reported hair shaft abnormalities include lack of pigment, trichoschisis, and absent medulla

hair is irregularly birefringent under polarizing microscopy

Discussion

some patients have trichothiodystrophy and may represent the most severe end of trichothiodystrophy spectrum (see Trichothiodystrophy)

REFERENCES

McK 248800

Norwood WF Jr. The Marinesco-Sjögren syndrome. J Pediatr 1964;65:431–437

Nyberg-Hansen R, Gronvik O. Hereditary cerebellar ataxia associated with congenital cataracts: 4 cases of the Marinesco-Sjögren syndrome with some unusual features. Acta Neurol Scand Suppl 1972;51:257–260

Rook A, Dawber R. Diseases of the Hair and Scalp. Oxford, Blackwell Scientific Publications, 1982;229–230

SABINAS BRITTLE HAIR SYNDROME

trichothiodystrophy causing brittle scalp hair and hypotrichosis from birth, especially in areas of friction; absent axillary and pubic hair

onychodysplasia

mental retardation and occasional ocular abnormalities including pigmentary retinopathy

AR

all affected trace ancestry to the town of Sabinas Hidalgo in Mexico

may be the same as BIDS (see Trichothiodystrophy)

McK 211390

Howell RR, Arbisser AI, Parsons DS, et al. The Sabinas syndrome. Am J Hum Genet 1981;33:957–967

ONYCHOTRICHODYSPLASIA AND NEUTROPENIA

sparse, curly scalp hair, eyebrows, and eyelashes

nail abnormalities include hyponychia, koilonychia, and onychorrhexis

chronic neutropenia

conjunctivitis

recurrent bacterial infections including otitis, tonsillitis, and sinusitis

variable mental retardation in some

AR

trichorrhexis nodosa and abnormal cuticular cells on microscopic examination

cysteine and sulfur content of hair decreased

alternating light and dark bands on polarizing microscopy

cuticular degeneration on electron microscopy

McK 258360

Cantu J-M, Arias J, Foncer-Rada M, et al. Syndrome of onychotrichodysplasia with chronic neutropenia in an infant from consanguineous parents. Birth Defects 1975;11:63–66

Hernandez A, Olivares F, Cantu J-M. Autosomal recessive onychotrichodysplasia, chronic neutropenia and mild mental retardation. Delineation of a syndrome. Clin Genet 1979;15:147–152

Itin PH, Pittelkow MR. Trichothiodystrophy with chronic neutropenia and mild retardation. J Am Acad Dermatol 1991;24:356–358

Verhage J, Habbema L, Vrensen GFJM, et al. A patient with onychotrichodysplasia, neutropenia, and normal intelligence. Clin Genet 1987;31:374–380

UNCOMBABLE HAIR SYNDROME

Synonyms

- pili trianguli et canaliculi
- spun-glass hair
- unruly hair
- cheveux incoiffables

Skin

silvery-blonde or straw-colored, glittery, frizzy, dry-appearing scalp hair that is disorderly and cannot be combed straight or flat (Fig. 9–9); no other body sites involved

usually seen in early childhood but may occur later on or at birth

hair grows slowly and may be brittle

Genetics

AD and AR inheritance suggested; many sporadic cases reported

Laboratory Data

see Figure 9–10

sulfur content is normal, and no light microscopy abnormalities noted

by scanning electron microscopy, hair shafts in cross-section resemble rounded triangles with a single longitudinal groove or canal on one surface; kidney-shaped hairs also noted; no twists or bends are present

a homogeneous band along one edge of the shaft is also seen under polarized light

histopathology: premature keratinization of inner root sheath

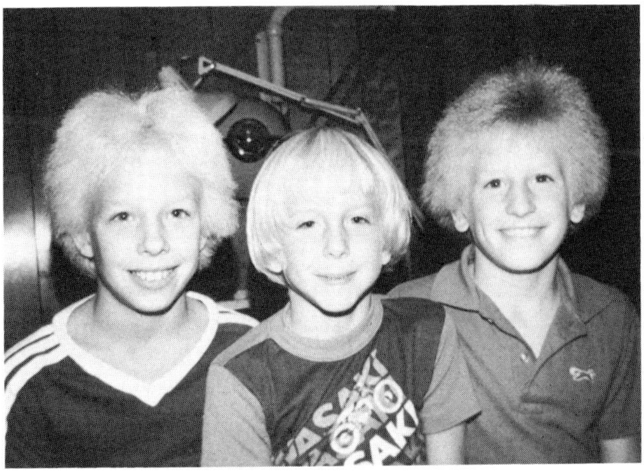

FIGURE 9–9
Three siblings, two of whom have the spangled, unruly hair of uncombable hair syndrome. (Courtesy of Robert Schoenfeld, MD, Birmingham, Michigan)

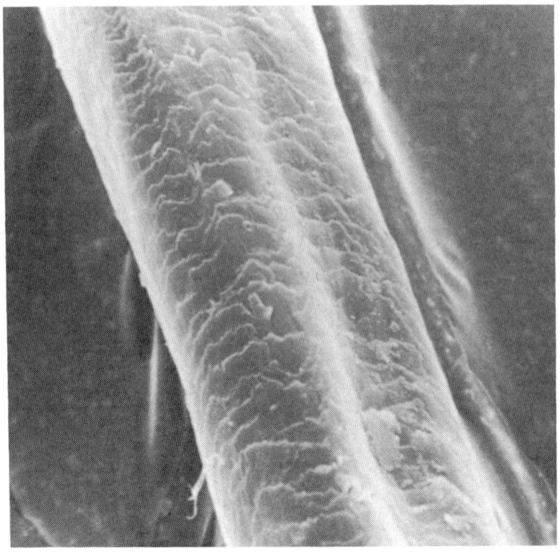

FIGURE 9–10
Scanning electron microscopy of a hair shaft from a patient in Figure 9–9. The longitudinal groove is characteristic of these hairs. (Courtesy of Robert Schoenfeld, MD, Birmingham, Michigan)

Prognosis

no effective treatment, but improved manageability may occur, even at an early age

Discussion

localized forms have been described, but most cases involve the entire scalp

AD inheritance may be more common than realized, since most studies have not examined hair from apparently normal relatives by scanning electron microscopy, in whom mild or spontaneously improved cases may otherwise escape detection

REFERENCES

McK 191480

Charuwichitratana S, Timpatanapong P, Sriurairatana S, et al. Pili trianguli et canaliculi: a nonfamilial case with eyebrow and eyelash involvement. Arch Dermatol 1986;122:977–978; see also erratum published in Arch Dermatol 1987;123:301

Garty B, Metzker A, Mimouni M, Varsano I. Uncombable hair: a condition with autosomal dominant inheritance. Arch Dis Child 1982;57:710–712

Hebert AA, Charrow J, Esterly NB, Fretzin DF. Uncombable hair (pili trianguli et canaliculi): evidence for dominant inheritance with complete penetrance based on scanning electron microscopy. Am J Med Genet 1987;28:185–193

Ravella A, Pujol RM, Noguera X, et al. Localized pili canaliculi and trianguli. J Am Acad Dermatol 1987;17:377–380

Whiting DA. Structural abnormalities of the hair shaft. J Am Acad Dermatol 1987; 16:1–125

HEREDITARY WOOLLY HAIR

Skin

thick unruly scalp hair that does not form locks, curling readily into spirals (Fig. 9–11); does not usually affect other body sites

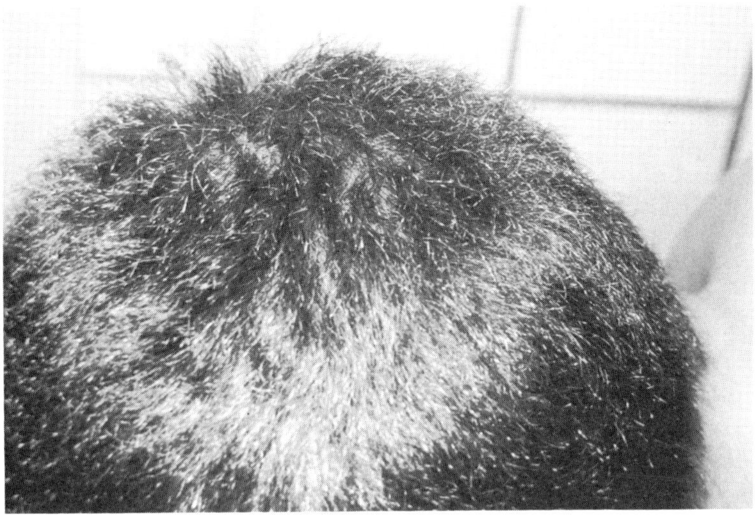

FIGURE 9–11
Woolly hair. This boy had his hair cropped short because the extreme curliness made it difficult to manage.

hair shows corrugations at intervals resembling the crimp in sheep's wool; fragility in some but particular color changes or alterations in growth rate not seen

seen at birth or in first months of life

condition may improve in adulthood

Non-Skin

eye abnormalities include cataracts

Genetics

AD

Discussion

confusion has arisen from difficulties in describing the appearance of unruly hair that does not fall into locks and that is difficult to brush; the terms *woolly, kinky, spun-glass-like, crimped, frizzly*, and *steely* are considered to be synonymous by many

- *woolly hair nevus*

  a rare, sporadically occurring condition with one or more patches of unruly, often lighter-colored hair that differs from surrounding, normal scalp hair in color, shape, and consistency

  hair is not fragile

  hairs twist along long axis

  usually noted in first few months of life but may be seen in young adulthood (some of the latter may be better classified as acquired progressive kinking of the hair) in 50% of cases, a linear epidermal or melanocytic nevus coexists elsewhere on skin, generally on the same side of body as the woolly hair nevus

the hair shaft may be flattened or fluted, or the cuticle may be absent

REFERENCES

McK 194300

Hutchinson PE, Cairns RJ, Wells RS. Woolly hair. Clinical and general aspects. Trans St Johns Hosp Dermatol Soc 1974;60:160–177

Jacobsen KU, Lowes M. Woolly hair naevus with ocular involvement: report of a case. Dermatologica 1975;151:249–252

Lantis SD, Pepper MC. Woolly hair nevus: two case reports and a discussion of unruly hair forms. Arch Dermatol 1978;114:233–238

McHenry PM, Nevin NC, Bingham EA. The association of keratosis pilaris atrophicans with hereditary woolly hair. Pediatr Dermatol 1990;7:302–304

Reda AM, Rogers RS III, Peters MS. Woolly hair nevus. J Am Acad Dermatol 1990; 22:377–380

Taylor AEM. Hereditary woolly hair with ocular involvement. Br J Dermatol 1990; 123:523–525

Verbov J. Woolly hair: study of a family. Dermatologica 1978;157:42–47

Whiting DA. Structural abnormalities of the hair shaft. J Am Acad Dermatol 1987; 16:1–25

FAMILIAL WOOLLY HAIR

thin, brittle, light-colored scalp hair at birth that is tightly curled; body hair and eyebrows also affected

length rarely exceeds 2 to 3 cm because of fragility and possibly a shortened growth cycle

probable AR

McK 278150

Hutchinson PE, Cairns RJ, Wells RS. Woolly hair: clinical and general aspects. Trans St John's Hosp Dermatol Soc 1974;60:160–177

DIFFUSE PARTIAL WOOLLY HAIR

a diffuse mix of woolly and straight hair on scalp

in one Scottish family, two thirds of scalp hairs were normal and one third were woolly

Ormerod AD, Main RA, Ryder ML, et al. A family with diffuse partial woolly hair. Br J Dermatol 1987;116:401–405

Hair Disorders—Abbreviated Entries

WOOLLY HAIR, HYPOTRICHOSIS, EVERTED LOWER LIP, OUTSTANDING EARS (SALAMON SYNDROME)

probable AR

do not confuse with another Salamon syndrome having hair findings (see main entry)

McK 278200

Salamon T. Ueber eine Familie mit recessiver Kraushaarigkeit, Hypotrichose und anderen Anomalien. Hautarzt 1963;14:540–544

FATAL INFANTILE DIARRHEA WITH ABNORMAL HAIR (TRICHORRHEXIS BLASTYSIS)

"rubbery" skin

woolly, easily removed black scalp hair

low birth weight, failure to thrive, and unexplained diarrhea

unusual facies with large, low-set ears

heredity undetermined; seen in two siblings who died by 3 months of age

hair mount shows pili torti, trichoschisis, trichoptilosis, and trichorrhexis nodosa

McK 222470

Stankler L, Lloyd D, Pollitt RJ, et al. Unexplained diarrhoea and failure to thrive in 2 siblings with unusual facies and abnormal scalp hair shafts: a new syndrome. Arch Dis Child 1982;57:212–216

ALOPECIA-CONTRACTURES-DWARFISM MENTAL RETARDATION SYNDROME

probable AR

McK 203550

Schinzel A. A case of multiple skeletal anomalies, ectodermal dysplasia and severe growth and mental retardation. Helv Paediat Acta 1980;35:243–251

van Gelderen HH. Syndrome of total alopecia, multiple skeletal anomalies, shortness of stature, and mental deficiency. Am J Med Genet 1982;13:383–387

CALCITRIOL-RESISTANT RICKETS WITH ALOPECIA

probable AR

McK 27744
Hochberg Z, Gilhar A, Haim S, et al. Calcitriol-resistant rickets with alopecia. Arch Dermatol 1985;121:646–647
Liberman UA, Halabe A, Samuel R, et al. End-organ resistance to 1,25-dihydroxycholecalciferol. Lancet 1980;1:504–507

KINKY HAIR, PHOTOSENSITIVITY, BROKEN EYEBROWS AND EYELASHES, AND NONPROGRESSIVE MENTAL RETARDATION

probable AR

hair was not tested for trichothiodystrophy

McK 234030
Calderon R, Gonzalez-Cantu N. Kinky hair, photosensitivity, broken eyebrows and eyelashes, and nonprogressive mental retardation. J Pediatr 1979;96:1007–1008

FAMILIAL CERVICAL HYPERTRICHOSIS WITH UNDERLYING KYPHOSCOLIOSIS

AD

McK 117850
Reed OM, Mellette JR, Jr, Fitzpatrick JE. Familial cervical hypertrichosis with underlying kyphoscoliosis. J Am Acad Dermatol 1989;20:1069–1072

HYPERTRICHOSIS OF THE PALMS AND SOLES

seen in a French-Canadian family

AD

McK 139650
Jackson CE, Callies QC, Krull EA, Mehregan A. Hairy cutaneous malformations of palms and soles. Arch Dermatol 1975;111:1146–1149

HAIRY NOSE TIP

heredity unclear

McK 139630
Goswami HK. Hairy tip of nose: a new trait in males. Am J Med Genet 1980;5:259–263

HYPERTRICHOSIS CUBITI (HAIRY ELBOWS)

hypertrichosis of the lower third of the upper arm and upper third of the forearm

probable AD but AR possible

McK 139600
Beighton PH. Familial hypertrichosis cubiti: hairy elbows syndrome. J Med Genet 1970;7:158–160
Flannery DB, Fink SM, Gilman PA. Hypertrichosis cubiti. Am J Med Genet 1989;32:482–483
MacDermot KD, Patton MA, Williams MJ, Winter RM. Hypertrichosis cubiti (hairy elbows) and short stature: a recognisable association. J Med Genet 1989;26:382–385

HAIRY EARS

growth of coarse hairs on the pinna, usually arising in the third decade

inheritance unknown except among the Bengali and Sinhalese, in whom it is YLD

McK 139500
Kamalam A, Thambiah AS. Genetics of hairy ears in South Indians. Clin Exp Dermatol 1990;15:192–194
Rao DC. A contribution to the genetics of hypertrichosis of the ear rims. Hum Hered 1970;20:486–492

TRICHOMEGALY WITH MENTAL RETARDATION, DWARFISM, AND PIGMENTARY DEGENERATION OF RETINA (OLIVER-MCFARLANE SYNDROME)

AR

McK 275400
Delleman JW, Van Walbeek K. The syndrome of trichomegaly, tapetoretinal degeneration and growth disturbances. Ophthalmologica 1975;171:313–315
Oliver GL, McFarlane DC. Congenital trichomegaly with associated pigmentary degeneration of the retina, dwarfism and mental retardation. Arch Ophthalmol 1965; 74:169–171
Patton MA, Harding AE, Baraitser M. Congenital trichomegaly, pigmentary retinal degeneration, and short stature. Am J Ophthalmol 1986;101:490–491
Sampson JR, Tolmie JL, Cant JS. Oliver-McFarlane syndrome: a 25-year follow-up. Am J Med Genet 1989;34:199–201

HYPERTRICHOTIC OSTEOCHONDRODYSPLASIA

generalized hypertrichosis at birth

dental abnormalities

macrosomy at birth

musculoskeletal abnormalities

cardiomegaly

probable AR

McK 239850
Cantu JM, Garcia-Cruz D, Sanchez-Corona J, et al. A distinct osteochondrodysplasia with hypertrichosis: individualization of a probable autosomal recessive entity. Hum Genet 1982;60:36–41

CONE-ROD CONGENITAL AMAUROSIS ASSOCIATED WITH CONGENITAL HYPERTRICHOSIS

hypertrichosis of face and body

trichomegaly, thick eyebrows and synophrys

cone-rod congenital amaurosis

probable AR

McK 204110
Jalili IK. Cone-rod congenital amaurosis associated with congenital hypertrichosis: an autosomal recessive condition. J Med Genet 1989;26:504–510

CATARACT, HYPERTRICHOSIS, AND MENTAL RETARDATION (CAHMR)

widespread hypertrichosis especially of face and back at birth

congenital cataracts

mental retardation

probable AR

McK 211770
Temtamy SA, Sinbawy AHH. Cataract, hypertrichosis, and mental retardation (CAHMR): a new autosomal recessive syndrome. Am J Med Genet 1991;41:432–433

MACROSTOMIA, ECTROPION, ATROPHIC SKIN, HYPERTRICHOSIS, AND GROWTH RETARDATION

possible AD
some consider this syndrome distinct from ablepharon-macrostomia syndrome (see below)

McK 200110
Barber N, Say B, Bell RF, Merveille OC. Macrostomia, ectropion, atrophic skin, hypertrichosis and growth retardation. Synd Ident 1982;8:6–9
Cesarino EJ, Pinheiro M, Freire-Maia N, Meira-Silva MC. Lid agenesis-macrostomia-psychomotor retardation-forehead hypertrichosis—a new syndrome? Am J Med Genet 1988;31:299–304
David A, Gordeeff A, Badounal J, Delaire J. Macrostomia, ectropion, atrophic skin, hypertrichosis: another observation. Am J Med Genet 1991;39:112–115

ABLEPHARON-MACROSTOMIA SYNDROME

absent eyelids, eyebrows, and eyelashes at birth

dry skin with redundant folds especially on neck, buttocks, knee flexures, and hands and feet

craniofacial abnormalities include fusion defects of the mouth, absence of zygomatic arches, and rudimentary external ears

other abnormalities include ambiguous genitalia and rudimentary or absent nipples

probable AR

McK 200110
Jackson IT, Shaw KE, del Pinal Matorras F. A new feature of the ablepharon macrostomia syndrome: zygomatic arch absence. Br J Plast Surg 1988;41:410–416
McCarthy GT, West CM. Ablepheron macrostomia syndrome. Dev Med Child Neurol 1977;19:659–672

DISTICHIASIS WITH CONGENITAL ANOMALIES OF THE HEART AND PERIPHERAL VASCULATURE

AD

McK 126320
Goldstein S, Qazi QH, Fitzgerald J, et al. Distichiasis, congenital heart defects and mixed peripheral vascular anomalies. Am J Med Genet 1985;20:283–294

ALOPECIA, PSYCHOMOTOR EPILEPSY, PYORRHEA, AND MENTAL SUBNORMALITY

AD

McK 104130
Shokeir MHK. Universal permanent alopecia, psychomotor epilepsy, pyorrhea and mental subnormality. Clin Genet 1977;11:13–17

ALOPECIA-MENTAL RETARDATION SYNDROME

probable AR

may be difficult to separate this disorder from congenital alopecia, seizures, and psychomotor retardation (see McK 203600 below)

McK 203650
Perniola T, Krajewska G, Carnevale F, Lospalluti M. Congenital alopecia, psychomotor retardation, convulsions in two sibs of a consanguineous marriage. J Inher Metab Dis 1980;3:49–53

CONGENITAL ALOPECIA, SEIZURES, AND PSYCHOMOTOR RETARDATION (MOYNAHAN SYNDROME)

probable AR

McK 203600
Moynahan EJ. Familial congenital alopecia, epilepsy, mental retardation with unusual electroencephalograms. Proc R Soc Med 1962;55:411–412

Pfeiffer RA, Völklein J. Congenital universal alopecia, mental deficiency, and microcephaly in two sibs. J Med Genet 1982;19:388–389 van Haeringen A, Hurst JA, Savidge R, Baraitser M. A familial syndrome of microcephaly, sparse hair, mental retardation and seizures. J Med Genet 1990;27:127–129

Wessel HB, Barmada MA, Hashida Y. Congenital alopecia, seizures, and psychomotor retardation in three siblings. Pediatr Neurol 1987;3:101–107

CONGENITAL ATRICHIA WITH NAIL DYSTROPHY, ABNORMAL FACIES, AND PSYCHOMOTOR RETARDATION

probable AR

Vogt BR, Traupe H, Hamm H. Congenital atrichia with nail dystrophy, abnormal facies, and retarded psychomotor development in two siblings: a new autosomal recessive syndrome? Pediatr Dermatol 1988;5:236–242

CILIARY AND SUPERCILIARY HYPOTRICHOSIS

AD

Garcia-Esquivel L, Hernandez A, Reynoso MC, et al. Ciliary and superciliary hypotrichosis: a distinct autosomal dominant trait. Ophthalmic Paediatr Genet 1986; 7:77–79

HYPOTRICHOSIS WITH LIGHT-COLORED HAIR AND FACIAL MILIA

probable AD

McK 146530

Parrish JA, Baden HP, Goldsmith LA, Matz MH. Studies of the density and the properties of the hair in a new inherited syndrome of hypotrichosis. Ann Hum Genet 1972;35:349–356

SPARSE BRITTLE HAIR AND SPONDYLOEPIMETAPHYSEAL DYSPLASIA

AD

McK 183849
Whyte MP, Petersen DJ, McAlister WH. Hypotrichosis with spondyloepimetaphyseal dysplasia in three generations: a new autosomal dominant syndrome. Am J Med Genet 1990;36:288–291

TRICHODYSPLASIA-XERODERMA

sparse, coarse, brittle scalp hair; eyebrows and eyelashes, axillary and pubic hair also sparse

moderate xeroderma

pili torti demonstrated on scanning electron microscopy

McK 190360
Pinheiro M, Freire-Maia N. Trichodysplasia-xeroderma: an autosomal dominant condition. Clin Genet 1987;31:337–342

THUMB DEFORMITY AND ALOPECIA

alopecia of scalp in infancy

generalized hyperpigmentation with superimposed hypopigmented macules

dental abnormalities

thumb hypoplasia

short stature

AD

McK 188150
Chiba A, Miura T. A family with hypotrichosis associated with congenital hypoplasia of the thumb. Jpn J Hum Genet 1979; 24:111–117
Lucky AW, Esterly NB, Tunnessen WW Jr. Ectodermal dysplasia and abnormal thumbs. J Am Acad Dermatol 1980;2:379–384
Winter RM, MacDermot KD, Hill FJ. Sparse hair, short stature, hypoplastic thumbs, single upper central incisor and abnormal skin pigmentation: a possible "new" form of ectodermal dysplasia. Am J Med Genet 1988;29:209–216

FAMILIAL ACNE CONGLOBATA, HIDRADENITIS SUPPURATIVA, PILI TORTI, AND CATARACTS

AD

Gold SC, Delaney TJ. Familial acne conglobata, hidradenitis-suppurativa, pili torti and cataracts. Br J Dermatol 1974;91(Suppl 10):54–57

HYPOTHYROIDISM, ATHYROIDAL, WITH SPIKY HAIR AND CLEFT PALATE

possible AR

McK 241850
Bamforth JS, Hughes IA, Lazarus JH, et al. Congenital hypothyroidism, spiky hair, and cleft palate. J Med Genet 1989;26:49–51

CONGENITAL TRIANGULAR ALOPECIA

triangular-shaped area of sparse vellus hairs located in temporal areas (unilateral or bilateral), usually noticed in childhood

sporadic; at least one familial report

Bargman H. Congenital temporal triangular alopecia. Can Med Assoc J 1984;131:1253–1254

Tosti A. Congenital triangular alopecia: report of fourteen cases. J Am Acad Dermatol 1987;16:991–993

REGIONAL CHOROIDAL ATROPHY AND ALOPECIA

congenital sparse scalp hair and thin eyebrows and eyelashes

nail dystrophy

regional choroidal atrophy

possible AR

Moloney J. Regional choroidal atrophy and alopecia: a new syndrome. Bull Soc Belge Ophthalmol 1987;224:39–41

HYPOGONADISM AND PRIMARY AND PARTIAL ALOPECIA

partial alopecia of scalp

hypogonadism

probable AR

McK 241090
Al-Awadi SA, Farag TI, Teebi AS, et al. Primary hypogonadism and partial alopecia in three sibs with Müllerian hypoplasia in the affected females. Am J Med Genet 1985;22:619–622

HYPOGONADISM, DIABETES MELLITUS, ALOPECIA, MENTAL RETARDATION, AND ELECTROCARDIOGRAPHIC ABNORMALITIES

probable AR

McK 241080
Woodhouse NJY, Sakati NA. A syndrome of hypogonadism, diabetes mellitus, mental retardation, deafness and ECG abnormalities. J Med Genet 1983;20:216–219

CHAPTER

10

Nail Disorders

Nail abnormalities are a common finding in many genetic skin diseases. However, only rarely are they a major manifestation of a particular syndrome or so distinctive that they constitute a specific and identifiable entity. For this reason, this chapter contains relatively few entries. The numerous syndromes in which nail changes are regarded as a minor or variable feature are discussed in other more appropriate chapters or are listed in Tables 10–1 through 10–4.

REFERENCES

Baran R, Dawber RPR, eds. Diseases of the Nails and Their Management. Oxford, Blackwell Scientific Publications, 1984

Scher RK, Daniel CR III, eds. Nails: Therapy, Diagnosis, Surgery. Philadelphia, WB Saunders, 1990

Zaias N. The Nail. New York, Spectrum Publications, 1980

Text continued on page 427

TABLE 10–1
NAIL FINDINGS IN DYSPLASIA AND MALFORMATION SYNDROMES

Disease (McK Number)	Inheritance	Nail Findings
Acrofacial dysostosis	AD	Hypoplasia or dysplasia
AEC syndrome (ankyloblepharon, ectodermal dysplasia, and cleft lip and palate syndrome) (McK 106260)	AD	Dystrophic or absent nails
Alopecia congenita with keratosis palmoplantaris (McK 104100)	AD	Dystrophy of fingernails
Apical dysplasia of fingers (McK 125540)	AD	Transverse depressions
Amelo-onychohypohidrotic dysplasia (McK 104570)	AD	Onycholysis and subungual hyperkeratosis
Jorgenson syndrome (McK 129200)	AD	Short and thick longitudinal ridges
CHANDS syndrome (McK 214350)	AR	Hypoplasia
Coffin-Siris syndrome (McK 135900)	AD	Usually absence or hypoplasia of fifth fingernails and toenails
Chondrodysplasia punctata (McK 302960)	XLD	Onychoschizia and platyonychia
Deafness and onychodystrophy syndrome (McK 124480, 220500)	AD and AR	Dysplasia and hypoplasia with furrows and cracks
Dento-oculocutaneous syndrome (McK 200970)	AD	Horizontal ridging and onychoschizia
Diffuse palmoplantar keratoderma (Unna-Thost) (McK 148400)	AD	Dystrophic changes
Dyskeratosis congenita (McK 305000)	XLR, AD, and AR	Hyponychia, paronychia, and occasional anonychia
EEC syndrome (ectrodactyly, ectodermal dysplasia, and cleft lip and palate syndrome) (McK 129900)	AD, AR, and many sporadic cases reported	Pitting, striations, brittleness and thinning
Chondroectodermal dysplasia (Ellis-van Creveld syndrome) (McK 225500)	AR	Brittle, furrowed, hypoplastic or absent
Tooth and nail syndrome of Fried	AR	Thin, small, and concave
Goltz syndrome (McK 305600)	XLD	Thin, narrow, spoon shaped; also may be normal or absent
Hypohidrotic ectodermal dysplasia with hypothyroidism syndrome (McK 225050)	AR	Dystrophy
Hypohidrotic ectodermal dysplasia (McK 305100)	XLR	Usually normal but occasionally brittle
Hidrotic ectodermal dysplasia (McK 129500)	AD	Onychauxis, longitudinal striations, paronychia, convex curvature, anonychia
Incontinentia pigmenti (McK 308300)	XLD	Nail dystrophy; occasional koilonychia; subungual tumors
KID syndrome (McK 148210)	AD (AR reported)	Anonychia, onychauxis, and leukonychia

TABLE 10–1
NAIL FINDINGS IN DYSPLASIA AND MALFORMATION SYNDROMES *Continued*

Disease (McK Number)	Inheritance	Nail Findings
Lacrimo-auriculo-dento-digital (LADD) syndrome (McK 149730)	AD	Ectopic nails, large thumb nail
Mal de Meleda syndrome (McK 248300)	AR	Koilonychia and subungual hyperkeratosis
Mikaelian syndrome (ectodermal dysplasia and neurosensory deafness) (McK 224800)	AR	Onychodystrophy
Naegeli-Franceschetti-Jadassohn syndrome (McK 161000)	AD	Onycholysis and subungual hyperkeratosis
Papillon-Lefèvre syndrome (McK 245000)	AR	Spoon shaped, striations, and onychogryphosis
Onychotrichodysplasia with neutropenia (McK 258360)	AR	Hyponychia, koilonychia, and onychorrhexis
Pachyonychia congenita, Jadassohn-Lewandowski type (McK 167200)	AD	Marked nail bed hyperkeratosis and associated distortion and brown discoloration of nail plate
Pachyonychia congenita, Jackson-Lawler type (McK 167210)	AD	Thick subungual hyperkeratosis
Rapp-Hodgkin syndrome (McK 129400)	probable AD	Small, narrow, and dystrophic
Rosselli-Gulienetti syndrome (McK 225000)	AR	Subungual hyperkeratosis, longitudinal striations, and distal plate chipping
Sabinas syndrome (McK 211390)	AR	Dystrophy
Salamon syndrome	AR	Dystrophy
Tricho-dento-osseous (TDO) syndrome (McK 190320)	AD	Brittle and white transverse banding
Tooth and nail syndrome (McK 189500)	AD	Nails, especially toenails, are hypoplastic and may be spoon shaped
Tricho-oculo-dermo-vertebral syndrome	AR	Fingernails thin and brittle; toenails broad, short, and dystrophic
Trichothiodystrophy (McK 234050)	AR but XLR also reported	Onychauxis, subungual hyperkeratosis, onychoschizia, longitudinal groove, koilonychia
Triphalangeal thumbs-onychodystrophy-deafness syndrome (deafness, onychodystrophy and digital anomalies; deafness-onycho-osteodystrophy-mental retardation; DOOR syndrome) (McK 220500, 124480)	Mostly AR cases, but AD also reported	Hypoplasia or absence
XTE (xeroderma, talipes, and enamel defect) syndrome	AD	Dystrophy

TABLE 10–2
INHERITED SYNDROMES WITH SKELETAL AND NAIL ABNORMALITIES

Disease (McKusick Number)	Inheritance	Nail Findings
Apert syndrome (McK 101200)	AD, most cases spontaneous mutations	Broad, short, fused nails and micronychia; lunulae may be absent
Brachydactyly with nail dysplasia	AD	Fourth digit nail absent, others dysplastic
Brachydactyly, type A5, with nail dysplasia (absent middle phalanges of digits 2 through 5 with nail dysplasia) (McK 112900)	AD	Hypoplasia
Carpenter syndrome (McK 201000)	AR	Short and broad
Cartilage-hair hypoplasia (McK 250250)	AR	Short and broad
CHILD syndrome (McK 308050)	XLD	Onychogryphosis and brittleness on affected side
Cleidocranial dysostosis (McK 119600)	AD	Down-curved and small
Cryptophthalmos (Fraser) syndrome (McK 219000)	AR	Hypoplasia
Keipert syndrome (McK 255980)	AR	Broad nails
Larsen syndrome (McK 150250, 245600)	AR	Short and broad
Leri pleonosteosis (McK 151200)	AD	Short and broad
Marfan syndrome (McK 154700)	AD	Pseudo-clubbing
Nail-patella-elbow syndrome (McK 161200)	AD	Hypoplasia or aplasia of nails generally with onset at birth; thumb nail and index fingernail are affected most severely, fifth finger least severely; the fingers are more severely affected than the toes; small remnants of nail may remain proximally; anonychia, especially of thumb, may result; rarely, only ulnar aspect of nail plate is absent; other nail plate abnormalities include hapalonychia, koilonychia, and onychorrhexis; lunulae are triangular or absent
Oculodentodigital syndrome (Meyer-Schwickerath syndrome; oculodento-osseous dysplasia) (McK 164200)	AD and possibly AR in some cases; also sporadic cases reported	Absent
Otopalatodigital syndrome I (McK 311300)	XLR	Short and broad
Pachydermoperiostosis (McK 167100)	AD	Clubbing, thin, and yellow discoloration
Popliteal web syndrome (McK 119500)	AD	Toenail dysplasia
Puretic syndrome (McK 265700)	? AR	Broad, pseudoclubbing, onycholysis

TABLE 10–2
INHERITED SYNDROMES WITH SKELETAL AND NAIL ABNORMALITIES *Continued*

Disease (McKusick Number)	Inheritance	Nail Findings
Pycnodysostosis (McK 265800)	AR	Short brittle nails with pseudoclubbing or platyonychia
Rubinstein-Taybi syndrome (McK 180849)	AD	Broad nails
Rudiger syndrome (McK 268650)	AR	Hypoplasia
Seckel syndrome (McK 210600)	AR	Clubbing
Sclerosteosis (McK 269500)	?	Absent or dysplastic second and third fingernails
Tricho-rhino-phalangeal syndrome (McK 190350)	AD, AR reported	Thin and short; koilonychia and leukonychia described
Williams syndrome (McK 194050)	AD	Hyponychia

TABLE 10–3
OTHER INHERITED SYNDROMES THAT MAY MANIFEST NAIL FINDINGS

Disease (McK Number)	Inheritance	Nail Findings
Acanthosis nigricans (McK 100600)	AD	Thick, friable, gray
Acrogeria (McK 201200)	Mostly sporadic; rare AR and AD cases reported	Atrophy, onychogryphosis, koilonychia
Anonychia (McK 206800)	AD	Total and occasionally partial absence of nails
Anonychia with ectrodactyly (McK 106900)	AD	Absence
Bart-Pumphrey syndrome (McK 149200)	AD	Total leukonychia
Congenital onychodysplasia of the index finger	Mostly sporadic but AD inheritance reported	Micronychia is the most common defect; radial aspect more often involved than ulnar
Curved nail of fourth toe (McK 219070)	Probably AR	Curved fourth toenail
Familial koilonychia (McK 149300)	AD	Nails thin and concave with everted edges
Familial mandibuloacral dysplasia (McK 248370)	AR	Broad nails
Hairy elbows syndrome (McK 139600)	Probable AD but AR also possible	Short nails
Hemochromatosis (McK 235200)	AR	White, gray or brownish; koilonychia
Hereditary onychodysplasia of fifth toenails	AD	Longitudinal furrows and distal onycholysis with splitting of fifth toenails after age 2
Hereditary onychogryposis	AD	Overcurved and laterally deviated
Hirschsprung disease with hypoplastic nails and dysmorphic facial features (McK 235760)	Probable AR	Hypoplastic nails
Leukonychia (McK 151600)	AD	Total, partial, striate, or punctate patterns may be seen

Table continued on following page

TABLE 10–3

OTHER INHERITED SYNDROMES THAT MAY MANIFEST NAIL FINDINGS *Continued*

Disease (McK Number)	Inheritance	Nail Findings
Leukonychia totalis, multiple sebaceous cysts, and renal calculi (McK 151600)	AD	Leukonychia totalis
Macular amyloidosis and familial nail dystrophy	AD	Yellow-brown
Multiple lentigines syndrome (LEOPARD syndrome) (McK 151100)	AD	Leukonychia; koilonychia
Onychodystrophy totalis (McK 161050)	AD	Onychodystrophy
Peutz-Jeghers syndrome (McK 175200)	AD	Brown discoloration
Progeria (McK 176670)	? AR, inheritance unclear	Brittle nail plate and thinning; yellowish discoloration
Rothmund-Thomson syndrome (McK 268400)	AR	Roughness and ridging; small and thin
Scleroatrophic and keratotic dermatosis of limbs (scleroatrophic syndrome of Huriez) (McK 181600)	AD	Hypoplasia; white
Tuberous sclerosis (McK 191100)	AD	Subungual and periungual fibromas (Koenen tumors); most commonly noted at or after puberty; distortion of nail plate
Werner syndrome (McK 277700)	AR	Nails are brittle, atrophic, or absent

TABLE 10–4

CHROMOSOMAL SYNDROMES WITH NAIL ABNORMALITIES

Disease	Nail Findings
Down syndrome	Clubbing with cardiac defects or macronychia
Trisomy 18 syndrome	Hypoplasia especially of fifth fingers and toes
Trisomy 13 syndrome	Narrow, hyperconvex or hypoplastic
Trisomy 9P syndrome	Dystrophic and claw-like
Monosomy 9p	Square shape, wide, and convex
Trisomy 8	Hypoplastic; may be absent at birth
Trisomy 8p	Hypoplastic or absent
Trisomy 7q	Hyperconvex
Monosomy 4p	Hyperconvex
Group G ring chromosome	Pachyonychia
Turner syndrome	Narrow, hyperconvex or deep set
Trisomy 3q	Hypoplastic or absent
Long arm 18 deletion syndrome	Narrow
Chromosome type C trisomy	Hypoplasia
Chromosome 21 long arm deletion syndrome (antimongolism)	Hypoplasia

References: Scher RK, Daniel CR III, eds. Nails: Therapy, Diagnosis, Surgery. Philadelphia, WB Saunders 1990; Baran R, Dawber RPR, eds. Diseases of the Nails and Their Management. Oxford, Blackwell Scientific Publications, 1984; and Zaias N. The Nail. New York, Spectrum Publications, 1980.

Pachyonychia Congenita

Pachyonychia congenita is a group of disorders with thickened nails. Extreme nail bed hyperkeratosis causes a characteristic brown discoloration and distortion of the nail plate, which is lifted from the nail bed and arched around its longitudinal axis, sometimes becoming cone shaped. Onset is usually in the first year of life but can be later.

The disorder has been subclassified on the basis of additional cutaneous and systemic findings. The two traditional subtypes are the Jadassohn-Lewandowsky and Jackson-Lawler forms. Gorlin describes pedigrees in which these subtypes overlap. Other variants have been described (e.g., Haber-Rose and Tidman-Wells-MacDonald types). Feinstein has reclassified pachyonychia congenita into four subtypes, as follows:

- *pachyonychia congenita, type I*

  hyperkeratosis of nail beds

  palmoplantar keratoderma

  follicular keratoses

  oral leukokeratosis

  AD

- *pachyonychia congenita, type II*

  features of type I, plus:

  - blisters of palms and soles
  - palmoplantar hyperhidrosis
  - neonatal (natal) teeth
  - steatocystoma multiplex or multiple epidermoid cysts
  - AD

- *pachyonychia congenita, type III*

  features of types I and II, plus:

  - angular cheilosis
  - corneal dyskeratosis and cataracts
  - AD

- *pachyonychia congenita, type IV*

  features of types I, II, and III, plus:

  - laryngeal lesions
  - hoarseness
  - mental retardation
  - hair anomalies and alopecia
  - AD

REFERENCES

Feinstein A, Friedman J, Schewach-Millet M. Pachyonychia congenita. [Review]. J Am Acad Dermatol 1988;19:705–711

Gorlin RJ, Cohen MM Jr, Levin LS. Syndromes affecting the skin and mucosa. In: Syndromes of the Head and Neck. 3rd ed. New York, Oxford University Press, 1990:445–448

PACHYONYCHIA CONGENITA, JADASSOHN-LEWANDOWSKY TYPE

Skin

nail units usually normal at birth

hyperkeratosis of nail bed, especially the distal half to two thirds, develops in first year of life (Figs. 10–1 and 10–2); rare onset in teens reported

all 20 nails involved; fingernails more severely affected than toenails

extreme nail bed hyperkeratosis causes a characteristic brown discoloration and distortion of the nail plate, which is lifted from the nail bed and arched around its longitudinal axis, sometimes becoming cone shaped

occasional shedding of nails, especially after trauma and recurrent paronychia; resultant scarring of the nail bed may cause further distortion

palmoplantar keratotic plaques, usually developing after onset of nail disease; soles more severely affected; plaques thicker over weight-bearing areas but may be diffuse

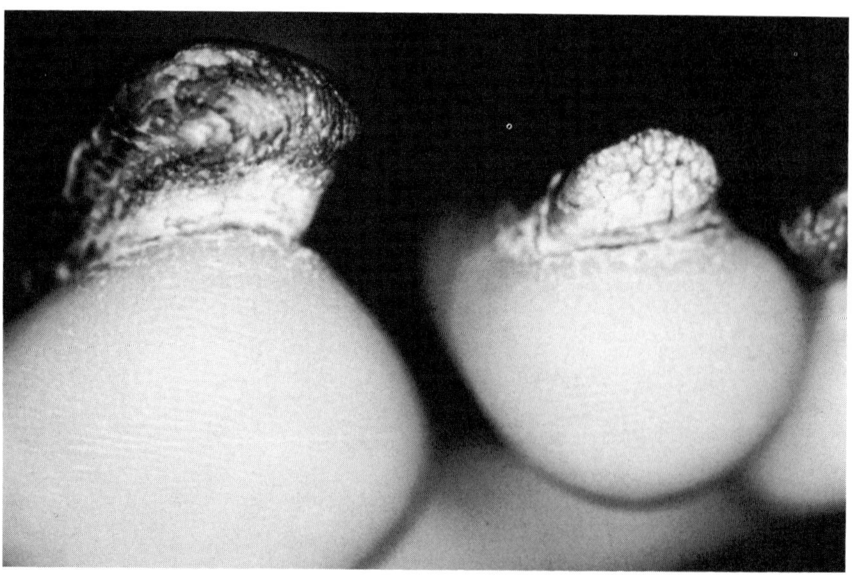

FIGURE 10–1
Close-up of the nails in a patient with pachyonychia congenita.

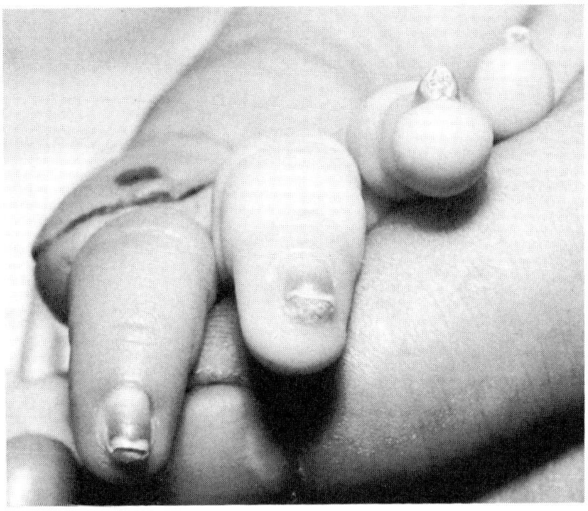

FIGURE 10–2
Discolored dystrophic nails of pachyonychia congenita. Note how the subungual hyperkeratosis causes arching and lifting from the nail bed.

palmoplantar hyperhidrosis in most; rest of skin dry and occasional generalized mild ichthyosiform eruption reported

occasional painful intraepidermal blisters and ulcers over sites of friction on palms and soles and rarely on elbows or knees; may worsen in summer; heal without scarring

occasional keratosis pilaris–like papules or verrucous plaques on extensor extremities, knees, elbows, popliteal spaces, buttocks, legs, and ankles

hyperkeratotic white striations or multiple plaques on buccal mucosa, labial mucosa, tongue, and gingiva (Fig. 10–3); occasional similar involvement of nasal mucosa, larynx (causing hoarseness), and tympanic membranes (causing deafness)

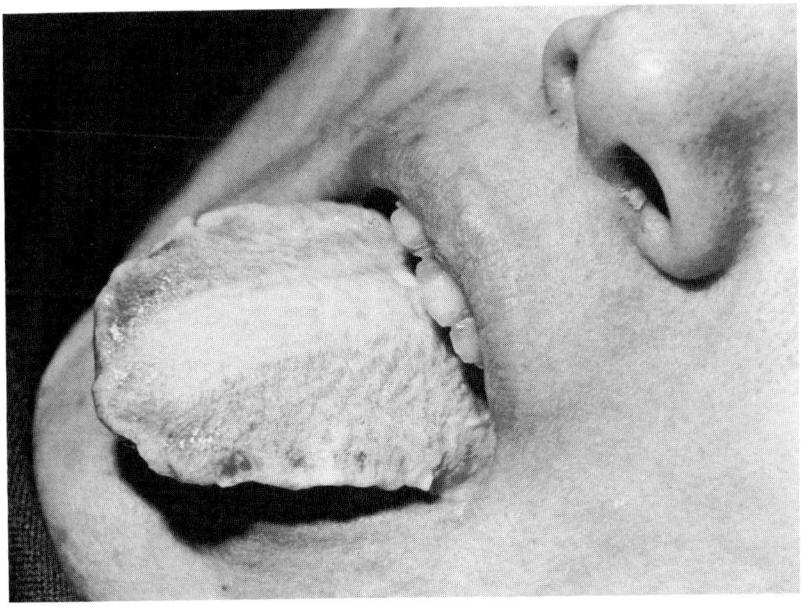

FIGURE 10–3
Pachyonychia congenita. There is marked leukokeratosis of the tongue.

oral white plaques not thought to have increased propensity for malignancy

sparse scalp hair occasionally

Non-Skin

ocular abnormalities occasionally present include corneal opacities (dyskeratosis), bilateral cataracts, and microphthalmos

Genetics

AD; possible AR

Prognosis

growth and development normal, but difficulty using hands and walking may handicap the patient

Discussion

occasionally, plantar keratoses are the only manifestation

nail changes alone in some pedigrees

REFERENCES

McK 167200

McK 260130

Paller AS, Moore JA, Scher R. Pachyonychia congenita tarda. Arch Dermatol 1991;127: 701–703

Su WPD, Chun SI, Hammond DE, et al. Pachyonychia congenita: a clinical study of 12 cases and review of the literature. [Review]. Pediatr Dermatol 1990;7:33–38

Thorman J, Kobayasi T. Pachyonychia congenita Jadassohn-Lewandowsky: a disorder of keratinization. Acta Derm Venereol 1977;57:63–67

PACHYONYCHIA CONGENITA, JACKSON-LAWLER TYPE

nail bed hyperkeratosis

palmoplantar keratoderma

follicular keratosis

cutaneous cysts (steatocytstoma multiplex and/or scalp epidermal cysts)

association with hidradenitis suppurativa reported

no oral leukokeratosis (cf. Jadassohn-Lewandowsky type)

natal teeth

AD

McK 167210
Clementi M, Cardin de Stefani E, Dei Rossi C, et al. Pachyonychia congenita Jackson-Lawler type: a distinct malformation syndrome. Br J Dermatol 1986;114:367–370
Jackson ADM, Lawler SD. Pachyonychia congenita: a report of six cases in one family. Ann Eugen 1951;16:141–146
Todd P, Garioch J, Rademaker M, et al. Pachyonychia congenita complicated by hidradenitis suppurativa: a family study. Br J Dermatol 1990;123:663–666

PACHYONYCHIA CONGENITA, HABER-ROSE TYPE

recurrent blisters primarily on hands and feet

keratotic papules on dorsa of fingers and toes; palmoplantar keratoderma

leukokeratosis on tongue and buccal mucosa

leukonychia

AR

some patients were originally classified as having epidermolysis bullosa

McK 260130
Haber RM, Rose TH. Autosomal recessive pachyonychia congenita. Arch Dermatol 1986;122:919–923

PACHYONYCHIA CONGENITA WITH HYPERPIGMENTATION AND AMYLOID DEPOSITS (TIDMAN-WELLS-MACDONALD PACHYONYCHIA CONGENITA)

nail dystrophy with onset in early childhood; improves with age

palmoplantar keratoderma

diffuse hyperpigmentation on neck and waist in early childhood; dappled appearance in axillae, popliteal fossae, thighs, buttocks, and lower abdomen

histopathology and electron microscopy: pigmentary incontinence and amyloid in papillary dermis

possible variant of Jadassohn-Lewandowsky type

AD

Tidman MJ, Wells RS, MacDonald DM. Pachyonychia congenita with cutaneous amyloidosis and hyperpigmentation: a distinct variant. J Am Acad Dermatol 1987;16:935–940

ODONTOONYCHODYSPLASIA

nail bed hypertrophy

natal teeth

no oral changes or palmoplantar keratoderma

AD

probably an ectodermal dysplasia, but some discuss this as a variant of pachyonychia congenita

do not confuse with odonto-onychodysplasia with alopecia (see main entry)

McK 167200

Murray FA. Congenital anomalies of the nails: four cases of hereditary hypertrophy of the nail bed associated with a history of erupted teeth at birth. Br J Dermatol 1921;33:409–412

NAIL-PATELLA-ELBOW SYNDROME

Synonyms

- osteo-onychodysplasia
- Fong syndrome

Skin

hypoplasia or aplasia of nails (Fig. 10–4); onset usually at birth

thumb and index fingernails are affected most severely, fifth finger least severely; fingers far more severely affected than toes

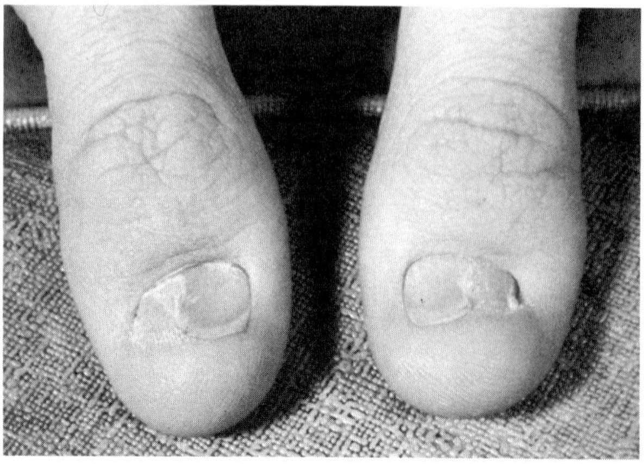

FIGURE 10–4
Abnormal nail plates on the thumbs of a patient with nail-patella-elbow syndrome. Asymmetry is due to more severe hypoplasia of the ulnar aspect of the nail plates. (Courtesy of Lester Weiss, MD, Detroit, Michigan)

small remnants of nail may remain proximally

rarely, only ulnar aspect of nail plate is absent

other nail plate abnormalities include hapalonychia, koilonychia, onychorrhexis, and pterygium

lunulae are triangular or absent

Non-Skin

hyperextensible joints of digits, caused by laxity of ligaments

knee abnormalities in nearly all (Fig. 10–5); resultant pain and gait abnormalities in childhood may call attention to the diagnosis

patellae are usually hypoplastic but occasionally absent; may be ovoid, triangular, or irregular

lateral subluxation of patella may be recurrent or permanent; complete dislocation is less common

genu valgum or lateral rotation of tibia may result

elbow abnormalities, less frequent than nail or knee abnormalities, include hypoplasia of lateral side of joint, including capitulum, epicondyle, and radial head; as a result, the carrying angle is increased and subluxation or dislocation may occur, usually posteriorly

disability often minimal, but gait may be abnormal and elbows may have contractures

iliac horns of the posterior aspect of pelvis in over half of patients; present early in life; may not be palpable or visible on radiographs

renal disease, especially chronic glomerulonephritis, is seen in one third of patients; proteinuria is a common presenting sign; renal failure may result

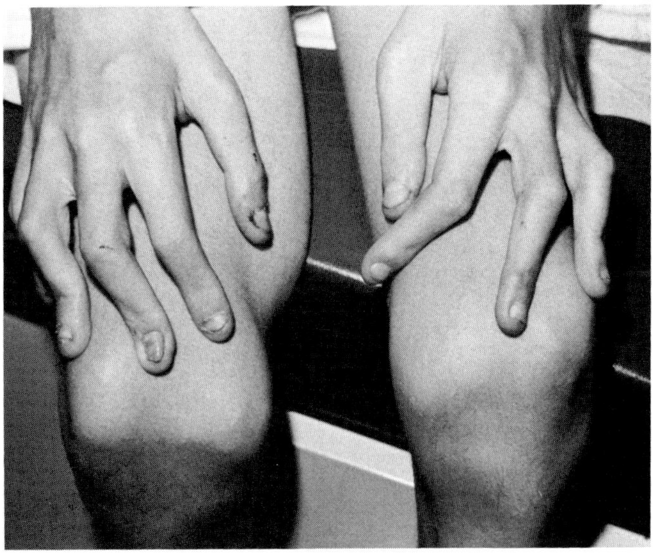

FIGURE 10–5
Nail-patella-elbow syndrome. Hypoplasia of the patellae and hypoplasia of the nails on the thumb and index fingers.

Lester's iris, an irregularly hyperpigmented pupillary border, is an important diagnostic sign; other eye abnormalities include glaucoma and microcornea

Genetics

AD; linked with gene locus for ABO blood group on long arm of chromosome 9

Prognosis

occasional death from renal failure in middle age

Discussion

severity varies greatly from patient to patient and from limb to limb

may be genetically linked with palmoplantar hyperhidrosis

triangular lunulae, though characteristic of nail-patella-elbow syndrome, may also be seen in acquired conditions or following trauma

in the trisomy 8 syndrome, patients often have nail hypoplasia or anonychia and absence of patellae

REFERENCES

McK 161200

Daniel CR III, Osment LS, Noojin RO. Triangular lunulae: a clue to nail-patella syndrome. Arch Dermatol 1980;116:448–449

Lucas GL, Opitz JM. The nail-patella syndrome: clinical and genetic aspects of 5 kindreds with 38 affected family members. J Pediatr 1966;68:273–288

Morita T, Laughlin O, Kawano K, Kimmelstiel P. Nail-patella syndrome. Arch Intern Med 1973;131:271–277

Pechman KJ, Bergfeld WF. Palmar-plantar hyperhidrosis occurring in a kindred with nail-patella syndrome. J Am Acad Dermatol 1980;3:627–632

ANONYCHIA

Skin

absence of nails of fingers and toes from birth (Fig. 10–6)

occasionally, partial nails are present at birth, which are subsequently shed permanently

Non-Skin

occasional absence of the distal phalanx of affected digits

Genetics

AD, AR, and sporadic cases reported

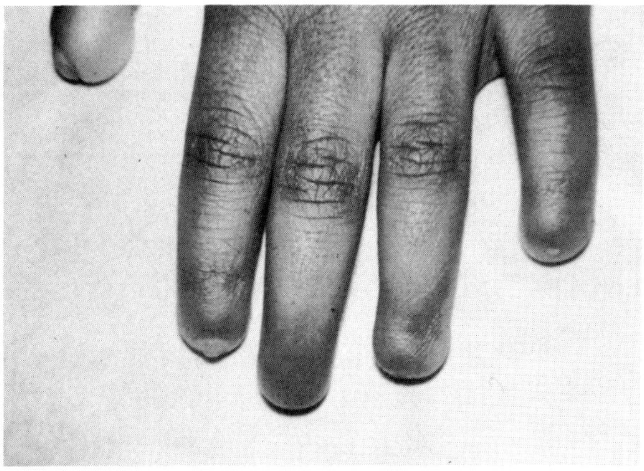

FIGURE 10–6
Anonychia. Absent and rudimentary nails of the hand of a child.

Discussion

in some cases, not all nails are affected

- *anonychia-onychodystrophy*

  absent or dystrophic nails without absence of digits (ectrodactyly) or other findings of the nail-patella-elbow syndrome

  AD

  McK 107000

REFERENCES

McK 206800
McK 106900
Hopsu-Havu VK, Jansen CT. Anonychia congenita. Arch Dermatol 1973;107:752–753
Littman A, Levin S. Anonychia as a recessive autosomal trait in man. J Invest Dermatol 1964;42:177–178
Mahloudji M, Amidi M. Simple anonychia. Further evidence for autosomal recessive inheritance. J Med Genet 1971;8:478–480
Rahbari H, Heath L, Chapel T. Anonychia with ectrodactyly. Arch Dermatol 1975;111:1482–1485
Timerman I, Museteanu C, Simionescu NN. Dominant anonychia onychodystrophy. J Med Genet 1969;6:105–106

ANONYCHIA WITH FLEXURAL PIGMENTATION

anonychia from birth

hypopigmentation and hyperpigmentation, especially of flexures (groins, axillae, and breasts)

dry and peeling palmoplantar skin

coarse, slow-growing hair

abnormal dermatoglyphics

AD

McK 106750
Verbov J. Anonychia with bizarre flexural pigmentation: an autosomal dominant dermatosis. Br J Dermatol 1975;92:469–474

CONGENITAL ONYCHODYSPLASIA OF THE INDEX FINGERS (ISO-KIKUCHI SYNDROME; COIF SYNDROME)

micronychia most common defect; radial aspect more often involved than ulnar; may be unilateral or bilateral

occasional minor abnormalities of other nails

occasional brachymesophalangia of index finger and minor abnormalities of other digits

AD reported; many sporadic cases

Baran R, Stroud JD. Congenital onychodysplasia of the index fingers: Iso and Kikuchi syndrome. Arch Dermatol 1984;120:243–244
Kitayama Y, Tsukada S. Congenital onychodysplasia: report of 11 cases. Arch Dermatol 1983;119:8–12
Millman AJ, Strier RP. Congenital onychodysplasia of the index fingers: report of a family. J Am Acad Dermatol 1982;7:57–65

ONYCHOMADESIS (UNGUINUM DEFLUVIUM; BOGAERT-SCHERER-EPSTEIN SYNDROME)

periodic shedding of nails beginning in childhood

nail separation initiates from proximal edge; because of onycholysis, the lunula appears dull yellow before nail is shed

growth of new nail follows immediately; new growth usually normal but long-standing cases or cases with onset early in life may result in nail atrophy or complete permanent anonychia

one, few, or all nails may be involved

rare association with amelogenesis imperfecta

AD

acquired recurrent onychomadesis has been described; most commonly, however, onychomadesis is not recurrent and secondary to factors including trauma and febrile illness

Martin S, Rudolph AH. Familial dystrophic periodic shedding of the nails. Cutis 1980;25:622–623
Montgomery DW. A case of hereditary and continuous shedding of the nails. J Cutan Dis 1897;15:252
Oliver WJ. Recurrent onychoptosis occurring as a family disorder. Br J Dermatol 1973;88:497

HEREDITARY KOILONCHIA

Synonym

- spoon nails

Skin

thin, concave nails with everted edges; onset at birth or early childhood

usually begins in one digit, especially the thumb, but may eventually involve all fingers

toenails usually less affected

persists lifelong

Genetics

AD

Prognosis

lifelong

Discussion

mild koilonychia often seen in normal children; this corrects with time; acquired koilonychia (e.g., in association with iron deficiency) is far more common than hereditary koilonychia

REFERENCES

McK 149300

Almager G, Haim S. Familial koilonychia. Dermatologica 1981;162:400–403

Bergeron JR, Stone OJ. Koilonychia: a report of familial spoon nails. Arch Dermatol 1967;95:351–353

Bumpers RD, Bishop ME. Familial koilonychia: a current case history. Arch Dermatol 1980;116:845

Hellier FF. Hereditary koilonychia. Br J Dermatol 1950;62:213–214

LEUKONYCHIA

Skin

striate (transverse), punctate, partial or total leukonychia; pattern may vary from nail to nail; all or some nails may be affected (Fig. 10–7)

onset from birth to childhood

in leukonychia totalis, nails may occasionally temporarily become normal in color

persists lifelong

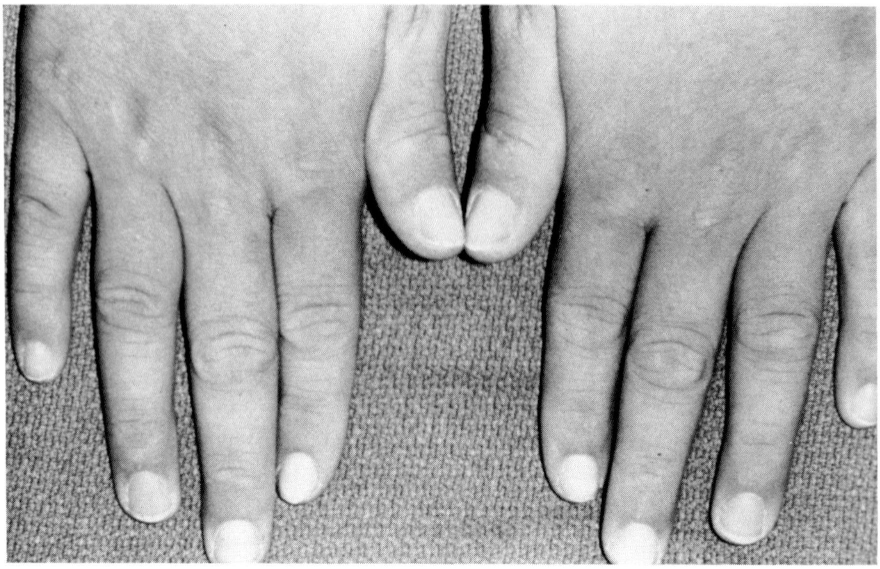

FIGURE 10–7
Total leukonychia.

Genetics

AD

Pathophysiology

white color due to presence of parakeratotic cells in nail plate, which is otherwise structurally normal

Discussion

in the Bart-Pumphrey syndrome (see main entry), leukonychia totalis is associated with knuckle pads and mixed hearing loss

association of leukonychia totalis, multiple sebaceous cysts, and renal calculi reported

REFERENCES

McK 151600

McK 151550

Bushkell LL, Gorlin RJ. Leukonychia totalis, multiple sebaceous cysts, and renal calculi: a new syndrome. Arch Dermatol 1975; 111:899–901

Juhlin L. Hereditary leukonychia. Acta Derm Venereol 1963;43:136–141

Medansky RS, Fox JM. Hereditary leukonychia totalis. Arch Dermatol 1960;82:412–414

RACQUET NAIL

Synonym

- nail en racquet

Skin

short and wide distal phalanx with a correspondingly short, broad, and flat (lateral curvature is lost) nail

thumb most commonly involved, left thumb twice as often as the right; rarely thumbnails normal

half of cases are bilateral

Genetics

probable AD

Discussion

there are a variety of causes of brachydactyly with shortened, broadened fingernails (McK 112410–113475)

REFERENCES

McK 113200

Goodman RM, Adam A, Sheba C. A genetic study of stub thumbs among various ethnic groups in Israel. J Med Genet 1965;2:116–121

Ronchese F. The racket thumb-nail. Dermatologica 1973;146:199–202

MALALIGNMENT OF THE GREAT TOENAILS, CONGENITAL

lateral deviation of nail plate on great toes

nail plates become discolored, ridged, onycholytic, and thickened secondary to trauma and may be shed

AD

may improve spontaneously or be treated surgically

complications include onychogryphosis, paronychia, and ingrown nails

Barth JH, Dawber RP, Ashton RE, et al. Congenital malalignment of great toenails in two sets of monozygotic twins. [Letter]. Arch Dermatol 1986;122:379–380

Cohen PR. Congenital malalignment of the great toenails: case report and literature review. Pediatr Dermatol 1991;8:43–45

Nail Disorders—Abbreviated Entries

YELLOW NAIL SYNDROME

slow-growing, abnormally shaped, yellow nails

lymphedema

chronic respiratory tract disease including chronic bronchiectasis and pleural effusions; chronic sinusitis

mostly sporadic but AD and probable AR cases reported

McK 153300
Govaert P, Leroy JG, Pauwels R, et al. Perinatal manifestations of maternal yellow nail syndrome. Pediatrics 1992;89:1016–1018
Kamatani M, Rai A, Hen H, et al. Yellow nail syndrome associated with mental retardation in two siblings. Br J Dermatol 1978;99:329–333
Magid M, Esterly NB, Prendiville J, Fujisaki C. The yellow nail syndrome in an 8-year-old girl. Pediatr Dermatol 1987;4:90–93
Samman PD, White WF. The "yellow nail" syndrome. Br J Dermatol 1964;76:153–157
Wells GC. Yellow nail syndrome with familial primary hypoplasia of lymphatics, manifest late in life. Proc R Soc Med 1966;59:447

ONYCHODYSTROPHY TOTALIS

AD

McK 161050
Pavone L, Li Volti S, Guarneri B, et al. Hereditary twenty-nail dystrophy in a Sicilian family. J Med Genet 1982;19:337–340

PARTIAL ONYCHOLYSIS WITH SCLERONYCHIA

nail abnormalities include distal partial onycholysis, scleronychia, absent lunulae, transverse overcurvature and slow growth; onset ranges from early childhood to adulthood

affects all nails

cold sensitivity and palmoplantar hyperhidrosis

AD

McK 164800
Bazex J, Baran R, Monbrun F, et al. Hereditary distal onycholysis: a case report. Clin Exp Dermatol 1990;15:146–148

OTO-ONYCHOPERONEAL SYNDROME

hypoplasia or aplasia of nails and fibulae

external ear deformity

joint contractures

possible AR

McK 259780

Pfeiffer RA. The oto-onycho-peroneal syndrome: a probably new genetic entity. Eur J Pediatr 1982;138:317–320

NAIL DYSPLASIA WITH ONYCHONYCHIA AND ABSENCE AND/OR HYPOPLASIA OF DISTAL PHALANGES

probable AD

Cooks RG, Hertz M, Katznelson MM, Goodman M. A new nail dysplasia syndrome with onychonychia and absence and/or hypoplasia of distal phalanges. Clin Genet 1985; 27:85–91

CHAPTER 11

Mucous Membrane Disorders

Mucous membrane lesions frequently accompany the skin lesions of heritable disorders and may involve the oropharynx, nose, eye, vagina, penis, and anus. In this chapter, we have included only those disorders in which the mucous membrane lesions represent the primary pathology and usually the feature for which the disease is named. Skin diseases in which the mucous membrane lesions represent a minor manifestation are found elsewhere in the book.

GINGIVAL FIBROMATOSIS

Synonyms

- hereditary gingival hyperplasia
- elephantiasis gingivae

Skin

painless enlargement of pale-appearing gingivae, most commonly the anterior attached maxillary gingiva

onset any age, most commonly around ages 6 to 7 years

delay in apparent eruption of permanent dentition may be first sign; teeth actually grow normally but are hidden by gingivae

mild to extremely marked hypertrichosis of scalp, eyebrows, forehead, back, and arms with onset usually around puberty and almost always after development of gingival hypertrophy

Non-Skin

occasional coarse facies, bony abnormalities of vertebrae and ribs

epilepsy and/or mental retardation

Genetics

AD and AR

Prognosis

speech and mastication may be impaired

Discussion

marked hypertrichosis may prompt an unnecessary evaluation for other conditions if the syndrome is not fully evident or recognized

some authors separate the entities of gingival fibromatosis alone from gingival fibromatosis with hypertrichosis

causes of acquired gingival hyperplasia include leukemic infiltrates, phenytoin or cyclosporine therapy, fetal hydantoin syndrome, fetal alcohol syndrome, and hormonal influences

REFERENCES

McK 135300
McK 135400
Anderson J, Cunliffe WJ, Roberts DF, Close H. Hereditary gingival fibromatosis. Br Med J 1969;3:218–219
Cuestas-Carnero R, Bornancini CA. Hereditary generalized gingival fibromatosis associated with hypertrichosis: report of five cases in one family. J Oral Maxillofac Surg 1988;46:415–420
Emerson TG. Hereditary gingival hyperplasia: a family pedigree of four generations. Oral Surg 1965;19:1–9
Gorlin RJ, Cohen MM Jr, Levin LS. Syndromes with gingival/periodontal components. In: Syndromes of the Head and Neck. 3rd ed. New York, Oxford University Press, 1990: 847–857
Horning GM, Fisher JG, Barker BF, Killoy WJ, Lowe JW. Gingival fibromatosis with hypertrichosis: a case report. J Periodontol 1985;56:344–347
Jorgenson RJ, Cocker ME. Variation in the inheritance and expression of gingival fibromatosis. J Periodontol 1974;45:472–477
Witkop CJ Jr. Heterogeneity in gingival fibromatosis? Birth Defects 1971;7:210–221
Zackin SJ, Weisberger D. Hereditary gingival fibromatosis. Oral Surg 1961;14:828–836

GINGIVAL FIBROMATOSIS WITH EAR, NOSE, BONE, AND NAIL DEFECTS AND HEPATOSPLENOMEGALY (ZIMMERMAN-LABAND SYNDROME)

gingival fibromatosis appearing in early childhood

absence or hypoplasia and dysplasia of nails

soft, bulky cartilage in ears and nose; occasional thick lips

absence or hypoplasia of terminal phalanges

AD

McK 135500
Chodirker BN, Chudley AE, Toffler MA, Reed MH. Zimmerman-Laband syndrome and profound mental retardation. Am J Med Genet 1986;25:543–547

RAMON SYNDROME (CHERUBISM, GINGIVAL FIBROMATOSIS, EPILEPSY, MENTAL DEFICIENCY, HYPERTRICHOSIS, AND STUNTED GROWTH)

AR

McK 266270
Pina-Neto JM, Moreno AFC, Silva LR, et al. Cherubism, gingival fibromatosis, epilepsy, and mental deficiency (Ramon syndrome) with juvenile rheumatoid arthritis. Am J Med Genet 1986;25:433–441

CONGENITAL HYPERTROPHY OF THE GINGIVA, ALTERED ERUPTION OF THE TEETH AND CORNEAL DYSTROPHY (RUTHERFURD SYNDROME)

AD

REFERENCES

McK 180900
Houston IB, Shotts N. Rutherfurd's syndrome: a familial oculo-dental disorders: a clinical and electrophysiologic study. Acta Paediatr Scand 1966;55:233–238

GINGIVAL FIBROMATOSIS WITH PROGRESSIVE DEAFNESS

McK 135550
Hartsfield JK Jr, Bixler D, Hazen RH. Gingival fibromatosis with sensorineural hearing loss: an autosomal dominant trait. Am J Med Genet 1985;22:623–627
Jones G, Wilroy RS Jr, McHaney V. Familial gingival fibromatosis associated with progressive deafness in five generations of a family. Birth Defects 1977;13:195–201

HEREDITARY BENIGN INTRAEPITHELIAL DYSKERATOSIS

Synonym

- Witkop syndrome

Skin

extensive white thickened plaques on oral mucosa, mainly the buccal, commissural, labial, ventral, lingual, and mouth floor surfaces (Fig. 11–1); folding of epithelium may occur in severe cases

scraping and stretching of mucosa reveals characteristic pinpoint elevations

appears in infancy or childhood and increases in severity until middle of second decade

no increased potential for malignancy

Non-Skin

intense conjunctivitis (first sign) and white gelatinous plaques develop in perilimbal distribution on the interpalpebral bulbar conjunctiva, usually within the first year of life

periodic overgrowth of ocular plaques causes temporary blindness; plaques shed spontaneously in late summer to fall

occasional marked photophobia

other mucous membranes are spared

Genetics

AD

seen in 22% to 34% of the Haliwa Indians, descendents of an inbred triracial (Indian, black, white) isolate originally from Halifax and Warren counties, North Carolina

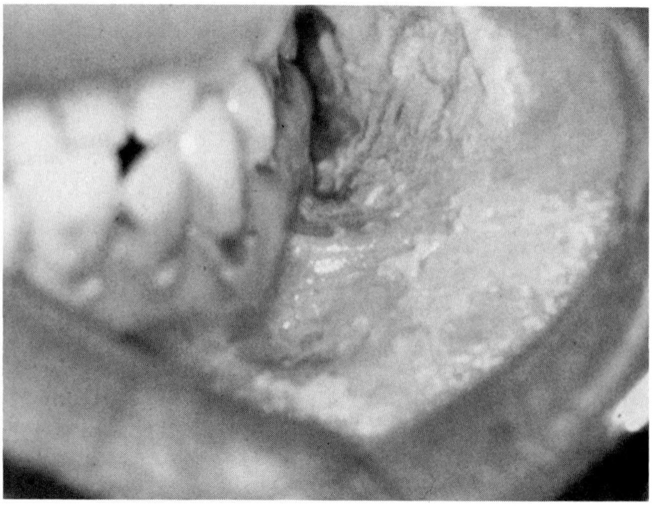

FIGURE 11–1
Hereditary benign intraepithelial dyskeratosis. A white plaque is seen on the oral vestibular mucosa of the lower lip. This is clinically indistinguishable from white sponge nevus, so other associated findings must be sought. (Courtesy of Robert J. Gorlin, DDS, MS, Minneapolis, Minnesota)

Laboratory Data

histopathology: eosinophilic dyskeratotic cells in an acanthotic epithelium

REFERENCES

McK 127600

Sadeghi EM, Witkop CJ Jr. Ultrastructural study of a hereditary benign intraepithelial dyskeratosis. Oral Surg 1977;44:567–577

Witkop CJ Jr, Gorlin RJ. Four hereditary mucosal syndromes. Arch Dermatol 1961; 84:762–771

Witkop CJ Jr, Shank LE, Graham JB, et al. Hereditary benign intraepidermal dyskeratosis. Arch Pathol Lab Med 1960;70:696–711

HEREDITARY MUCOEPITHELIAL DYSPLASIA

Skin

intense erythema of mucous membranes of mouth (Color Fig. 11–1), nose, vagina, urethra, anus, and bladder occurs by age 1 year and persists throughout life

rough, dry skin with follicular keratoses on trunk and extremities

easy burning on sun exposure

coarse, scanty scalp hair

clubbing of digits

Non-Skin

photophobia, excessive tearing, nystagmus, keratitis, corneal vascularization, and cataracts develop during early to middle of first decade; may lead to blindness before puberty

pyuria, hematuria, melena, diarrhea, and hemoptysis common

increased susceptibility to infections, particularly involving respiratory tract, bladder, and eyes

fibrocystic lung disease with spontaneous pneumothoraces and cor pulmonale

esophageal webs

Genetics

AD; sporadic cases reported

Laboratory Data

mucosal biopsy specimens from all sites show lack of epithelial cohesion, dyskeratosis, incomplete keratinization, and unusual cytoplasmic inclusions and vacuoles

ultrastructural findings suggest defects in desmosomes and gap junctions

Prognosis

life expectancy may be shortened by lung disease and cor pulmonale

REFERENCES

Scheman AJ, Ray DJ, Witkop CJ Jr, et al. Hereditary mucoepithelial dysplasia: case report and review of the literature. [Review]. J Am Acad Dermatol 1989;21:351–357

Urban MD, Schosser R, Spohn W, et al. New clinical aspects of hereditary mucoepithelial dysplasia. Am J Med Genet 1991; 39:338–341

Witkop CJ Jr, White JG, King RA, et al. Hereditary mucoepithelial dysplasia: a disease apparently of desmosome and gap junction formation. Am J Hum Genet 1979;31:414–427

VAN DER WOUDE SYNDROME

Synonyms

- congenital pits and sinuses of the lips
- lip pits

Skin

pits of the vermillion surface of the lips, usually bilaterally on each side of the midline, almost always on the lower lip (Fig. 11–2)

small accessory salivary glands empty into sinuses; clear or viscid saliva fluid may drain or be expressed

sinuses lined by squamous epithelium; end blindly in orbicularis oris muscle

second premolars may be missing

Non-Skin

cleft palate in two thirds; of these, half also have cleft lip

Genetics

AD

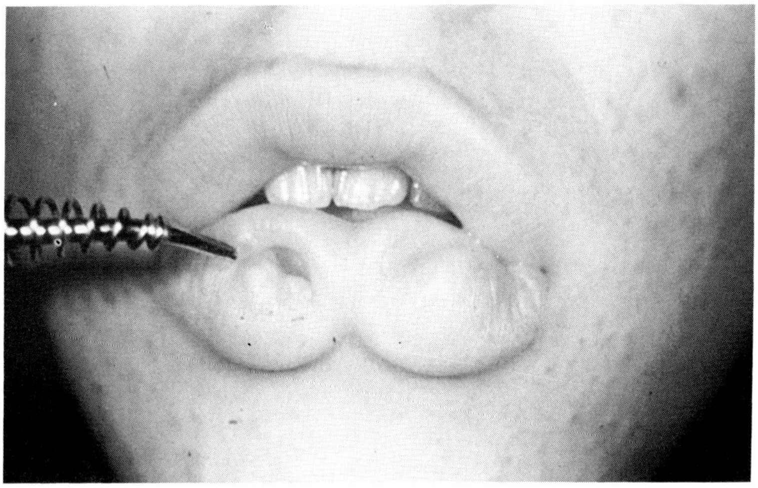

FIGURE 11–2
Van der Woude syndrome. The lower lip has bilateral paramedian pits. (Courtesy of Robert J. Gorlin, DDS, MS, Minneapolis, Minnesota)

Prognosis

fistulae may be excised surgically

Discussion

variations include single median pit or involvement of the upper lip

REFERENCES

McK 119300

Burdick AB, Bixler D, Puckett CL. Genetic analysis in families with van der Woude syndrome. J Craniofac Genet Dev Biol 1985;5:181–208

Rintala HE, Ranta R. Lower lip sinuses: epidemiology, microforms and transverse sulci. Br J Plast Surg 1980;34:25–30

Schinzel A, Kläusler M. The van der Woude syndrome (dominantly inherited lip pits and clefts). J Med Genet 1986;23:291–294

Srivastava S, Bang RL. Congenital sinuses of the lower lip: reappraisal of Van der Woude syndrome on the basis of nine patients. Ann Plast Surg 1989;22:316–320

Taylor WB, Lane DK. Congenital fistulas of the lower lip. Arch Dermatol 1966;94:421–424

COMMISSURAL LIP PITS

Skin

located at the corners of the mouth

Genetics

probable AD; genetics are confusing because condition is so common

Discussion

- *commissural lip pits with congenital conductive or mixed deafness, preauricular sinus, and external ear anomaly*

  AD

  McK 120502

REFERENCES

McK 120500
Baker BR. Pits of the lip commissures in caucasoid males. Oral Pathol 1966;21:56–60
Everett FG, Wescott WB. Commissural lip pits. Oral Pathol 1961;14:202–209
Marres HAM, Cremers CWRJ. Congenital conductive or mixed deafness, preauricular sinus, external ear anomaly, and commissural lips pits: an autosomal dominant inherited syndrome. Ann Otol Rhinol Laryngol 1991;100:928–932

WHITE SPONGE NEVUS OF THE MUCOSA

Synonyms

- hereditary leukokeratosis
- oral white sponge nevus of Cannon

Skin

thickened, folded, white, slightly shaggy plaques on mucosal surfaces (Fig. 11–3); usually asymptomatic

buccal mucosa involved in virtually every case; other oral mucosae (e.g., floor of mouth) and other mucous membranes including laryngeal,

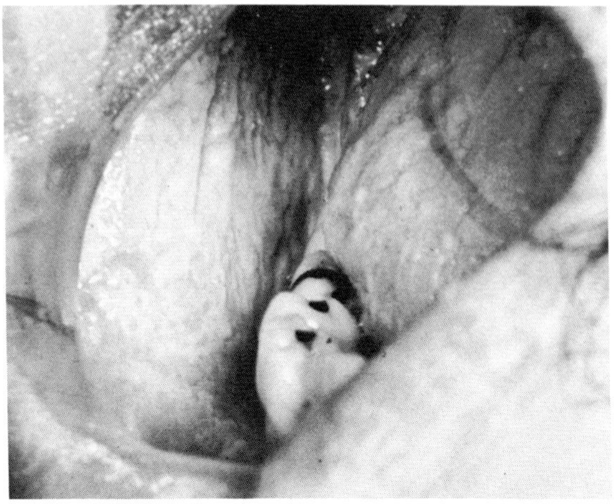

FIGURE 11–3
White sponge nevus. A permanent thickened hyperkeratotic white plaque of the buccal mucosa. (Courtesy of Robert J. Gorlin, DDS, MS, Minneapolis, Minnesota)

esophageal, nasal, anal, rectal, vaginal, and penile surfaces may be affected

unilateral involvement rare

onset ranges from birth to adolescence in most cases, but rarely up to the fifth decade

usually reaches full severity in adolescence and persists; no increased potential for malignancy

Genetics

AD

Laboratory Data

histopathology: acanthosis with marked but focal intraepithelial edema that spares the basal layer

Discussion

acquired conditions in the differential diagnosis include leukoedema (minimally elevated whitish gray oral plaques, usually in black men) and oral focal epithelial hyperplasia (Heck disease; oral papillomas due to human papillomavirus 13 and others, common in Navajos and Eskimos)

REFERENCES

McK 193900

Geist ET, Gross BD. Third and fourth generation white sponge nevus; report of a case. J Oral Surg 1981;39:457–458

Jorgenson RJ, Levin S. White sponge nevus. Arch Dermatol 1981;117:73–76

Reaves CE. White sponge nevus of the tongue. South Med J 1975;68:1170–1172

Wright S, Levy IS. White sponge naevus and ocular coloboma. Arch Dis Child 1991; 66:514–516

Zegarelli EV, Everett FG, Kutscher AH, et al. Familial white folded dysplasia of the mucous membranes. Arch Dermatol 1959; 80:59–65

Mucous Membrane Disorders—Abbreviated Entries

MELKERSSON-ROSENTHAL SYNDROME (MELKERSSON SYNDROME; GRANULOMATOUS CHEILITIS)

chronic, recurrent swelling of lip and face

recurrent facial palsy

scrotal tongue

mostly sporadic; AD cases reported

McK 155900
Carr RD. Is the Melkersson-Rosenthal syndrome hereditary? Arch Dermatol 1966; 93:426–427
Lygidakis C, Tsankanikas C, Ilias A, Vassilopoulos D. Melkersson-Rosenthal's syndrome in four generations. Clin Genet 1979;15:189–192

FOUNTAIN SYNDROME

progressive swelling of the lips

mental retardation, sensorineural deafness, and musculoskeletal abnormalities

probable AR

McK 229120
Fountain RB. Familial bone abnormalities, deaf mutism, mental retardation and skin granuloma. Proc R Soc Med 1974;67:878–879
Fryns JP, Dereymaeker AM, Hoefnagels M, Van den Berghe H. Mental retardation, deafness, skeletal abnormalities, and coarse face with full lips: confirmation of the Fountain syndrome. Am J Med Genet 1987;26:551–555

CHAPTER

12

Neurocutaneous Disorders

The diseases collectively known as the neurocutaneous disorders are evidenced by a wide spectrum of cutaneous lesions and also have prominent, if variable, neurologic findings such as seizures, developmental delay, and hemiplegia. Although other major organ systems may be involved as well, in most instances it is the specific cutaneous abnormalities that signal the presence of a potentially serious multisystemic disorder. Recognition of these skin lesions also permits identification of mildly affected individuals, an important benefit for genetic counseling.

Neurofibromatosis

Neurofibromatosis is a group of heterogeneous disorders that can be classified in several ways. We favor Riccardi's scheme, which classifies neurofibromatosis into at least eight subtypes in three classes:

Type A neurofibromatosis is of congenital onset with total-body involvement; neurofibromas are a constant feature. There are four subtypes:

- neurofibromatosis (NF-I or von Recklinghausen neurofibromatosis; 85% to 90% of all cases of neurofibromatosis)
- central neurofibromatosis (NF-II or acoustic neurofibromatosis)
- mixed neurofibromatosis (NF-III)
- variant neurofibromatosis (NF-IV)

Type B neurofibromatosis is limited in distribution or late in onset; neurofibromas are not a necessary feature. Subtypes are:

- segmental neurofibromatosis (NF-V)
- café-au-lait macule neurofibromatosis (NF-VI)
- late-onset neurofibromatosis (NF-VII)

Type C neurofibromatosis is neurofibromatosis not classifiable into the other categories:

- unspecified neurofibromatosis (NF-VIII)

Neurofibromatosis I is the most important subtype. Two or more of the following seven criteria establish a diagnosis of NF-I:

1. Six or more café-au-lait spots over 5 mm in greatest diameter in prepubertal individuals and over 15 mm in greatest diameter in postpubertal individuals
2. Two or more neurofibromas of any type or one plexiform neurofibroma
3. Freckling in the axillary or inguinal regions
4. Optic pathway glioma
5. Two or more Lisch nodules
6. A distinctive osseous lesion (e.g., sphenoid dysplasia or thinning of long-bone cortex with or without pseudoarthrosis)
7. A first-degree relative (parent, sibling, or offspring) with NF-I by the above criteria

REFERENCES

Neurofibromatosis. Conference statement. National Institutes of Health Consensus Development Conference. Arch Neurol 1988; 45:575–578

Riccardi VM. Neurofibromatosis: Phenotype, Natural History, and Pathogenesis. 2nd ed. Baltimore, Johns Hopkins University Press, 1992

NEUROFIBROMATOSIS I

Synonyms

- von Recklinghausen disease
- NF-I

Skin

see introduction for diagnostic criteria of NF-I

café-au-lait spots: brown, evenly pigmented and sharply demarcated macules and patches (Fig. 12–1)

- present in most patients with NF-I; variable or absent in some forms of NF (e.g., NF-II and NF-VII); seen in small numbers (one to three) in 10% of the general population
- present at birth or within first few years of life
- usually widely distributed over body, except on scalp, palms, soles, or oral mucosa
- may increase in number and size with age, puberty, or pregnancy

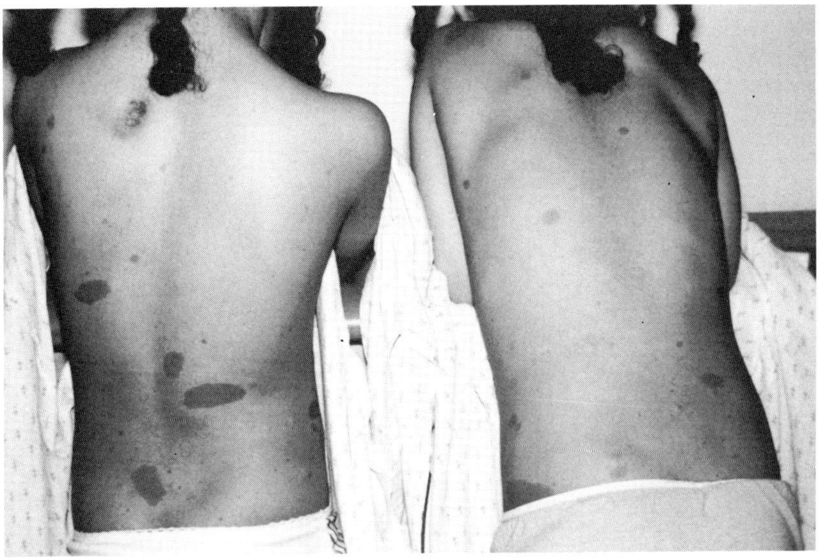

FIGURE 12–1
Twin girls with neurofibromatosis, type 1. Multiple café-au-lait macules are visible on the backs of both of these children.

diffuse "freckling" often seen in axillae and/or in other body folds, usually in childhood or adulthood; axillary freckling called Crowe's sign (Fig. 12–2)

rare diffuse grayish or bronze hyperpigmentation of skin, resembling argyria

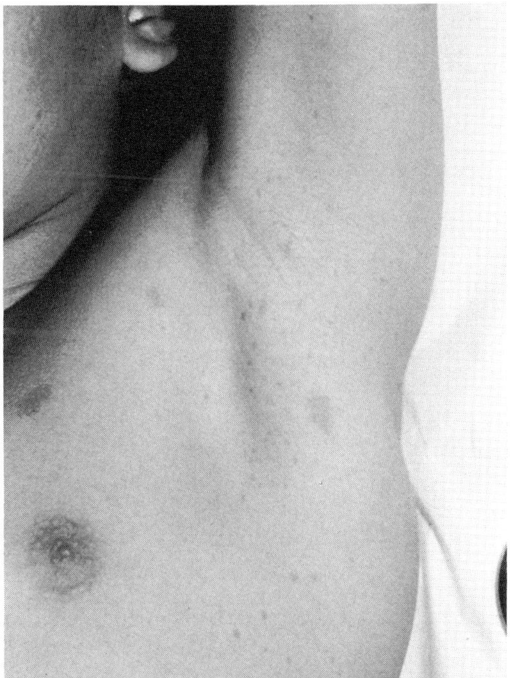

FIGURE 12–2
Crowe's sign (axillary freckling) as well as multiple larger café-au-lait macules in neurofibromatosis, type 1.

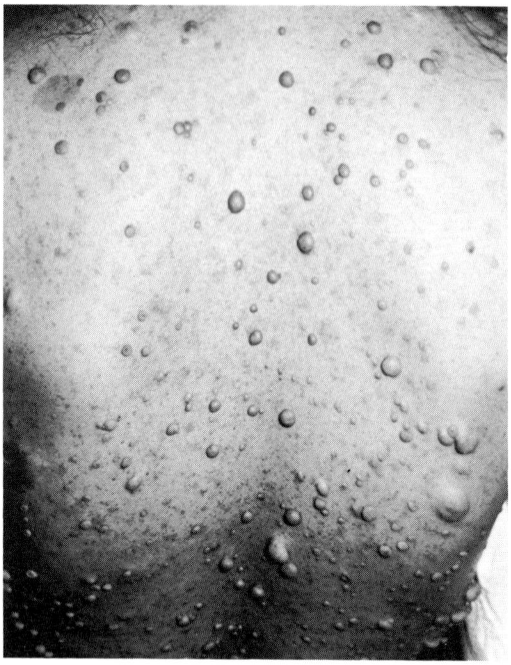

FIGURE 12–3
Numerous dermal neurofibromas of varying sizes scattered over the back. Several café-au-lait macules are also visible. (Courtesy of Benjamin K. Fisher, MD, Toronto, Ontario)

neurofibromas (and other tumors including schwannomas)

- soft, pink to skin-colored papules, nodules, and tumors (Fig. 12–3); lesions may be sessile or pendunculated
- few to hundreds, cutaneous or subcutaneous, most commonly on trunk
- onset of neurofibromas usually during puberty but may occur from infancy to fourth decade or later
- increase in size and number during adulthood, sometimes later becoming quiescent; pruritus associated with growth of neurofibromas may be very distressing; subcutaneous lesions occasionally painful
- occasionally involve scalp, extremities, or oral or rectal mucosae
- when rapidly growing and closely spaced, result in massive, pendulous masses of skin termed *elephantiasis neuromatosa*
- other variants include blue-red or pseudoatrophic macules
- occasional plexiform neurofibromas of the skin and subcutis usually present at birth, sometimes quite firm, almost cartilaginous in consistency; large plexiform neurofibromas have been likened to a "bag of worms" (Figs. 12–4 and 12–5); may progress to involve adjacent structures
- plexiform neurofibromas may have overlying hyperpigmentation and hypertrichosis; if the midline of the body is crossed, involvement of the neuroaxis (e.g., vertebral erosion and/or spinal cord compression) should be presumed until proven otherwise

occasional hypertrichosis (besides that overlying plexiform neurofibromas) and/or hypopigmented macules

increased incidence of juvenile xanthogranulomas, which may be a harbinger of the development of juvenile chronic myelogenous leukemia

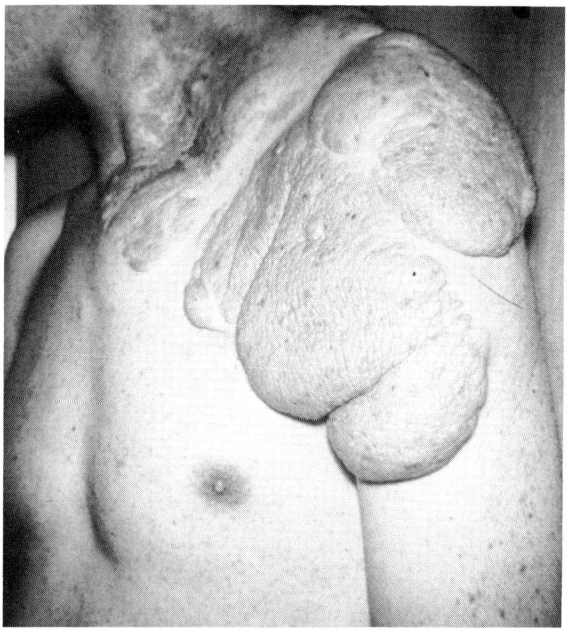

FIGURE 12–4
Plexiform neurofibroma over the shoulder and neck.

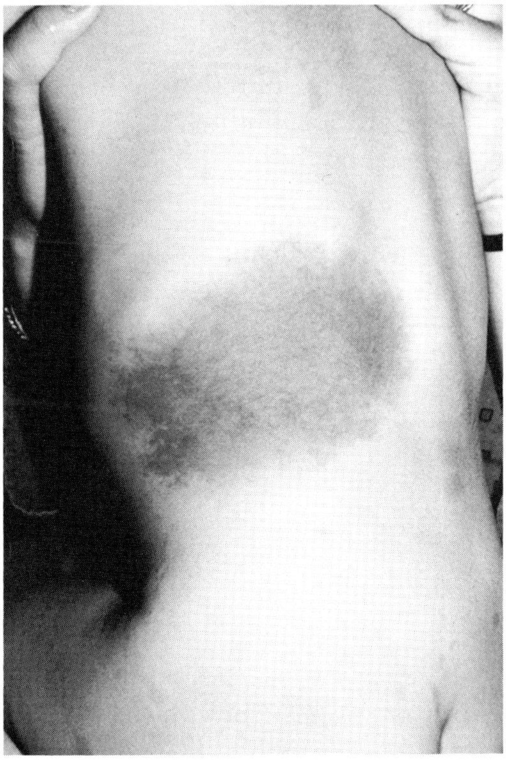

FIGURE 12–5
Plexiform neurofibroma on the flank with overlying characteristic gray-brown hyperpigmentation and hypertrichosis. Note the multiple café-au-lait macules on the back, buttocks, and thigh.

Non-Skin

a variety of organ systems are affected

nervous system abnormalities include

- optic pathway gliomas, onset probably congenital; may result in blindness
- other intracranial tumors, including single or multiple glial or meningeal tumors
- spinal gliomas and meningiomas
- intellectual impairment in at least 40% of patients, with frank mental retardation in 2% to 5% of patients
- seizures in infancy and childhood

ocular abnormalities include

- Lisch nodules (melanocytic hamartomas of the iris); pathognomonic for NF-I when multiple; seen in at least 90% of patients with NF-I by the second decade but in only about 30% before age 6; slit-lamp examination necessary to rule out their presence, although they frequently can be seen without magnification, especially in adults; rarely, may be the only sign of NF-I
- neurofibromas of optic nerve, eyelids, conjunctiva, and iris
- corneal opacities and glaucoma, which may be congenital (buphthalmos)
- retinal phacomas
- eyelid neurofibromas

skeletal abnormalities, which may or may not be related to neurofibromas, include

- macrocephaly
- congenital pseudoarthrosis of tibia and/or fibula; quite characteristic but seen only in 0.5% of patients
- scoliosis, usually of cervical and/or upper thoracic spine with kyphosis
- erosive changes or scalloping of vertebrae
- characteristic skull abnormalities include congenital sphenoid wing dysplasia or round bony defect of lambdoidal suture, almost always on left
- twisted, ribbon-like ribs
- short stature, pectus excavatum, and genu valgum or varum

neoplasias of increased frequency

- pheochromocytomas, usually occurring in adulthood, found in 1%; conversely, up to 20% of patients in general population with pheochromocytoma(s) have neurofibromatosis

- neurofibrosarcomas, usually in plexiform or subcutaneous neurofibromata, in 3% to 6% of adults
- leukemia (usually juvenile chronic myelogenous leukemia)
- rhabdomyosarcoma

other findings include

- diffuse interstitial pulmonary fibrosis reported in adulthood
- renovascular hypertension, especially in adolescents and pregnant females, in addition to hypertension related to pheochromocytomas
- diffuse hepatic disease ("hepatopathy")
- endocrine abnormalities include acromegaly and menstrual irregularities
- a variety of developmental abnormalities including hypospadias and cryptorchidism
- gastrointestinal tumors including neurofibromas, adenomatous polyps, carcinoid tumors, and leiomyomas
- genitourinary neurofibromas of bladder and uterus
- cardiovascular abnormalities including pulmonary valve and artery stenoses

Genetics

AD; at least 50% of cases are spontaneous mutations

highly variable expression within and between pedigrees but almost complete penetrance

NF-I gene assigned to chromosome 17; frequency around 1 in 3000 to 4000

Laboratory Data

computed tomography or magnetic resonance imaging in affected infants and young children may help detect optic pathway gliomas

chest radiographs for newborns with or at risk for NF-I may detect mediastinal plexiform neurofibromas

giant melanosomes seen by electron microscopy biopsy specimens of café-au-lait spots most commonly in NF-I but are not pathognomonic

Prognosis

NF-I is a progressive disorder with significant morbidity and increased likelihood of premature death

serial eye examinations recommended from birth onward

developmental milestone delays, learning disabilities, speech impediments, and school performance problems must be recognized and addressed in a large percentage of affected children close surveillance for scoliosis and/or kyphosis in second half of first decade of life; internal fixation may be beneficial in preventing or decreasing deformities

screening for hypertension is especially important during adolescence

pregnancy and puberty are associated with worsening of NF but latter may be overstated

increased incidence of spontaneous abortion

increased incidence of malignancy, especially of the central nervous system; true incidence unknown; women more prone and have lower survival

ketotifen, an S2 serotoninergic blocker, may be beneficial in the treatment of pruritus

appropriateness of birth control pill use in NF-I is determined on an individual basis

Discussion

optic glioma is the most common central nervous system tumor in NF-I, while acoustic schwannomas and meningiomas are most common central nervous system tumors in other forms of NF

■ *McCune-Albright syndrome*

shares presence of pigmentary and skeletal abnormalities with neurofibromatosis (see main entry)

characteristically described as having large pigmented macules with an irregular outline in contrast to café-au-lait spots in neurofibromatosis, which are reported to be of greater number, smaller size, and more uniform pigmentation; this distinction, however, has largely been abandoned

café-au-lait spots contain few or no giant melanosomes

■ *neurilemmomatosis (schwannomatosis)*

multiple neurilemmomas, most commonly on the trunk, extremities, and head, usually first appearing in first and second decades (range, birth to adulthood)

central nervous system tumors and associated neurologic defects may be seen; distinguished from neurofibromatosis by absence of café-au-lait spots and neurofibromas and lack of hereditary component

REFERENCES

McK 162200

Ackerman CD, Cohen BA. Juvenile xanthogranuloma and neurofibromatosis. Pediatr Dermatol 1991;8:339–340

Cooper PH, Frierson HF, Kayne AL, Sabio H. Association of juvenile xanthogranuloma with juvenile myeloid leukemia. Arch Dermatol 1984;120:371–375

Crowe FW. Axillary freckling as a diagnostic aid in neurofibromatosis. Ann Intern Med 1964;61:1142–1143

Dunn DW. Neurofibromatosis in childhood. Curr Probl Pediatr 1987;17:445–497

Huson SM. The different forms of neurofibromatosis. Br Med J (Clin Res) 1987; 394:1113–1114

Johnson BL, Charneco DR. Café-au-lait spot in neurofibromatosis and in normal individuals. Arch Dermatol 1970;102:442–446
Lubs ME, Bauer MS, Formas ME, Djokic B. Lisch nodules in neurofibromatosis type 1. N Engl J Med 1991;324:1264–1266
Mulvihill JJ, Parry DM, Sherman JL, et al. NIH conference. Neurofibromatosis 1 (Recklinghausen disease) and neurofibromatosis 2 (bilateral acoustic neurofibromatosis): an update. Ann Intern Med 1990;113:39–52
Purcell SM, Dixon SL. Schwannomatosis: an unusual variant of neurofibromatosis or a distinct clinical entity? Arch Dermatol 1989;125:390–393
Romero MJ, Ortega M, Camacho F. Is chronic diffuse hepatopathy a manifestation of neurofibromatosis? J Am Acad Dermatol 1989;21:1026
Rongioletti F, Drago F, Rebora A. Multiple cutaneous plexiform schwannomas with tumors of the central nervous system. [Letter]. Arch Dermatol 1989;125:431–432
Sorensen SA, Mulvihill JJ, Nielsen A. Long-term follow-up of von Recklinghausen neurofibromatosis: survival and malignant neoplasms. N Engl J Med 1986;314:1010–1015
Stern HJ, Sall HM, Lee JS, et al. Clinical variability of type 1 neurofibromatosis: is there a neurofibromatosis-Noonan syndrome? J Med Genet 1992;29:184–187
Wasserteil V, Bruce S, Riccardi VM. Non–von Recklinghausen's neurofibromatosis presenting as hemifacial neurofibromas and contralateral café au lait spots. J Am Acad Dermatol 1987;16:1090–1096
Westerhof W, Konrad K. Blue-red macules and pseudoatrophic macules: additional cutaneous signs in neurofibromatosis. Arch Dermatol 1982;118:577–581
Zehavi C, Romano A, Goodman RM. Iris (Lisch) nodules in neurofibromatosis. Clin Genet 1986;29:51–55

CENTRAL NEUROFIBROMATOSIS (NF-II; ACOUSTIC NEUROFIBROMATOSIS)

few café-au-lait spots or cutaneous neurofibromas

onset of symptoms frequently not until second decade or later

presence of acoustic neuromas, bilateral in over 90% of patients, which are not typically seen in other forms of neurofibromatosis

frequent spinal astrocytomas, paraspinal neurofibromas, and spinal and cranial meningiomas

posterior subcapsular cataracts relatively specific for NF-II

no Lisch nodules, pseudoarthroses, or optic gliomas

AD

genetically distinct from NF-I; gene localized to chromosome 22

pregnancy highly undesirable (due to worsening of disease), but oral contraceptives contraindicated

swimming and diving are contraindicated since patients tend to lose orientation under water and may drown

McK 101000
Kanter WR, Eldridge R, Fabricant R, et al. Central neurofibromatosis with bilateral acoustic neuroma: genetic, clinical and biochemical distinctions from peripheral neurofibromatosis. Neurology 1980;30:851–859
Martuza RL, Eldridge R. Neurofibromatosis 2. N Engl J Med 1988;318:684–688
Pastores GM, Michels VV, Jack CR Jr. Early childhood diagnosis of acoustic neuromas in presymptomatic individuals at risk for neurofibromatosis 2. Am J Med Genet 1991;41:325–329
Rouleau GA, Wertelecki W, Haines JL, et al. Genetic linkage of bilateral acoustic neurofibromatosis to a DNA marker on chromosome 22. Nature 1987;329:246–248

MIXED NEUROFIBROMATOSIS (NF-III)

mixture of features of NF-I and NF-II

café-au-lait spots, fewer in number than NF-I

cutaneous neurofibromas; palmar location characteristic

nervous system neoplasms include acoustic neuromas, spinal and or paraspinal neurofibromas, and meningiomas

no Lisch nodules or optic gliomas

AD

McK 162260
Riccardi VM. Neurofibromatosis: Phenotype, Natural History, and Pathogenesis. 2nd ed. Baltimore, Johns Hopkins University Press, 1992

VARIANT NEUROFIBROMATOSIS (NF-IV)

café-au-lait spots and neurofibromas present diffusely

may or may not have central nervous system tumors or Lisch nodules

AD

McK 162270

SEGMENTAL NEUROFIBROMATOSIS (NF-V)

cutaneous or internal neurofibromas and/or café-au-lait spots limited to a body segment; head and neck usually not involved

mostly sporadic; postzygotic somatic mutation proposed; because of familial cases, additional germ line mosaicism speculated

occurrence in families with full-blown NF-I reported

patients with segmental distribution of neurofibromas and/or café-au-lait spots who have bilateral Lisch nodules have NF-I, not NF-V

some patients may have unilateral Lisch nodules; the genetic implications of this occurrence are not known

Jaakkola S, Muona P, James WD, et al. Segmental neurofibromatosis: immunocytochemical analysis of cutaneous lesions. J Am Acad Dermatol 1990;22:617–621
Roth RR, Martines R, James WD. Segmental neurofibromatosis. Arch Dermatol 1987; 123:917–920
Sanchez Conejo-Mir J, Herrera Saval A, Camacho Martinez F. Segmental neurofibromatosis. J Am Acad Dermatol 1989; 20:681–682
Sloan JB, Fretzin DF, Bovenmyer DA. Genetic counseling in segmental neurofibromatosis. [Review]. J Am Acad Dermatol 1990; 22:461–467

CAFÉ-AU-LAIT MACULE NEUROFIBROMATOSIS (NF-VI)

development of café-au-lait spots in first year of life; inguinal and axillary freckling absent

no neurofibromas or Lisch nodules

AD in some cases

patients with more than six café-au-lait spots 1.5 cm or greater in diameter who do not have NF-I most likely have NF-VI

Riccardi VM. Pathophysiology of neurofibromatosis: IV. Dermatologic insights into heterogeneity and pathogenesis. J Am Acad Dermatol 1980;3:157–166
Charrow J, Listernick R, Ward K. Autosomal dominant multiple café-au-lait spots and neurofibromatosis-I: Evidence of non-linkage. Am J Med Genet 1993;45:606–608.

LATE-ONSET NEUROFIBROMATOSIS (NF-VII)

onset in third decade or later of neurofibromas in the absence of other stigmata or familial transmission

inheritance unclear; heritability doubted but not excluded

UNSPECIFIED NEUROFIBROMATOSIS (NF-VIII)

neurofibromatosis not classifiable into the other categories

Rare Syndromes That May Overlap With Neurofibromatosis

WATSON SYNDROME (CAFÉ-AU-LAIT MACULES AND PULMONARY STENOSIS)

freckling, especially axillary and perineal, and café-au-lait macules

mental retardation

pulmonary stenosis

AD

may be a variant of NF-I or the multiple lentigines syndrome

McK 193520
Allanson JE, Upadhyaya M, Watson GH, et al. Watson syndrome: is it a subtype of type 1 neurofibromatosis? J Med Genet 1991; 28:752–756
Partington MW, Burggraf GW, Fay JE, Frontini E. Pulmonary stenosis, café au lait spots and dull intelligence: the Watson syndrome revisited. [Abstract]. Proc Greenwood Genet Center 1985;4:105
Watson GH. Pulmonary stenosis, café-au-lait spots, and dull intelligence. Arch Dis Child 1967;42:303–307

DUODENAL CARCINOID, PHEOCHROMOCYTOMA, AND NEUROFIBROMAS

cutaneous neurofibromas

AD reported; most cases sporadic

may comprise a distinct multiple endocrine neoplasia (MEN) syndrome

McK 162240
Griffiths DFR, Williams GT, Williams ED. Multiple endocrine neoplasia associated with von Recklinghausen's disease. Br Med J 1983;287:1341–1343
De Angelis LM, Kelleher MB, Post KD, Fetell MR. Multiple paragangliomas in neurofibromatosis: A new neuroendocrine neoplasia. Neurology 1987;37:129–133

CAFÉ-AU-LAIT MACULES AND TEMPORAL DYSRHYTHMIA

café-au-lait macules but no other signs or family history of neurofibromatosis

neurologic findings include headaches, depression, syncope, impaired memory, temporal lobe electroencephalographic abnormalities, and cortical atrophy

AD

Verner JVJ, Johnson JH, Merritt FL. Café au lait spots, temporal dysrhythmia, and emotional instability. Int J Neuropsychiatry 1966;2:179–187

WESTERHOF SYNDROME

hypomelanotic and hypermelanotic (café-au-lait) macules on trunk and extremities; onset at birth

growth and mental retardation in some

probable AD; extremely rare

ultrastructurally, hyperpigmented lesions showed large melanosomes, singly distributed in keratinocytes

McK 154000
Westerhof W, Beemer FA, Cormane RH, et al. Hereditary congenital hypopigmented and hyperpigmented macules. Arch Dermatol 1978;114:931–936

TUBEROUS SCLEROSIS

Synonyms

- Bourneville disease
- epiloia

Skin

clavate hypopigmented (ash-leaf) macules seen at birth in half, eventually in 80% or more (onset rarely delayed until mid childhood); any part of the body may be involved, but trunk is favored; Wood's light helpful in detection; may number from 1 to more than 100 (Fig. 12–6)

angiofibromas (Pringle tumors; adenoma sebaceum), initially involving nasolabial folds, then progressing to the face and forehead symmetrically, usually spare upper lip (Fig. 12–7); rarely seen below clavicles; onset in first decade, usually from 4 to 9 years; rarely present at birth; number and size increase during puberty

yellowish red forehead plaques (Fig. 12–8); may be variants of connective tissue nevi

connective tissue nevi (collagenous plaques; shagreen patches) with a pigskin-like appearance typically occur in later childhood or adolescence but may be present at birth (Figs. 12–9 and 12–10); favor lumbosacral area but may occur anywhere; often precede onset of angiofibromas

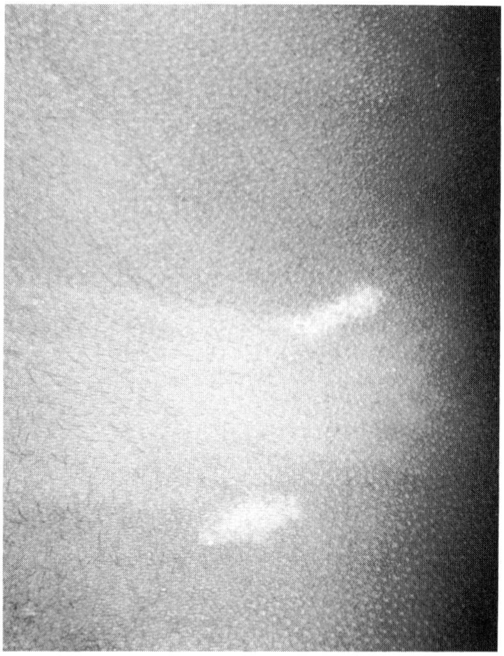

FIGURE 12–6
Ash-leaf macules on the back of a child with tuberous sclerosis.

occasional scalp fibromas and fibrous polyps of the skin folds around the neck or in axillae

poliosis may be another presenting sign

occasional café-au-lait macules

confetti-like white spots usually on trunk (not ash-leaf macules) in childhood

occasional fibrous nodules of the gingiva, buccal mucosa, hard palate, tongue, and nasal mucosa (Fig. 12–11)

subungual and periungual fibromas (Koenen tumors); onset usually at or after puberty (Fig. 12–12)

specific pit-shaped enamel defects in permanent and deciduous teeth

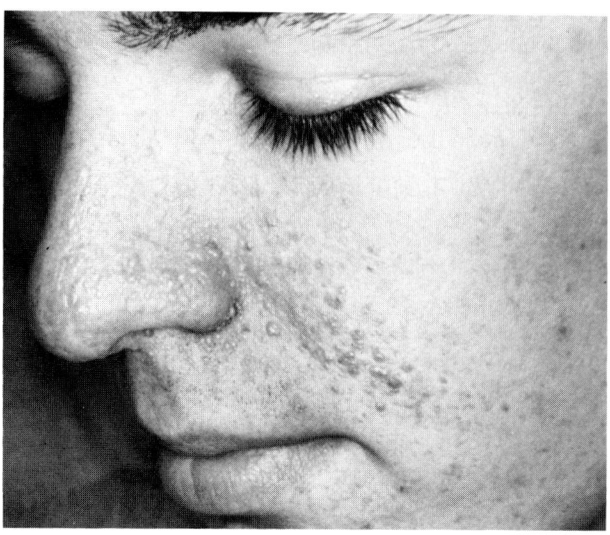

FIGURE 12–7
Tuberous sclerosis. Clustered angiofibromas (so-called adenoma sebaceum) over the nose, paranasal skin, and cheeks. (Courtesy of Edward A. Krull, MD, Detroit, Michigan)

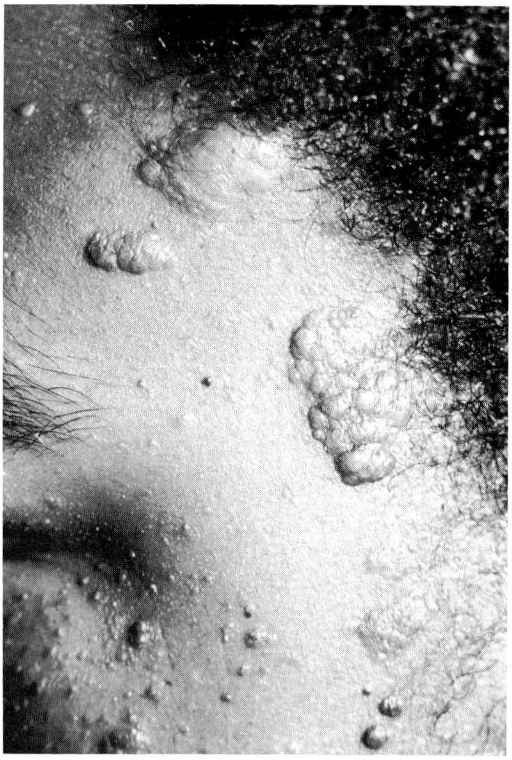

FIGURE 12–8
Multiple fibrous plaques and angiofibromas on the periorbital area and temple of a young man with tuberous sclerosis.

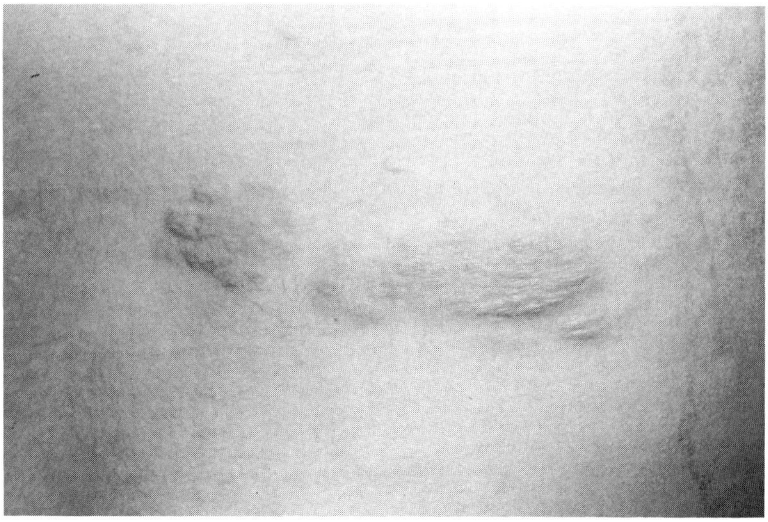

FIGURE 12–9
Reddish cobblestone plaque (shagreen patch) in the lumbosacral area.

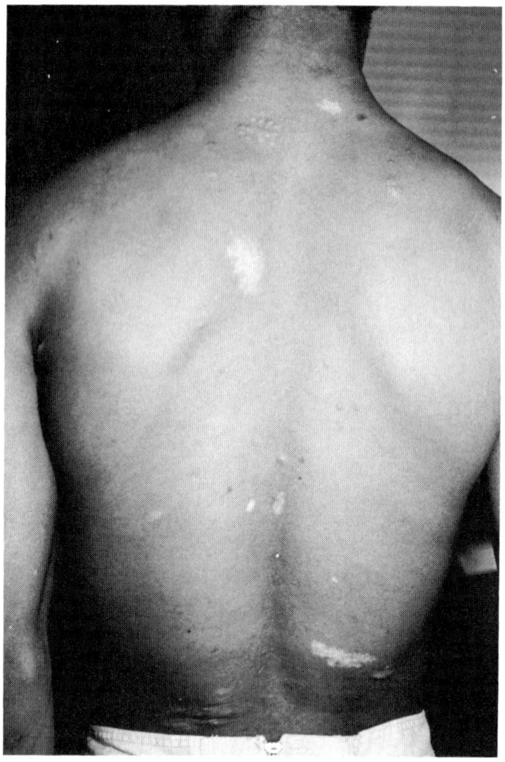

FIGURE 12–10
Back of a young man with tuberous sclerosis showing ash-leaf macules, multiple fibrotic papules, and a shagreen patch at the waist.

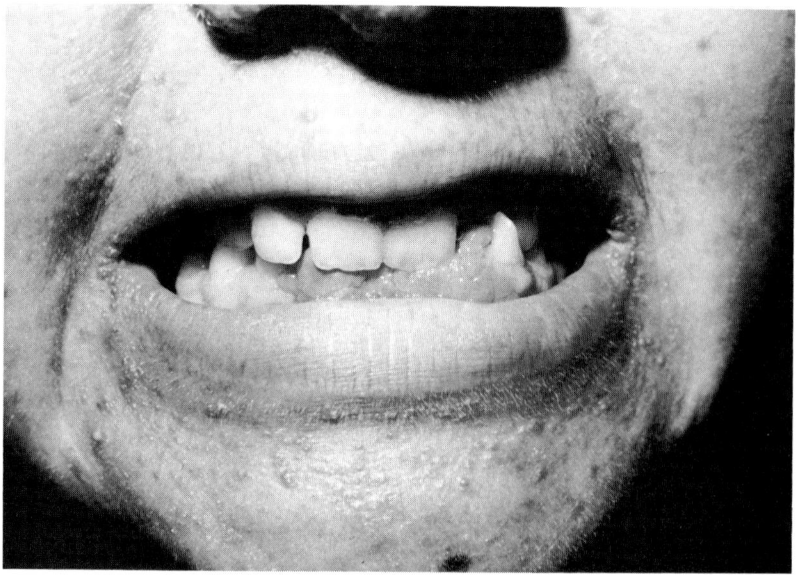

FIGURE 12–11
Gingival fibromas and multiple angiofibromas on the nose, cheeks, and chin of a patient with tuberous sclerosis.

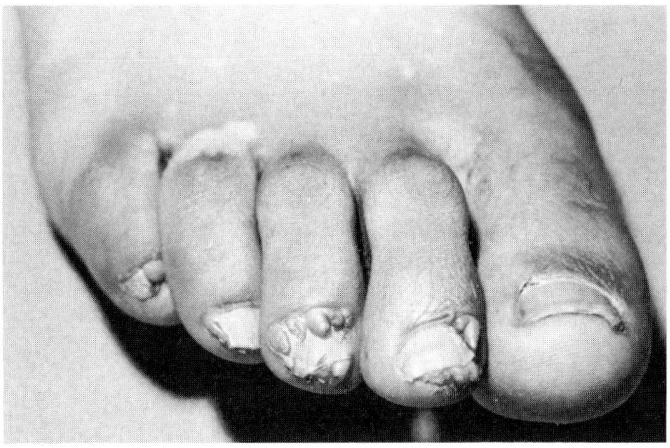

FIGURE 12–12
Multiple clove-like fibromatous periungual tumors (Koenen tumors).

Non-Skin

mental deficiency and/or seizure disorder in many but up to 25% of affected individuals have normal intellect; onset in infancy or early childhood

hamartomas of almost any internal organ

renal disease seen in up to 80% of cases: polycystic kidneys and/or hamartomas (characteristically angiomyolipomas), often multiple and bilateral; usually asymptomatic but occasional hematuria and pain

rhabdomyomas (usually multiple and asymptomatic) and/or congenital malformations of the heart

glial hamartomas, producing white tumors of the retina (phakomata), are characteristic and also produce potato-like (thus, "tuberous") nodules of glial proliferation usually in the cerebral cortex, basal ganglia, and ventricular walls

other findings include pulmonary disease (e.g., honeycomb lung on radiography) and bony changes (e.g., periosteal bone formation and/or phalangeal pseudocysts)

Genetics

AD; up to 85% represent new mutations

defective gene on chromosome 16 in two thirds of patients and chromosome 9 in about one third of patients

markedly variable expression; skip generations not uncommon (unlike NF, where skip generations are rare)

male to female ratio is 1:1

Pathophysiology

ash-leaf macules are due to abnormal melanin synthesis and impaired melanosome transfer from melanocyte to keratinocyte

Laboratory Data

radiographs: bilateral multiple sites of calcification of brain may give early clue to diagnosis; occasional "cotton ball"-like densities in older patients; calvarial thickening (noted after puberty); phalangeal cysts; flat bone cortical thickening

electroencephalographic abnormalities

glial "tubers" detected on computed tomography (CT) scan and magnetic resonance imaging; head CT scan of parents and siblings of patients with tuberous sclerosis may detect those with minimal disease

Prognosis

life expectancy decreased due to increased incidence of status epilepticus, intercurrent infections, cardiac failure, pulmonary fibrosis, or tumors of heart, kidney or brain; death occurs from infancy to early adulthood in more severely affected individuals, while those with less severe disease (e.g. predominantly cutaneous manifestations)

triad of adenoma sebaceum, mental retardation, and seizures is usually present, but expression quite variable

Wood's lamp examination to aid in detection of ash-leaf macules should be performed in any infant with otherwise undiagnosed seizures or mental retardation

epiloia, an archaic term for tuberous sclerosis, is a contraction of *epi*lepsy, *lo*w *i*ntelligence, and *a*denoma sebaceum

REFERENCES

McK 191100

Bell SD, MacDonald DM. The prevalence of café-au-lait patches in tuberous sclerosis. Clin Exp Dermatol 1985;10:562–565

Fryer AE, Osborne JP, Schutt W. Forehead plaque: a presenting skin sign in tuberous sclerosis. Arch Dis Child 1987;62:292–304

Gomez MR, ed. Tuberous Sclerosis. 2nd ed. New York, Raven Press, 1988

Hausser I, Anton-Lamprecht I. Electron microscopy as a means for carrier detection and genetic counseling in families at risk of tuberous sclerosis. Hum Genet 1987; 76:73–80

Hunt A. Tuberous sclerosis: a survey of 97 cases: II: Physical findings. Dev Med Child Neurol 1983;25:350–352

McWilliam RC, Stephenson JBP. Depigmented hair: the earliest sign of tuberous sclerosis. Arch Dis Child 1978;53:961–963

Mlynarczyk G. Enamel pitting: common symptom of tuberous sclerosis. Oral Surg 1991; 71:63–67

Oppenheimer EY, Rosman NP, Dooling EC. The late appearance of hypopigmented maculae in tuberous sclerosis. Am J Dis Child 1985;139:408–409

Reed WB, Nickel WR, Campion G. Internal manifestations of tuberous sclerosis. Arch Dermatol 1963;87:715–728

Sampson JR, Attwood D, Al Mughery AS, Reid JS. Pitted enamel hypoplasia in tuberous sclerosis. Clin Genet 1992;42:50–52

ATAXIA-TELANGIECTASIA

Synonyms

- Louis-Bar syndrome
- cephalo-oculocutaneous telangiectasia

Skin

onset of telangiectases of exposed bulbar conjunctivae (peripheral to limbus); occurs around age 4 or 5 years (i.e., usually after ataxia is present), sometimes later in first decade and rarely at birth or during infancy (Fig. 12–13)

telangiectases develop elsewhere on head later in first decade, especially on the auricle and periorbital skin; also on trunk and extremities, and occasionally in nonexposed body folds (e.g., popliteal and antecubital fossae) (Color Fig. 12–1)

mucous membranes may be involved; hemorrhage occurs rarely

occasionally skin becomes sclerodermoid, especially on face and ears

persistent erythematous, scaly, sometimes tender and atrophic, papules, plaques, and nodules on the extremities and less often trunk; frequently ulcerate; onset mostly in first and second decade

other cutaneous manifestations include hirsutism of arms and legs in women, seborrheic dermatitis, café-au-lait macules, poliosis; poikiloderma develops with continued sun exposure and aging

Non-Skin

cerebellar ataxia including characteristic peculiar eye movements and cerebellar dysarthria are earliest signs; onset usually at 12 to 18 months of age but may occur later in childhood

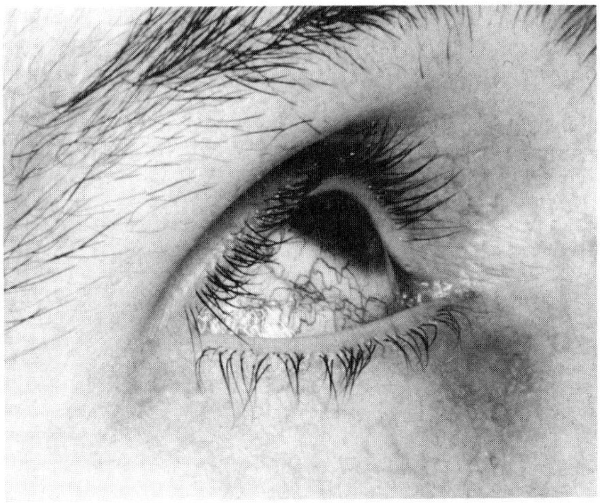

FIGURE 12–13
Ataxia-telangiectasia. Striking telangiectases of the sclera. Note the involvement of the periorbital skin as well. (Courtesy of Benjamin K. Fisher, MD, Toronto, Ontario)

other neurologic abnormalities include choreoathetoid movements, progressive hypotonia, decreased deep tendon reflexes, intention tremor, constant drooling, and muscle atrophy due to disuse and peripheral neuropathy

intelligence normal early in life, but usually declines in late childhood

frequent sinopulmonary infections in three fourths; onset usually between ages 3 and 8 years; sequelae include chronic obstructive pulmonary disease, bronchiectases, finger clubbing, respiratory failure, and death

frequent hypoplasia or aplasia of thymus, growth retardation, hypogonadism, and poor secondary sexual development

insulin-resistant diabetes mellitus in about half of patients

occasional generalized lymphadenopathy and hepatosplenomegaly

Genetics

AR

in the United States, gene frequency estimated to be 1 in 100, with an incidence of homozygotes of 1 in 40,000

Pathophysiology

characteristic DNA defects include increased spontaneous and x-ray–induced chromosomal breaks, rearrangements, translocations, and ring formations; demonstrable in peripheral lymphocytes

sister chromatid exchanges are not increased

Laboratory Data

histopathology: papules, plaques, and nodules show granulomatous inflammation

lymphocytopenia and mild anemia common

total IgA deficiency in half and partial deficiency in 30%

serum IgE and IgG2 deficiency in most

most patients have an abnormal low molecular weight 8S IgM in serum

cell-mediated immunity and cytoxicity are impaired owing to hypoplasia or aplasia of thymus and lymphoid tissues

increased number of T cells with gamma/delta chains in the T-cell receptors, rather than the alpha/beta chains seen on mature T-cells; in normal individuals, gamma/delta chains are most often found on immature T-cells; may relate to defects in cell-mediated immunity

alpha-fetoprotein or carcinoembryonic antigen levels may be elevated

in vitro hypersensitivity (decreased cell survival) following x-ray irradiation, paralleling clinical hypersensitivity to x-rays prenatal diagnosis by demonstration of clastogenic factor in amniotic fluid and high spontaneous chromosomal breakage rate of amniotic fluid cells with translocation

Prognosis

most affected individuals wheel-chair bound by age 10

gamma globulin immunotherapy may be beneficial

severe respiratory infections and chronic pulmonary disease cause death in about half

lymphoreticular malignancies, including Hodgkin disease, lymphocytic leukemia, and undifferentiated sarcoma, develop in those who survive into adolescence

Discussion

ultraviolet irradiation does not damage DNA, which contrasts to xeroderma pigmentosum in which cells are sensitive to ultraviolet irradiation but not x-rays

heterozygotes reported to have an increased incidence of malignancy, especially of breast, ovary, biliary tract, and stomach; if true, this would account for some "sporadic" carcinomas in the "general" population

REFERENCES

McK 208900

Carbonari M, Cherchi M, Paganelli R, et al. Relative increase of T cells expressing the gamma/delta rather than the alpha/beta receptor in ataxia-telangiectasia [see comments]. N Engl J Med 1990;322:73–76

Cohen LE, Tanner DJ, Schaefer HG, Levis WR. Common and uncommon cutaneous findings in patients with ataxia-telangiectasia. J Am Acad Dermatol 1984;10:431–438

McFarlin DE, Strober W, Waldmann TA. Ataxia-telangiectasia. Medicine 1972; 51:281–314

Oxelius V, Berkel AI, Hanson LA. IgG2 deficiency in ataxia-telangiectasia. N Engl J Med 1982;306:515–517

Paller AS, Massey RB, Curtis MA, et al. Cutaneous granulomatous lesions in patients with ataxia-telangiectasia. J Pediatr 1991;119:917–922

Smith LL, Conerly SL. Ataxia-telangiectasia or Louis-Bar syndrome. [Review]. J Am Acad Dermatol 1985;12:681–696

Swift M, Morrell D, Massey RB, Chase CL. Incidence of cancer in 161 families affected by ataxia-telangiectasia. N Engl J Med 1991;325:1831–1836

Waldmann TA, Misiti J, Nelson DL, Kraemer KH. Ataxia-telangiectasia: a multisystem hereditary disease with immunodeficiency, impaired organ maturation, x-ray hypersensitivity and a high incidence of neoplasia. Ann Intern Med 1983;99:367–369

Welshimer K, Swift M. Congenital malformations and developmental disabilities in ataxia-telangiectasia, Fanconi anemia, and xeroderma pigmentosum families. Am J Hum Genet 1982;34:781–793

Yount WJ. IgG2 deficiency and ataxia-telangiectasia. N Engl J Med 1982;306:541–543

Hereditary Sensory Neuropathies

There are a number of disorders, poorly defined and rare, in which pain and other sensations are impaired leading to cutaneous injury from trauma, heat,

TABLE 12–1
HEREDITARY SENSORY SYNDROMES

Name	Inheritence	Onset	Mucocutaneous Findings	Comments
HSAN-1 (hereditary radicular neuropathy)	AD	Adolescence or adulthood	Indolent, painless nonhealing neurotropic ulcers of feet with hyperkeratotic borders; onset in adolescence or adulthood	Peroneal muscular atrophy; RTe + +; RTo +; AxR −; sweat loss distally, DTR may be decreased
HSAN-II (congenital sensory neuropathy)	AR	Birth		Universal pain loss; RTe+; RTo+ +; AxR −; DTR: decreased or absent; sweat loss distally
HSAN-III (familial dysautonomia; Riley-Day syndrome)	AR	Birth	Oral ulcerations and ankyloglossia; livedo reticularis and acrocyanosis; vasomotor instability	Abnormal and erratic sweating; RTe +/−; AxR+; DTR: decreased
HSAN-IV (congenital sensory neuropathy with anhidrosis)	AR	Birth	Hypohidrosis anhidrosis, self-mutilation	Congenital insensitivity to pain; RTe +/−; RTo +/− or normal; AxR+; sweating decreased or absent; mental retardation in some
HSAN-V	AR	Birth	Similar to type IV	Similar to type IV but normal DTR and mentation
HNNA (congenital indifference to pain; congenital insensitivity to pain)	AR	Birth	Trophic ulcers rare	Universal pain loss; AxR+; normal temperature, touch, DTR, autonomic function, sweating, and nerve histology

AxR, axon reflex (+, present; −, absent); DTR, deep tendon reflexes; HNNA, hereditary nonneuropathic analgia; HSAN, hereditary sensory and autonomic neuropathy; RTe, reduced temperature sensation; RTo, reduced touch sensation; RDTR, reduced deep tendon reflexes.

From Gorlin RJ, Cohen MM Jr, Levin LS. Syndromes of the Head and Neck. 3rd ed. New York, Oxford University Press, 1990:599.

cold and other factors. Skin findings depend on the site and nature of the neurologic abnormalities. Of these entities, Riley-Day syndrome is the most clearly defined. Table 12–1 lists the salient features of other such syndromes.

Gorlin RJ, Cohen MM Jr, Levin LS. Syndromes of the Head and Neck. 3rd ed. New York, Oxford University Press, 1990:598–601

FAMILIAL DYSAUTONOMIA

Synonyms

- Riley-Day syndrome
- HSAN type III

Skin

sharply defined erythematous patches greater than 2 cm in size, most commonly on face and upper trunk, occurring during eating or periods of excitement (vasomotor disturbance); disappear within 10 to 15 minutes

profuse hyperhidrosis, especially of trunk, elicited by excitement

frequent livedo reticularis and acrocyanosis of extremities

ankyloglossia and/or ulcerations of tongue, lips, or mucous membranes in some

absence of fungiform papillae and, less consistently, circumvallate papillae, resulting in deficient taste perception

Non-Skin

abnormalities of the autonomic, motor, and somatic sensory nervous systems

indifference to pain in newborns

swallowing difficulties and episodic vomiting soon after birth

characteristic facial features include hypertelorism, almond-shaped eyes, large and low-set ears, pointed chin, and a generally thin-appearing face with an "apprehensive" expression

small stature due to retarded bone growth and kyphoscoliosis developing late in first decade

persistent drooling beyond infancy

recurrent pneumonia and sleep apnea

lack of normal lacrimation is especially evident with crying

corneal hypesthesia or anesthesia results in punctate keratitis, ulcers, and opacities

intermittent hypertension, postural hypotension, unexplained febrile episodes, and cold hands and feet (erratic thermoregulation)

decreased or absent deep tendon reflexes

dysarthria, dysphagia, constipation, or diarrhea

other neurologic abnormalities include occasional mental retardation, breath-holding spells, and ataxia

Genetics

AR

mostly affects Ashkenazi Jews

Laboratory Data

increased urinary homovanillic acid and decreased vanillylmandelic acid

intradermal injection of histamine fails to produce pain or erythematous flare

methylcholine drops in eye causes prompt meiosis

prolonged hypoglycemic response to insulin

exaggerated rise in systolic blood pressure and pulse with norepinephrine injection

Schirmer's test demonstrates lacrimal dysfunction

Prognosis

emotional and vasomotor instability persist throughout life; sensory loss is slowly progressive

death in infancy and early childhood common; causes include aspiration or infectious pneumonia, cardiac and respiratory arrest secondary to hypotension, and respiratory arrest during sleep; however, at least one third of patients are older than 20 and the proportion surviving into fourth decade is increasing

Discussion

the most common and most extensively studied of the hereditary neuropathies

REFERENCES

McK 223900

Axelrod FB, Abularrage JJ. Familial dysautonomia: a prospective study of survival. J Pediatr 1982;101:234–236

Axelrod FB, Porges RF, Sein ME. Neonatal recognition of familial dysautonomia. J Pediatr 1987;110:946–948

Brunt PW, McKusick VA. Familial dysautonomia: a report of genetic and clinical studies, with a review of the literature. Medicine 1970;49:343–373

PERIPHERAL MOTOR NEUROPATHY WITH DYSAUTONOMIA

cold-induced profuse sweating in two sisters

McK 252320

Lisker R, Garcia-Ramos G, de la Rosa-Laris C, Diaz-Mitoma F. Peripheral motor neuropathy associated with autonomic dysfunction in two sisters: new hereditary syndrome? Am J Med Genet 1981;9:255–259

Sato K, Kang WH, Saga K, et al. Biology of sweat glands and their disorders: II. Disorders of sweat gland function. [Review]. J Am Acad Dermatol 1989;20:713–726

Nonhereditary Congenital Neurologic Disorders

There are a number of congenital, mostly sporadic neurologic disorders that are sometimes mistakenly regarded as hereditary. Although there are occasional familial case reports, the great majority of cases are not hereditary. Therefore, genetic counseling is straightforward, although frequently sought.

CORNELIA DE LANGE SYNDROME

Synonym

- Brachmann-de Lange syndrome

Skin

generalized hypertrichosis; onset at birth

low occipital and frontal hairlines, with occasional "widow's peak"; synophrys and characteristic, long, upturned eyelashes

hair on lateral elbows and sacral areas often very long and lanugo-like

generalized livedo reticularis, except for palms and soles, which are erythematous; decreases with age

late eruption of small, widely spaced teeth

frequent dermatoglyphic abnormalities

Non-Skin

small for gestational age; physical retardation and short stature throughout life

feeding difficulties, increased susceptibility to infection and aspiration pneumonia early in life

distinctive, low-pitched, raucous, "growling" cry; becomes less typical with age

micromelia and phocomelia reported

distinctive craniofacies including microbrachycephaly, hypertelorism, antimongolian slant of palpebral fissures, low nasal bridge, anteverted nostrils, long philtrum, thin lips, micrognathia, and low-set ears

occasional blue sclerae

frequent high-arched and cleft palate

severe mental retardation

musculoskeletal abnormalities include clinodactyly of fifth fingers, proximally placed short thumbs, webbing of second and third toes, small hands, pectus excavatum, flexural contractures, and elbow webbing

genital abnormalities in most males include cryptorchidism and hypospadias

Genetics

mostly sporadic; AR and AD inheritance speculated in some cases, but others claim AD cases are examples of the Coffin-Siris syndrome

Prognosis

decreased life expectancy; mortality due to pulmonary infection and aspiration pneumonia, severe heart disease and cerebral hemorrhage; death usually before adulthood

Discussion

phenotypic similarities with the dup(3q) syndrome and Coffin-Siris syndrome

REFERENCES

McK 122470

Bankier A, Haan E, Birrell R. Familial occurrence of Brachmann-de Lange syndrome. Am J Med Genet 1986;25:163–165

Fryns J. On the nosology of the Cornelia de Lange and Coffin-Siris syndromes. Clin Genet 1986;29:263–264

Robinson LK, Wolfsberg E, Jones KL. Brachmann-de Lange syndrome: evidence for autosomal dominant inheritance. Am J Med Genet 1985;22:109–115

Salazar FN. Dermatological manifestations of the Cornelia de Lange syndrome. Arch Dermatol 1966;94:38–43

RUBINSTEIN-TAYBI SYNDROME

Synonyms

- broad thumb–great toe syndrome
- Rubinstein syndrome

Skin

nevus flammeus of lumbar area, forehead, or nape of neck in 50%

hypertrichosis of trunk, limbs, and face in two thirds of infants

increased tendency to form hypertrophic scars or keloids

racquet nails

teeth irregularily shaped and overcrowded

abnormal dermatoglyphics and simian crease in patients and relatives

Non-Skin

broad terminal phalanges of thumbs and great toes; present at birth

radial deviation of thumb and great toe in one fourth of cases (in these cases, proximal phalanx is triangular)

50% have clinodactyly of fifth finger

bony abnormalities of ribs, vertebrae, and sternum

distinctive facies including prominent forehead, low-set ears, high-arched eyebrows, long eyelashes, broad and beaked nasal bridge, and frequent extension of nasal septum below alae

eye abnormalities include strabismus (75%), antimongoloid slant of eyes, and cataracts

mental retardation in most cases and epilepsy in 25%

short stature and overweight

Genetics

almost all cases sporadic (chromosomal microdeletion speculated), but possible AD and AR cases reported

Laboratory Data

prominent foramen magnum in 60% and skeletal abnormalities demonstrable radiographically

electroencephalogram abnormal in two thirds

normal chromosomal studies

Discussion

variable expressivity characteristic

patients with trisomy 13 syndrome may also present with mental retardation and broad thumbs and great toes, so cytogenetic studies are recommended in all patients with the diagnosis of Rubinstein-Taybi syndrome

REFERENCES

McK 180849

Gillies DR, Roussounis SH. Rubinstein-Taybi syndrome: further evidence of a genetic aetiology. Dev Med Child Neurol 1985; 27:751–755

Hennekam RC, Stevens CA, Van de Kamp JJ. Etiology and recurrence risk in Rubinstein-Taybi syndrome. Am J Med Genet 1990;6:56–64

Kurwa AR. Rubinstein-Taybi syndrome and spontaneous keloids. Clin Exp Dermatol 1979;4:251–254

Selmanowitz VJ, Stiller MJ. Rubinstein-Taybi syndrome: cutaneous manifestations and colossal keloids. Arch Dermatol 1981; 117:504–506

Siraganian PA, Rubinstein JH, Miller RW. Keloids and neoplasms in the Rubinstein-Taybi syndrome. Med Pediatr Oncol 1989;17:485–491

Neurocutaneous Disorders—Abbreviated Entries

FAMILIAL CONGENITAL ANTERIOR CERVICAL HYPERTRICHOSIS ASSOCIATED WITH PERIPHERAL SENSORY AND MOTOR NEUROPATHY

probable AR

McK239840

Trattner A, Hodak E, Sagie-Lerman T, et al. Familial congenital anterior cervical hypertrichosis associated with peripheral sensory and motor neuropathy—a new syndrome? J Am Acad Dermatol 1991; 25:767–770

NOTALGIA PARESTHETICA (HEREDITARY LOCALIZED PRURITUS)

pruritus or dysesthesia of posterior upper thorax; onset in adulthood

affected area may be hyperpigmented

only some cases hereditary, possibly XLD

predominantly a sensory neuropathy of posterior primary rami of spinal nerves T2–T6

McK 177100

Comings DE, Comings SN. Hereditary localized pruritus. Arch Dermatol 1965;92:236–237

Weber PJ, Poulos EG. Notalgia paresthetica: case reports and histologic appraisal. J Am Acad Dermatol 1988;18:25–30

MENTAL RETARDATION, SEIZURES, AND PSORIASIS

possible XLR

McK 309480

Tranebjaerg L, Svejgaard A, Lykkesfeldt G. X-linked mental retardation associated with psoriasis: a new syndrome? Am J Med Genet 1988;30:263–273

KABUKI MAKE-UP SYNDROME

distinctive facial abnormalities reminiscent of the make-up used in Kabuki theatre

mild to moderate mental retardation and progressive postnatal growth retardation

short stature, short fifth fingers, scoliosis, and hip dislocation

mostly sporadic; AD cases reported

McK 147920
Gorlin RJ, Cohen MM Jr, Levin LS. Syndromes of the Head and Neck. 3rd ed. New York, Oxford University Press, 1990:762–763
Niikawa N, Kuroki Y, Kajii T, et al. Kabuki make-up (Niikawa-Kuroki) syndrome: a study of 62 patients. Am J Med Genet 1988;31:565–589

CHAPTER

13

Vascular and Hematologic Disorders

This chapter includes the heritable disorders of the cutaneous vasculature and the lymphatic system. In many instances, the terminology is confusing since it reflects old nomenclature in which no distinction was made between hemangiomas and vascular malformations. Hemangiomas are proliferative lesions that almost always regress spontaneously; malformations are structural defects and represent errors in morphogenesis. We have tried to indicate which type of lesion characterizes each disorder, but the reader must bear in mind that reference titles may fail to make this distinction and may use incorrect terminology to describe a particular vascular lesion. We have also included the hereditary angioedemas and urticarias in this chapter.

REFERENCE

Mulliken JB, Young AE, eds. Vascular Birthmarks: Hemangiomas and Malformations. Philadelphia, WB Saunders, 1988

Hereditary Angioedemas and Urticarias

HEREDITARY ANGIOEDEMA

Synonyms

- Quincke edema
- hereditary angioneurotic edema
- C1-esterase inhibitor deficiency

Skin

attacks of cutaneous and mucosal nonpitting angioedema usually appearing in childhood or early in second decade; however, they may not appear until early or late adult life

reticulate erythema frequently precedes attacks, but angioedema may also appear in isolation

commonly affects extremities, face (especially periorbital areas), and genitalia; buttocks and trunk involved less often

pharyngeal and laryngeal edema in half; lips and tongue also affected

premonitory pruritus, pricking sensation, or dysuria may herald attacks

attacks last hours to days, recur at regular or irregular intervals, and are often provoked by trauma or stress; complete resolution between attacks

Non-Skin

attacks of abdominal pain, vomiting, diarrhea, and/or obstipation may simulate an acute abdomen, but rigidity is absent; abdominal attacks may occur separately or simultaneously with cutaneous or oropharyngeal attacks and have similar timing and frequency

occasional joint effusions

Genetics

AD

Pathophysiology

C1-esterase inhibitor (alpha-2-globulin) deficiency (85% of patients) or dysfunction (15% of patients)

C2 kinin (may be a fragment of C2) mediates angioedema

Laboratory Data

screening test: low serum C2 or C4 levels during attacks; C4 may be low between attacks

C1q levels are not decreased

Prognosis

before institution of therapy (e.g., in undiagnosed patients) laryngeal edema may result in asphyxiation unless intervention is prompt; incidence of this complication varies widely between kindreds; some individuals require tracheostomies

acute attacks preferably treated with transfusion of fresh-frozen plasma or purified C1-esterase inhibitor; traditional therapies for anaphylaxis including corticosteroids, epinephrine, and antihistamines are generally ineffective

ethinyl testosterone (danazol) and modified androgen therapy (e.g., stanozolol) therapy raises C1-esterase levels through increased liver production but are only effective prophylactically

epsilon-aminocaproic acid and tranexamic acid (inhibitors of plasminogen activation) may be used preoperatively to decrease attacks induced by surgery

exogenous estrogens and menses may worsen attacks, whereas improvement may be noted during pregnancy

attacks less frequent and milder with age and occasionally cease

Discussion

hereditary angioneurotic edema accounts for far less than 10% of all cases of angioedema

angioedema may occur with deficiencies of other protease inhibitors including alpha-1-antitrypsin and plasma kallikrein inhibitor

■ *episodic angioedema with eosinophilia*

severe cyclic angioedema of face, neck, and trunk

urticaria may also be seen

onset from childhood to adulthood

fever and weight gain

leukocytosis with marked eosinophilia

acquired

REFERENCES

McK 106100
Brickman CM, Hosea SW. Hereditary angioedema. Int J Dermatol 1983;141:141–147
Cicardi M, Bergamaschini L, Marasini B, et al. Hereditary angioedema: an appraisal of 104 cases. Am J Med Sci 1982;284:2–9
Cullmann W, Opferkuch W. Deficiencies in regulator proteins 1: C1 inhibitor. Progr All 1986;39:311–334
Davis A III. Hereditary and acquired deficiencies of C1 inhibitor. Immunodefic Rev 1989;1:207–226
Gleich GJ, Schroeter AL, Marcoux MP, et al. Episodic angioedema associated with eosinophilia. N Engl J Med 1984;310:1621–1626
Massa MC, Connolly SM. An association between C1 esterase inhibitor deficiency and lupus erythematosus: report of two cases and review of the literature. J Am Acad Dermatol 1982;7:255–264
Williamson DM. Reticulate erythema—a prodrome in hereditary angio-oedema. Br J Dermatol 1979;101:549–552
Wolf C, Pehamberger H, Breyer S, et al. Episodic angioedema with eosinophilia. J Am Acad Dermatol 1989;20:21–27

HEREDITARY VIBRATORY ANGIOEDEMA

pruritic, erythematous and edematous cutaneous and subcutaneous plaques elicited by mechanical vibration and/or friction; tendency noted at birth pruritus is unusual in most other types of angioedema

flushing and/or generalized erythema may accompany severe attacks

angioedema may persist for hours or days, depending on the strength of stimulus

potentiated by prior exposure to cold

tracheal or laryngeal edema do not occur

AD

McK 193050

Epstein PA, Kidd KK. Dermo-distortive urticaria: an autosomal dominant dermatologic disorder. Am J Med Genet 1981;9:307–315

Patterson R, Mellies CJ, Blankenship ML, Pruzansky JJ. Vibratory angioedema: a hereditary type of physical hypersensitivity. J Allergy Clin Immun 1972;50:174–182

FAMILIAL COLD URTICARIA

Skin

one half to several hours after exposure to cold, sites develop erythema and urticarial plaques; petechial lesions also reported; lesions last 4 to 5 hours to several days, usually in proportion to length of cold exposure

in severe attacks, lesions may also involve skin not exposed to cold

onset usually in early childhood but may begin at birth or infancy; attacks may worsen with age

pruritus is not present, but lesions may sting or burn

ingestion of cold foods and drinks do not cause symptoms

Non-Skin

stiff, swollen, painful, often erythematous joints (most commonly of hands, feet, and knees) in proportion to degree of urticaria

malaise, chills, and mild fever accompany joint and skin attacks

occasional headache, nausea, extreme thirst, conjunctivitis, and photophobia

Genetics

AD; more common in females

Laboratory Data

leukocytosis may precede and/or accompany signs and symptoms, as distinct from acquired cold urticaria

ice cube test is negative (positive in idiopathic acquired cold urticaria)

passive transfer test is negative

Prognosis

generally persists lifelong

Discussion

- *idiopathic acquired cold urticaria*

  more common than familial cold urticaria

  presents in childhood or adulthood, with urticaria occurring immediately on exposure to cold; reaction mediated by histamine

  lesions pruritic

  ice cube test positive

  passive transfer tests are positive in about half of cases

  symptoms usually disappear after months to years

REFERENCES

McK 120100
Derbes VJ, Coleman WP. Familial cold urticaria. Ann Allergy 1972;30:335–341
Doeglas HMG, Bleumink E. Familial cold urticaria. Arch Dermatol 1974;110:382–388
Ormerod AD, Smart L, Reid TMS, Milford-Ward A. Familial cold urticaria. Arch Dermatol 1993;129:343–346

DELAYED COLD-INDUCED URTICARIA

erythema, edema, and induration develop 9 to 18 hours after exposure to cold

AD

Soter NA, Joshi NP, Twarog FJ, et al. Delayed cold-induced urticaria: a dominantly inherited disorder. J Allergy Clin Immunol 1977;59:294–297

FAMILIAL LOCALIZED HEAT URTICARIA

development of wheals 1 to 2 hours after heat exposure; a delayed-onset form has also been reported

wheals last 12 to 14 hours

onset in childhood, persists

AD

McK 191950

Michaelsson G, Ross A. Familial localized heat urticaria of a delayed type. Acta Derm Venereol 1971;51:279–283

MUCKLE-WELLS SYNDROME (URTICARIA, DEAFNESS, AND AMYLOIDOSIS)

during adolescence, attacks of malaise, chills, fever, lassitude, and pain in limbs and joints; these flu-like symptoms are sometimes called "aguey bouts"

attacks last 1 to 2 days and recur about every 3 weeks indefinitely

episodic, geographic urticarial lesions accompany attacks

lesions may be pruritic and are worsened by heat

deafness develops from second to sixth decades

amyloidosis of kidney and occasionally other viscera

AD

hypergammaglobulinemia and elevated erythrocyte sedimentation rate during and between attacks

decreased life expectancy due to amyloid nephropathy and renal failure in some

---

McK 191900

Black JT. Amyloidosis, deafness, urticaria, and limb pains: a hereditary syndrome. Ann Intern Med 1969;70:989–994

Muckle TJ. The Muckle-Wells syndrome. Br J Dermatol 1979;100:87–92

Hereditary Lymphedema

CONGENITAL HEREDITARY LYMPHEDEMA

Synonym

- Milroy disease

Skin

pitting edema, usually symmetrical, involves the feet, ankles, and legs (Fig. 13–1); occasionally, the thighs (up to Poupart's ligament) and rarely the upper extremities involved

onset at birth or shortly thereafter

in time, firm, pale nonpitting areas may develop

severity and course of disease vary widely; findings range from slight postural swelling to an elephantiasis-like appearance with hyperkeratotic, occasionally fissured, warty excrescences ("mossy foot")

development of lymphangiosarcoma occurs rarely and is heralded by purple macular or papular lesions in affected limbs

yellow nails in some

hypodontia, hypotrichosis or hypertrichosis, and/or xerosis rarely

Genetics

AD

AR form also reported (McK 247440)

Pathophysiology

hypoplasia or aplasia of lymphatics

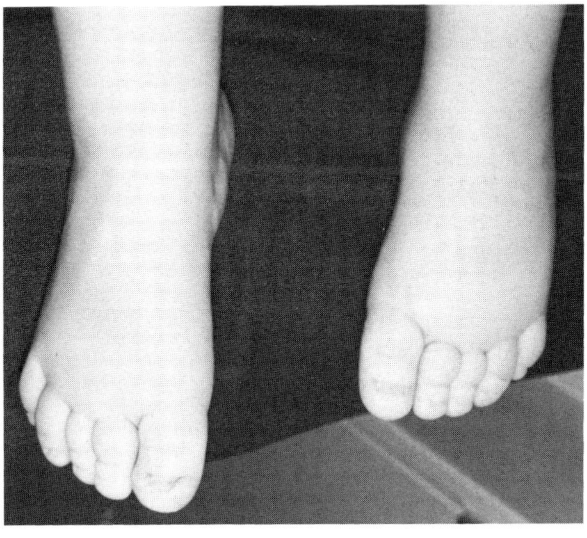

FIGURE 13–1
Congenital hereditary lymphedema. Edema of the toes, dorsa of the feet, and ankles of a young child whose father also had lymphedema.

Prognosis

normal life span, but some degree of disability

recurrent secondary infection (frequently streptococcal) of limb is common

Discussion

lymphedema has been reported with a variety of abnormalities including spina bifida, distichiasis (extra row of eyelashes), ptosis, and extradural cysts in various combinations

lymphedema may have late onset as well; some authors use the term *lymphedema praecox* (see later) for noncongenital lymphedema with onset before age 35 years and *lymphedema tarda* for cases with onset after age 35 years

REFERENCES

McK 153100
McK 247440
Brostrom LA, Nilsonne U, Kronberg M, Soderberg G. Lymphangiosarcoma in chronic hereditary oedema (Milroy's disease). Ann Chir Gynaecol 1989;78:320–323
Esterly JR. Congenital hereditary lymphoedema. J Med Genet 1965;2:93–98
Milroy WF. Chronic hereditary edema: Milroy's disease. JAMA 1928;91:1172–1175

LYMPHEDEMA PRAECOX (LATE-ONSET HEREDITARY LYMPHEDEMA; MEIGE LYMPHEDEMA)

lymphedema beginning in second to fourth decades, usually of the lower extremities

onset is abrupt and often accompanied by inflammation

frequent secondary streptococcal infection of limb

a "mossy foot" appearance may develop

laryngeal and intestinal lymphangiectasia reported

mostly affects women

AR

McK 153200
Goodman RM. Familial lymphedema of the Meige's type. Am J Med 1962;32:651–656
Herbert FA, Bowen PA. Hereditary late-onset lymphedema with pleural effusion and laryngeal edema. Arch Intern Med 1983;143:913–915
Holmes LB, Fields JP, Zabriskie JB. Hereditary late-onset lymphedema. Pediatrics 1978;61:575–579
Wheeler ES, Chan V, Wassman R, et al. Familial lymphedema praecox: Meige's disease. Plast Reconstr Surg 1981;67:362–364

DISTICHIASIS-LYMPHEDEMA SYNDROME

distichiasis (extra row of eyelashes)

lymphedema of legs and feet, onset usually between mid-first and third decades

AD

McK 153400

Jester HG. Lymphedema-distichiasis. Hum Genet 1977;39:113–116

Pap Z, Biro T, Szabo L, Papp Z. Syndrome of lymphoedema and distichiasis. Hum Genet 1980;53:309–310

CONGENITAL ABSENCE OF VENOUS VALVES

lower extremity edema begins around puberty and worsens with age

characteristically appears after standing during the day, disappearing at night

varicosities develop in most patients

stasis dermatitis and supramalleolar ulceration may develop

occasional syncopal episodes due to hypotension

AD

male to female ratio: 1:1

total or partial absence of valves in the deep and superficial veins of the lower extremities

phlebography required to confirm diagnosis

Friedman EI, Taylor LM Jr, Porter JM. Congenital venous valvular aplasia of the lower extremities. Surgery 1988;103:24–26

Hereditary Disorders of Red Blood Cells

There are a group of congenital hemolytic anemias due to abnormalities in the red blood cells that may be associated with leg ulcers without accompanying venous or lymphatic disease. Some of these disorders are listed below.

- *hereditary spherocytosis (familial hemolytic anemia)*

  leg ulcers, usually developing in adulthood, uncommonly in adolescence

  AD

- *hereditary elliptocytosis*

  leg ulcers occasionally

  AD

- *hereditary nonspherocytic hemolytic anemia*

  leg ulcers occasionally

  AR

- *sickle cell anemia*

  indolent, slow or nonhealing ulcers on shins commonly

  AR

- *thalassemia*

  indolent, slow or nonhealing ulcers on shins

  AR

McK 182900, 182870

Agre P, Asimos A, Casella JF, McMillan C. Inheritance pattern and clinical response to splenectomy as a reflection of erythrocyte spectrin deficiency in hereditary spherocytosis. N Engl J Med 1986;315:1579–1583

Bannerman RM, Renwick JH. The hereditary elliptocytoses: clinical and linkage data. Ann Hum Genet 1962;26:23–38

Gabuzda TG. Sickle cell leg ulcers: current pathophysiologic concepts. Int J Dermatol 1975;14:322–325

Lawrence P, Aronson I, Saxe N, Jacobs P. Leg ulcers in hereditary spherocytosis. Clin Exp Dermatol 1991;16:28–30

Vascular Tumors and Malformations

HEREDITARY HEMORRHAGIC TELANGIECTASIA

Synonym

- Osler-Weber-Rendu syndrome

Skin

telangiectases of skin and mucous membranes, with first manifestations usually being frequent epistaxis in childhood and visible telangiectases in adolescence

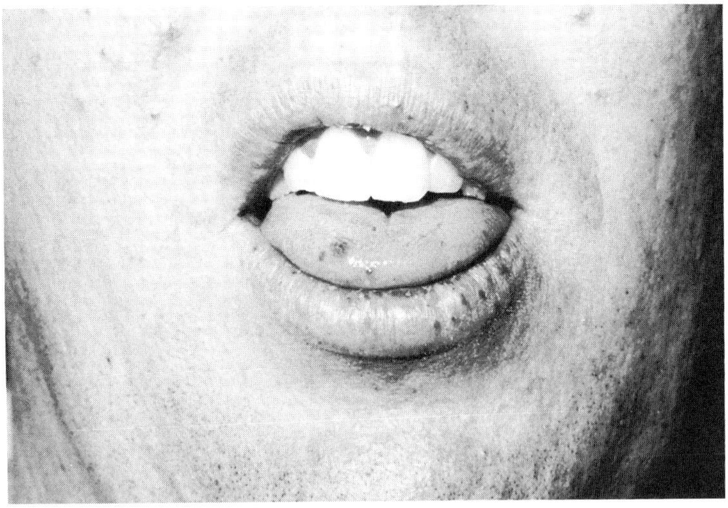

FIGURE 13–2
Multiple papular telangiectases on the tongue, lips, and face of this man with hereditary hemorrhagic telangiectasia.

commonly involved sites include the oral cavity, nasal septum, face, acral areas (e.g., ears, tips of fingers and nail beds), chest, and arms (Figs. 13–2 and 13–3)

tongue characteristically shows dilated capillaries within fungiform papilla

telangiectases increase during third and fourth decades and are usually punctate or linear, less commonly nodular; rarely they develop a stellate or spider-like appearance

increased incidence of epistaxis and telangiectases during pregnancy

occasional clubbing of digits

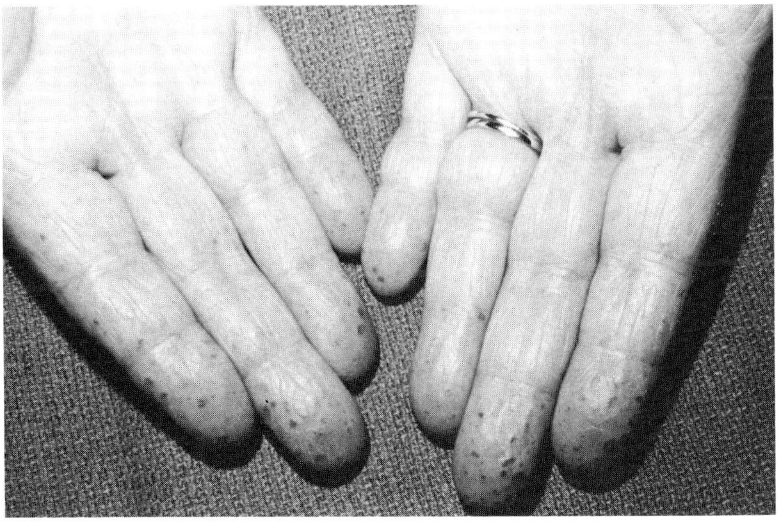

FIGURE 13–3
Numerous telangiectatic papules on the fingertips of the same patient as in Figure 13–2. (Courtesy of Benjamin K. Fisher, MD, Toronto, Ontario)

Non-Skin

multiple pulmonary arteriovenous fistulae (hereditary hemorrhagic telangiectasia is the most common cause of this lesion); septic emboli from these foci are a major cause of morbidity and mortality

telangiectases of the gastrointestinal and genitourinary tracts as well as lungs, brain, conjunctivae, and retinae

aneurysms of other vessels, aortic arch, and splenic artery occasionally

significant hemorrhage may occur from mucosal lesions; skin lesions seldom bleed

Genetics

AD

less common in darker-skinned races

Laboratory Data

bleeding and clotting studies are usually normal, but abnormalities of coagulation similar to von Willebrand disease have been documented

Prognosis

overall, the life span is not shortened, except in the 4% who die of hemorrhage (especially intracranial or spinal) or high-output cardiac failure due to pulmonary arteriovenous fistulae

intra-arterial balloon embolization of pulmonary arteriovenous malformations has been successful

Discussion

cutaneous telangiectases not always present

- *generalized essential telangiectasia*

  onset of telangiectases in late childhood or early adulthood, usually linear and most commonly on the extremities

  recurrent hemorrhages from skin or mucous membranes may occur and be misdiagnosed as atypical hereditary hemorrhagic telangiectasia

  acquired

REFERENCES

McK 187300

Bean WB. Vascular Spiders and Related Lesions of the Skin. Springfield, IL, Charles C Thomas, 1958

Buillen B, Guizar J, De La Cruz J, Salamanca F. Hereditary hemorrhagic telangiectasia: report of 15 affected cases in a Mexican family. Clin Genet 1991;39:214–218

Cox KL, Frates RC Jr, Wong A, Gandhi G. Hereditary generalized juvenile polyposis associated with pulmonary arteriovenous malformation. Gastroenterology 1980; 78:1566–1570

Hodgson CH, Burchell HB, Good CA, Clagett OT. Hereditary hemorrhagic telangiectasia and pulmonary arteriovenous fistula. N Engl J Med 1959;261:625–636

Porteous MEM, Burn J, Proctor SJ. Hereditary haemorrhagic telangiectasia: a clinical analysis. J Med Genet 1992;29:527–530
Press OW, Ramsey PG. Central nervous system infections associated with hereditary hemorrhagic telangiectasia. Am J Med 1984;77:86–92
Reilly PJ, Nostrant TT. Clinical manifestation of hereditary hemorrhagic telangiectasia. Am J Gastroenterol 1984;79:363–367

HEREDITARY BENIGN TELANGIECTASIA

Skin

telangiectases, usually spider-like, of vermilion border of lips, neck, trunk (Color Fig. 13–1), forearms, dorsal hands, and knees; begins in childhood

Non-Skin

lesions do not involve viscera, and hemorrhagic complications not seen

Genetics

AD

REFERENCES

McK 187260
Gold MH, Eramo L, Prendiville JS. Hereditary benign telangiectasia. Pediatr Dermatol 1989;6:194–197
Ryan TJ, Wells RS. Hereditary benign telangiectasia. Trans St John's Hosp Dermatol Soc 1971;57:148–156

HEREDITARY PHLEBECTASIA OF THE LIPS

swelling of the lower lip and varicosities; onset after age 40 years

AD

McK 171450
Reed WB. Hereditary phlebectasia of the lips. Arch Dermatol 1976;112:712–714

ANGIOMA SERPIGINOSUM

asymptomatic, 1-mm bright red to purple punctate lesions arranged in annular or serpiginous patterns; groups of lesions spread peripherally with central clearing initially present on lower limbs and buttocks unilaterally, but may spread to other areas except for mucous membranes and rarely palms and soles

diffuse or reticulate backround erythema may be seen, but no purpura

usually involves females, beginning in late childhood or adolescence

disease is progressive over months to a few years, and further spread occasionally occurs in adulthood

mostly sporadic; possible AD cases reported

McK 106050

Marriott PJ, Munro DD, Ryan T. Angioma serpiginosum—familial incidence. Br J Dermatol 1975;93:701–706

BLUE RUBBER BLEB NEVUS SYNDROME

Skin

soft, compressible, rubbery, tender bluish 0.1- to 5.0-cm nodules, representing venous malformations; usually on trunk or upper arms (Color Fig. 13–2)

onset at birth or during childhood, very rarely during adulthood

nodules can be blanched with pressure, temporarily leaving a folded, nipple-like sac

number of lesions ranges from one to numerous; lesions do not involute

spontaneous nocturnal pain associated with hyperhidrosis of lesions (usually not manifest until puberty)

characteristic blue nodular lesions on and under tongue

Non-Skin

venous malformations of gastrointestinal mucosa, especially small intestine; bleeding (e.g., hematemesis and melena) may result in anemia or shock; may not manifest until adulthood

may have venous malformations in central nervous system, liver, spleen, heart, lungs, urinary tract, muscles, and joints

Genetics

AD; many sporadic cases

Prognosis

complications mostly occurring after first decade include anemia (from bleeding of visceral lesions especially gastrointestinal) and consumption coagulopathy

Discussion

the term *blue rubber bleb nevus syndrome* may be misleading; patients with this syndrome may have cutaneous vascular malformations with gastrointestinal lesions and bleeding without having bluish compressible lesions

REFERENCES

McK 112200
Fretzin DG, Potter B. Blue rubber bleb nevus. Arch Dermatol 1965;116:924–929
Munkvad M. Blue rubber bleb nevus syndrome. Dermatologica 1983;167:307–309
Oranje AP. Blue rubber bleb nevus syndrome. Pediatr Dermatol 1986;3:304–310
Rice JS, Fisher DS. Blue rubber bleb nevus syndrome. Arch Dermatol. 1962;86:503–511
Sumi Y, Taguchi N, Kaneda T. Blue rubber bleb nevus syndrome with oral hemangiomas. Oral Surg 1991;71:84–86

MULTIPLE GLOMUS TUMORS

Synonym

- glomangioma

Skin

generally nontender, bluish 0.5- to 4.0-cm nodules, present at birth or within the first 2 decades of life

lesions are usually distributed regionally, but there is no particular site predilection; occasionally, lesions generalized

no malignant potential reported

Non-Skin

rarely hypoplasia and osteoporosis of affected extremity

Genetics

AD

Pathophysiology

benign hyperplasia of Suquet-Hoyer canal (arteriovenous anastomosis)

Discussion

solitary glomus tumors are usually tender and of adult onset (later than in multiple glomus tumors); usually on extremities, especially subungually; acquired

REFERENCES

McK 138000

Beasley SW, Mel J, Chow CW, Jones PG. Hereditary multiple glomus tumours. Arch Dis Child 1986;61:801–802

Nishimoto K, Nishimoto M, Yamamoto S, et al. Multiple glomus tumors: successful treatment with electron-beam irradiation. Br J Dermatol 1990;123:657–661

Rycroft RJG, Menter MA, Sharvill DE, et al. Hereditary multiple glomus tumours: report of four families and a review of literature. Trans St John's Hosp Dermatol Soc 1975;61:70–81

VON HIPPEL-LINDAU SYNDROME (HEMANGIOBLASTOMA OF CEREBELLUM AND RETINA)

occasional port wine stains of face or occipitocervical region (5%)

retinal angiomas in up to half; may result in blindness if not treated

cerebellar, medullary (medulla oblongata), or spinal hemangioblastoma

pheochromocytoma, usually bilateral, in some kindreds

renal cell carcinoma in about one fourth of patients

other reported findings include polycythemia, polycystic disease of numerous organs including pancreas and kidneys, and vascular lesions of the adrenal glands, lungs, and liver

occasional seizures and mental retardation

AD

hypertension and cerebellar hemangioblastomas may lead to subarachnoid hemorrhage

McK 193300

Horton WA, Wong V, Eldridge R. von Hippel-Lindau disease. Arch Intern Med 1976; 136:769–777

Jennings AM, Smith C, Cole DR, et al. Von Hippel-Lindau disease in a large British family: clinicopathological features and recommendations for screening and follow-up. Q J Med 1988;66:233–249

Lamiell JM, Salazar FG, Hsia YE. Von Hippel-Lindau disease affecting 43 members of a single kindred. Medicine 1989;68:1–29

Melmon KL, Rosen SW. Lindau's disease review of the literature and study of a large kindred. Am J Med 1964;36:595–617

Nonhereditary Congenital Vascular Disorders

There are a number of vascular disorders that are erroneously perceived as genetic in etiology. This confusion may be perpetuated by rare case reports of familial occurrence. Although these conditions are not hereditary in the vast majority of cases, genetic counseling is often sought by families in which there is one afflicted member. For this reason, we have included these disorders in a subsection of this chapter but wish to emphasize that we believe these conditions to be sporadic rather than heritable.

CUTIS MARMORATA TELANGIECTATICA CONGENITA

Synonyms

- reticulate vascular nevus
- congenital phlebectasia

Skin

fixed, flat, reticulated blue-violet cutaneous vascular malformations, venous and capillary, sometimes with telangiectases, most commonly on limbs (Fig. 13–4); frequent underlying subcutaneous atrophy

onset at birth

distribution usually asymmetrical, segmental, or unilateral

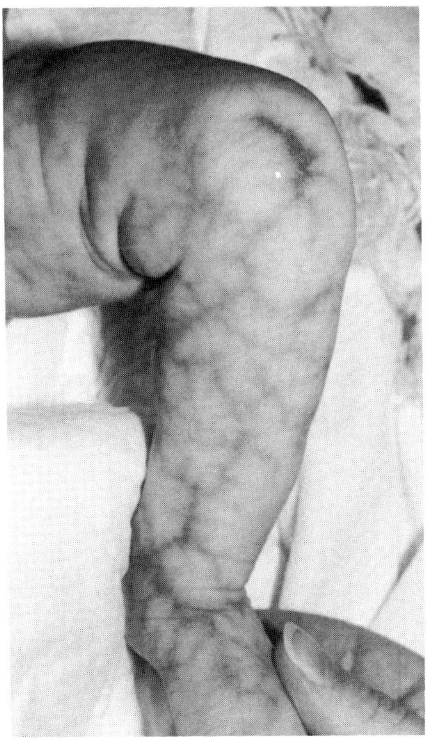

FIGURE 13–4
Cutis marmorata telangiectatica congenita. Reticulated red-purple bands representing dilated vessels involving the thigh, lower leg, and foot of this newborn. This syndrome is not hereditary.

lesions may be large; occasionally the face may be involved

may have atrophic areas or linear erosions of affected skin

occasional associated port wine stains

Non-Skin

associated abnormalities, usually minor, reported in about 50% of patients

atrophy or hypertrophy of the affected limb is the most frequent associated finding; rarely facial hemiatrophy

musculoskeletal abnormalities include short stature and syndactyly of toes and short fingers

craniofacial abnormalities include micrognathia, a triangular face, high-arched palate, and asymmetrical skull shape

increased incidence of congenital glaucoma, especially if a facial nevus flammeus is associated; if diffuse, glaucoma may be bilateral

Genetics

mostly sporadic

male to female ratio: 1:2

Prognosis

gradual spontaneous improvement (most rapid in first year) of vascular abnormalities

ophthalmologic examination is indicated in patients with an associated facial port wine stain

Discussion

some argue the high incidence of associated abnormalities is due to biased reporting

cutis marmorata (livedo reticularis) is a physiologic response to cold in infants

REFERENCES

McK 219250

Del Giudice SM, Nydorf ED. Cutis marmorata telangiectatica congenita with multiple congenital anomalies. Arch Dermatol 1986; 122:1060–1061

Kurczynski TW. Hereditary cutis marmorata telangiectatica congenita. Pediatrics 1982; 70:52–53

Picascia DD, Esterly NB. Cutis marmorata telangiectatica congenita: report of 22 cases. J Am Acad Dermatol 1989;20:1098–1104

MAFFUCCI SYNDROME

Synonyms

- dyschondroplasia with hemangiomatosis
- Ollier disease with hemangiomatosis

Skin

bluish, vascular nodules (venous malformations) appearing at birth or in early life on fingers and toes

lymphangiomas may occur concurrently or even as the only cutaneous finding

Non-Skin

multiple enchondromas and exostoses involve the metaphyses of long bones and hands and feet; develop simultaneously with cutaneous lesions

enchondromas may result in pathologic fractures or disrupt epiphyseal cartilage

fractures and disruption of normal tissue by enchondromas result in bending and shortening of long bones of hands, feet, and extremities, asymmetrical growth rates and other grotesque skeletal deformities

various benign and malignant ovarian tumors may develop

visceral vascular malformations reported

Genetics

sporadic

Laboratory Data

enchondromas are radiolucent

phlebectasias may be seen in lymphangiograms

Prognosis

vascular lesions do not resolve

20% develop malignancies including chondrosarcomas and, more rarely, angiosarcomas, malignant lymphangiomas, and gliomas

Discussion

- *Ollier disease*

  enchondromatosis without cutaneous findings, with development of chondrosarcomas in some lesions

  rare reports of visceral vascular lesions or nonmesodermal tumors in association with Ollier disease have led some to speculate that it forms a continuum with Maffucci syndrome

REFERENCES

McK 166000

Anderson IF. Maffucci's syndrome. S Afr Med J 1965;39:1066–1070

Loweinger RJ, Lichtenstein JR, Dodson WE, Eisen AZ. Maffucci's syndrome: a mesenchymal dysplasia and multiple tumour syndrome. Br J Dermatol 1977;96:317–322

Mellon CD, Carter JE, Owen DB. Ollier's disease and Maffuci's syndrome: distinct entities or a continuum. J Neurol 1988; 235:376–378

KLIPPEL-TRENAUNAY AND PARKES WEBER SYNDROMES

These syndromes are often grouped under the designation of Klippel-Trenaunay-Weber syndrome. They share sporadic occurrence and the following triad of findings, which involve the lower extremities more frequently than the upper, and the trunk and head less commonly (Fig. 13–5):

cutaneous vascular malformation, usually capillary (port wine stain) but sometimes angiokeratoma-like lesion

congenital venous varicosities, usually not apparent until later in childhood

hypertrophy of soft tissue and/or bone

Separation of the Klippel-Trenaunay-Weber syndrome into Klippel-Trenaunay and Parkes Weber syndromes is supported by the following differences:

- *Klippel-Trenaunay syndrome*

concomitant lymphatic abnormalities, particularly hypoplastic lymphatics

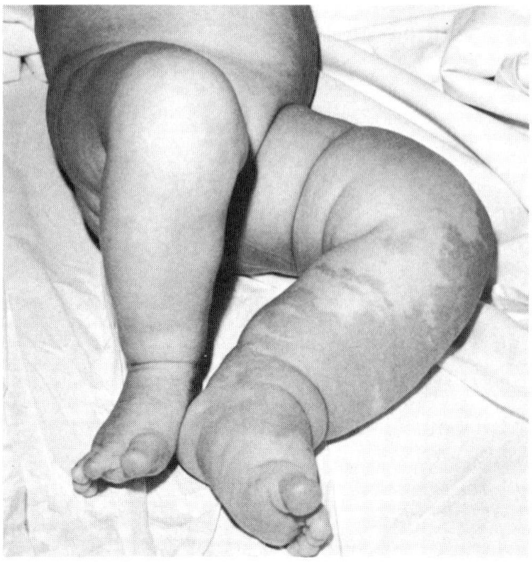

FIGURE 13–5
Klippel-Trenaunay syndrome. Soft tissue and skeletal hypertrophy in association with a port wine stain of the left lower limb. The venous varicosities are not apparent at this age. This syndrome is not hereditary.

lateral venous anomaly and atresia/hypoplasia of deep veins

good prognosis with stabilization after childhood

disproportionate gigantism; macrodactyly common

usually minor lengthening of limb

common associated anomalies

- *Parkes Weber syndrome*

arteriovenous fistula

marked lengthening of limb; pain and swelling of involved limb moderately common

progressive and unstable ulceration and hemorrhage

McK 149000

Aelvoet GE, Jorens PG, Roelen LM. Genetic aspects of the Klippel-Trenaunay syndrome. Br J Dermatol 1992;126:603–607

Happle R. Lethal genes surviving by mosaicism: a possible explanation for sporadic birth defects involving the skin. J Am Acad Dermatol 1987;16:899–906

Mulliken JB, Young AE, eds. Vascular Birthmarks: Hemangiomas and Malformations. Philadelphia, WB Saunders, 1988

Viljoen D, Saxe N, Pearn J, Beighton P. The cutaneous manifestations of the Klippel-Trenaunay-Weber syndrome. Clin Exp Dermatol 1987;12:12–17

STURGE-WEBER SYNDROME

Synonyms

- Sturge-Weber-Dimitri syndrome
- encephalotrigeminal angiomatosis
- encephalofacial angiomatosis

Skin

cutaneous capillary malformations (port wine stain), present at birth; often unilateral, usually following distribution of the ophthalmic and maxillary branches (V1, V2) of trigeminal nerve but may involve skin innervated by all branches of the trigeminal nerve and other nerves (Fig. 13–6)

may be bilateral or even involve the neck, trunk, or limbs

oral involvment of lips, tongue, nasal and buccal mucosa and maxillary gingiva in up to a third of cases; usually stops at midline

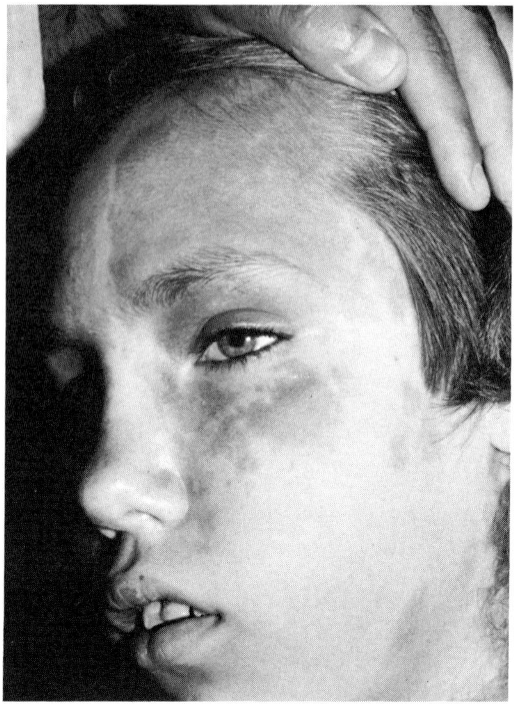

FIGURE 13–6
Bilateral port wine stain (involving skin innervated by the first and second branches of the sensory portion of the trigeminal nerve) in a patient with Sturge-Weber syndrome. This syndrome is not hereditary.

Non-Skin

neurologic findings include vascular malformation of cerebral meninges and calcification of subjacent cortex ipsilateral to port wine stain, usually detectable radiographically by late childhood but earlier by computed tomography scan (double-contoured curvilinear "tram tracks")

epilepsy in most, usually focal motor (contralateral to vascular malformation and less frequently generalized); onset in early infancy or childhood

many cases of mental retardation and contralateral hemiplegia reported

may find capillary malformation of the conjunctiva, iris, and choroid ("tomato catsup" fundus) ipsilateral to the port wine stain; other ocular findings include congenital glaucoma (buphthalmos) and megalocornea; may sustain retinal detachment with progression to blindness

visceral vascular malformations occasionally

hypertrophy of soft tissues and bone underlying port wine stain

Genetics

sporadic

Prognosis

prognosis variable and mostly dependent on extent of cerebral lesions

treatment of the seizure disorder is especially important to avoid further neurologic deficit

REFERENCES

McK 185300
Enjolras O, Riche MC, Merland JJ. Facial port-wine stains and Sturge-Weber syndrome. Pediatrics 1985;76:48–51
Paller AS. The Sturge-Weber syndrome. [Review]. Pediatr Dermatol 1987;4:300–304

Vascular and Hematologic Disorders—Abbreviated Entries

FAMILIAL NEVUS FLAMMEUS (FAMILIAL PORT WINE STAIN)

port wine stains, single or multiple, most often on glabella (Color Fig. 13–3)

AD

McK 163000
Merlob P, Reisner SH. Familial nevus flammeus of the forehead and Unna's nevus. Clin Genet 1985;27:165–166
Pasyk KA. Familial multiple lateral telangiectatic nevi (port wine stains or nevi flammei). Clin Genet 1992;41:197–201
Selmanowitz VJ. Nevus flammeus of the forehead. J Pediatr 1968;73:755
Shelley WB, Livingood CS. Familial multiple nevi flammei. Arch Dermatol Syphilol 1949;59:343–345
Shuper A, Merlob P, Garty B, Varsano I. Familial multiple naevi flammei. J Med Genet 1984;21:112–113

ERYTHEMA PALMARE HEREDITARIUM (LANE DISEASE)

bright erythema on thenar and hypothenar eminences, distal palm, and tips of terminal phalanges

onset in childhood

triangular area in center of palm is spared

rarely, soles are involved, usually to a milder degree

probable AD

McK 133000
Lane JE. Erythema palmare hereditarium. Arch Dermatol Syphilol 1929;20:445–448

ERYTHEMA OF ACRAL REGIONS

red papules and plaques on ears and distal extremities in infancy

dental abnormalities

clubfoot

probable AR

REFERENCES

McK 227000
Bryan HG, Coskey RJ. Familial erythema of acral regions. Arch Dermatol 1967;95:483–486

FAMILIAL ANNULAR ERYTHEMA

pruritic, erythematous urticarial plaques; anywhere on body

lesions evolve in 4- to 5-day cycles; enlarge, clear centrally, then disappear

onset varies from shortly after birth to adolescence

dermatographism

AD

McK 106500
Beare JM, Froggatt P, Jones JH, Neill DW. Familial annular erythema, an apparently new dominant mutation. Br J Dermatol 1966;78:59–68

ERYTHROMELALGIA

mostly sporadic; AD reported

McK 133020
Finley WH, Lindsey JR Jr, Fine JD, et al. Autosomal dominant erythromelalgia. Am J Med Genet 1992;42:310–315

HEREDITARY NEUROCUTANEOUS ANGIOMA

scattered circumscribed cutaneous vascular lesions, probably malformations

cerebrospinal arteriovenous malformations

neurologic sequelae with onset from infancy to adulthood include hemiparesis and epilepsy

AD

McK 106070
Hurst J, Baraitser M. Hereditary neurocutaneous angiomatous malformations: autosomal dominant inheritance in two families. Clin Genet 1988;33:44–48

CORTICOMENINGEAL ANGIOMATOSIS

prominent livedo reticularis on trunk and extremities from birth

leptomeningeal angiomatosis leads to abnormalities including headaches, visual field defects, epilepsy, and progressive dementia

probable AR

McK 206570
Divry P, Van Bogaert L. Une maladie familiale caracterisée par une angiomatose diffuse cortico-meningée noncalcificante et une demyelinisation progressive de la substance blanche. J Neurol Neurosurg Psychiatry 1946;64:1042–1063
Martin JJ, Navarro C, Roussel JM, Michielssen P. Familial capillarovenous leptomeningeal angiomatosis. Eur Neurol 1973;9:202–215

SNEDDON SYNDROME (LIVEDO RETICULARIS AND CEREBROVASCULAR ACCIDENTS)

AD reported but mostly sporadic

McK 182410
Berciano J. Sneddon syndrome: another mendelian etiology of stroke. [Letter]. Ann Neurol 1988;24:586–587
Bruyn RPM, van der Veen JPW, Donker AJM, Valk J, Wolters EC. Sneddon's syndrome: case report and literature review. J Neurol Sci 1987;79:243–253.
Sneddon IB. Cerebrovascular lesions and livedo reticularis. Br J Dermatol 1965; 77:180–185.

HEREDITARY ACROLABIAL TELANGIECTASIA

bluish discoloration of lips, areolae, and nail beds in first year of life

telangiectases of dorsa of hands, chest, and elbows

AD

Millns JL, Dicken CH. Hereditary acrolabial telangiectasia: a report of familial blue lips, nails, and nipples. Arch Dermatol 1979;115:474–478

TELANGIECTASES, SPONDYLOEPIPHYSEAL DYSPLASIA, HYPOTHYROIDISM, NEOVASCULARIZATION, AND TRACTIONAL RETINAL DETACHMENTS

possible AR

Lavin MP, Olson JC, Ruttum MS, et al. Two sisters with telangiectases, spondyloepiphyseal dysplasia, hypothyroidism, neovascularization, and tractional retinal detachments: a new entity? Pediatr Dermatol 1989;6:178–184; published erratum appears in Pediatr Dermatol 1989;6:360

CONGENITAL LYMPHEDEMA, HYPOPARATHYROIDISM, NEPHROPATHY, PROLAPSING MITRAL VALVE, AND BRACHYTELEPHALANGY

lymphedema of upper and lower extremities with onset in early infancy; worsens with ambulation inheritance unclear; XLR vs AR

McK 247410

Dahlberg PJ, Borer WZ, Newcomer KI, Yutuc WR. Autosomal or X-linked recessive syndrome of congenital lymphedema, hypoparathyroidism, nephropathy, prolapsing mitral valve, and brachytelephalangy. Am J Med Genet 1983;16:99–104

HENNEKAM LYMPHANGIECTASIA-LYMPHEDEMA SYNDROME

lymphedema of face, extremities, and genitals

severe mental retardation

intestinal lymphangiectasia

craniofacial abnormalities

probable AR

McK 235510
Gabrielli O, Catassi C, Carlucci A, Coppa GV, Giorgi P. Intestinal lymphangiectasia, lymphedema, mental retardation, and typical face: confirmation of the Hennekam syndrome. Am J Med Genet 1991;40:244–247
Hennekam RCM, Geerdink RA, Hamel BCJ, et al. Autosomal recessive intestinal lymphangiectasia and lymphedema, with facial anomalies and mental retardation. Am J Med Genet 1989;34:593–600

LYMPHEDEMA AND CEREBRAL ARTERIOVENOUS ANOMALY

AD

McK 152900
Avasthey P, Roy SB. Primary pulmonary hypertension, cerebrovascular malformation, and lymphoedema feet in a family. Brit Heart J 1968;30:769–775

LYMPHEDEMA AND MICROCEPHALY

AD

McK 152950
Leung AKC. Dominantly inherited syndrome of microcephaly and congenital lymphedema. Clin Genet 1985;27:611–612

LYMPHEDEMA AND PTOSIS

AD

lymphedema and ptosis also occurs in the Noonan syndrome

McK 153000
Bloom D. Hereditary lymphedema (Nonne-Milroy-Meige): report of a family with hereditary lymphedema associated with ptosis of the eyelids in several generations. NY J Med 1941;41:856–863

CHOLESTASIS-LYMPHEDEMA SYNDROME (AAGENAES SYNDROME)

probable AR

McK 214900
Aagenaes O, Sigstad H, Bjorn-Hansen R. Lymphoedema in hereditary recurrent cholestasis from birth. Arch Dis Child 1970;45:690–695
Aagenaes O. Hereditary recurrent cholestasis with lymphoedema—two new families. Acta Paediatr Scand 1974;63:465–471

FAMILIAL NEVUS ANEMICUS

usually sporadic; AD reported

McK 163050
Cardaso H, Vignale R, Abreu de Sastre H. Familial naevus anemicus. [Abstract]. Am J Hum Genet 1975;27:24A

CHAPTER

14

Immunodeficiency Disorders

The immunodeficiency diseases are a complex group of disorders that are rarely diagnosed by their cutaneous manifestations. Indeed, these disorders share a proclivity for a variety of mucocutaneous skin changes as well as recurrent cutaneous infections caused by all types of organisms. These nonspecific features point the clinician in the right direction but are almost never helpful in arriving at a precise diagnosis. Immunologic investigations are invariably required to sort out these entities; likewise, management is difficult, is not always successful, and requires the input of an immunologist.

CHRONIC GRANULOMATOUS DISEASE

Skin

recurrent bacterial and fungal infections and chronic dermatitis; usual onset by 1 year of age

dermatitis, a common presenting sign, often involves scalp, face, and/or postauricular region

furunculosis, subcutaneous abscesses, recurrent ulcerative stomatitis, and suppurative lymphadenopathy are frequent findings

severely impaired wound healing

Non-Skin

persistent fever and failure to thrive

recurrent bacterial and fungal infections develop in lungs, lymph nodes, liver, and/or bone; numerous other sites affected less frequently

chronic rhinitis

ocular abnormalities include conjunctivitis and, less commonly, destructive chorioretinal disease

hepatosplenomegaly

Genetics

XLR in about two thirds, AR in one third

male to female ratio: 9:1

Pathophysiology

this is a heterogenous group of disorders associated with inability of neutrophils to kill certain organisms, particularly catalase-positive bacteria and fungi, most commonly, *Staphylococcus aureus*, enteric bacteria, *Candida albicans*, and *Aspergillus* species

neutrophils unable to generate superoxide anion and other reactive oxygen species

XLR-inherited form associated with absence of cytochrome b, a membrane-associated component of the NADPH oxidase system

some X-linked inherited cases do not have decreased cytochrome b activity, suggesting that another defect is operative

additionally, autosomally inherited forms may show normal membrane oxidase components but have defective functional cytosolic activity due to the absence of cytosolic proteins (molecular weights of 47 and 67 kd) required for oxidase activation

other biochemical abnormalities include abnormal flavoproteins, low affinity NADPH oxidase, and deficiency of glucose-6-phosphate dehydrogenase

Laboratory Data

leukocytosis and hypergammaglobulinemia

neutrophils have impaired ability to reduce nitroblue tetrazolium dye due to absence of oxidative burst; this is a screening test while confirmation requires neutrophil chemiluminescence or quantitative bactericidal assays

prenatal diagnosis possible

Prognosis

immunodeficiency worsens with age

death usually occurs in late first or early second decade, but longer survival as well as later onset of disease have been reported

subcutaneous gamma-interferon may be beneficial (corrects defective respiratory burst) prompt and adequate treatment of infection and sequelae improves prognosis and length of disease-free intervals

sulfonamide antibiotics may be especially beneficial

Discussion

clinical severity and age at onset vary

genetic heterogeneity for the chronic granulomatous phenotype produced by familial deficiencies of myeloperoxidase and glucose-6-phosphate dehydrogenase

- *female carriers of chronic granulomatous disease*

have diminished ability to reduce nitroblue tetrazolium dye, but not as severely as in homozygous individuals

severe bacterial infections not seen

may develop photosensitivity, severe aphthous stomatitis, and/or cutaneous lesions resembling discoid lupus erythematosus, Jessner's lymphocytic infiltrate, or erythema annulare centrifugum

cutaneous eruption is a distinct entity deserving its own designation (e.g., "chronic granulomatous disease carrier dermatosis")

REFERENCES

McK 306400

McK 233690; McK 233700; McK 233710; McK 138990 (AD type)

Clark RA, Malech HL, Gallin JI, et al. Genetic variants of chronic granulomatous disease: prevalence of deficiencies of two cytosolic components of the NADPH oxidase system. N Engl J Med 1989;321:647–652

Ezekowitz RAB, Dinauer MC, Jaffe HS, Orkin SH. Partial correction of the phagocyte defect in patients with X-linked chronic granulomatous disease by subcutaneous interferon gamma. N Engl J Med 1988;319:146–151

Finn A, Morgan NHG, Strobel S, Levinsky RJ. Prognosis of chronic granulomatous disease. Arch Dis Child 1990;65:942–945

Garioch JJ, Sampson JR, Seywright M, Thomson J. Dermatoses in five related female carriers of X-linked chronic granulomatous disease. Br J Dermatol 1989;121:391–396

Hitzig WH, Seger RA. Chronic granulomatous disease, a heterogeneous syndrome. Hum Genet 1983;64:207–215

Schapiro BL, Newburger PE, Klempner MS, Dinauer MC. Chronic granulomatous disease presenting in a 69-year-old man. N Engl J Med 1991;325:1786–1790

Tauber AI, Borregaard N, Simons E, Wright J. Chronic granulomatous disease: a syndrome of phagocyte oxidase deficiencies. Medicine 1983;62:286–309

Yeaman GR, Froebel K, Galea G, Ormerod A, Urbaniak SJ. Discoid lupus erythematosus in an X-linked cytochrome positive carrier of chronic granulomatous disease. Br J Dermatol 1992;126:60–65

HYPERIMMUNOGLOBULINEMIA-E SYNDROME

Synonyms

- staphylococcal abscess syndrome
- Buckley syndrome
- Hill-Quie syndrome
- Job syndrome

Skin

recurrent pyogenic infections of skin and large to massive abscesses without warmth, tenderness, or erythema ("cold abscesses"); irregular scarring may result

occasional recurrent urticaria, mucocutaneous candidiasis, and other fungal infections

chronic atopic-like dermatitis or papulopustular eruption of scalp and flexures including neck, axillae, and groin (Fig. 14–1)

dystrophic nails

Non-Skin

recurrent pyogenic sinopulmonary infections, sometimes resulting in pneumatoceles in which *Aspergillus* organisms are found

absence of fever in presence of major abscesses

distinctive, coarse craniofacies include broad nasal bridge, bulbous nose, and irregular facial scars from previous infections

hyperextensible joints in some

Genetics

mostly sporadic, but familial cases reported, which are probably AD with incomplete penetrance

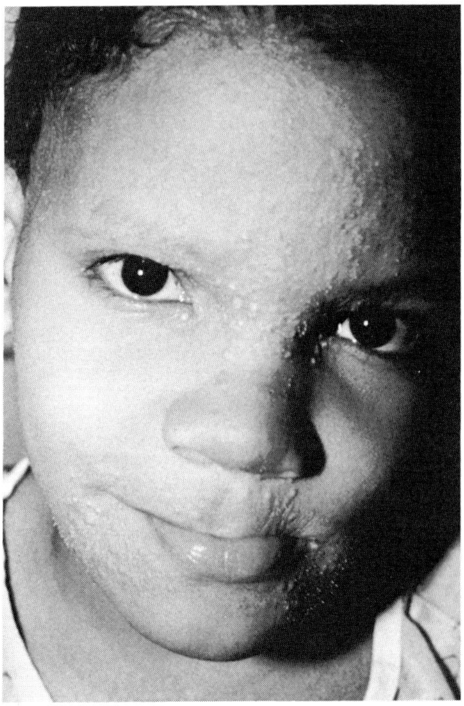

FIGURE 14–1
Young boy with a chronic recalcitrant eczematous dermatitis involving the face, with extremely high serum IgE levels, and with the "coarse facies" of hyperimmunoglobulinemia-E syndrome.

Laboratory Data

extreme elevation in serum IgE with high levels of antistaphylococcal IgE is characteristic

deficient salivary and serum antistaphylococcal IgA

eosinophilia

often impairment of neutrophil and monocyte chemotaxis

T-cell defects

Discussion

laboratory abnormalities, such as hyperimmunoglobulinemia-E, may not be present in first year of life

a history of recurrent sinopulmonary and cutaneous infections and deep abscesses is essential for the diagnosis of hyperimmunogloublinemia-E syndrome; many children with dermatitis, recurrent skin infections, and elevated levels of IgE simply have severe secondarily infected atopic dermatitis

patients in initial case reports of Job syndrome were red-haired girls, but the majority of subsequent reports are not limited to this group

REFERENCES

McK 147060; 243700

Donabedian H, Gallin JI. The hyperimmunoglobulin E recurrent infection (Job's) syndrome: a review of the NIH experience and the literature. Medicine 1983;62:195–208

Dreskin SC, Gallin JI. Evolution of the hyperimmunoglobulin E and recurrent infection (HIE, Job's) syndrome in a young girl. J Allergy Clin Immunol 1987;80:746–751

Dreskin SC, Goldsmith PK, Gallin JI. Immunoglobulins in the hyperimmunoglobulin E and recurrent infection (Job's) syndrome. J Clin Invest 1985;75:26–34

Kamei R, Honig PJ. Neonatal Job's syndrome featuring a vesicular eruption. Pediatr Dermatol 1988;5:75–82

Lavoie A, Rottem M, Grodofsky MP, Douglas SD. Anti–*Staphylococcus aureus* IgE antibodies for diagnosis of hyperimmunoglobulinemia-E recurrent infection syndrome in infancy. Am J Dis Child 1989;143:1038–1041

Leung DYM, Geha RS. Clinical and immunologic aspects of the hyperimmunoglobulin E syndrome. Hematol Oncol Clin North Am 1988;2:81–100

Mucocutaneous Candidiasis

Candidial infection of the skin or mucous membranes is seen in a variety of immunodeficiencies. *Chronic mucocutaneous candidiasis* (CMC) is a term used to describe persistent candidal infection of the mucous membranes, skin, and nails that is only partially responsive to therapy. Clinical findings include the following:

widespread erythematous, hyperkeratotic, annular or serpiginous plaques of the skin, especially flexures, face, scalp, and hands

marked hyperkeratotic and nodular lesions, which have been referred to as "*Candida* granuloma"

persistent oral thrush and, in females, vulvovaginitis

paronychia and nail dystrophy; may be marked

There are a small but heterogeneous group of diseases in which CMC is the predominant feature. Immunologic abnormalities occurring in this group of patients are not well defined and may be temporarily reversed with therapy. There is considerable clinical overlap among these diseases, but features that help to distinguish them, though not invariably, are listed under specific diseases, which follow this entry.

CMC is seen as a variable and often minor component of well-defined immunodeficiency disorders, including severe combined immunodeficiency (and its individual causes), selective IgA deficiency, IgG subclass deficiency, congenital thymic aplasia, myeloperoxidase deficiency, and multiple carboxylase deficiency. Some of these disorders are described elsewhere in the text.

Hay RJ, Roberts SOB, Mackenzie DWR. Chronic mucocutaneous candidiasis. In: Champion RH, Burton JL, Ebling FJG, eds. Textbook of Dermatology. Oxford, Blackwell Scientific Publications, 1992:1191–1193

Hebert AA, Esterly NB. Bacterial and candidal cutaneous infections in the neonate. Dermatol Clin 1986;4:1–21

Jorizzo JL. Chronic mucocutaneous candidosis: an update. Arch Dermatol 1982;118:963–965

Kirkpatrick CH, Rich RB, Bennett JE. Chronic mucocutaneous candidiasis: model building in cellular immunology. Ann Intern Med 1971;74:955–978

Ro BI. Chronic mucocutaneous candidosis. Int J Dermatol 1988;27:457–462

CHRONIC MUCOCUTANEOUS CANDIDIASIS WITH ENDOCRINOPATHY (POLYGLANDULAR AUTOIMMUNE SYNDROME TYPE I; AUTOIMMUNE POLYENDOCRINOPATHY CANDIDOSIS–ECTODERMAL DYSTROPHY [APECED])

see Figures 14–2 and 14–3

CMC in early childhood

broad clinical spectrum; mucocutaneous findings may occur years before endocrine abnormalities

occasional alopecia totalis and/or vitiligo

occasional dental enamel hypoplasia

endocrinopathies, most commonly, hypoparathyroidism and hypoadrenocorticism (Addison disease); others include diabetes mellitus and hypothyroidism

occasional keratopathy, thyroiditis, chronic hepatitis, intestinal malabsorption, pernicious anemia, or gonadal failure

AR

endocrinopathies may develop after CMC; severity does not necessarily parallel severity of CMC; may be life threatening

treating endocrinopathies generally does not improve candidiasis

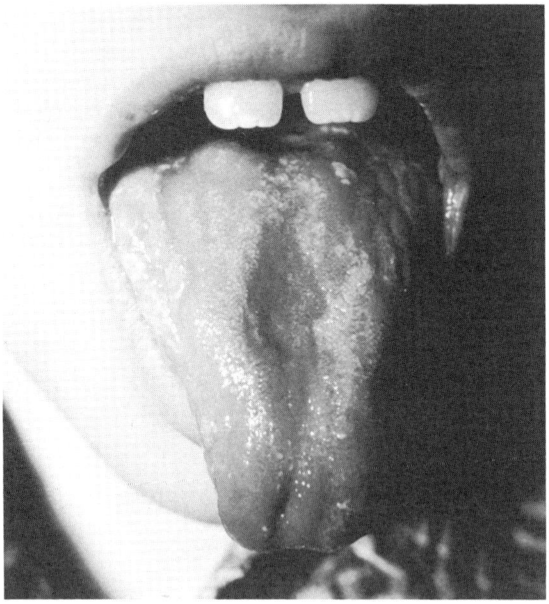

FIGURE 14–2
Chronic candidiasis of the tongue in a boy with mucocutaneous candidiasis and hypoparathyroidism.

■ *chronic candidiasis with thymoma*

candidal involvement of mucous membranes, skin, and nails arising after third decade

in most cases, candidiasis precedes the presentation of thymoma

myasthenia gravis is commonly associated; rarely seen in patients with systemic lupus erythematosus and certain sporadic infections

aplastic anemia, neutropenia, and hypogammaglobulinemia also reported

the presence of thymoma should be considered in patients with late-onset mucocutaneous candidiasis

acquired

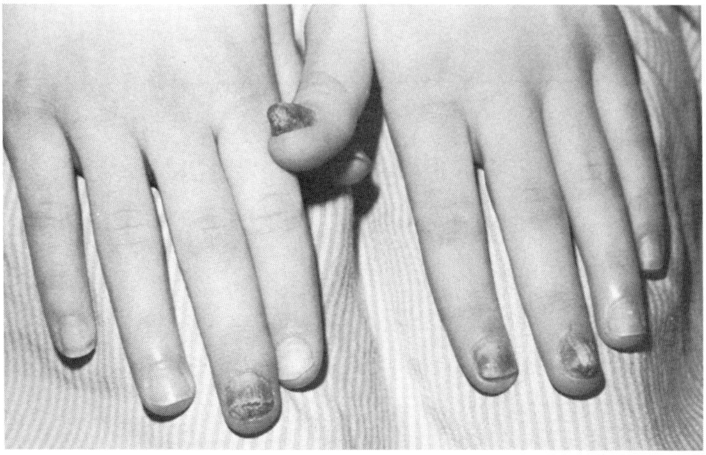

FIGURE 14–3
Nail dystrophy due to chronic candidiasis of the nails in a girl with mucocutaneous candidiasis and hypoparathyroidism.

McK 240300
Ahonen P. Autoimmune polyendocrinopathy–candidosis–ectodermal dystrophy (APECED): autosomal recessive inheritance. Clin Genet 1985;27:535–542
Ahonen P, Myllarniemi S, Sipila I, Perheentupa J. Autoimmune polyendocrinopathy–candidiasis–ectodermal dystrophy (APECED) in a series of 68 patients. N Engl J Med 1990;322:1829–1836
Gorlin RJ, Cohen MM Jr, Levin LS. Syndromes affecting the skin and mucosa. In: Syndromes of the Head and Neck. 3rd ed. New York, Oxford University Press, 1990:498–501
Feingold KR, Elias PM. Endocrine–skin interactions. J Am Acad Dermatol 1988;19:1–20
Leshin M. Southwestern internal medicine conference: polyglandular autoimmune syndromes. Am J Med Sci 1985;290:77–88
Rycroft RJG, Valdimarsson H, Bannister LH, Wells RS. Chronic mucocutaneous candidiasis of late onset, thymoma and myopathy. Clin Exp Dermatol 1976;1:59–74

CHRONIC MUCOCUTANEOUS CANDIDIASIS WITHOUT ENDOCRINOPATHY

mucocutaneous findings of CMC

good general health

low iron stores frequent

AR

improve with age

McK 212050
Hay RJ, Roberts SOB, MacKenzie DWR. Chronic mucocutaneous candidiasis. In: Champion RH, Burton JL, Ebling FJG, eds. Textbook of Dermatology. Oxford, Blackwell Scientific Publications, 1992:425–426
Wells RS, Higgs JM, McDonald A, et al. Familial chronic mucocutaneous candidiasis. J Med Genet 1972;9:302–310

CHRONIC CANDIDIASIS AND DERMATOPHYTOSIS WITHOUT ENDOCRINOPATHY

CMC of childhood onset

alopecia, loss of teeth, and recurrent viral infections

dermatophytosis may be especially severe

childhood onset

AD

McK 114580
Sams WM Jr, Jorizzo JL, Snyderman R, et al. Chronic mucocutaneous candidiasis: immunologic studies of three generations of a single family. Am J Med 1979;67:948–959
Shama SK, Kirkpatrick CH. Dermatophytosis in patients with chronic mucocutaneous candidiasis. J Am Acad Dermatol 1980;2:285–294

MYELOPEROXIDASE DEFICIENCY

some patients have CMC or disseminated candidiasis

AR; myeloperoxidase gene localized to chromosome 17

partial or complete absence of myeloperoxidase (a lysosomal enzyme) in neutrophils and monocytes

no increase in bacterial infections

most patients do not have increased numbers of infections

interestingly, most other diseases with CMC are due to defects of cell-mediated immunity, not defects of phagocyte function as in myeloperoxidase deficiency

McK 254600
Nauseef WM. Myeloperoxidase deficiency. Hematol Oncol Clin North Am 1988;2:135–158

SELECTIVE IgA DEFICIENCY

reputed to be associated with a host of infections and autoimmune diseases (including CMC, collagen vascular disease, and atopy), but this may be due to other associated immunologic abnormalities, specifically IgG2 and/or IgG4 deficiency, in symptomatic cases

usually sporadic; AD and AR cases reported

may be due to a maturational defect of B cells

low serum levels of IgA (less than 5 mg/dL), IgE (in over half of patients), IgG2 (in 20%), and an abnormal low-molecular-weight, nonpentameric IgM (in some patients) are reported; otherwise, levels of IgM and total IgG are usually normal

anaphylaxis following administration of human serum globulin may occur due to failure to develop tolerance to one's own IgA and/or IgE anti-IgA antibody

most with selective IgA deficiency are healthy, unless associated with lack of IgG subtypes

McK 137100

Ammann AJ, Hong R. Selective IgA deficiency: presentation of 30 cases and a review of the literature. Medicine 1971;52:223–236

de Laat PC, Weemaes CM, Bakkeren JA, et al. Familial selective IgA deficiency with circulating anti-IgA antibodies: a distinct group of patients? Clin Immunol Immunopathol 1991;58:92–101

Nell PA, Ammann AJ, Hong R, Stiehm ER. Familial selective IgA deficiency. Pediatrics 1972;49:71–79

Oxelius V, Laurell A, Lindquist B, et al. IgG subclasses in selective IgA deficiency: importance of IgG2-IgA deficiency. N Engl J Med 1981;304:1476–1477

Plebani A, Ugazio AG, Monafo V. Selective IgA deficiency: an update. Curr Probl Dermatol 1989;18:66–78

COMPLEMENT DEFICIENCIES

Almost every deficiency of the various components of complement has been associated with a lupus-like syndrome; frequently, these patients lack antinuclear antibodies or antibody to DNA. However, the incidence of clinical disease in individuals with complement deficiencies is low, being especially rare in heterozygotes.

In general, the disease associations with homozygous complement component deficiencies include

1. C1-esterase inhibitor:

    see main entry (see Chapter 13)

    angioedema

    about 2% of these patients also develop systemic lupus erythematosus

2. Deficiency of C1, C2, or C4 (classical pathway components):

    immune complex diseases, especially systemic lupus erythematosus; increased infections including pneumonia, meningitis, and septicemia

3. C3 or C3 inactivator (I) deficiency:

    infections with encapsulated bacteria, especially gram-negative bacteria, including *Neisseria* and *Haemophilus*

    opsonization is defective, but immune adherence is normal

4. C5, C6, C7, or C8 deficiency:

    generally these patients are well, but they may develop recurrent, disseminated infections with *Neisseria* and pneumococci

    opsonization and immune adherence are normal

    in cases with meningococcemia, onset is later, severity is decreased, and rate of recurrence is higher than in sporadically occurring cases without complement deficiency

Salient features of individual complement and related protein deficiencies are listed in Table 14–1.

TABLE 14–1
COMPLEMENT AND COMPLEMENT RECEPTOR DISORDERS

Deficient Protein or Receptor or Disease Name	Inheritance and McKusick Number	Disease Associations	Other Findings and Comments
C1q	Autosomal co-dominant; 120550, 120560, 120570	Cutaneous vasculitis; DLE; SLE; GN; infections	C1 is a calcium-dependent complex that is composed of three subunits: C1q binds immunoglobulin complexes; C1r is an enzyme; C1s is a proenzyme
C1r	Probable autosomal co-dominant	Cutaneous vasculitis; DLE; SLE; GN; infections	Often accompanied by C1s deficiency
C1s	Possibly autosomal co-dominant; 120580	SLE	Usually accompanied by C1r deficiency
C2	Autosomal co-dominant; 217000	Cutaneous vasculitis; DLE; SLE; GN; infections	Most common complement deficiency; most patients asymptomatic
C3	Autosomal co-dominant 120700	Cutaneous vasculitis; SLE; GN; infections	
C3 hypercatabolism (complement factor 1 (C3b/C4b inactivator))	Autosomal co-dominant; 120700	Infections including pyoderma	
C4	Autosomal co-dominant; 120970	Raynaud phenomenon; SLE; GN; vasculitis	
C5	Autosomal co-dominant; 120900	Infections *(Neisseria);* SLE; GN	
C6	Autosomal co-dominant	Infections *(Neisseria)*	
C7	Autosomal co-dominant	Infections *(Neisseria)*; SLE; CRST; Raynaud syndrome	
C8, alpha and beta chain	Autosomal co-dominant; 120950, 120960	Infections *(Neisseria)*; SLE	
C9	Autosomal co-dominant	Infections *(Neisseria)*	
CR-1 (membrane C3b receptor)	Probable autosomal co-dominant; 120620	Possible SLE and/or GN	
CR-2 (membrane C3d; Epstein-Barr virus receptor)	Possible autosomal co-dominant; 120650		
CR-3 (human leukocyte adhesion deficiency)	Possible autosomal co-dominant; 120980	Delayed umbilical cord separation; infections; pyoderma gangrenosum-like lesions	
Properdin deficiency	X-linked recessive 312060	Infections *(Neisseria);* DLE	
Factor H (complement factor H deficiency)	Autosomal co-dominant 134370	Possible association with IgA nephropathy or vasculitis	

CRST, calcinosis, Raynaud phenomenon, sclerodactyly, telangiectasias; SLE, systemic lupus erythematosus; DLE, discoid lupus erythematosus; GN, glomerulonephritis; C, complement; CR1, complement receptor type 1 protein; CR2, complement receptor type 2 protein; CR3, complement receptor type 3 protein.

Reference: Johnston RB Jr. Disorders of the complement system. In: Stiehm ER, ed. Immunologic Disorders in Infants and Children. 3rd ed. Philadelphia, WB Saunders, 1989:384–399.

Fries LF, O'Shea JJ, Frank MM. Inherited deficiencies of complement and complement-related proteins. Clin Immunol Immunopathol 1986;40:37–49
Liszewski MK, Atkinson JP. The role of complement in autoimmunity. Immunol Ser 1991;54:13–37
Rother K. Summary of reported deficiencies. Prog Allergy 1986;39:202–211
Tappeiner G. Immunodeficiency and complement deficiency states. Curr Prob Dermatol 1989;18:116–119

LEINER DISEASE

erythroderma, failure to thrive, recurrent infections, and diarrhea can be associated with different immunodeficiencies; thus, the constellation of findings seen under what has been called Leiner disease is nonspecific; opsonization defect is also an unreliable sign

we no longer use the name Leiner disease

McK 227100
McK 120900
Glover MT, Atherton DJ, Levinsky DJ. Syndrome of erythroderma, failure to thrive, and diarrhea in infancy: a manifestion of immunodeficiency. Pediatrics 1988;81:66–72
Leiner C. Erythroderma desquamativa (universal dermatitis of children at the breast). Br J Dis Child 1908;5:244–251
Soothill JF, Harvey BAM. Defective opsonization: a common immunity deficiency. Arch Dis Child 1976;51:91–99

Combined Immunodeficiency

Combined immunodeficiency disease (CID) is a heterogeneous group of congenital disorders of both genetic and sporadic etiology. Patients have both T- and B-cell immunodeficiency associated with thymic dysplasia and lymphoid aplasia and may have lymphopenia and/or absence of immunoglobulins. These diseases are associated with severe bacterial, viral, and fungal infections that may involve the skin. Some disorders are associated with known biochemical abnormalities, including adenosine deaminase deficiency, bare lymphocyte syndrome, nucleoside phosphorylase deficiency, and a defect in interleukin-2 production. Other patients with CID without known biochemical markers have been separated along clinical or genetic grounds under the rubrics of severe combined immunodeficiency disease (SCID), Swiss agammaglobulinemia, Omenn syndrome, reticular dysgenesis, immunodeficiency with short-limbed dwarfism (see main entry), and cellular immunodeficiency with immunoglobulins (Nezelof syndrome). Some of these individual entities are described in the following pages or elsewhere in this book.

Amman AJ, Hong R. Disorders of the T-cell system. In: Stiehm ER, ed. Immunologic Disorders in Infants and Children. 3rd ed. Philadelphia, WB Saunders, 1989:257–315

Atherton DJ. Severe combined immunodeficiency. In: Champion RH, Burton JL, Ebling FJG, eds. Textbook of Dermatology. Oxford, Blackwell Scientific Publications, 1992:425–426

Llorente CP, Amoros JI, Ortiz de Frutos, et al. Cutaneous lesions in severe combined immunodeficiency: two case reports and a review of the literature. Pediatr Dermatol 1991;8:314–321

Weinberg K, Parkman R. Severe combined immunodeficiency due to a specific defect in the production of interleukin-2. N Engl J Med 1990;322:1718–1723

SEVERE COMBINED IMMUNODEFICIENCY

Synonyms

- SCID
- Swiss-type agammaglobulinemia

Skin

see Figures 14–4 and 14–5

mucocutaneous candidiasis beginning at 3 to 6 months of age; the most common presenting sign is persistent oral thrush; severe esophageal candidiasis may complicate disorder

necrotic bacterial skin infections resembling ecthyma gangrenosum

various cutaneous eruptions including exfoliative erythroderma, seborrheic-like dermatitis, and epidermal necrolysis; eruptions may represent graft-versus-host disease

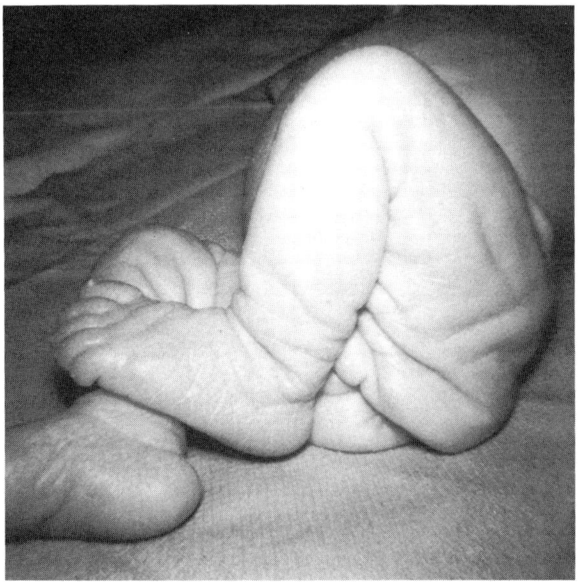

FIGURE 14–4
Dermatomegaly involving the buttocks and lower extremities in an infant with severe combined immunodeficiency and short-limbed dwarfism.

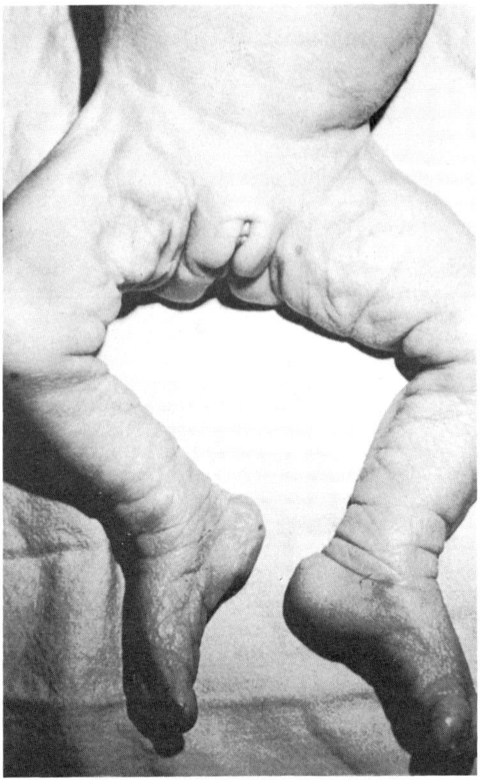

FIGURE 14–5
Severe combined immunodeficiency. Same patient as in Figure 14–4 showing massive enlargement of the inguinal lymph nodes.

Non-Skin

onset by 3 months

intractable diarrhea, malabsorption, and failure to thrive

recurrent infections, most commonly of the lungs, noted by 6 months of age; organisms include viruses, bacteria, yeast, fungi, and other microorganisms, including *Pneumocystis carinii*

severe viral infections, herpesvirus infections such as varicella are invariably severe or fatal

histiocytic infiltration of tissue may result in hepatosplenomegaly

Genetics

XLR (50% of cases), AR (Swiss-type agammaglobulinemia), and sporadic cases reported

Laboratory Data

severe lymphopenia with markedly decreased numbers of T lymphocytes; often the only lymphocytes present are of maternal origin or are immature (thymocytes)

absent delayed hypersensitivity skin tests; depressed response to mitogens low to absent quantitative immunoglobulins (noted after disappearance of maternal antibody); absence of specific antibodies

possible absence of HLA antigens

thymus histology is pathognomonic, consisting of islands of endodermal cells that have not become lymphoid cells; also, Hassall's corpuscles are absent

Prognosis

death often by 2 years of age, usually in first year, unless bone marrow reconstitution is successful

Discussion

graft-versus-host-disease may result from receiving blood products that have not been irradiated, from intrauterine transplacental transfusion, or following bone marrow reconstitution; skin manifestations are invariably seen

cases of SCID with histiocytic infiltration in multiple organs may simulate Langerhans cell histiocytosis

a possible milder variant of SCID has been reported (McK 312863)

REFERENCES

McK 202500

Bortin MM, Rimm AA. Severe combined immunodeficiency. JAMA 1977;238:591–600

De Raeve L, Song M, Levy J, Mascart-Lemone F. Cutaneous lesions as a clue to severe combined immunodeficiency. Pediatr Dermatol 1992;9:49–51

Rosen FS, Cooper MD, Wedgwood RJP. The primary immunodeficiencies (second of two parts). N Engl J Med 1984;311:300–310

Schmalstieg FC, Wirt DP, Adkins LT, et al. Postnatal development of T lymphocytes in a novel X-linked immunodeficiency disease. Clin Immunol Immunopathol 1992;64:71–77

Sillevis Smitt JH, Weening RS, Krieg SR, Bos JD. The skin in severe combined immunodeficiency: a case with transient cutaneous presence of gamma/delta (TRC1+) T cells. Br J Dermatol 1992;127:281–285

BARE LYMPHOCYTE SYNDROME

candidiasis and other cutaneous infections

occasional generalized unremitting dermatitis

increased incidence of infections, including pneumonia, gastroenteritis, and septicemia

lymph nodes are easily palpable, in contrast to the usual situation in a child with severe forms of CID

persistent diarrhea and profound failure to thrive

AR

complete or partial deficiency of class I and, in some cases, class II antigens on lymphocytes

hypogammaglobulinemia in infants with class II deficiency

should be able to respond to bone marrow transplantation but need ablation first owing to sufficient T-cell immunity

a type of combined immunodeficiency with variable but frequently severe clinical and immunologic findings

McK 209920

Amman AJ, Hong R. Disorders of the T-cell system. In: Stiehm ER, ed. Immunologic Disorders in Infants and Children. 3rd ed. Philadelphia, WB Saunders, 1989:267–268

Griscelli C, Lisowska-Grospierre B, Mach B. Combined immunodeficiency with defective expression in MHC class II genes. Immunodefic Rev 1989;1:135–153

Will N, Seger RA, Betzler C, et al. Bare lymphocyte syndrome: combined immunodeficiency and neutrophil dysfunction. Eur J Pediatr 1990;149:700–704

NUCLEOSIDE PHOSPHORYLASE DEFICIENCY

predominantly recurrent viral, fungal, and bacterial infections

AD (co-dominant)

less severe than myeloperoxidase deficiency, starting at later age, but patients may develop aplastic anemia; absent or severely depressed T-cell immunity while B-cell immunity normal

McK 164050

Edwards NI. Immunodeficiencies associated with errors in purine metabolism. Med Clin North Am 1985;69:505–518

Gibblet ER, Ammann AJ, Wara DW, et al. Nucleoside-phosphorylase deficiency in a child with severely defective T-cell immunity and normal B-cell immunity. Lancet 1972;1:1010–1013

Hirschhorn R, Ratech H. Genetic deficiencies of adenosine deaminase and purine nucleoside phosphorylase and their implications for therapy of leukemias. Curr Top Hematol 1983;4:1–35

Markert ML. Purine nucleoside phosphorylase deficiency. Immunodefic Rev 1991;3:45–81

Rosen FS, Cooper MD, Wedgwood RJP. The primary immunodeficiencies (second of two parts). N Engl J Med 1984;311:300–310

Sandman R, Ammann AJ, Grose C, Wara DC. Cellular immunodeficiency associated with nucleoside phosphorylase deficiency. Clin Immunol Immunopathol 1977;8:247–253

ADENOSINE DEAMINASE DEFICIENCY

SCID presenting in first weeks of life with severe diarrhea, pneumonia, otitis media, and failure to thrive

increased viral, candidal, bacterial, and protozoal infections

bony abnormalities

AR; accounts for 50% of AR forms of SCID

absent adenosine deaminase activity (important in purine nucleotide reutilization pathways, deoxyadenosine detoxification) measured in lymphocytes and red blood cell lysates

impaired cellular and humoral immunity

although bone marrow transplantation gives best results, some benefit may be obtained by enzyme replacement therapy using irradiated red blood cells

gene insertion therapy promising

McK 102700
Amman AJ, Hong R. Disorders of the T-cell system. In: Stiehm ER, ed. Immunologic Disorders in Infants and Children. 3rd ed. Philadelphia, WB Saunders 1989:268–274
Hirschhorn R, Ellenbogen A. Genetic heterogeneity in adenosine deaminase (ADA) deficiency: five different mutations in five new patients with partial ADA deficiency. Am J Hum Genet 1986;38:13–25
Hirschhorn R, Papageorgiou PS, Kesarwala HH, Taft LT. Amelioration of neurologic abnormalities after "enzyme replacement" in adenosine deaminase deficiency. N Engl J Med 1980;303:377–380
Kantoff PW, Cillio AP, McLachlin JR et al. Expression of human adenosine deaminase in nonhuman primates after retrovirus-mediated gene transfer. J Exp Med 1987;166:219–234
Rosen FS, Cooper MD, Wedgwood RJP. The Primary immunodeficiencies (second of two parts). N Engl J Med 1984;311:300–310
Vega MA. Adenosine deaminase deficiency: a model system for human somatic cell gene correction therapy. Biochim Biophys Acta 1992;14:253–260

CELLULAR IMMUNODEFICIENCY WITH IMMUNOGLOBULINS (NEZELOF SYNDROME)

may have findings of SCID, but usually less severe, at least initially; long-term prognosis poor

recurrent pyoderma and mucocutaneous candidiasis

fever and diarrhea

thymic aplasia

lymphadenopathy

AR

no graft-versus-host disease (in contrast to SCID)

generally normal or elevated serum levels of immunoglobulins, especially increased IgM

McK 242700
Amman AJ, Hong R. Disorders of the T-cell system. In: Stiehm ER, ed. Immunologic Disorders in Infants and Children. 3rd ed. Philadelphia, WB Saunders, 1989:261–263
Lawlor GJ Jr, Ammann AJ, Wright WC, et al. The syndrome of cellular immunodeficiency with immunoglobulins. J Pediatr 1974;84:183–192
Nezelof C, Jammet ML, Lortholary P, Labrune B, Lamy M. L'hypoplasie hereditaire du thymus: sa place et sa responsabilité dans une observation d'aplasie lymphocytaire, normoplasmocytaire et normoglobulinemique du nourrisson. Arch Fr Pediatr 1964;21:897–920
Rosen FS, Cooper MD, Wedgwood RJP. The primary immunodeficiencies (second of two parts). N Engl J Med 1984;311:300–310

OMMEN SYNDROME

Synonym

- familial reticuloendotheliosis with eosinophilia

Skin

onset in early infancy, frequently with skin findings

severe widespread erythroderma and thickening of the skin in first few weeks of life; recalcitrant to therapy

occasional diffuse alopecia of scalp and eyebrows

Non-Skin

recurrent infections, especially bacterial and fungal

fever, diarrhea, and failure to thrive

hepatosplenomegaly and lymphadenopathy

Genetics

AR

Pathophysiology

unclear whether immunodeficiency is the primary abnormality; the phenotype may be nonspecific resulting from more than one biochemical defect

Laboratory Data

histopathology: histiocytic infiltration of enlarged lymph nodes

eosinophilia, anemia, granulocytopenia, and thrombocytopenia

occasional hyperlipidemia

T- and B-cell immune defects demonstrated

Prognosis

lifesaving bone marrow transplantation and chemotherapy reported

death occurs within weeks to months without therapy

Discussion

some have postulated a pathophysiology similar to a graft-versus-host reaction

REFERENCES

McK 267700

Dyke MP, Marlow N, Berry PJ. Ommen's disease. Arch Dis Child 1991;66:1247–1248

Jouan H, Le Deist F, Nezelof C. Omenn's syndrome-pathologic arguments in favor of a graft versus host pathogenesis: a report of nine cases. Hum Pathol 1987;18:1101–1108

Omenn GS. Familial reticuloendotheliosis with eosinophilia. N Eng J Med 1965;273:427–432

Schofer O, Blaha I, Mannhardt W, et al. Omenn phenotype with short-limbed dwarfism. J Pediatr 1991;118:86–89

Velders AJ, Kuis W, van Dijk HA, et al. Omenn syndrome: familial reticuloendotheliosis with eosinophilia and combined immunodeficiency. Br J Dermatol 1983;108:118–120

FAMILIAL ERYTHROPHAGOCYTIC LYMPHOHISTIOCYTOSIS (FAMILIAL HEMOPHAGOCYTIC RETICULOSIS)

onset in early infancy to childhood

nonspecific rashes in some

jaundice and purpura may develop with progression of illness

fever, hepatosplenomegaly, cytopenia (in at least two thirds of lineages)

neurologic abnormalities include seizures, hemiparesis, and altered consciousness

AR

may be defect in immunoregulation permitting uncontrolled proliferation of histiocytes

laboratory abnormalities include hemophagocytosis in bone marrow, spleen, and lymph nodes; histiocytes and lymphocytes in bone marrow and multiple viscera; multiple immune defects

uniformly fatal if untreated; chemotherapy and corticosteroids may produce long-term remission

McK 267700

Blaese RM, Muchmore AV, Poplack DG. Disorders of the mononuclear phagocytic system. In: Stiehm ER, ed. Immunologic Disorders in Infants and Children. 3rd ed. Philadelphia, WB Saunders, 1989:367

Henter J, Elinder G, Soder O, Ost A. Incidence in Sweden and clinical features of familial hemophagocytic lymphohistiocytosis. Acta Paediatr Scand 1991;80:428–435

Henter JI, Elinder G, Finkel Y, Soder O. Successful induction with chemotherapy in-

cluding teniposide in familial erythrophagocytic lymphohistiocytosis. [Letter]. Lancet 1986;2:1402
Henter JI, Elinder G, Ost A, et al. Diagnostic guidelines for hemophagocytic lymphohistiocytosis. Semin Oncol 1991;18:29–33
Ladisch S, Poplack DG, Holiman B, Blaese RM. Immunodeficiency in familial erythrophagocytic lymphohistiocytosis. Lancet 1978;1:581–583

WISKOTT-ALDRICH SYNDROME

Skin

extensive and severe eczematous dermatitis appearing in early infancy, most commonly affecting scalp, face, flexures, and diaper area (Fig. 14–6)

petechiae and purpura commonly appear in dermatitic areas or on mucosae

extensive warts occasionally

Non-Skin

thrombocytopenia, frequently the first sign of disease, common from birth onward; severe bleeding from circumcision site often initial presentation

hemorrhagic sequelae occur early and include bloody diarrhea, hematemesis, hematuria, epistaxis, and purpura of mucous membranes

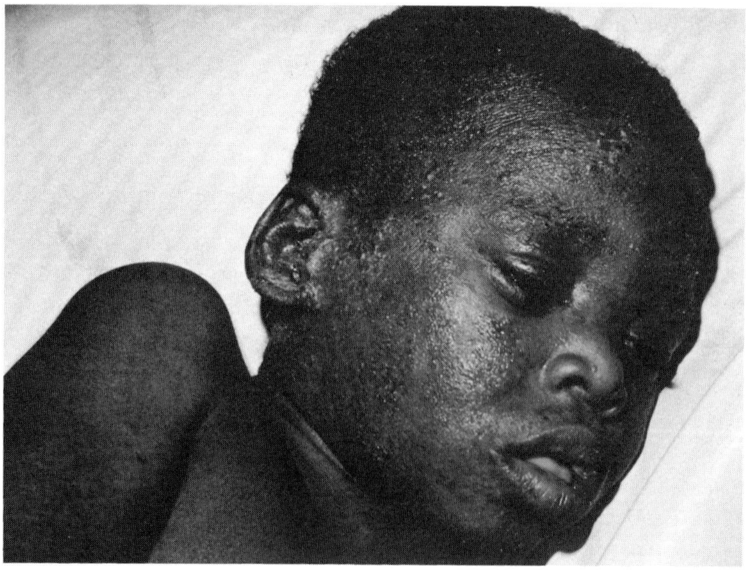

FIGURE 14–6
Extensive facial eczematous dermatitis in a boy with Wiskott-Aldrich syndrome. This boy had frequent recurrent episodes of widespread eczema herpeticum.

intracranial, pulmonary, or gastrointestinal hemorrhage may be life threatening

increased susceptibility to bacteria having polysaccharide capsules (e.g., *Streptococcus pneumoniae, Neisseria meningitis, Haemophilus influenzae,* and *Salmonella* species)

in addition, there are increased numbers of infections due to *Staphylococcus* species, protozoa (including *Pneumocystis carinii*), and viruses (especially herpesviridae such as cytomegalovirus)

typical infections include pneumonia, meningitis, sinusitis, otitis media, pyodermas, and furuncles

bronchiectasis may result from recurrent pneumonia

increased incidence of malignancy, most commonly lymphoreticular or leukemia

other findings that may relate to abnormal immune response include nonseptic arthritis, renal disease, and autoimmune hemolytic anemia

Genetics

XLR (males only)

Pathophysiology

inability to produce immunoglobulins to polysaccharide antigens

defective glycosylation of surface protein CD43 on lymphocytes, neutrophils, and platelets; relevance to primary defect in Wiskott-Aldrich syndrome unknown

Laboratory Data

platelet size, number, and function all decreased

hemolytic anemia

immunoglobulin abnormalities including decreased serum IgM levels (although these may be normal during the first year of life), absent isohemagglutinins, and often increased levels of IgA and IgE; IgG levels are usually normal

decreased T-cell–mediated and phagocytic functions

identification of carrier females is possible by DNA analysis

Prognosis

infection and hemorrhage are prominent causes of death in addition to leukemias and lymphoreticular malignancies

death usually occurs in infancy or childhood, but overall survival is improving, with more cases of survival into adulthood

splenectomy has improved platelet size, function, and number, but with increased risk of fatal septicemia infusions of immunoglobulin may help prevent infection in selected patients

drugs impairing platelet function should not be used

all blood products should be irradiated

bone marrow transplantation has been used with success; also reverses skin findings

Discussion

two possible variants of Wiskott-Aldrich syndrome are described:

"attenuated" forms have been reported in which both thrombocytopenia and immunodeficiency have been milder; may be identical with X-linked thrombocytopenia (McK 313900)

a possible variant with minimal susceptibility to infection and longer survival has been reported; other features include thrombocytopenia, dermatitis, elevated serum IgA, and glomerulonephritis (McK 314000); XLR

REFERENCES

McK 301000

Aldrich RA, Steinberg AG, Campbell DC. Pedigree demonstrating a sex-linked recessive condition characterised by draining ears, eczematoid dermatitis and bloody diarrhea. Pediatrics 1954;13:133–139

Brochstein JA, Gillio AP, Ruggiero M, et al. Marrow transplantation from human leukocyte antigen–identical or haploidentical donors for correction of Wiskott-Aldrich syndrome. J Pediatr 1991;119:907–912

Canales L, Mauer AM. Sex-linked hereditary thrombocytopenia as a variant of Wiskott-Aldrich syndrome. N Engl J Med 1967;277:899–901

Di Lernia V, Patrizi A, Ricci G, Masi M. Wiskott-Aldrich syndrome. Pediatr Dermatol 1991;8:250–252

Fearon ER, Kohn DB, Winkelstein JA, et al. Carrier detection in the Wiskott-Aldrich syndrome. Blood 1988;72:1735–1739

Gutenberger J, Trystad CW, Stiehm ER, et al. Familial thrombocytopenia, elevated serum IgA and renal disease. Am J Med 1970;49:729–741

Peacocke M, Siminovitch KA. Wiskott-Aldrich syndrome: new molecular and biochemical insights. J Am Acad Dermatol 1992;27:507–519

Perry GS, Spector BD, Schuman LM, et al. The Wiskott-Aldrich syndrome in the United States and Canada (1892–1979). J Pediatr 1980;97:72–78

Standen GR, Lillicrap DP, Matthews N, et al. Inherited thrombocytopenia, elevated serum IgA and renal disease: identification as a variant of Wiskott-Aldrich syndrome. Q J Med 1986;59:401–408

Standen GR. Wiskott-Aldrich syndrome: new perspectives in pathogenesis and management. J R Coll Physicians Lond 1988; 22:80–83

X-LINKED HYPOGAMMAGLOBULINEMIA

Synonyms

- X-linked agammaglobulinemia
- Bruton agammaglobulinemia
- infantile agammaglobulinemia

Skin

cutaneous bacterial infections including furunculosis, abscesses, and impetigo seen in about 25%

occasional atopic dermatitis–like eruption unresponsive to gamma globulin therapy

Non-Skin

maternal antibodies provide protection in early life; onset of disease in most patients between ages 18 months and 3 years

recurrent, mostly bacterial infections develop before second year of life, occasionally later

infections of the upper and lower respiratory and gastrointestinal tracts are the most common, especially otitis media, sinusitis, pneumonitis, and acute gastroenteritis

tonsillar, adenoid, and other lymphoid tissue is absent or scant

occasional monoarticular or oligoarticular arthritis, mainly of large joints; can be septic or aseptic

occasional meningitis, encephalitis, and/or septicemia

rare dermatomyositis-like or polymyositis-like syndrome; possibly related to chronic disseminated echovirus infection

Genetics

XLR (at least two genetically distinct forms of the disease reported)

female carriers can be distinguished by immunologic assays, but genetic heterogeneity may complicate carrier detection and prenatal diagnosis

Pathophysiology

arrest of B-lymphocyte maturation at the level of the precursor B cell

most infections are due to encapsulated bacteria

cell-mediated immunity is intact, but some viral infections are not well tolerated, particularly echoviruses and other enteroviruses

variable adverse responses to live virus vaccines reported

Laboratory Data

diagnosis made by examining lymph node biopsy after immunization: plasma cells are characteristically absent and B cells are not detected by tests for surface immunoglobulin markers

there is decrease to virtual absence of IgG, IgA, IgM, IgD, and IgE, isohemagglutinins, and certain complement components

T-cell immunity is intact

the Schick test often results in induration, even after DPT immunization

adenoids are absent on lateral x-ray film of pharynx

defective gene can be identified by molecular genetic techniques

Prognosis

prophylactic gamma globulin replacement therapy is of benefit and has even been used in patients diagnosed before onset of signs or symptoms of the disease

major causes of death are cardiorespiratory failure due to recurrent pulmonary infections and multiorgan failure accompanying disseminated enterovirus infection, frequently in second and third decades of life

Discussion

variable expressivity; almost any one of the clinical features listed may be the presenting sign

REFERENCES

McK 300300
McK 300310
Journet O, Durandy A, Doussau M, et al. Carrier detection and prenatal diagnosis of X-linked agammaglobulinemia. Am J Med Genet 1992;43:885–887
Lederman HM, Winkelstein JA. X-linked agammaglobulinemia: an analysis of 96 patients. Medicine 1985;64:145–156
Liese JG, Wintergerst U, Tympner KD, Belohradsky BH. High- vs low-dose immunoglobulin therapy in the long-term treatment of X-linked agammaglobulinemia. Am J Dis Child 1992;146:335–339
Mease PJ, Ochs HD, Wedgwood RJ. Successful treatment of echovirus meningoencephalitis and myositis-fasciitis with intravenous immune globulin therapy in a patient with X-linked agammaglobulinemia. N Engl J Med 1981;304:1278–1281
Mensink EJBM, Thompson A, Schot JDI, et al. Genetic heterogeneity in X-linked agammaglobulinemia complicates carrier detection and prenatal diagnosis. Clin Genet 1987;31:91–96

X-LINKED IMMUNODEFICIENCY WITH HYPERIMMUNOGLOBULINEMIA-M

Synonym

- immunodeficiency with hyperimmunoglobulinemia-M

Skin

recurrent pyodermas

atopic-like dermatitis

cyclic indolent oral ulcerations in patients with neutropenia

generalized verrucae in some

Non-Skin

recurrent bacterial infections beginning after 6 months of age

otitis media, tonsillitis, lower respiratory and gastrointestinal tract infections

frequent cervical lymphadenopathy and hepatosplenomegaly

Genetics

usually XLR, but AR, AD, and sporadic cases also reported

Pathophysiology

B-lymphocytes fail to make immunoglobulins other than IgM owing to a defect in "switch" T cells

Laboratory Data

histopathology: lack of lymphoid follicles in lymphoid tissue

elevated serum IgM levels

serum IgG and IgA are severely deficient

recurrent cyclic or persistent neutropenia, hemolytic anemia, and thrombocytopenia

Prognosis

prognosis generally better than X-linked hypogammaglobulinemia; major cause of death is chronic pulmonary disease

regular gamma globulin injections beneficial

Discussion

female carriers with similar findings reported

sporadic cases may be transitory

a similar clinical disease may occur as a late-onset acquired form or secondary to intrauterine rubella infection

REFERENCES

McK 308230

Brahmi Z, Lazarus KH, Hodes ME, Baehner RL. Immunologic studies of three family members with the immunodeficiency with hyper-IgM syndrome. J Clin Immunol 1983;3:127–134

Hong R. Update on the immunodeficiency diseases. Am J Dis Child 1990;144:983–992

Kyong CU, Virella G, Fudenberg HH, Darby CP. X-linked immunodeficiency with increased IgM: clinical, ethnic, and immunologic heterogeneity. Pediatr Res 1978;12:1024–1026

Mayer L, Kwan SP, Thompson C, et al. Evidence for a defect in "switch" T cells in patients with immunodeficiency and hyperimmunoglobulinemia M. N Engl J Med 1986;314:409–413

Ochs HD, Wedgwood RJ. Disorders of the B-cell system. In: Stiehm ER, ed. Immuno-

logic Disorders in Infants and Children. 3rd ed. Philadelphia, WB Saunders, 1989:236–237
Rosen FS, Kevy SV, Merler E, et al. Recurrent bacterial infections and dysgammaglobulinemia: deficiency of 7S gamma-globulins in the presence of elevated 19S gamma-globulins. Pediatrics 1961;28:182–195
Schimke RN, Bolano C, Kirkpatrick CH. Immunologic deficiency in the congenital rubella syndrome. Am J Dis Child 1969;118:626–633

Immunodeficiency Disorders—Abbreviated Entries

TUFTSIN DEFICIENCY

severe, repeated infections, including multiple skin abscesses

dermatitic eruptions reported

lung infections including bronchitis, bronchiolitis, and pneumonia

tonsilitis and otitis media

fluctuant and enlarged lymph nodes

septicemia

probable AD; acquired cases occur in splenectomized patients or sickle cell anemia patients due to "autosplenectomy"

decreased or absent tuftsin, a tetrapeptide derived from the immunoglobulin heavy chain that is activated in the spleen; stimulates the phagocytic activity of polymorphonuclear leukocytes

susceptibility to infection diminishes with age

splenectomized patients also have absent tuftsin levels and increased incidence of infection

McK 191150
Constantopoulos A, Najjar VA, Smith JW. Tuftsin deficiency: a new syndrome with defective phagocytosis. J Pediatr 1972; 80:564–572
Constantopoulos A, Najjar VA. Tuftsin deficiency syndrome: a report of two new cases. Acta Paediatr Scand 1973;62:645–648

SPECIFIC GRANULE DEFICIENCY (LACTOFERRIN-DEFICIENT NEUTROPHILS)

severe recurrent bacterial cutaneous and soft tissue infections

AR

CHAPTER 15

Metabolic Disorders

Many of the metabolic diseases are named for their most prominent biochemical abnormality. Whereas this type of nomenclature may be suitable for a minority of metabolic errors, in many cases it is misleading, since it focuses on only one of several enzymatic defects characterizing that disorder. Clinical diagnosis is complicated by the fact that more than one enzymatic defect may cause the same phenotype; conversely, a single metabolic error may produce a variety of phenotypes. This has led to considerable confusion and made it difficult to keep pace with the rapid developments in this field and the discovery of multiple variants and subtypes of some of these conditions.

Few of the metabolic disorders have specific cutaneous features. Nevertheless, we have tried to include those disorders for which a cutaneous abnormality may provide a clinical clue to the correct diagnosis.

Porphyrias

The porphyrias are a group of disorders caused by abnormalities in porphyrin metabolism. They are all inherited, although the expression of the genotype is subject to environmental modification. Some porphyrias have no cutaneous findings, but most are characterized by some degree of photosensitivity (Table 15–1). Often used abbreviations for these disorders are listed below:

AIP = acute intermittent porphyria

ALA = delta-aminolevulinic acid

COPRO = coproporphyrin

COPROGENO = coproporphyrinogen oxidase

EP = erythropoietic porphyria

EPP = erythropoietic protoporphyria

HCP = hereditary coproporphyria

TABLE 15–1
PORPHYRIAS

Disease	Inheritance	Cutaneous Findings	Neurovisceral Findings	Principal Enzyme Defect (Postulated)	Red Blood Cells	Plasma	Urine	Stool
Erythropoietic porphyria (EP)	AR	Severe photosensitivity beginning in infancy or early childhood; blisters and erosions; hypertrichosis; sclerodermoid changes; scarring alopecia; scarring and mutilating deformities	–	Uroporphyrinogen III cosynthase (UROCOSYN-III)*	URO> COPRO	URO> COPRO	URO>COPRO pink to red color	COPRO>>URO; PROTO
Erythropoietic protoporphyria (EPP)	AD	Mild to severe photosensitivity beginning in early childhood; erythema, edema and rare bullae, sometimes only stinging and burning; shallow waxy scars of nose and dorsal hands	–	Ferrochelatase	PROTO	PROTO		PROTO>COPRO
Hepatoerythropoietic porphyria (HEP)	AD	Severe photosensitivity beginning in infancy; blisters and erosions; fragility; hypertrichosis; sclerodermoid changes; scarring alopecia; scarring and mutilating deformities	+/–	Uroporphyrinogen decarboxylase (UROGEND)	PROTO	URO; PROTO	URO>COPRO; ISOCOPRO; pink red urine	COPRO; ISOCOPRO

Acute intermittent porphyria (AIP)	AD	None	+	Porphobilinogen deaminase (PBGD)	URO	ALA; PBG (red to purple urine)	
Variegate porphyria (VP)	AD	See PCT	+/−	Protoporphyrinogen oxidase (PROTOGENO)	Porphyrin-protein	COPRO; URO; ALA; PBG	PROTO>COPRO> URO; X-porphyrin
Porphyria cutanea tarda (PCT)	AD	Moderate to severe photosensitivity beginning in adulthood; blisters and erosions with milia; fragility; hyperpigmentation and sclerodermoid changes; scarring alopecia	−	Uroporphyrinogen decarboxylase (UROGEND)	URO>COPRO	URO>>COPRO	COPRO>URO; ISOCOPRO
Hereditary coproporphyria (HCP)	AD	Blisters and photosensitivity may be seen	+/−	Coproporphyrinogen oxidase (COPROGENO)	COPRO	COPRO>URO; ALA; PBG	COPRO>URO; PROTO

*Cohen and DeLeo postulate defect as uroporphyrinogen III synthetase.

Note: See introduction to porphyrias for explanation of abbreviations.

Data from Cohen PR, DeLeo VA. Disorders of porphyrin metabolism. In: Alper JC, ed. Genetic Disorders of the Skin. St. Louis, Mosby–Year Book, 1991:79–104; and Bickers DR, Pathak MA. The porphyrias. In: Cutaneous lesions in nutritional, metabolic, and heritable disorders. In: Fitzpatrick TB, Eisen AZ, Wolff K, Freedberg IM, Austen KF, eds. Dermatology in General Medicine. New York, McGraw-Hill, 1987:1666–1715.

HEP = hepatoerythropoietic porphyria

HP = harderoporphyria

ISOCOPRO = isocoproporphyrin

PBG = porphobilinogen

PBGD = porphobilinogen deaminase

PCT = porphyria cutanea tarda

PROTO = protoporphyrin

PROTOGENO = protoporphyrinogen oxidase

URO = uroporphyrin

UROGEND = uroporphyrinogen decarboxylase

UROCOSYN-III = uroporphyrinogen-III cosynthase

VP = variegate porphyria

REFERENCE

Moore MR, McColl KEL, Rimington C, Goldberg A. Disorders of Porphyrin Metabolism. New York, Plenum Medical Book Company, 1987

ERYTHROPOIETIC PORPHYRIA

Synonyms

- Günther disease
- EP

Skin

see Figure 15–1

early in life, on exposure to light, blisters develop on face, ears, and dorsa of hands; lesions often crust or ulcerate; may heal with scarring and milia

repeated exposure to light results in scarring mutilation of ears, nose, face, scalp, and digits; characteristic linear scars around mouth resemble rhagades; scarring may be sclerodermoid

hypertrichosis, hypopigmentation and hyperpigmentation of affected areas are common, leading to the so-called werewolf or wolfman appearance; the increased hair is of lanugo type and fair over the extremities but may be coarse and dark on the face

scarring alopecia

cutaneous malignancies may develop in scars

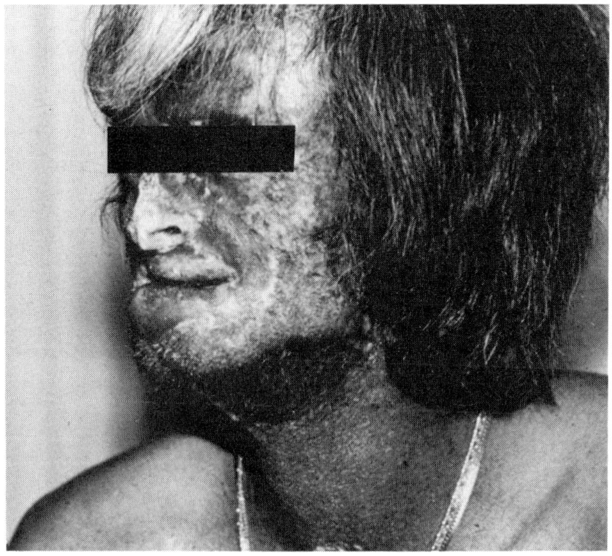

FIGURE 15–1
Congenital erythropoietic porphyria (Günther disease). Patient had marked photosensitivity and scarring and later developed several aggressive squamous cell carcinomas on his face and extremities.

Non-Skin

red urine is noted shortly after birth

teeth are brownish red to lavender and fluoresce bright red under Wood's lamp; bones are similarly discolored

ectropion, conjunctivitis, keratitis, and photophobia develop and may result in blindness

hemolytic anemia and splenomegaly; sequelae include porphyrin gallstones, bone marrow expansion, and resulting pathologic fractures with vertebral compression and shortness of stature

Genetics

AR

Pathophysiology

deficiency of UROCOSYN-III; other possible enzymatic abnormalities include increased PBGD; decreased UROGEND, and increased ALA synthetase

Laboratory Data

red blood cell and marrow normoblasts have a stable red fluorescence under Wood's lamp due to increased URO I, COPRO I, and PROTO

urine: increased URO I and COPRO I; pink to port wine in color; fluoresces red under Wood's lamp

feces: increased URO I and COPRO I

liver porphyrin levels slightly elevated

porphyrin maximal absorption: light wavelengths 400 to 410 nm (Soret band)

histopathology: subepidermal bullae; immunofluorescence shows occasional IgG deposits in basement membrane and vascular walls

Prognosis

sepsis or severe anemia usually cause death by fifth decade or earlier

beta-carotene therapy has been helpful in some

other therapies of reported benefit include oral charcoal, cholestyramine, pyridoxine, splenectomy, transfusions, and bone marrow transplantation

Discussion

some newborns have been diagnosed in the nursery after exposure to phototherapy lamps for hyperbilirubinemia

a delayed-onset adult form has been reported that may be confused with porphyria cutanea tarda, but red urine is a helpful clue

hepatoerythropoietic porphyria (see later) has similar clinical findings, but the biochemical findings more closely resemble porphyria cutanea tarda

REFERENCES

McK 263700

Horiguchi Y, Horio T, Yamamoto M, et al. Late onset erythropoietic porphyria. Br J Dermatol 1989;121:255–262

Kauffman L, Evans DI, Stevens RF, Weinkove C. Bone-marrow transplantation for congenital erythropoietic porphyria. Lancet 1991;337:1510–1511

Murphy GM, Hawk JL, Nicholson DC, Magnus IA. Congenital erythropoietic porphyria (Günther disease). Clin Exp Dermatol 1987;12:61–65

Pimstone NR, Gandhi SN, Mukerji SK. Therapeutic efficacy of oral charcoal in congenital erythropoietic porphyria. N Engl J Med 1987;316:390–393

Piomelli S, Poh-Fitzpatrick MB, Seaman C, et al. Complete suppression of the symptoms of congenital erythropoietic porphyria by long-term treatment with high-level transfusions. N Engl J Med 1986;314:1029–1031

Warner CA, Poh-Fitzpatrick MB, Zaider EF, et al. Congenital erythropoietic porphyria: a mild variant with low uroporphyrin I levels due to a missense mutation (A66V) encoding residual uroporphyrinogen III synthase activity. Arch Dermatol 1992;128:1243–1248

ERYTHROPOIETIC PROTOPORPHYRIA

Synonyms

- erythrohepatic protoporphyria
- EPP

Skin

onset in infancy or early childhood with first exposure to sunlight; tingling, burning, or otherwise painful sensation in skin accompanied by erythema and edema of sun-exposed areas; occurs within minutes of sun exposure; often followed by pruritus

small vesicles and subsequent crusting may be seen; erythema, swelling, or urticaria, however, may be the only manifestations

symptoms worsen in summer

lesions heal with hypopigmentation, hyperpigmentation, and superficial linear or depressed scarring with a "waxy" or "worm-eaten" appearance; especially prominent on cheeks, nose, and dorsa of hands (Figs. 15–2 and 15–3)

skin may be dry and taut; occasional perioral furrowing

occasional onycholysis and onychomadesis

Non-Skin

cholelithiasis with stones containing protoporphyrins is a common finding and may appear early in life

mild nonhemolytic anemia is common, but hemolytic anemia is rare

occasional cirrhosis and hepatic failure

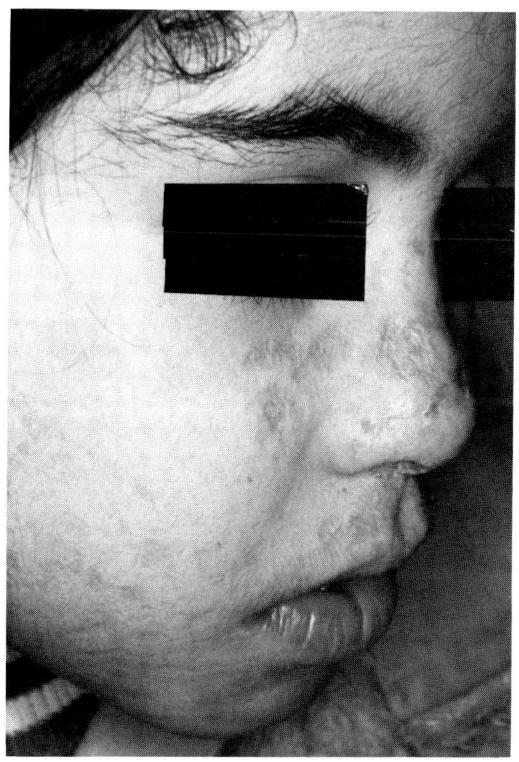

FIGURE 15–2
Erythropoietic protoporphyria. Multiple atrophic scars scattered over the nose, cheeks, and upper lip.

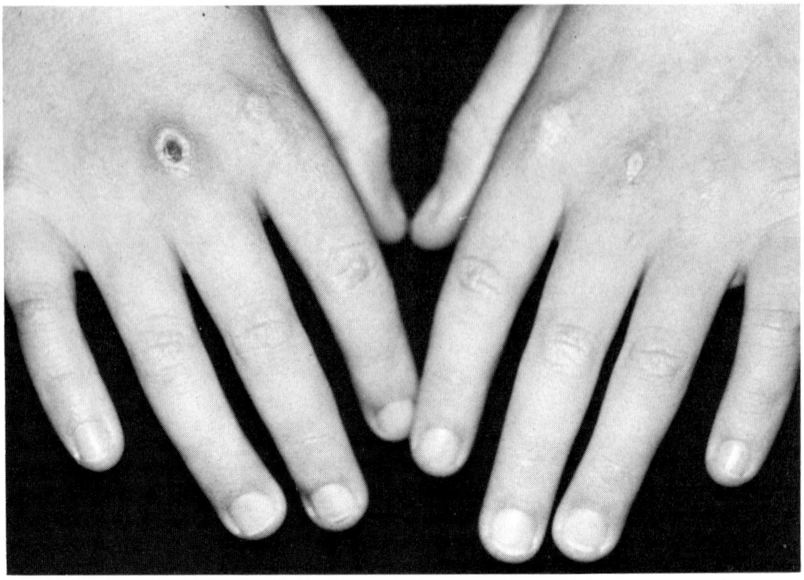

FIGURE 15–3
Erythropoietic protoporphyria. Healing erosions and scars on the dorsum of the hands with predilection for the knuckles. (Courtesy of Edward A. Krull, MD, Detroit, Michigan.)

Genetics

AD

most commonly seen in whites

Laboratory Data

ferrochelatase deficiency in red blood cells, bone marrow, skin fibroblasts, and liver

urine: normal porphyrins

feces: increased PROTO

red blood cells and plasma: increased PROTO; fluorescence under Wood's lamp during attacks

histopathology: eosinophilic homogeneous material in and around vessel walls (periodic acid–Schiff positive); immunofluorescence shows IgG in basement membrane and vascular walls

Prognosis

variable response of photosensitivity to beta-carotene but should be tried

photosensitivity may spontaneously abate with age

some patients develop fatal hepatic failure; cholestyramine may be of benefit in early liver disease, but liver failure requires liver transplantation for survival

some patients are misdiagnosed as having psychiatric illness because symptoms seem out of proportion to clinical signs

Discussion

rarely presents in adulthood, thus may be confused with porphyria cutanea tarda

much more common than erythropoietic porphyria

may be confused with idiopathic photodermatoses (e.g., hydroa aestivale and polymorphous light eruption); red blood cell porphyrin screens are therefore part of any photosensitivity workup

REFERENCES

McK 177000

Baart de la Faille H, Bylmer-Iest JC, van Hattum J, et al. Erythropoietic protoporphyria: clinical aspects with emphasis on the skin. Curr Probl Dermatol 1991;20:123–134

Corbett MF, Herxheimer A, Magnus IA, et al. The long-term treatment with beta-carotene in erythropoietic protoporphyria: a controlled trial. Br J Dermatol 1989; 97:655–662

DeLeo VA, Poh-Fitzpatrick M, Mathews-Roth M, Harber LC. Erythropoietic protoporphyria: ten years experience. Am J Med 1976;60:8–22

Fallon JD, Kvedar JC, Margolis RJ, et al. Erythropoietic protoporphyria presenting in adulthood. [Letter]. Arch Dermatol 1989;125:1286–1287

Johnson JA, Fusaro RM. Prognosis of liver transplantation in patients with erythropoietic protoporphyria. [Letter]. Transplantation 1989;48:175–176

Ross JB, Moss MA. Relief of the photosensitivity of erythropoietic protoporphyria by pyridoxine. J Am Acad Dermatol 1990;22:340–342

ERYTHROPOIETIC COPROPORPHYRIA

photosensitivity beginning in childhood; clinically resembles erythropoietic protoporphyria

inheritance unclear

defect: not established

urine: normal porphyrins

feces: increased PROTO and COPRO

red blood cells: increased PROTO and COPRO and small amounts of URO

extremely rare; very few cases described

differentiation from erythropoietic protoporphyria may be quantitative only; in fact, in many cases of erythropoietic protoporphyria red blood cells may contain small amounts of COPRO

Gordon M, Stern W. Erythropoietic coproporphyria and protoporphyria. Arch Dermatol 1969;99:770–773

Topi GC, D'Alessandro GL, Fazio M, Mariani L. [Congenital erythropoietic coproporphyria observed in a brother and a sister (new form of hereditary erythropoietic coproporphyria)]. Ann Dermatol Venereol (Paris) 1977;104:68–70

PORPHYRIA CUTANEA TARDA

Synonyms

- acquired hepatic porphyria
- chemical porphyria
- PCT

Skin

vesicles and bullae form on light-exposed areas, especially hands and face, and heal with depressed scars and milia (Fig. 15–4)

skin fragility is increased; predilection for dorsa of hands

gray-brown discoloration of exposed skin

onset usually in the fourth to sixth decades for the more common type I form; onset of type II form is during childhood or infancy (see later)

hypertrichosis of the face, especially upper face, is common (Fig. 15–5); subsequent spread to back, arms, and trunk is less common

scarring alopecia in areas of repeated trauma or blister formation may be pronounced

sclerodermoid thickening of face, back of neck, and other sun-exposed areas may be seen, sometimes also in nonexposed areas

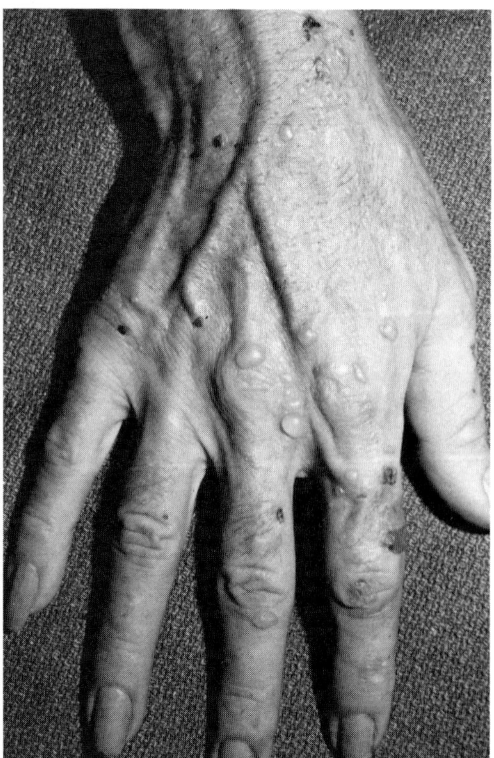

FIGURE 15–4
Porphyria cutanea tarda. Multiple blisters, crusted erosions, and atrophic scars on the dorsum of the hand and fingers. (Courtesy of Benjamin K. Fisher, MD, Toronto, Ontario.)

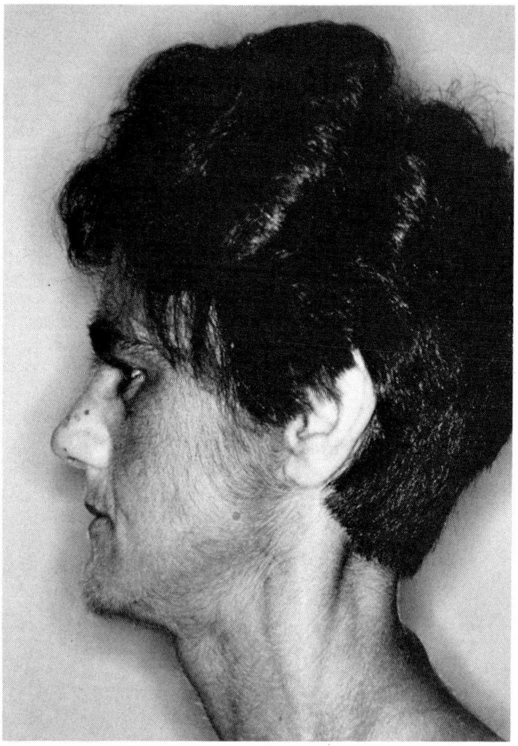

FIGURE 15–5
Hypertrichosis of the face characteristic of porphyria cutanea tarda.

Non-Skin

increased incidence of diabetes mellitus

increased incidence of cirrhosis and/or hepatoma, at least in some racial groups

Genetics

AD

Laboratory Data

iron accumulation in tissues, especially liver, is related to development of diabetes and expression of porphyria; hepatic siderosis in virtually all and increased plasma iron in one third to one half

decreased UROGEND in liver

urine: increased URO (I > III), 7-carboxyl porphyrins (III > I), and ISOCOPRO; orange to red-brown; fluoresces red under Wood's lamp

feces: increased ISOCOPRO, COPRO, PROTO, and URO

histopathology: noninflammatory subepidermal bullae with hyalin-like thickening of blood vessel walls of superficial dermal plexus

Prognosis

liver cirrhosis and carcinoma may develop

hemochromatosis may be a complicating factor

phlebotomy is the treatment of choice, but low doses of chloroquine are an alternative

hepatotoxins should be avoided, including alcohol

Discussion

although PCT is an inherited disorder, acquired liver disease (e.g., alcoholic liver disease) is needed to trigger the condition

asymptomatic relatives have decreased hepatic UROGEND

many patients with chronic renal failure on dialysis who had blisters were later discovered to have PCT; other disease states associated with PCT include systemic lupus erythematosus and acquired immunodeficiency syndrome

PCT is a heterogeneous group of disorders that can be roughly divided into two types:

- *porphyria cutanea tarda, type I:*

  the "sporadic" form of PCT and the cause of the majority of cases

  onset in adulthood, usually in association with alcohol or estrogen use

  other triggering agents, mostly hepatotoxins, include hexachlorobenzene (an antifungal agent that caused a large PCT epidemic in Turkey), chlorinated phenols, iron, and tetrachlorodibenzodioxin

  liver UROGEND activity is 50% of normal

  at least a proportion, if not most, of the "sporadic" cases are being recognized as having a genetic basis; enzyme deficiency is latent until hepatic siderosis, caused by a variety of hepatotoxins, is advanced enough to cause porphyria

- *porphyria cutanea tarda, type II:*

  the "familial" form of PCT

  onset in childhood

  AD

  UROGEND is decreased to 50% of normal in a variety of tissues, not just the liver

  in some familial cases the enzyme levels are normal; referred to as PCT type III by some

REFERENCES

McK 176090

McK 176100

Brunsting L. Observations on porphyria cutanea tarda. Arch Dermatol 1954;70:551–564

Grossman ME, Bickers DR, Poh-Fitzpatrick MB, et al. Porphyria cutanea tarda: clinical features and laboratory findings in 40 patients. Am J Med 1979;67:277–286

Grossman ME, Poh-Fitzpatrick MB. Porphyria

cutanea tarda: diagnosis, management, and differentiation from other hepatic porphyrias. Dermatol Clin 1986;4:297–309
Kappas A, Sassa, S, Galbraith RA, Nordmann Y. The porphyrias. In: Scriver CR, Beaudet AL, Sly WS, Valle D, eds. The Metabolic Basis of Inherited Disease. 6th ed. New York, McGraw-Hill, 1989:1305–1365
Nip-Sakamoto CJ, Wong RH, Izumi AK. Porphyria cutanea tarda and AIDS. Cutis 1989;44:470–471

HEPATOERYTHROPOIETIC PORPHYRIA (HEP)

marked cutaneous photosensitivity with vesicles, bullae, burning, and pruritus in sun-exposed areas, usually during first summer of life; photosensitivity decreases with age

blistering may heal with hyperpigmentation and sclerodermoid changes, with mutilated scarred deformities of acral areas (e.g., hands, ears, face, and nose), and with scarring alopecia

hypertrichosis

ocular findings include ectropion and scleromalacia perforans

dark urine is present from birth

occasional splenomegaly and/or hemolytic anemia

AR; usually requires homozygous defect for clinical problems to occur, but some obligate heterozygotes have clinical manifestations

markedly decreased red blood cell and liver UROGEND; probably homozygous UROGEND deficiency

urine: increased ISOCOPRO, URO (I and III), and 7-carboxylporphyrin; dark color

feces: increased COPRO, ISOCOPRO

red blood cells: increased PROTO (most characteristic porphyrin abnormality in HEP)

clinical manifestations are similar to erythropoietic porphyria

biochemical findings are similar to severe porphyria cutanea tarda, but HEP has PROTO present in red blood cells and COPRO instead of ISOCOPRO present in feces

some consider HEP like a "homozygous porphyria cutanea tarda," but there are only rare examples of porphyria cutanea tarda–like clinical expression in heterozygotes

only biochemical findings allow infantile familial porphyria cutanea tarda to be distinguished from HEP and also allow differentiation from incompletely expressed, forme fruste examples of erythropoietic porphyria

McKusick includes this entity with familial porphyria cutanea tarda
Bundino S, Topi GC, Zina AM, et al. Hepatoerythropoietic porphyria. Pediatr Dermatol 1987;4:229–233
Czarnecki DB. Hepatoerythropoietic porphyria. Arch Dermatol 1980;116:307–311
Toback AC, Sassa S, Poh-Fitzpatrick MB, et al. Hepatoerythropoietic porphyria: clinical, biochemical, and enzymatic studies in a three-generation family lineage. N Engl J Med 1987;316:645–650

VARIEGATE PORPHYRIA

Synonyms

- mixed porphyria
- South African porphyria
- protocoproporphyria

Skin

cutaneous lesions identical to porphyria cutanea tarda; onset usually between 15 and 30 years of age

skin signs precede onset of abdominal and neurologic symptoms in two thirds of cases and may be more common in men

Non-Skin

neurologic and abdominal symptoms similar to acute intermittent porphyria; may be more common in women

Genetics

AD

found in South Africa and Finland, rarely elsewhere (e.g., New England)

Laboratory Data

enzyme: decreased PROTOGENO, increased ALA synthetase, possible decreased ferrochelatase

urine: increased ALA and PBG during attacks only; pink to red on standing during attacks only

feces: increased PROTO, COPRO (and URO during attacks only), and X-porphyrin

Prognosis

provocation by drugs and prognosis similar to acute intermittent porphyria (see main entry)

Discussion

asymptomatic family members may have increased fecal COPRO

homozygotes have onset of skin findings in infancy or early childhood; high red blood cell protoporphyrin levels

REFERENCES

McK 176200

Corey TJ, DeLeo VA, Christianson H, Poh-Fitzpatrick MB. Variegate porphyria: clinical and laboratory features. J Am Acad Dermatol 1980;2:36–43

Fromke VL, Bossenmaier BA, Cardinal R, Watson CJ. Porphyria variegata: study of a large kindred in the United States. Am J Med 1978;65:80–88

Logan GM, Weimer MK, Ellefson M, et al. Bile porphyrin analysis in the evaluation of variegate porphyria. N Engl J Med 1991;324:1408–1411

Muhlbauer JE, Pathak MA, Tishler PV, Fitzpatrick TB. Variegate porphyria in New England. JAMA 1982;247:3095–3102

Mustajoki P, Tenhunen R, Niemi KM, et al. Homozygous variegate porphyria: a severe skin disease of infancy. Clin Genet 1987;32:300–305

ACUTE INTERMITTENT PORPHYRIA (AIP; SWEDISH PORPHYRIA)

the only major porphyria without consistent skin findings; nondiagnostic hyperpigmentation has been reported, but there is no photosensitivity

onset between third and sixth decades, rarely before puberty

acute and severe abdominal pain, colic, and vomiting, probably due to autonomic neuropathy; neither rigidity nor ileus on examination

other neurologic sequelae range from peripheral neuropathy to localized weakness to generalized paralysis; may resemble poliomyelitis or amyotrophic lateral sclerosis

psychiatric symptoms, including frank psychosis or delirium, are common during attacks

patients are frequently normal between attacks

more frequent in women than men and in Scandinavians

AD

decreased PBGD (formerly known as uroporphyrinogen synthetase) activity in liver (as well as red blood cells, lymphocytes, and skin fibroblasts), increased ALA synthetase, and decreased hepatic 5-alpha-reductase

urine: increased ALA and PBG levels during and between attacks; increased URO and COPRO during attacks

urine is colorless when voided, but becomes wine-red on standing owing to oxidization (in erythropoietic porphyria, urine is already red without standing)

feces: normal

the Watson-Schwartz test distinguishes COPRO from PBG during attacks; a qualitative procedure, it depends on the insolubility of 7 PBG aldehyde in chloroform and butanol

family members may excrete increased urinary PBG

many drugs may precipitate attacks (e.g., barbiturates, hydantoin, griseofulvin, sulfonamides, ethanol, exogenous estrogens, and progestins)

may be mimicked by paroxysmal nocturnal hemoglobinuria or lead poisoning

death may result from respiratory failure due to neurologic, especially medullary, paralysis

muscle weakness associated with acute attacks may persist

pregnancy and menses may exacerbate disease

increased dietary iron or carbohydrates may be beneficial

McK 176000
Gawkrodger DJ. Porphyrias. In: Champion RH, Burton JL, Ebling FJG, eds. Textbook of Dermatology. Oxford, Blackwell Scientific Publications, 1992:2295–2313

CHESTER PORPHYRIA

no cutaneous photosensitivity

an acute porphyria with neurovisceral symptomatology including abdominal pain and psychiatric symptoms

AD

reduced activity of PBGD (as in acute intermittent porphyria) and PROTOGENO (as in variegate porphyria)

porphyrin excretion pattern in different individuals may be similar to that for variegate porphyria or acute intermittent porphyria or both

appears to be limited to Great Britain, where a large kindred lives in the Chester area

may ultimately represent a variant of variegate porphyria

McK 176010
McColl KE, Thompson GG, Moore MR, et al. Chester porphyria: biochemical studies of a new form of acute porphyria. Lancet 1985;2:796–799

Qadiri MR, Church SE, McColl KE, et al. Chester porphyria: a clinical study of a new form of acute porphyria. Br Med J [Clin Res] 1986;292:455–459

HEREDITARY COPROPORPHYRIA

infrequent cutaneous photosensitivity, blistering, and scarring

symptoms resembling acute intermittent porphyria may occur at any age

hypertension and tachycardia are most common physical signs during attacks

occasionally, patients may show only psychiatric symptoms

AD; rare

enzyme: decreased COPROGENO (lymphocytes, skin fibroblasts), increased ALA synthetase

urine: increased ALA, PBG, COPRO III, and URO during attacks and in lesser quantities between attacks; urine red during attacks

feces: increased COPRO, URO (and hepta-, hexa-, and pentacarboxylic porphyrins) during and between attacks

may be exacerbated by pregnancy

provocation by drugs and prognosis similar to acute intermittent porphyria

asymptomatic family members may have increased urine and fecal COPRO

genetic heterogeneity is suspected, since differences in porphyrin excretion are seen between some homozygotes with hereditary coproporphyria and those with harderoporphyria

McK 121300

Andrews J, Erdjument H, Nicholson DC. Hereditary coproporphyria: incidence in a large English family. J Med Genet 1984;21:341–349

Hunter JAA, Khan SA, Hope E, et al. Hereditary coproporphyria: photosensitivity, jaundice and neuropsychiatric manifestations associated with pregnancy. Br J Dermatol 1971;84:301–310

HARDEROPORPHYRIA

photosensitivity, hypertrichosis, and jaundice due to hemolytic anemia in childhood

occasionally homozygotes for COPROGENO deficiency occur (heterozygotes are patients with HCP), and they excrete high levels of harderoporphyrin (an intermediate product in the conversion of COPRO to PROTO) in stools

Nordmann Y, Grandchamp B, de Verneuil H, et al. Harderoporphyria: a variant hereditary coproporphyria. J Clin Invest 1983;72:1139–1149

ACTINIC PRURIGO OF NATIVE AMERICANS

Synonyms

- hereditary polymorphic light eruption of American Indians
- hereditary photosensitivity of American Indians

Skin

pruritic erythematous, scaling, exudative and crusted papules on face and sun-exposed dorsa of hands and forearms (Fig. 15–6); onset most commonly in childhood

characteristic crusted cheilitis of lips, predominantly lower lip

no vesicles, bullae, or scarring

worse in spring and summer

improves with age

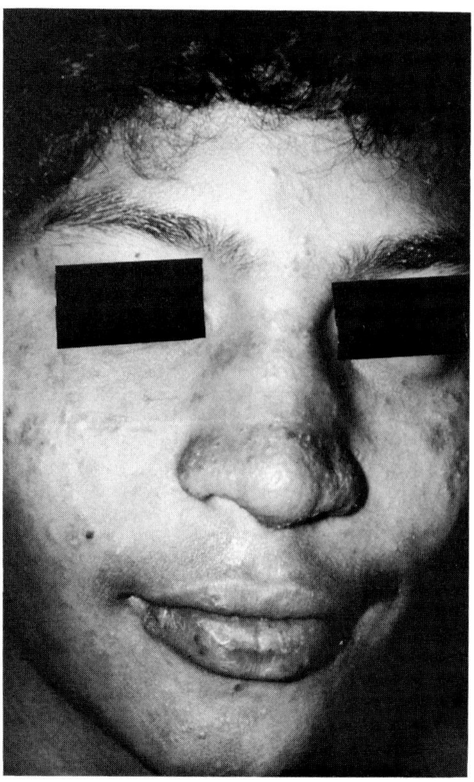

FIGURE 15–6
Actinic prurigo of Native Americans. Young Native American child from Arizona has blisters and erosions on the nose and lips as well as a papular rash on the face. (Courtesy of Ronald C. Hansen, MD, Tucson, Arizona.)

Genetics

AD

Pathophysiology

photosensitizing wavelengths usually in ultraviolet A range

Laboratory Data

laboratory workup for porphyria and lupus erythematosus is negative

REFERENCES

McK 174770
Birt AR, Davis RA. Hereditary polymorphic light eruption of American Indians. Int J Dermatol 1975;14:105–111
Draelos ZK, Hansen RC. Polymorphic light eruption in pediatric patients with American Indian ancestry. Pediatr Dermatol 1986;3:384–389
Lane PR, Hogan DJ, Martel MJ, et al. Actinic prurigo: clinical features and prognosis. J Am Acad Dermatol 1992;26:683–692

HEMOCHROMATOSIS

Synonyms

- bronze diabetes
- pigmentary cirrhosis

Skin

metallic-gray to brown hyperpigmentation, sometimes termed *bronzing*, in most; first involves sun-exposed areas and flexural creases, then becomes generalized

hyperpigmentation may involve ocular, conjunctival, or genital mucosae

hyperpigmentation more likely as disease progresses but may precede other symptoms by years

spider angiomata, palmar erythema, hypotrichosis (axillae and other body hair), and a female-pattern pubic escutcheon may develop due to hyperestrogenemia

Non-Skin

earliest symptoms are usually weakness, lassitude, and weight loss, most often occurring between the fifth and seventh decades

hepatomegaly and frequent abdominal pain and diarrhea; hepatomegaly and abdominal pain may precede other symptoms

cirrhosis variably reported in half to nearly all patients, especially as the disease progresses; ascites may result

splenomegaly in about half

diabetes mellitus, regarded as a classic feature, in about two thirds, usually late in the disease course

myocardial hemosiderosis may result in cardiomyopathy and myocardial conduction abnormalities, with subsequent heart failure or arrhythmias, which may cause death

occasional painful neuropathy in extremities

decreased libido, hypogonadism, atrophic testes, and gynecomastia in up to two thirds of patients; probably related to increased estrogen levels caused by liver disease

arthralgia occurs in up to half of patients; may be the presenting sign

Genetics

AR

compared with women, clinical disease in men is 5 to 10 times more common, is of greater severity, and is of earlier onset; among other factors, menstruation and differences in dietary iron and alcohol intake may explain some of these differences

among a normal white population, about 10% are heterozygous and 0.3% are homozygous for this gene

the gene is closely linked to the HLA locus on the short arm of chromosome 6 and is especially associated with HLA-A3, HLA-B7, and HLA-B14

Laboratory Data

histopathology: hyperpigmentation of skin is mainly due to increased epidermal melanin; liver biopsy has greatest diagnostic specificity, but serum iron studies may be helpful

iron deposits in eccrine sweat glands may occur late in the course of the disease but cause no color changes

Prognosis

survival is variable; those with younger age at onset have a worse prognosis

common causes of death include heart failure, hepatic coma, hepatic carcinoma, hemorrhage, and pneumonia

serial phlebotomies help deplete excess iron stores

Discussion

diagnosis may be difficult since findings may be subtle or variable; some have suggested the workup of any patient with unexplained elevations in iron or serum transferrin levels

environmental factors play an important role in modifying the expression of the phenotype; increased dietary iron and increased alcohol intake will increase the likelihood of disease

heterozygotes are clinically asymptomatic, but laboratory iron abnormalities are seen in up to one fourth; with a normal diet and low alcohol intake, these heterozygotes will have only a modest excess of total body iron

in secondary (i.e., nongenetic) hemochromatosis (secondary hemosiderosis), causes include excessive iron intake, repeated blood transfusions, and alcoholic liver disease; pigmentation is similar, but visceral fibrosis and diabetes are rare; total body iron stores are much less than in the genetic variety

REFERENCES

McK 235200

Bothwell TH, Charlton RW, Motulsky AG. Hemochromatosis. In: Scriver CR, Beaudet AL, Sly WS, Valle D, eds. The Metabolic Basis of Inherited Disease. 6th ed. New York, McGraw-Hill, 1989:1433–1462

Chevrant-Breton J, Simon M, Bourel M, Ferrand B. Cutaneous manifestations of idiopathic hemochromatosis. Arch Dermatol 1977;113:161–165

Edwards CQ, Carroll M, Bray P, Cartwright GE. Hereditary hemochromatosis diagnosis in siblings and children. N Engl J Med 1977;297:7–13

Edwards CQ, Cartwright GE, Skolnick MH, Amos DB. Homozygosity for hemochromatosis: clinical manifestations. Ann Intern Med 1980;93:519–525

Kaikov Y, Wadsworth LD, Hassall E, et al. Primary hemochromatosis in children: report of three newly diagnosed cases and review of the pediatric literature. Pediatrics 1992;90:37–42

Leyden JJ, Lockshin NA, Kriebel S. The black keratinous cyst: a sign of hemochromatosis. Arch Dermatol 1972;106:379–381

Milman N, Graudal N, Nielsen LS, et al. Family studies of hereditary hemochromatosis in Denmark and the Faroe Islands. Hum Genet 1990;85:228–232

Yaouanq J, El Kahloun A, Chorney M, et al. Familial screening for genetic haemochromatosis by means of DNA markers. J Med Genet 1992;29:320–322

ALPHA-1-ANTITRYPSIN DEFICIENCY

Skin

red, painful, tender subcutaneous nodules that may ulcerate and drain; found on trunk and proximal extremities and may be precipitated by trauma

usually begins in adulthood but onset in first 2 decades of life reported

Non-Skin

chronic obstructive pulmonary disease is most common clinical manifestation, with emphysema predominating over bronchitic presentations; onset usually in adulthood with most by sixth decade

liver disease in 10% to 20%, usually manifesting as obstructive jaundice in infancy that resolves; some eventually develop cirrhosis

Genetics

autosomal co-dominant

partial deficiency (heterozygote state) found in 1 of 50 North Americans

Pathophysiology

alpha-1-antitrypsin is a serum protease inhibitor; the main physiologic substrate it protects is elastase, particularly in the lower respiratory tract

Laboratory Data

histopathology: lobular panniculitis

plasma alpha-1-antitrypsin level usually less than 20% of normal in those with ZZ genotype (see Discussion)

antineutrophil cytoplasmic antibody may be positive

Prognosis

avoidance of smoking may greatly delay onset of clinical symptoms of lung disease and retard course of pulmonary deterioration

intravenous infusions of human alpha-1-antitrypsin concentrates from donors and dapsone reportedly successful in treating panniculitis

Discussion

at least 60 alleles, or protease inhibitor (PI) types, are known, the majority of which result in quantitatively and qualitatively normal alpha-1-antitrypsin; PI M is the most common normal allele; PI ZZ (homozygous for the Z allele) patients have the most serious disease.

heterozygotes are less severely affected but are still predisposed to emphysema

any panniculitis not involving the legs, especially in those with pulmonary disease, may warrant evaluation for alpha-1-antitrypsin deficiency

REFERENCES

McK 107400

Edmonds BK, Hodge JA, Rietschel RL. Alpha-1-antitrypsin deficiency-associated panniculitis: case report and review of the literature. Pediatr Dermatol 1991;8:296–299

Ibarguen E, Gross CR, Savik SK, Sharp HL. Liver disease in alpha-1-antitrypsin deficiency: prognostic indicators. J Pediatr 1990;117:864–870

Morse JO. Alpha-1-antitrypsin deficiency. N Engl J Med 1978;299:1045–1048, 1099–1105

Smith KC, Pittelkow MR, Su WP. Panniculitis associated with severe alpha-1-antitrypsin deficiency: treatment and review of the literature. [Review]. Arch Dermatol 1987;123:1655–1661

Smith KC, Su WP, Pittelkow MR, et al. Clinical and pathologic correlations in 96 patients with panniculitis, including 15 patients with deficient levels of alpha-1-antitrypsin. J Am Acad Dermatol 1989;21:1192–1196

Su WPD, Smith KC, Pittelkow MR, Winkelmann RK. Alpha-1-antitrypsin deficiency panniculitis: a histopathologic and immunopathologic study of four cases. Am J Dermatopathol 1987;9:483–490

Multiple Carboxylase Deficiency

Multiple carboxylase deficiency is divided into two forms, both of autosomal recessive inheritance: (1) holocarboxylase synthetase deficiency and (2) biotinidase deficiency. These enzyme deficiencies involve metabolic pathways requiring biotin, an essential coenzyme needed in a variety of carboxylation reactions related to metabolism of nucleic acids, fatty acids, carbohydrates, and branched-chain amino acids. Nutritional biotin deficiency mimics the clinical and biochemical features of these inherited disorders.

Holocarboxylase synthetase binds biotin to an inactive apocarboxylase, converting it into an active holocarboxylase that fixes carbon dioxide. In holocarboxylase synthetase deficiency, at least three carboxylases are functionally deficient: beta-methylcrotonyl (or 3-methylcrotonyl) CoA carboxylase, propionyl-CoA carboxylase, and pyruvate carboxylase. Since levels of all three carboxylases are deficient, the condition is termed *multiple* carboxylase deficiency. Biotinidase is required to degrade the individual carboxylases into biotin and apocarboxylase.

Decreased B- and T-cell immunity are presumed to follow from the biochemical abnormalities. Delayed hypersensitivity skin testing is usually negative. Diagnosis is made by demonstrating elevation of specific organic acids in plasma and urine and confirmed by demonstrating enzyme deficiency in cultured leukocytes or fibroblasts. Treatment is with oral biotin.

REFERENCES

McK 210200

Sweetman L, Nyhan WL. Inheritable biotin-treatable disorders and associated phenomena. Ann Rev Nutr 1986;6:317–343

Williams ML. Biotin-responsive multiple carboxylase deficiency and immunodeficiency. Curr Probl Dermatol 1989;18:89–92

HOLOCARBOXYLASE SYNTHETASE DEFICIENCY

Skin

the neonatal variant of multiple carboxylase deficiency

dermatitis is not a prominent feature in the early stages but later may become generalized

alopecia, when present, is usually generalized

Non-Skin

severe vomiting, metabolic acidosis, seizures, hypotonia and hypertonia, and coma in first days to weeks of life

severe bacterial and viral infections; various immune defects described in some patients

Genetics

AR

Laboratory Data

increased urinary excretion of 3-hydroxyisovaleric acid and 3-methylcrotonylglycine are hallmark features

prenatal diagnosis possible (markedly elevated 3-hydroxyisovaleric acid levels in amniotic fluid)

Prognosis

death occurs in absence of prompt diagnosis and therapy with biotin

Discussion

hair loss but no cutaneous eruption reported in isolated deficiency of 3-methylcrotonyl-CoA carboxylase

REFERENCES

McK 253270

Charles BM, Hosking G, Green A, et al. Biotin-responsive alopecia and developmental regression. Lancet 1979;2:118–120

Sweetman L, Nyhan WL. Inheritable biotin-treatable disorders and associated phenomena. Ann Rev Nutr 1986;6:317–343

Williams ML. Biotin-responsive multiple carboxylase deficiency and immunodeficiency. Curr Probl Dermatol 1989;18:89–92

BIOTINIDASE DEFICIENCY

Skin

the infantile variant of multiple carboxylase deficiency

periorificial scaling and erythema, sometimes crusted; perioral and periorbital areas most involved; onset in infancy (usually after several months of life) or early childhood

sparse scalp hair; occasional alopecia of eyebrows and eyelashes

alopecia and periorificial dermatitis may resemble findings in acrodermatitis enteropathica

Non-Skin

neurologic abnormalities include seizures and ataxia

intermittent metabolic acidosis

recurrent infections; various immune defects described in some patients

sensorineural hearing loss

eye abnormalities include keratoconjunctivitis, corneal ulcers, and optic atrophy

Genetics

AR

Laboratory Data

patients have less than 10% of mean normal biotinidase activity

neonatal screening using a rapid colorimetric method (biotinidase assay)

increased urinary excretion of 3-hydroxyisovaleric acid, 3-methylcrotonylglycine, 3-hydroxypropionic acid, and 2-methylcitric acid

low levels of biotin in blood and urine

increased biocytin in urine

parents have 50% of mean normal biotinidase activity

prenatal diagnosis may be possible through measurement of biotinidase activity of amniocytes

Prognosis

early biotin therapy may reverse disease course except for some neurologic abnormalities, including sensorineural hearing loss and optic atrophy

Discussion

- *partial biotinidase deficiency*

  possible variant of profound biotinidase deficiency

  may have hair loss, cutaneous eruption, and hypotonia

  AR in most

  10% to 30% of mean normal biotinidase activity (cf. <10% of mean normal activity in profound biotinidase deficiency)

  resolves with biotin therapy

REFERENCES

McK 253260

Packman S, Sweetman L, Yoshino M, et al. Biotin-responsive multiple carboxylase deficiency of infantile onset. J Pediatr 1981;99:421–423

McVoy JR, Levy HL, Lawler M, et al. Partial biotinidase deficiency: clinical and biochemical features. J Pediatr 1990; 116:78–83

Sweetman L, Nyhan WL. Inheritable biotin-treatable disorders and associated phenomena. Ann Rev Nutr 1986;6:317–343

Williams ML. Biotin-responsive multiple carboxylase deficiency and immunodeficiency. Curr Probl Dermatol 1989;18:89–92

Wolf B, Heard GS, Jefferson LG, et al. Clinical findings in four children with biotinidase deficiency detected through a statewide neonatal screening program. N Engl J Med 1985;313:16–19

OXALOSIS I

Synonyms

- glycolic aciduria
- L-glyceric aciduria

Skin

skin findings include calcinosis cutis, acrocyanosis, livedo reticularis, vasospasm, Raynaud phenomenon, and peripheral gangrene, especially late in course

Non-Skin

renal oxalosis causes nephrolithiasis and renal colic in two thirds of patients by age 5 years

other organs may be involved, including the heart (causing arrhythmias), liver, joints (causing arthritis), and nerves (causing progressive peripheral neuropathy)

Genetics

AR; many sporadic cases reported

Pathophysiology

type I (glycolic aciduria): deficiency of 2-hydroxy-3-oxoadipate carboxylase

type II (L-glyceric aciduria): deficiency of D-glyceric dehydrogenase

Laboratory Data

widespread deposition of calcium oxalate crystals in many tissues

skin biopsy specimens show granulomatous inflammation with birefringent crystals in dermal and subcutaneous blood vessel walls and extravascularly

Prognosis

renal failure ensues in childhood or adulthood; 80% of patients die of renal failure by age 20 years

Discussion

milder adult onset forms have been reported

causes of acquired (secondary) oxalosis include ingestion of ethylene glycol, glycerol, large doses of ascorbic acid and excessive dietary intake; other causes include increased intestinal oxylate absorption (seen in ileal resection or other intestinal diseases), methoxyflurane anesthesia, glycerol or xylitol infusions, pyridoxine deficiency, and impaired renal excretion (acute or chronic renal failure)

REFERENCES

McK 259900

Greer KE, Cooper PH, Campbell F, Westervelt FBJ. Primary oxalosis with livedo reticularis. Arch Dermatol 1980;116:213–214

Spiers EM, Sanders DY, Omura EF. Clinical and histologic features of primary oxalosis. J Am Acad Dermatol 1990;22:952–956

PROLIDASE DEFICIENCY

Skin

most patients have cutaneous manifestations, usually before puberty

increased fragility and, in some areas, atrophic-appearing skin; leg ulcers are common and heal with scarring (Fig. 15–7)

occasional photosensitivity, telangiectasia, poliosis, and erythematous scaling plaques, most notably on the face

Non-Skin

chronic recurrent infections, including otitis media and sinusitis

craniofacial abnormalities, splenomegaly, and variable mental retardation also common

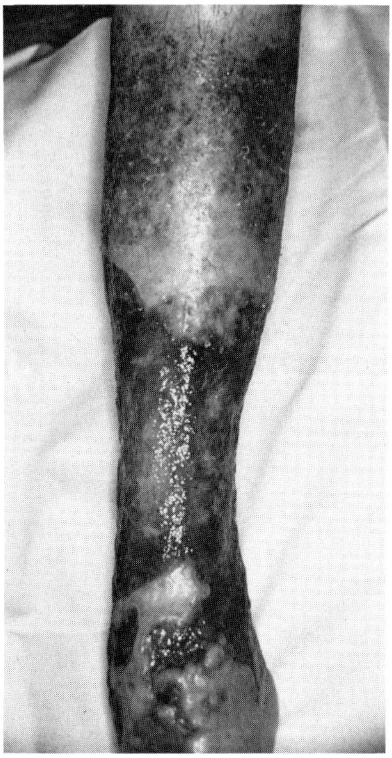

FIGURE 15–7
Prolidase deficiency. This woman had chronic ulcerations of both legs for many years. She was diagnosed as having factitial ulcers and was treated by a psychiatrist. Once prolidase deficiency was diagnosed, her legs were amputated and she did well. Ulceration is almost always limited to below the knee in prolidase deficiency.

Genetics

AR

Pathophysiology

deficiency of prolidase (imidodipeptidase or proline dipeptidase), which is essential for normal metabolism of proline and hydroxyproline residues abundant in collagen and elastin

Laboratory Data

enzyme deficiency can be measured in erythrocytes, leukocytes, and fibroblasts

Prognosis

proline topically may be beneficial

enzyme replacement therapy may be possible

Discussion

some patients have the metabolic abnormality but are asymptomatic

REFERENCES

McK 170100

Arata J, Hatakenaka K, Oono T. Effect of topical application of glycine and proline on recalcitrant leg ulcers of prolidase deficiency. Arch Dermatol 1986;122:626–627

Arata J, Umemura S, Yamamoto Y, et al. Prolidase deficiency: its dermatological manifestations and some additional biochemical studies. Arch Dermatol 1979;115:62–67

Hechtman P, Richter A, Corman N, Leong Y-M. In situ activation of human erythrocyte prolidase: potential for enzyme replacement therapy in prolidase deficiency. Pediatr Res 1988;24:709–712

Leoni A, Cetta G, Tenni R, et al. Prolidase deficiency in two siblings with chronic leg ulcerations. Clinical, biochemical, and morphologic aspects. Arch Dermatol 1987;123:493–499

Milligan A, Graham-Brown RA, Burns DA, Anderson I. Prolidase deficiency: a case report and literature review. Br J Dermatol 1989;121:405–409

PROTEIN C DEFICIENCY, TYPE I

Skin

see Figure 15–8

ecchymoses, purpura, and occasionally gangrenous plaques or body parts (e.g., toes) in later childhood to adulthood; many asymptomatic

Non-Skin

recurrent deep venous thromboses, pulmonary emboli, and/or portal vein thromboses begin in early or middle adult life; thromboembolic phenomena are usually venous and rarely arterial

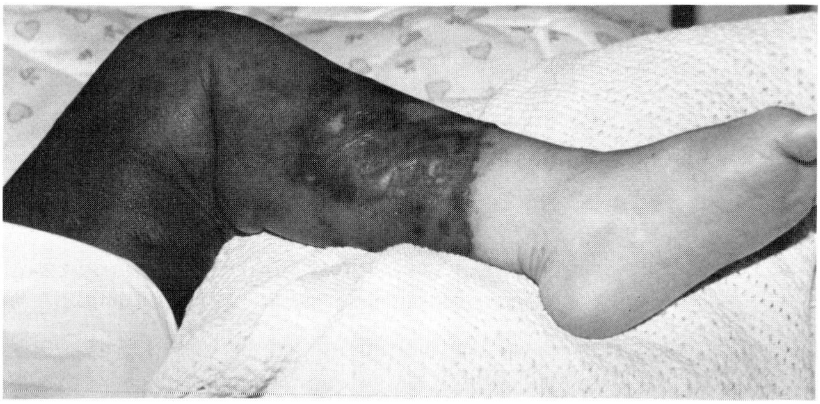

FIGURE 15–8
Protein C deficiency. This young child suffered a massive area of purpura fulminans and deep necrosis. A sibling had died of a stroke in infancy.

thromboembolic phenomena are occasionally precipitated by trauma, including surgery, pregnancy, or oral contraceptive use

Genetics

AD; prevalence 1:15,000

Pathophysiology

protein C is 62-kd vitamin K–dependent serum protease zymogen; when activated, it is a natural anticoagulant, inactivating clotting factors V and VIII; it is also profibrinolytic

protein S, another vitamin K–dependent serum protein, enhances the anticoagulant activity of protein C

mechanism of thromboses due to warfarin therapy involves decrease in protein C faster than warfarin's depression of vitamin K–dependent procoagulants

Laboratory Data

protein C concentration reduced in plasma in both functional and immunologic assays

Prognosis

acute cases accompanied by disseminated intravascular coagulation are treated with fresh frozen plasma; treatment with purified protein C concentrate also reported

long-term treatment with warfarin may minimize occurrence of thrombosis, but initiation of therapy may paradoxically cause thrombosis in a small proportion (1% or less of heterozygotes) of patients (see Pathophysiology)

warfarin-induced thrombosis may be preventable with initial heparin loading or, if it occurs, be treated with fresh-frozen plasma

Discussion

acquired protein C deficiency may be seen in disseminated intravascular coagulation and multiple myeloma

- *homozygous type I protein C deficiency*

an extremely variable phenotype

some suffer recurrent, moderately severe thromboses while others die in infancy of overwhelming thromboses and embolism involving both the skin (purpura fulminans) and internal organs

some individuals remain entirely unaffected

initial treatment is with plasma; once lesions have healed either protein C replacement or oral anticoagulant therapy may be used for long-term treatment

beneficial liver transplantation reported

McK 176860.0005

- *type II protein C deficiency*

antigenically normal but functionally abnormal protein C activity; less common than type I protein C deficiency

REFERENCES

McK 176860

Clouse LH, Comp PC. The regulation of hemostasis: the protein C system. N Engl J Med 1986;314:1298–1304

Dreyfus M, Magny JF, Bridey F, et al. Treatment of homozygous protein C deficiency and neonatal purpura fulminans with a purified protein C concentrate. N Engl J Med 1991;325:1565–1568

Gladson CL, Groncy P, Griffin JH. Coumarin necrosis, neonatal purpura fulminans, and protein C deficiency. [Review]. Arch Dermatol 1987;123:1701a–1706a

Manco-Johnson MJ, Mariar RA, Jacobson LJ, et al. Severe protein C deficiency in newborn infants. J Pediatr 1988;113:359–363

Marlar RA, Montgomery RR, Broekmans AW. Diagnosis and treatment of homozygous protein C deficiency: report of the Working Party on Homozygous Protein C Deficiency of the Subcommittee on Protein C and Protein S, International Committee on Thrombosis and Haemostasis. J Pediatr 1989; 114:528–534

Peters C, Casella JF, Marlar RA, et al. Homozygous protein C deficiency: observations on the nature of the molecular abnormality and the effectiveness of warfarin therapy. Pediatrics 1988;81:272–276

PROTEIN S DEFICIENCY

most patients are asymptomatic

leg ulcers reported

a homozygous patient presented in infancy with purpuric and necrotic skin lesions

recurrent thromboembolic disease including deep venous thromboses, superficial thrombophlebitis, and pulmonary embolism occurring in early adulthood; onset ranges from second to seventh decade

AD

warfarin therapy is effective and has not been associated with skin necrosis

protein S is a vitamin K–dependent serum protein that enhances the anticoagulant activity of protein C

McK 176880

Comp PC, Esmon CT. Recurrent venous thromboembolism in patients with a partial deficiency of protein S. N Engl J Med 1984;311:1525–1528

Engesser I, Broekmans AW, Briet E, et al. Hereditary protein S deficiency: clinical manifestations. Ann Intern Med 1987;106:677–682

Mahasandana C, Suvatte V, Chuansumrit A, et al. Homozygous protein S deficiency in an infant with purpura fulminans. J Pediatr 1990;117:750–753

Pegelow CH, Ledford M, Young J, Zilleruelo G. Severe protein S deficiency in a newborn. Pediatrics 1992;89:674–676

Vicente V, Alberca I, Tabernero MD, Lopez BAL. Ulcer necrotic legs as first manifestation of protein S deficiency. [Letter]. Blut 1987;54:253–254

LIPOID PROTEINOSIS

Synonyms

- hyalinosis cutis et mucosae
- Urbach-Wiethe disease

Skin

yellowish white indurated papules, plaques, and nodules on skin and oral, rectal, and genital mucosae (Fig. 15–9); cutaneous lesions may be present at birth but usually develop later than mucosal lesions, which commonly begin in infancy or early childhood

lesions typically found on face, forehead, eyelids, dorsa of hands and feet, extremities, and axillae; eyelid lesions usually on upper lids with a characteristic "string of pearls" appearance; occasional linear groups of papules in axillary folds (Fig. 15–10)

varioliform or "worm-eaten" scarring resulting from dark, crusted blisters and pustules in early life (typically, a history of "impetigo" or "infection" is given); grooves radiate from the corners of the mouth onto cheeks and chin

occasional yellowish verrucous plaques on the elbows, knees, hands, feet, and buttocks

hypotrichosis of scalp and eyelashes, less often involving eyebrows or beard

thickened and indurated lips, especially lower lip

nodules or grooves may form on the tongue, which becomes thickened and indurated; lingual papillae are atrophic and the frenulum shortens; protrusion of the tongue is difficult

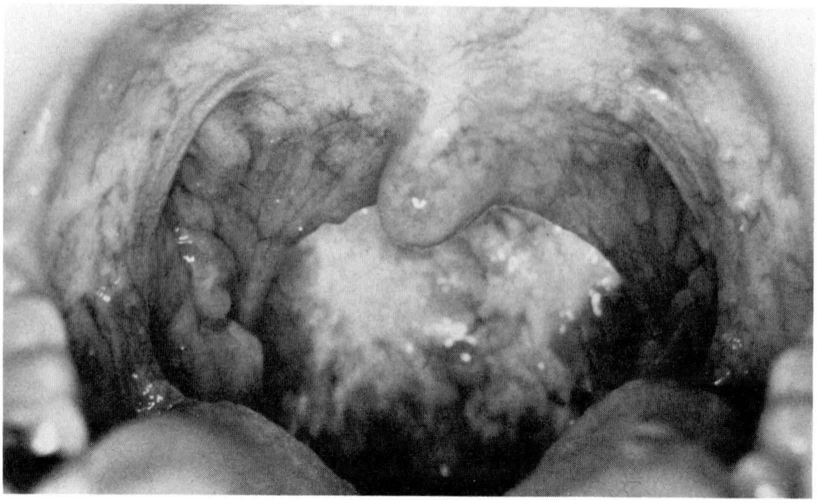

FIGURE 15–9
Lipoid proteinosis. Infiltrative plaques are seen covering much of the palate. They also involve the larynx and lead to hoarseness. (Courtesy of Dr. Miklos Simon, Erlangen, Germany; reprinted with permission from Simon M Jr, Zobe A, Fartasch M. Hyalinosis cutis et mucosae [Urbach-Wiethe] in 2 sisters. Hautarzt 1990;41:458–460.)

involvement of Stenson's papillae may cause recurrent parotitis

nails normal

dental abnormalities common

Non-Skin

involvement of almost any organ may occur

mucosal lesions may involve the larynx (causing a hoarse cry, frequently the first sign of the disease at birth or in early infancy, or stenosis, which rarely requires tracheostomy), lacrimal system (lacrimation may not develop), esophagus, possibly causing dysphagia, or the stomach

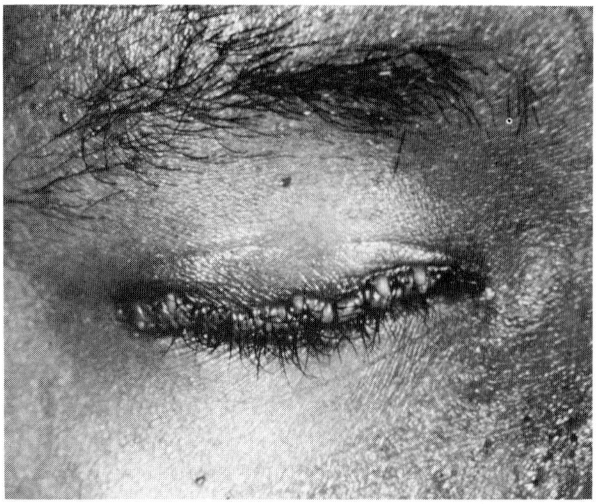

FIGURE 15–10
Lipoid proteinosis. Multiple yellowish white papules on the eyelid with the characteristic "string of pearls" appearance.

frequent bilateral cerebral calcification (the sickle-shaped calcifications may be pathognomonic), sometimes associated with epilepsy

eye abnormalities include drusen of Bruch's membrane in about half (seen later in life), retinal degenerative changes, corneal opacities, and pseudomembranous conjunctivitis

Genetics

AR

greater incidence in whites with patients mostly of Dutch and German ancestry; large pedigrees in South Africa and Sweden

Laboratory Data

histopathology: in early lesions, hyaline material in and around the basement membranes of superficial blood vessels, eccrine sweat glands, smooth muscle, and nerves; in older lesions, diffuse hyaline material in dermis or submucosa

exact chemical composition of the hyaline material is unknown; mixtures of normal and abnormal collagen, lipids, glycoproteins, and proteoglycans reported; the material is periodic acid–Schiff positive (sudanophilic) and diastase resistant

decreased type I procollagen mRNA reported

Prognosis

life expectancy usually normal, but early death may result from uncommon systemic involvement or infection

hyaline deposits increase until adult life, then stabilize

dramatic response to oral dimethyl sulfoxide reported

Discussion

cutaneous and mucosal findings variably absent (e.g., tongue may not be indurated), hoarseness may be absent, and different presentations of the disease may not manifest until adult life

REFERENCES

McK 247100

Harper JI, Duance VC, Sims TJ, Light ND. Lipoid proteinosis: an inherited disorder of collagen metabolism? Br J Dermatol 1985; 113:145–151

Hofer PA. Urbach-Wiethe disease (lipoglycoproteinosis; lipoid proteinosis; hyalinosis cutis et mucosae): a review. Acta Derm Venereol Suppl 1973;53:1–52

Moy LS, Moy RL, Matsuoka LY, et al. Lipoid proteinosis: ultrastructural and biochemical studies. J Am Acad Dermatol 1987; 16:1193–1201

Pierard GE, Van Cauwenberge D, Budo J, Lapiere CM. A clinicopathologic study of six cases of lipoid proteinosis. Am J Dermatopathol 1988;10:300–305

Urbach E, Wiethe C. Lipoidosis cutis et mucosae. Virchows Arch [Pathol Anat] 1929; 273:285–319

Wong CK, Lin CS. Remarkable response of lipoid proteinosis to oral dimethyl sulphoxide. Br J Dermatol 1988;119:541–544

Hereditary Amyloidosis Syndromes

The amyloidoses are a heterogeneous group of disorders characterized by the extracellular deposition of straight, beta-pleated protein fibrils 7.5 to 10 nm in diameter and of varying length. The fibrils are formed from a variety of proteins, including immunoglobulin light chains, serum acute-phase proteins, and keratin degradation products. The beta-pleated structure leads to birefringence, certain histochemical properties, and lack of degradability. Persistence of amyloid deposits disrupts normal tissue function; for example, amyloid deposits in nerves causes neuropathy.

There are many ways to classify amyloidoses. When classified by amyloid protein type, the two main amyloidoses are

1. Amyloid AA (AA = amyloid A protein); seen in reactive amyloidoses, familial Mediterranean fever, and Muckle-Wells syndrome
2. Amyloid AL (AL = amyloid immunoglobulin light chain); seen in idiopathic (primary) myeloma or macroglobulinemia-associated amyloidosis

The great majority of cases of hereditary amyloidosis are due to abnormal transthyretin (TTR), also known as prealbumin, a plasma protein. The name "prealbumin" refers to electrophoretic behavior, since prealbumin has no structural relationship to albumin. The abnormal amyloid protein is designated ATTR. Most types of hereditary systemic amyloidosis can be classified chemically according to amino acid substitutions in the abnormal prealbumin molecules. These molecules are not often deposited in the skin in sufficient quantity to produce clinical lesions; findings may include carpal tunnel syndrome, neuropathy, and abnormalities related to deposition of amyloid in organs, including the eye, heart, bowel, and kidney. Thus, skin biopsy is relatively unhelpful in most familial amyloidoses. The reader is referred to a review of hereditary amyloidosis syndromes by Benson and Wallace (1989) (see References).

There are hereditary syndromes presented elsewhere in this book in which amyloidosis may be seen and these include

familial Mediterranean fever
Muckle-Wells syndrome
Sipple syndrome
pachyonychia congenita, Tidman-Wells-MacDonald type

REFERENCES

Benson MD, Wallace MR. Amyloidosis. In: Scriver CR, Beaudet AL, Sly WS, Valle D, eds. The Metabolic Basis of Inherited Disease. 6th ed. New York, McGraw-Hill, 1989:2439–2460

Benson MD. Inherited amyloidosis. J Med Genet 1991;28:73–78

Cohen AS. Amyloidosis. Bull Rheum Dis 1991;40:1–12

Newton JA, Jagjivan A, Bhogal B, et al. Familial primary cutaneous amyloidosis. Br J Dermatol 1985;112:201–208

Varga J, Wohlgethan JR. The clinical and biochemical spectrum of hereditary amyloidosis. Semin Arthritis Rheum 1988;18:14–28

Vasily DB, Bhatia SG, Uhlin SR. Familial primary cutaneous amyloidosis: clinical, genetic, and immunofluorescent studies. Arch Dermatol 1978;114:1173–1176

FAMILIAL PRIMARY CUTANEOUS AMYLOIDOSIS (FAMILIAL LICHEN AMYLOIDOSIS)

pruritic, discrete yellowish to yellowish brown papules, usually developing in childhood but also occurring in adults

lesions gradually progressive; may become hyperkeratotic

usually involve the shins, especially initially, but may also involve the thighs, trunk, neck, and/or upper extremities

hyperpigmented macules or swirled hyperpigmentation in some

AD

histopathology: amyloid deposits in the papillary dermis

indistinguishable from the sporadic form; amyloid deposits are localized to the skin

McK 105250

Le Boit PH, Greene I. Primary cutaneous amyloidosis: identically distributed lesions in identical twins. Pediatr Dermatol 1986; 3:244–246

Newton JA, Jagjivan A, Bhogal B, et al. Familial primary cutaneous amyloidosis. Br J Dermatol 1985;112:201–208

Ozaki M. Familial lichen amyloidosis. Int J Dermatol 1984;23:190–193

Partington MW, Marriott PJ, Prentice RSA, et al. Familial cutaneous amyloidosis with systemic manifestations in males. Am J Med Genet 1981;10:65–75

Vasily DB, Bhatia SG, Uhlin SR. Familial primary cutaneous amyloidosis: clinical, genetic and immunofluorescence studies. Arch Dermatol 1978;114:1173–1176

AMYLOIDOSIS OF GINGIVA AND CONJUNCTIVA WITH MENTAL RETARDATION

possible AR

McK 204850

Hornova J, Dlurosova O. Primary amyloidosis of gingiva and conjunctiva and mental disorder in a brother and sister. Oral Surg 1968;25:457–464

FAMILIAL MEDITERRANEAN FEVER

Synonyms

- benign paroxysmal peritonitis
- familial recurrent polyserositis
- periodic disease

Skin

occasional erysipelas-like eruption on lower extremities (Color Fig. 15–1); may rarely be the only sign besides fever

occasional mobile subcutaneous periarticular nodules

infrequent generalized or localized urticaria between or during attacks

Non-Skin

recurrent bouts of self-limited, low-grade fever usually lasting 1 to 3 days; onset at any age, most commonly first or second decades

febrile attacks initially infrequent but become more frequent, often every 1 to 4 weeks

abdominal pain, either preceding (by hours) or coincident with febrile attacks, occurs in 95% of cases

acute abdominal findings are common, including board-like rigidity, tenderness, and absence of bowel sounds

pain and abdominal findings last 1 to 2 days, rarely as long as 1 week; diarrhea often follows the attacks

attacks may decrease during pregnancy, but the opposite has also been reported

synovitis with arthralgia, especially knee, ankle, hip, and shoulder, occurs in 75%; effusion is sterile, but symptoms may mimic septic arthritis (fever and arthralgia)

pleuritis, often unilateral and inferior, occurs in 40% of cases, most commonly in children, either in isolation or in conjunction with fever and abdominal pain

physical and sexual development is commonly retarded

amyloidosis of the kidney with nephrotic syndrome and uremia in one fourth of patients

Genetics

AR; possible AD cases also reported

male to female ratio: 3:2

mostly in persons of Mediterranean origin, especially Arabs, Sephardic Jews, and Armenians

defective gene localized to short arm of chromosome 16

Prognosis

life expectancy shortened due to renal failure in about one fourth of patients

colchicine ameliorates or prevents nephropathy if used early enough in the course of the disease

Discussion

in one variant, amyloidosis is the first manifestation of the disease, preceding the onset of the febrile attacks

the Muckle-Wells syndrome (see main entry) also has periodic constitutional symptoms ("aguey bouts" occurring every few weeks) and renal amyloidosis; however, polyserositis not seen

REFERENCES

McK 249100

Azizi E, Fisher BK. Cutaneous manifestations of familial Mediterranean fever. Arch Dermatol 1976;112:364–366

Barakat MH, Karnik AM, Majeed HW, et al. Familial Mediterranean fever (recurrent hereditary polyserositis) in Arabs—a study of 175 patients and review of the literature. Q J Med 1986;60:837–847

Meyerhoff J. Familial Mediterranean fever: report of a large family, review of the literature, and discussion of the frequency of amyloidosis. Medicine 1980;59:66–77

Pras E, Akseutijevich I, Gruberg L, et al. Mapping of a gene causing familial Mediterranean fever to the short arm of chromosome 16. N Engl J Med 1992;326:1509–1513

Zemer D, Pras M, Sohar E, et al. Colchicine in the prevention and treatment of the amyloidosis of familial Mediterranean fever. N Engl J Med 1986;314:1001–1005

ALBRIGHT HEREDITARY OSTEODYSTROPHY

Synonyms

- pseudohypoparathyroidism
- pseudopseudohypoparathyroidism

Skin

ectopic bone formation in skin, subcutaneous tissue, along fascial planes, in tendons, and in periarticular areas (e.g., calcified nodules of scalp or distal extremities); onset in first few years of life; unrelated to serum phosphorus or calcium levels

attached earlobes; low occipital hairline

short wide nails in about half

dental abnormalities include enamel hypoplasia and delayed dentition

Non-Skin

short stature, obesity, and round facies are apparent by infancy or early childhood

craniofacial abnormalities include brachycephaly or (rarely) microcephaly, prominent forehead, low nasal bridge, and a short neck; cranial hyperostosis in about one third

anosmia in patients deficient in coupling protein (Gs protein [stimulatory guanine nucleotide-binding protein]) brachymetacarpalism and brachymetatarsalism (short, stubby fingers and toes) particularly of the fourth and fifth digits due to premature epiphyseal closure; results in dimpling over metacarpophalangeal joint ("Albright's sign," sometimes called "knuckle-knuckle-dimple-dimple" sign)

short distal thumb with a wide thumbnail is also characteristic

mild to moderate mental retardation in about 70% of those with low calcium levels, less commonly in normocalcemic patients

cataracts in about one fourth of patients; blue sclerae

frequent hypogonadism and hypothyroidism

Genetics

AD; AR cases reported

more frequent and severe in females

Pathophysiology

kidneys and bones fail to respond to parathyroid hormone; in type I pseudohypoparathyroidism there is an absence of the normally increased urinary excretion of both cyclic adenosine monophosphate and phosphate in response to exogenous parathyroid hormone, while in type II there is increased cyclic adenosine monophosphate excretion and only phosphate excretion is blunted; type I is further divided into type Ia in which there is a defect in a receptor-cyclase coupling protein Gs, and type Ib in which this defect is not manifest; pseudopseudohypoparathyroidism is a normocalcemic variant

Laboratory Data

laboratory evaluation is confusing because calcium levels vary throughout life and cannot be used for screening

in pseudohypoparathyroidism, serum calcium level is decreased, serum phosphorus level is increased, and immunoreactive parathyroid hormone is increased; patients do not respond to exogenous parathyroid hormone

pseudopseudohypoparathyroidism has phenotype of pseudohypoparathyroidism, but serum calcium and phosphorus levels are normal

radiographs reveal bony deposits and calcification of basal ganglia, choroid plexus, and falx cerebri

Prognosis

early diagnosis through recognition of skin manifestations important in prevention of hypocalcemia-related side effects

measurement of Gs coupling-protein detects type Ia subgroup identifying those at greatest risk for endocrine disturbances

in later life, patients become normocalcemic and disease seems to abate

REFERENCES

McK 300800
McK 203330
Barranco VP. Cutaneous ossification in pseudohypoparathyroidism. Arch Dermatol 1971; 104:643–647
Eyre WG, Reed WB. Albright's hereditary osteodystrophy with cutaneous bone formation. Arch Dermatol 1971;104:636–642
Fitch N. Albright's hereditary osteodystrophy: a review. Am J Med Genet 1982;11:11–29
Gorlin RJ, Cohen MM Jr, Levin LS. Syndromes of the Head and Neck. 3rd ed. New York, Oxford University Press, 1990:139–143
Prendiville JS, Lucky AW, Mallory SB, et al. Osteoma cutis as a presenting sign of pseudohypoparathyroidism. Pediatr Dermatol 1991;8:11–8
Spiegel AM. Albright's hereditary osteodystrophy and defective G proteins. N Engl J Med 1990;322:1461–1462

LESCH-NYHAN SYNDROME

Skin

violent self-mutilation of lips (lower lip more commonly than upper lip), buccal mucosa, fingers, and shoulders in 85% of patients (Fig. 15–11)

onset usually in first 4 years of life but rarely up until second decade

Non-Skin

normal at birth, but motor retardation evident later in first year of life; few patients ever walk or sit unassisted; postnatal growth retardation

"orange sand" or "orange crystals" may be noted in infant diapers before neurologic problems manifest

moderate to severe mental retardation in most; dysarthric speech

choreoathetosis and spastic paralysis by 1 year of age, with subsequent hypertrophy of some muscles due to spasms; frequent head-banging is characteristic

stigmata of gout due to hyperuricemia, include renal stones, acid crystal nephropathy, tophi formation, and a form of gouty arthritis

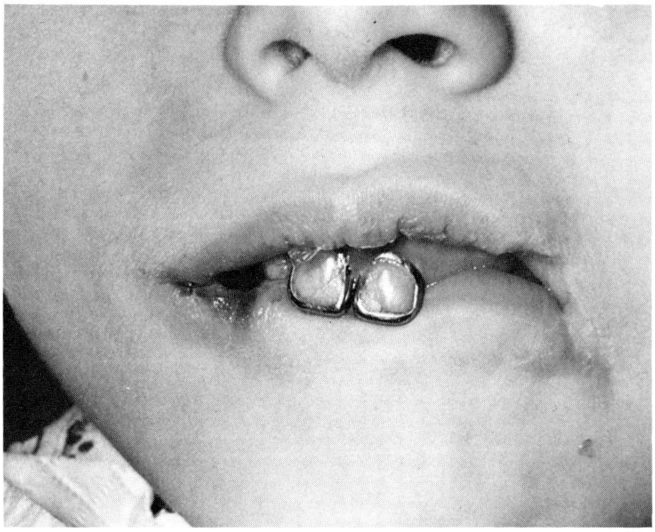

FIGURE 15–11
Lesch-Nyhan syndrome. Distortion of the lips with angular scars due to self-mutilation.

Genetics

XLR; males only; marked genetic heterogeneity

Pathophysiology

deficiency of hypoxanthine-guanine phosphoribosyltransferase (HGPRT), causing a fivefold increase in uric acid production

Laboratory Data

prenatal diagnosis possible by enzyme assay in amniocytes or chorionic villus tissue

urinary uric acid/creatinine ratio is a useful screening test to detect individuals with undifferentiated neurologic signs

Prognosis

death occurs early, usually due to renal failure, inanition, aspiration pneumonia, or neurologic damage

uric acid–lowering drugs decrease most of the sequelae of hyperuricemia but do not prevent neurologic abnormalities

Discussion

rarely, some individuals lack self-mutilating behavior despite having the biochemical defect and the other clinical features

patients with partial deficiency of HGPRT may develop only hyperuricemia and gouty arthritis without neurologic sequelae

the Lesch-Nyhan phenotype with normal HGPRT reported (McK 308950)

REFERENCES

McK 308000

Christie R, Bay C, Kaufman IA, et al. Lesch-Nyhan disease: clinical experience with nineteen patients. Dev Med Child Neurol 1982;24:293–306

Hoefnagel D, Andrew ED, Mireault NG, Berndt WO. Hereditary choreoathetosis, self-mutilation and hyperuricemia in young males. N Engl J Med 1965;273:130–135

Lesch M, Nyhan WL. A familial disorder of uric acid metabolism and central nervous system function. Am J Med 1964;36:561–570

Stout JT, Caskey CT. The Lesch-Nyhan syndrome: clinical, molecular and genetic aspects. Trends Genet 1988;4:175–178

ACATALASEMIA

Synonyms

- Takahara disease

Skin

increased susceptibility to peroxide-generating bacteria such as streptococci and pneumococci

spectrum of disease ranges from painful gingival ulcers to alveolar bone necrosis with loss of teeth and jawbone resorption

onset is in childhood and condition is progressive until puberty, after which disease activity is rare

Non-Skin

occasional aniridia

Genetics

AR

mostly in Japanese

Pathophysiology

catalase deficiency most evident in red blood cells (e.g., activity in homozygotes is less than 1% of normal)

variable catalase levels in other tissues, including skin, mucosa, liver, muscle, and bone marrow

Laboratory Data

blood turns dark brown due to methemoglobin formation and does not foam after hydrogen peroxide is added

Prognosis

life expectancy normal if infections are avoided or appropriately treated

Discussion

at least half of homozygotes are asymptomatic; this proportion appears to be increasing

asymptomatic (heterozygous) carriers have hypocatalasia; red blood cell catalase activity is about half of normal

REFERENCES

McK 115500

Eaton JW. Acatalasemia. In: Scriver CR, Beaudet AL, Sly WS, Valle D, eds. The Metabolic Basis of Inherited Disease. 6th ed. New York, McGraw-Hill, 1989:1551–1561

Takahara S. Progressive oral gangrene probably due to lack of catalase in the blood (acatalasemia): report of nine cases. Lancet 1952;2:1101–1104

Lipoproteinemias

The best known classification of hyperlipidemias is on the basis of electrophoretic patterns (Fredrickson system); the World Health Organization uses this nomenclature. However, the genetic and biochemical causes of these disorders are now better understood, and classification based on this information is, in general, more useful. For the most part, our discussion uses the new terminology, but the old terminology is also referred to for the sake of completeness. The major hyperlipidemias and abbreviations used in this chapter are presented in Table 15–2.

REFERENCE

Seymour CA, Xanthomas and abnormalities of lipid metabolism and storage. In: Champion RH, Burton JL, Ebling FJG, eds. Textbook of Dermatology. Oxford, Blackwell Scientific Publications, 1992:2314–2325

FAMILIAL LIPOPROTEIN LIPASE DEFICIENCY

Synonyms

- Bürger-Grütz disease

Skin

eruptive xanthomas on the extensor surfaces and buttocks (Color Fig. 15–2) but may involve entire body, including the scalp or oral mucosa

xanthomas wax and wane with fluctuations in serum triglyceride level

onset usually before age 10 years but ranges into adulthood

Non-Skin

hepatosplenomegaly in nearly all children and in half of adults

intermittent recurrent attacks of abdominal pain in about half of patients; frequency ranges from days to weeks; during attacks, rapid enlargement of spleen and liver and engorgement of abdominal veins occurs

pancreatitis may occur with triglyceride levels greater than 1500 to 2000 mg/dL

lipemia retinalis, which does not affect the vision, is present when serum triglyceride level is 3000 to 4000 mg/dL; its presence may give clue to diagnosis, especially during acute abdominal attacks

occasional growth retardation

higher incidence of respiratory infections

no increased incidence of myocardial infarctions

TABLE 15–2

FAMILIAL LIPOPROTEINEMIAS

Name (McKusick Number)	Biochemical Abnormality	Inheritance	Predominant Electrophoretic Pattern	Lipoprotein	Plasma Cholesterol	Plasma LDL Cholesterol	Plasma Triglyceride	Serum Supranatant After Standing	Serum Infranatant After Standing
Familial lipoprotein lipase deficiency (McK 238600)	Deficiency of lipoprotein lipase (or Apo C-II deficiency)	AR	IA V	Excess CM (and VLDL if type V pattern)	Elevated	Low to elevated	Elevated	Clear (creamy if type V pattern)	Creamy (turbid if type V pattern)
Familial hyper-cholesterolemia (McK 143890)	Defect of number or function of LDL receptor	AD	IIA	Excess LDL	Markedly elevated	Elevated	Moderately elevated	Clear	Clear
Familial combined hyperlipidemia (McK 144250)	Unknown		IIB IV IIA	Excess LDL Excess VLDL	Usually elevated	Elevated	Usually elevated	Slightly turbid	Clear
Familial type III hyperlipoprotein-emia (McK 107741)	Abnormal or absent apolipoprotein E (variety of defects)	AR	III	Excess IDL Excess VLDL	Elevated	Low or normal	Elevated	Turbid (rarely creamy)	Turbid
Familial hyper-triglyceridemia (McK 145750)	Unknown	AD	IV (occas. V)	Excess VLDL (and CM if type V pattern)	Normal or slightly elevated	Normal	Elevated	Milky, cloudy (creamy if type V pattern)	Milky, cloudy (turbid if type V pattern)

Modified from Gawkrodger DJ. Metabolic and nutritional disorders. In: Champion RH, Burton JL, Ebling FJG, eds. Textbook of Dermatology. Oxford, Blackwell Scientific Publications, 1992:2314; and Kane JP, Havel RJ. Introduction: structure and metabolism of plasma lipoproteins. In: Scriver CR, Beaudet AL, Sly WS, Valle D, eds. The Metabolic Basis of Inherited Disease. 6th ed. New York, McGraw-Hill, 1989:1129–1138.

CM = chylomicrons; LDL = low-density lipoprotein; VLDL = very low-density lipoprotein; HDL = high-density lipoprotein; IDL = intermediate-density lipoprotein; Apo = apolipoprotein.

Genetics

AR

males affected more than females

mostly occurs in whites

Laboratory Data

chylomicrons: 85% triglycerides, 9% cholesterol, 5% phospholipids, and 1% to 2% protein

freshly drawn blood is creamy; when sample is left standing, infranatant is clear, supernatant is creamy

increased apo-B48 and apo-B100 in triglyceride-rich lipoproteins (i.e., chylomicrons and very low-density lipoproteins)

Prognosis

pancreatitis is the greatest threat to life

restriction of dietary fats, especially long-chain triglycerides, is advised

Discussion

excessive ingestion of alcohol or carbohydrates causes increased triglyceride levels and may lead to serious sequelae

causes of acquired or secondary chylomicronemia include severe diabetes (which causes an acquired lipoprotein lipase deficiency), paraproteinemias, pancreatitis, acute alcoholism, and hypothyroidism

- *apolipoprotein C-II (apo C-II) deficiency*

  in homozygote, functional lipoprotein deficiency due to absence of apo C-II, a lipoprotein lipase cofactor

  lacks eruptive xanthomas and hepatosplenomegaly; manifestations are not as severe as in lipoprotein lipase deficiency with adult onset

  AR; very rare

REFERENCES

McK 238600

Baggio G, Manzato E, Gabelli C, et al. Apolipoprotein C-II deficiency. J Clin Invest 1986;77:520–527

Brunzell JD. Familial lipoprotein lipase deficiency and other causes of the chylomicronemia syndrome. In: Scriver CR, Beaudet AL, Sly WS, Valle D, eds. The Metabolic Basis of Inherited Disease. 6th ed. New York, McGraw-Hill, 1989:1165–1180

Cruz PD, East C, Bergstresser PR. Dermal, subcutaneous, and tendon xanthomas: diagnostic markers for specific lipoprotein disorders. J Am Acad Dermatol 1988; 19:95–111

Seymour CA. Xanthomas and abnormalities of lipid metabolism and storage. In: Champion RH, Burton JL, Ebling FJG, eds. Textbook of Dermatology. Oxford, Blackwell Scientific Publications, 1992:2314–2325

FAMILIAL HYPERCHOLESTEROLEMIA

Skin

tendon xanthomas are very common (especially on Achilles tendon) and increase with age (Color Fig. 15–3); tendon thickening is usually detectible in adolescence and is often the presenting sign (Color Fig. 15–4)

cutaneous xanthelasmas, tuberous xanthomas (especially on knuckles, elbows, knees, and buttocks) and corneal arcus also seen, usually with onset in second or third decades but may occur earlier or later

Non-Skin

coronary artery disease; onset in third to fourth decades in men, fourth to fifth decades in women

occasional recurrent polyarthritis and tenosynovitis

Genetics

AD

affects 1 in 500 of North Americans and Europeans

Pathophysiology

defective number or function of low density lipoprotein receptors

Laboratory Data

serum electrophoresis: increased low density lipoproteins (beta-lipoprotein)

serum supernatant: clear

serum infranatant: clear

serum cholesterol: markedly increased

serum triglycerides: moderately increased

plasma cholesterol and low density lipoproteins are elevated from birth, reaching 300 to 400 mg/dL in adult heterozygotes and 700 to 1200 mg/dL in homozygous children; high-density lipoproteins decreased

prenatal diagnosis of the homozygous condition possible

Prognosis

myocardial infarction usually occurs by sixth decade in men and by seventh decade in women

cholesterol-lowering drugs including lovastatin, cholestyramine, and nicotinic acid may be beneficial

Discussion

the majority of hypercholesterolemic patients in the general population have a type IIa lipoprotein pattern but do not have tendinous xanthomas or family history of lipoproteinemia; this hypercholesterolemic disorder is common and believed to be polygeneic

tendon xanthomas may be seen secondarily in other disorders including Cushing disease and hypothyroidism

- *familial hypercholesterolemia, homozygous*

very rare; patients present in the first year of life with plane xanthomas (which rarely occur in heterozygotes) at sites of trauma and on palms, buttocks, and extremities; the first interdigital web space of the hand is a characteristic location

tendon and tuberous xanthomas, corneal arcus (commonly before age 10 years), and xanthelasmas

coronary artery atherosclerosis, myocardial infarction, and supravalvular aortic stenosis develop before age 20

patients usually die by end of third decade of cardiovascular disease

REFERENCES

McK 143890

Bulkley BH, Buja M, Ferrans VJ, et al. Tuberous xanthoma in homozygous type II hyperlipoproteinemia: a histologic, histochemical and electron microscopical study. Arch Pathol 1975;99:203–300

Goldstein JL, Brown MS. Familial hypercholesterolemia. In: Scriver CR, Beaudet AL, Sly WS, Valle D, eds. The Metabolic Basis of Inherited Disease. 6th ed. New York, McGraw-Hill, 1989:1215–1250

Thompson GR, Seed M, Niththyananthan S, et al. Genotypic and phenotypic variation in familial hypercholesterolemia. Arteriosclerosis 1989;9:175–180

Yamamoto A, Kamiya T, Yamamura T, et al. Clinical features of familial hypercholesterolemia. Arteriosclerosis 1989;9:166–174

FAMILIAL COMBINED HYPERLIPIDEMIA

Synonyms

- familial multiple-type hyperlipoproteinemia

Skin

tendinous, tuberous, and eruptive xanthomas as well as xanthelasmas and corneal arcus

onset in fourth to fifth decades

Non-Skin

increased incidence of coronary artery disease (similar to heterozygote familial hypercholesterolemia), diabetes mellitus, and hyperuricemia; onset in fourth to fifth decades

Genetics

inheritance unclear; AD versus polygeneic

occurs in about 1% of the North American population

Pathophysiology

marked elevation in plasma apo-B lipoprotein

Laboratory Data

electrophoresis: variable increases in cholesterol and triglycerides (variable LDL and VLDL, i.e., beta and pre-beta lipoproteins)

supernatant: slightly turbid (not creamy)

infranatant: clear

serum cholesterol: usually elevated

serum triglycerides: usually elevated

one third of patients have elevated triglyceride levels, one third have elevated cholesterol levels, and the other third have both elevated triglyceride and cholesterol levels; homozygotes may have severe hypertriglyceridemia

Discussion

this is the most common familial lipid abnormality (30% of all patients with hereditary lipoproteinemias) and the most common known metabolic cause of premature atherosclerosis

only 10% to 20% have hyperlipidemia in childhood (familial hypercholesterolemia)

REFERENCES

McK 144250

Cortner JA, Coates PM, Gallagher PR. Prevalence and expression of familial combined hyperlipidemia in childhood. J Pediatr 1990;116:514–519

Glueck CJ, Fallat R, Buncher CR, et al. Familial combined hyperlipoproteinemia: studies in 91 adults and 95 children from 33 kindreds. Metabolism 1973;22:1403–1428

Goldstein JI, Schrott HG, Hazzard WR, et al. Hyperlipidemia in coronary heart disease: II. Genetic analysis of lipid levels in 176 families and delineation of a new inherited disorder, combined with hyperlipidemia. J Clin Invest 1973;52:1544–1568

Kane JP, Havel RJ. Disorders of the biogenesis and secretion of lipoproteins containing the B apolipoproteins. In: Scriver CR, Beaudet AL, Sly WS, Valle D, eds. The Metabolic Basis of Inherited Disease. 6th ed. New York, McGraw-Hill, 1989:1139–1164

FAMILIAL TYPE III HYPERLIPOPROTEINEMIA

Synonyms

- familial dysbetalipoproteinemia

Skin

tuberous or characteristic tuberoeruptive xanthomas in over 80% of patients, most commonly on knuckles, elbows, knees, and buttocks; onset in second or third decade

xanthoma striatum palmare in about two thirds of patients (Color Fig. 15–5); virtually pathognomonic

tendon xanthomas, especially on Achilles tendon, in about one fourth of patients

xanthelasmas uncommon

Non-Skin

cardiovascular complications include peripheral vascular occlusive disease, especially of femoral and popliteal vessels, severe claudication, and coronary artery disease

obesity (70%), glucose intolerance (50%), and hyperuricemia (40%)

Genetics

autosomal co-dominant; manifestation of disease, however, appears to require additional genetic, environmental, or other secondary influences (e.g., presence of familial hypercholesterolemia or diabetes mellitus)

rare

Pathophysiology

apoprotein E is required for uptake of intermediate density lipoprotein in liver; a variety of abnormal apoprotein E states may cause this disease (e.g., it may be caused by the absence of apoprotein E or the presence of abnormal apoprotein E); the most common abnormal expression is apoprotein E2/E2, while apoprotein E3/E3 is the predominant normal apoprotein E expression in the normolipemic general population

Laboratory Data

electrophoresis: increased intermediate-density lipoprotein; also increased very low-density lipoprotein (broad-beta band)

supranatant: turbid (rarely creamy)

infranatant: turbid

serum cholesterol: elevated

serum triglycerides: elevated

very low- and intermediate-density lipoproteins have abnormal composition, being cholesterol rich and triglyceride poor, owing to apoprotein E abnormalities; thus, the very low-density lipoprotein–cholesterol/plasma triglyceride ratio is greater than 0.3, normally being less than 0.3

decreased serum low density and high-density lipoproteins

Prognosis

life expectancy decreased due to peripheral vascular and coronary artery occlusive disease, but not as severely as in familial hypercholesterolemia

treatment of coexistent and aggravating factors such as alcohol ingestion, diabetes mellitus, systemic lupus erythematosus, paraproteinemias, and hypothyroidism is important

dietary treatment is beneficial, as well as drug therapy including clofibrate, nicotinic acid, and gemfibrozil

Discussion

heterozygotes are asymptomatic unless accompanied by other genetic or metabolic disorders (e.g., familial hypercholesterolemia or diabetes mellitus)

tuberous and tendinous xanthomas are less common than in familial hypercholesterolemia

REFERENCES

McK 107741
McK 224020 (defective apoprotein E)
Mahley RW, Rall SC Jr. Type III hyperlipoproteinemia (dysbetalipoproteinemia): the role of apolipoprotein E in normal and abnormal lipoprotein metabolism. In: Scriver CR, Beaudet AL, Sly WS, Valle D, eds. The Metabolic Basis of Inherited Disease. 6th ed. New York, McGraw-Hill, 1989:1195–1213
Morganroth J, Levy RI, Fredrickson DS. The biochemical, clinical, and genetic features of type III hyperlipoproteinemia. Ann Intern Med 1975;82:158–174
Schaefer EJ, Gregg RE, Ghiselli G, et al. Familial apolipoprotein E deficiency. J Clin Invest 1986;78:1206–1219

FAMILIAL HYPERTRIGLYCERIDEMIA

Synonyms

- familial endogenous hypertriglyceridemia

Skin

eruptive xanthomas are only seen in patients with severe forms of familial hypertriglyceridemia or when accompanied by exacerbating factors

rare xanthelasmas, tuberous xanthomas, and xanthoma striatum palmare

Non-Skin

lipemia retinalis or pancreatitis may be seen with markedly increased triglyceride levels

increased obesity, hypertension, glucose intolerance, hyperuricemia, and gallbladder disease, including cholelithiasis

Genetics

AD

Pathophysiology

glucose intolerance, hyperinsulinemia, and obesity result in increased very low-density lipoprotein due to increased triglyceride production by liver

decreased lipoprotein lipase activity, frequently related to glucose intolerance, further impairs very low-density lipoprotein and chylomicron clearance

Prognosis

life expectancy may be shortened by atherosclerotic disease or from complications of diabetes or obesity

markedly worsened by large intake of carbohydrates or alcohol

Discussion

patients with familial hypertriglyceridemia not associated with another disease are usually asymptomatic; only when associated with a secondary cause of hypertriglyceridemia do xanthomatosis and atherosclerosis result; secondary causes of hypertriglyceridemia include diabetes mellitus, pancreatitis, alcohol or heavy carbohydrate ingestion, von Gierke disease (glycogenosis type I), hypercalcemia, hypothyroidism, nephrotic syndrome, gout, Niemann-Pick disease, Gaucher disease, total lipodystrophy, Werner syndrome, and estrogen use

termed *endogenous* hypertriglyceridemia because high serum triglycerides are hepatic, not dietary, in origin

■ *familial type V hyperlipoproteinemia*

uncommon

patients develop severe hypertriglyceridemia, usually in the fourth and fifth decades of life, without any known defect in lipoprotein metabolism (e.g., deficiencies in apoprotein C-II or lipoprotein lipase); increase in very low-density lipoprotein and chylomicrons

eruptive xanthomas, abdominal pain, and pancreatitis

neuropsychiatric symptoms may occur with severe triglyceride elevation

a combination of the findings seen in familial lipoprotein lipase deficiency and familial hypertriglyceridemia

may be seen in some patients with familial hypertriglyceridemia

inheritance unclear

REFERENCES

McK 145750

Archer CB, MacDonald DM. Eruptive xanthomata in type V hyperlipoproteinaemia associated with diabetes mellitus. Clin Exp Dermatol 1984;9:312–316

Brunzell JD. Familial lipoprotein lipase deficiency and other causes of the chylomicronemia syndrome. In: Scriver CR, Beaudet AL, Sly WS, Valle D, eds. The Metabolic Basis of Inherited Disease. 6th ed. New York, McGraw-Hill, 1989:1165–1180

François J, Lentini F, Hoste P, Rottiers R. Genetic study of hyperlipoproteinaemia types IV and V. Clin Genet 1977;12:202–207

Glueck CJ, Tsang R, Fallat R, et al. Familial hypertriglyceridemia: studies in 130 children and 45 siblings of 36 index cases. Metabolism 1973;22:1287–1301

Schreibman PH, Wilson DE, Arky RA. Familial type IV hyperlipoproteinemia. N Engl J Med 1969;281:981–985

CEREBROTENDINOUS XANTHOMATOSIS

Skin

tendon xanthomas, most commonly on Achilles tendon, usually first noted in second or third decades but may be noted as early as first decade

xanthelasmas and tuberous xanthomas reported

Non-Skin

mild to moderate mental retardation in many but not all patients

xanthomas may occur in sites including cerebrum, cerebellum, bones, and lungs

neurologic abnormalities include spasticity, ataxia, and dementia, with onset in adolescence or early adulthood; may lead to incapacitation in fourth or fifth decade

juvenile cataracts may precede neurologic abnormalities by decades

premature atherosclerotic cardiovascular disease

Genetics

AR

Pathophysiology

biochemical defect: bile acid synthesis abnormalities, resulting in decreased cholic and chenodeoxylic bile acids and increased cholestanol and glucuronide c27 alcohols in bile; feedback inhibition of hepatic cholesterol and cholestanol production is lost

Laboratory Data

increased cholestanol (5,6-dihydroxy cholesterol; derived from cholesterol and transported in low-density lipoprotein) in plasma lipoproteins and tissues

serum cholesterol is normal or only slightly elevated

carriers may be identified by the presence of a characteristic cholestane metabolite in the urine after ingesting cholestyramine

Prognosis

prognosis is variable; patients die of progressive neurologic disease, especially pseudobulbar paralysis, or myocardial infarction, mostly in the fourth to sixth decade, but sometimes as early as the third decade

chenodeoxycholic acid and mevinolin therapies are beneficial

Discussion

in familial hypercholesterolemia, xanthomas absent from cerebrum, cerebellum, bones, and lungs

REFERENCES

McK 213700

Berginer VM, Salen G, Shefer S. Cerebrotendinous xanthomatosis. Neurol Clin 1989; 7:55–74

Berginer VM, Salen G, Shefer S. Long-term treatment of cerebrotendinous xanthomatosis with chenodeoxycholic acid. N Engl J Med 1984;311:1649–1652

Björkhem I, Skrede S. Familial diseases with storage of sterols other than cholesterol: cerebrotendinous xanthomatosis and phytosterolemia. In: Scriver CR, Beaudet AL, Sly WS, Valle D, eds. The Metabolic Basis of Inherited Disease. 6th ed. New York, McGraw-Hill, 1989:1283–1302

Hwang SY, Lee KH, Ahn JI. Cerebrotendinous xanthomatosis. J Dermatol 1990;17:115–119

Koopman BJ, Waterreus RJ, Van Den Brekel HWC. Detection of carriers of cerebrotendinous xanthomatosis. Clin Chim Acta 1986;158:179–186

PHYTOSTEROLEMIA

Synonyms

- sitosterolemia with xanthomatosis
- beta-sitosterolemia

Skin

tendon xanthomas, especially of the Achilles tendon and the extensor tendons of the hands, appear in early childhood to second decade of life

occasional xanthelasmas and tuberous xanthomas

Non-Skin

premature atherosclerosis and sequelae

occasional hemolytic anemia, platelet abnormalities, and hypersplenism

Genetics

AR

Pathophysiology

accumulation of phytosterols (plant sterols) in plasma and tissues; xanthomas contain 90% cholesterol and 10% plant sterols

increased absorption of sterols from gut, including cholesterol and plant and fish sterols; may be important in pathogenesis

phytosterols are transported by low-density lipoproteins

Laboratory Data

normal or mildly elevated serum cholesterol levels

unusual fecal bile acid pattern: contains deoxycholic and lithocholic acids

Prognosis

a diet low in plant and shellfish sterols is recommended

cholestyramine causes increased excretion and lowered levels of phytosterols

death by myocardial infarction in males as early as second decade

Discussion

since low-density lipoprotein receptor function is normal, this disease is sometimes referred to as pseudo–familial hypercholesterolemia

phytosterolemia should be considered in the differential diagnosis of a young patient with tendon xanthomas and hypercholesterolemia (in most patients with phytosterolemia, however, cholesterol levels are normal)

REFERENCES

McK 210250

Björkhem I, Skrede S. Familial diseases with storage of sterols other than cholesterol: cerebrotendinous xanthomatosis and phytosterolemia. In: Scriver CR, Beaudet AL, Sly WS, Valle D, eds. The Metabolic Basis of Inherited Disease. 6th ed. New York, McGraw-Hill, 1989:1283–1302

Shulman RS, Bhattacharyya AK, Connor WE, Fredrickson DS. Beta-sitosterolemia and xanthomatosis. N Engl J Med 1976; 294: 482–483

TANGIER DISEASE (ALPHA-LIPOPROTEIN DEFICIENCY)

characteristic enlarged tonsils with orange-yellow striations

excess cholesterol and cholesteryl ester storage in tissues occurs, especially tonsils, rectal mucosa, spleen, thymus, and bone marrow, less often in lymph nodes and liver

more than 50% of patients have neurologic abnormalities, including recurrent neuropathies

asymptomatic corneal infiltrates are frequently present

atherosclerosis is uncommon despite high-density lipoprotein deficiency

AR; named for the high prevalence among the inhabitants of Tangier Island in Chesapeake Bay, most of whom are descendants of the original 17th century settlers

decreased HDL and apo A-I

cholesterol and phospholipid levels are markedly decreased while plasma triglyceride levels may be slightly elevated

histopathology: focal collections of foamy histiocytes have been described in otherwise normal skin

heterozygotes in families of known homozygotes can usually be identified by low high-density lipoprotein concentrations

REFERENCES

McK 205400

Assmann G, Herbert PN, Fredrickson DS, et al. Isolation and characterization of an abnormal high density lipoprotein in Tangier disease. J Clin Invest 1977;60:242–252

Ferrans VJ, Fredrickson DS. The pathology of Tangier disease. Am J Pathol 1975;78:101–158

Waldorf DS, Levy RI, Fredrickson DS. Cutaneous cholesterol ester deposition in Tangier disease. Arch Dermatol 1967;95:161–165

APOLIPOPROTEIN A-I DEFICIENCY

planar xanthomas of neck, arms, trunk, and eyelids beginning in childhood

no tonsillar abnormalities

corneal clouding, premature atherosclerotic cardiovascular disease, and hepatosplenomegaly

markedly decreased high density lipoprotein cholesterol levels and absent apolipoproteins A-I

in one kindred, apolipoprotein C-III was also absent

McK 107680

Breslow JL. Familial disorders of high density lipoprotein metabolism. In: Scriver CR, Beaudet AL, Sly WS, Valle D, eds. The Metabolic Basis of Inherited Disease. 6th ed. New York, McGraw-Hill, 1989:1251–1266

Norum RA, Lakier JB, Goldstein S, et al. Familial deficiency of apolipoproteins A-I and C-III and precocious coronary-artery disease. N Engl J Med 1982;306:1513–1519

WATSON-ALAGILLE SYNDROME

Synonym

- arteriohepatic dysplasia

Skin

intense pruritus

widespread plaque-like and tuberous xanthomas

rare photosensitivity

Non-Skin

jaundice may be present around birth or develops later in infancy

characteristic craniofacies in two thirds of patients with prominent forehead, deep-set eyes, straight nose, and small, pointed chin

musculoskeletal abnormalities include short stature and vertebral, ulnar, and distal phalangeal anomalies

ocular abnormalities include posterior embryotoxon and retinal pigmentary changes

cardiovascular abnormalities include pulmonary valve and peripheral artery stenoses

Genetics

AD

Pathophysiology

congenital cholestasis due to intrahepatic ductal atresia; extrahepatic bile ducts may also be abnormal

Prognosis

in one report, 16 of 69 patients died by age 5 years of cardiac and hepatic complications

Discussion

distinctive facies occasionally occurs in relatives without any of the other features of the disease; also may occur in patients with other forms of congenital cholestasis

REFERENCES

McK 118450

Alagille D, Estrada A, Hadchovel, M et al. Syndromic paucity of interlobular bile ducts (Alagille syndrome or arteriohepatic dysplasia): review of 80 cases. J Pediatr 1987;110:195–200

Mueller RF, Pagon RA, Pepin MG, et al. Arteriohepatic dysplasia: phenotypic features and family studies. Clin Genet 1984; 25:323–331

Mueller RF. The Alagille syndrome. J Med Genet 1987;24:621–626

Weston CF, Burton JL. Xanthomas in the Watson-Alagille syndrome. J Am Acad Dermatol 1987;16:1117–1121

Disorders of Amino Acid Metabolism

The primary disorders of amino acid metabolism (aminoacidurias) are a group of inherited metabolic defects with aminoaciduria as a constant clinical finding. They are traditionally divided into three etiologic types. *Overflow aminoaciduria* develops when an enzyme deficiency causes elevated plasma levels of amino acids with resulting "overflow" into the urine once the amino acid concentration exceeds the threshold for renal reabsorption (e.g., phenylketonuria). In *no-threshold aminoaciduria*, as in arginosuccinic aciduria, even minimally elevated plasma levels of amino acid result in aminoaciduria, because the substrate amino acid is nonmetabolizable and cannot be reabsorbed by the kidney. The third type of primary aminoaciduria is *renal* or *transport aminoaciduria*, which results when renal reabsorption of an amino acid is defective, for example, when there is an abnormality of the transport or carrier protein for the amino acid. Hartnup disease is due to such an abnormality.

There are other ways to classify the aminoacidurias, such as by their biochemical role in normal metabolism (e.g., the urea cycle enzymes).

The clinical findings and treatment of the urea cycle enzyme deficiencies are almost identical; arginosuccinic aminoaciduria can be regarded as the model. Other deficiencies of dermatologic interest include arginosuccinic acid synthetase deficiency (which causes citrullinemia) and carbamoyl phosphate synthetase deficiency.

Prenatal diagnosis is possible in some of these diseases.

ARGINOSUCCINIC AMINOACIDURIA

Skin

short, dull, brittle, sparse scalp hair; about half have microscopic findings of trichorrhexis nodosa; pili torti also reported

Non-Skin

two patterns of onset:

neonatal onset: normal-appearing infant develops hyperammonemia within 24 to 48 hours of birth; progressive lethargy, hypothermia, and apnea due to encephalopathy; may be fatal

infancy, childhood, or adulthood onset: chronic neurologic findings include mental retardation, epilepsy, and cerebellar ataxia, as well as episodic mental status changes; in children, this may be accompanied by vomiting

occasional liver disease and aversion to food high in protein

Genetics

AR; rare

Pathophysiology

high renal clearance aminoaciduria (no threshold)

Laboratory Data

enzyme defect: arginosuccinase

elevated plasma and urine arginosuccinic acid levels

elevated serum ammonia

Prognosis

protein restriction with arginine and benzoate supplementations may be beneficial

REFERENCES

McK 207900

Brusilow SW, Horwich AL. Urea cycle enzymes. In: Scriver CR, Beaudet AL, Sly WS, Valle D, eds. The Metabolic Basis of Inherited Disease. 6th ed. New York, McGraw-Hill, 1989:629–663

Kvedar JC, Baden HP, Baden LA, et al. Dietary management reverses grooving and abnormal polarization of hair shafts in argininosuccinase deficiency. Am J Med Genet 1991;40:211–213

Levin B. Arginosuccinic aciduria. Am J Dis Child 1967;113:162–165

Phillips ME, Barrie H, Cream JJ. Arginosuccinic aciduria with pili torti. J R Soc Med 1981;74:221–222

Potter JL, Timmon GD, Silvidi AA. Arginosuccinic aciduria: the hair abnormality revisited. Am J Dis Child 1980;134:1095–1096

CITRULLINEMIA (NEONATAL CITRULLINEMIA)

generalized moist, red, scaly plaques accentuated on genitalia, lower abdomen, buttocks, and perioral skin

other findings are as in arginosuccinic aminoaciduria (see main entry)

AR

arginosuccinic acid synthetase is deficient; it normally catalyzes the formation of arginosuccinic acid from citrulline and aspartic acid

elevated plasma and urine citrulline, as well as decreased serum arginine levels (characteristic of neonatal form)

heterozygotes may be detected by measuring fasting plasma citrulline levels

protein restriction with arginine and benzoate supplementations may be beneficial

clearing of cutaneous eruption reported when normalization of serum arginine levels achieved

McK 215700
McK 238970
Brusilow SW, Horwich AL. Urea cycle enzymes. In: Scriver CR, Beaudet AL, Sly WS, Valle D, eds. The Metabolic Basis of Inherited Disease. 6th ed. New York, McGraw-Hill, 1989:629–663
Burgess EA, Oberholzer VG, Semmens JM, et al. Acute neonatal and benign citrullinemia in one sibship. Arch Dis Child 1978;53:179–182
Goldblum OM, Brusilow SW, Maldonado YA, et al. Neonatal citrullinemia associated with cutaneous manifestations and arginine deficiency. J Am Acad Dermatol 1986;14:321–326
Thoene J, Batshaw M, Spector E, et al. Neonatal citrullinemia: treatment with ketoanalogues of essential amino acids. J Pediatr 1977;90:218–224
Whelan DT, Brusso T, Spate M. Citrullinemia: phenotypic variations. Pediatrics 1976;57:936–941

CARBAMYL PHOSPHATE SYNTHETASE DEFICIENCY

cutaneous findings similar to citrullinemia

clearing of cutaneous eruption reported when normal serum arginine levels achieved

McK 237300
Brusilow SW, Horwich AL. Urea cycle enzymes. In: Scriver CR, Beaudet AL, Sly WS, Valle D, eds. The Metabolic Basis of Inherited Disease. 6th ed. New York, McGraw-Hill, 1989:629–663
Farriaux JP, Ponte C, Pollitt RJ, et al. Carbamyl-phosphate-synthetase deficiency with neonatal onset of symptoms. Acta Paediatr Scand 1977;66:529–534
Kline JJ, Hug G, Schubert WK, Berry H. Arginine deficiency syndrome: its occurrence in carbamyl phosphate synthetase deficiency. Am J Dis Child 1981;135:437–442

HARTNUP DISEASE

Synonym

- H disease

Skin

pellagra-like photosensitive symmetrical erythematous scaling plaques on face, neck, hands, and legs are often the first sign of the disease, usually appearing in mid to late first decade, but can start from infancy to early adolescence

eruption varies from mild erythema to acute vesicular dermatitis, with each episode lasting weeks

sites of eruption become hyperpigmented later in life

alopecia, premature graying, and fragility of hair reported

Non-Skin

severe but reversible cerebellar ataxia in more than two thirds of patients; onset usually between ages 5 and 10 years

neuropsychiatric signs, which often parallel severity of cutaneous eruption, include involuntary movements of the hand and tongue, nystagmus, eyelid ptosis, diplopia, delusions, and emotional lability

Genetics

AR

Pathophysiology

defective renal tubular and intestinal transport of neutral amino acids (e.g., decreased intestinal absorption of tryptophan; may be basic defect, resulting in decreased tryptophan and nicotinic acid; occasionally the renal or intestinal defects occur in isolation)

Laboratory Data

increased urinary excretion of indolic compounds, especially indican (indoxyl sulfate); these compounds are products of degradation of unabsorbed tryptophan by bacteria in the gut

however, when only the kidneys have an absorption defect, urinary indolic compound excretion is normal

increased fecal protoporphyrin

Prognosis

improves with age

nicotinamide therapy results in prompt improvement in skin disease; neurologic disease improves less reliably, and aminoaciduria is not affected

avoid sunlight

Discussion

most persons with the metabolic defects of Hartnup disease are asymptomatic (those detected by newborn metabolic screening programs and affected siblings of symptomatic patients)

variability in phenotype may be due to the interaction of the known monogeneic transport defect with other (poly)genetic and environmental factors

patients with pellagra may have similar cutaneous findings but differ by absence of neurologic findings and in dietary history

- pellagra-like syndrome

  reports of several families in which affected individuals manifested a pellagra-like rash in infancy or early childhood

  other findings included developmental retardation, cerebellar ataxia, dysarthria, but, unlike Hartnup disease, an absence of a transport defect in the kidney and characteristic pattern of urinary amino acid excretion, and in one family the presence of cataracts

  defects in tryptophan catabolism postulated

  AR

  McK 260650

REFERENCES

McK 234500

Fenton DA, Wilkinson JD, Toseland PA. Family exhibiting cerebellar-like ataxia, photosensitivity and shortness of stature: a new inborn error of tryptophan metabolism. J R Soc Med 1983;76:736–739

Freundlich E, Statter M, Yatziv S. Familial pellagra-like skin rash with neurological manifestations. Arch Dis Child 1981; 56:146–148

Levy HL. Hartnup disorder. In: Scriver CR, Beaudet AL, Sly WS, Valle D, eds. The Metabolic Basis of Inherited Disease. 6th ed. New York, McGraw-Hill, 1989:2515–2527

Salih MAM, Bender DA, McCreanor GM. Lethal familial pellagra-like skin lesions associated with neurologic and developmental impairment and the development of cataracts. Pediatrics 1985;76:787–793

Scriver CR, Mahon B, Levy HL, et al. The Hartnup phenotype: mendelian transport disorder, multifactorial disease. Am J Hum Genet 1987;40:401–412

Sneddon W, Mellor CS, Martin JR. Hypertryptophanemia and indolketonuria in two mentally retarded subnormal siblings. N Engl J Med 1982;302:1405

Wilcken B, Yu JS, Brown DA. Natural history of Hartnup disease. Arch Dis Child 1977;52:38–40

KYNURENINASE DEFICIENCY (XANTHURENICACIDURIA)

photosensitive rash resembling pellagra

occasional stomatitis and gingivitis

frequent mental retardation and ataxia

AR

block in tryptophan degradation, limiting nicotinic acid synthesis, is possible etiology

McK 278600

Levy HI. Hartnup disorder. In: Scriver CR, Beaudet AL, Sly WS, Valle D, eds. The Metabolic Basis of Inherited Disease. 6th ed. New York, McGraw-Hill, 1989:2515–2527

Reddi OS, Reddy MV, Reddy KR. Familial hydroxykynureninuria. Hum Hered 1978; 28:238–240

HOMOCYSTINURIA

Skin

hair is fair, fragile, and sparse

malar flush and/or a livedo reticularis–like eruption of trunk and limbs (especially legs) in about half of patients; onset in infancy to early childhood

superficial thrombophlebitis common

Non-Skin

musculoskeletal abnormalities include arachnodactyly, marfanoid habitus, dolichostenomelia, and osteoporosis

ectopia lentis, usually downwardly displaced, in most; onset usually in childhood, but ranging from infancy to adulthood; resultant ocular abnormalities include myopia, iridodonesis, and glaucoma

spontaneous arterial and venous thromboses and embolism may occur, resulting in sequelae including cerebrovascular accidents and pulmonary and coronary artery occlusion

neurologic abnormalities include developmental delay, seizures, and variable mental retardation

Genetics

AR

Pathophysiology

most common cause is deficiency of cystathionine synthetase, which catalyzes formation of cystathionine from homocystine and serine

methyltetrahydrofolate-homocysteine methyltransferase deficiency produces many of the findings but does not result in skin disease

Laboratory Data

diagnosis is established by nitroprusside cyanide urine screening and demonstration of enzyme deficiency in fibroblast culture; prenatal diagnosis using cultured amniocytes is possible

increased plasma levels of homocysteine and methionine

heterozygotes identified by elevated serum methionine levels after methionine loading or by enzyme determinations in cultured fibroblasts

Prognosis

dietary treatment with low methionine, high cystine, and large doses of vitamin B_6 (a cofactor for cystathionine synthetase) may be beneficial, especially when initiated early in life; those that respond to vitamin B_6 have a better prognosis

those with no enzyme activity are essentially unresponsive to vitamin B_6, while those with residual enzyme activity are usually responsive in proportion to residual activity

vitamin B_6 responders regardless of treatment are less likely to suffer lens dislocation, but early treatment appears to give added protection; osteoporosis appears to be less severe in the vitamin B_6 responders

90% survive to mid second decade and 75% to fifth decade

Discussion

patients with Marfan syndrome also may have scoliosis, pectus excavatum, and genu valgum, as well as ectopia lentis but with lens displaced upward; however, they have normal hair, no mental retardation, nor homocysteine in urine

REFERENCES

McK 236200

Boers GH, Fowler B, Smals AG, et al. Improved identification of heterozygotes for homocystinuria due to cystathionine synthetase deficiency by the combination of methionine loading and enzyme determination in cultured fibroblasts. Hum Genet 1985; 69:164–169

Carey MC, Donovan DE, FitzGerald O, McAuley FD. Homocystinuria: a clinical and pathological study of nine subjects in six families. Am J Med 1968;45:7–25

Gorlin RJ, Cohen MM Jr, Levin LS. Syndromes of the Head and Neck. 3rd ed. New York, Oxford University Press, 1990:132–135

OCHRONOSIS

Synonym

- alkaptonuria

Skin

see Figures 15–12 and 15–13

dusky, grayish brown or bluish hyperpigmentation, most easily seen in forehead, malar areas, ears, axillae, and/or groin

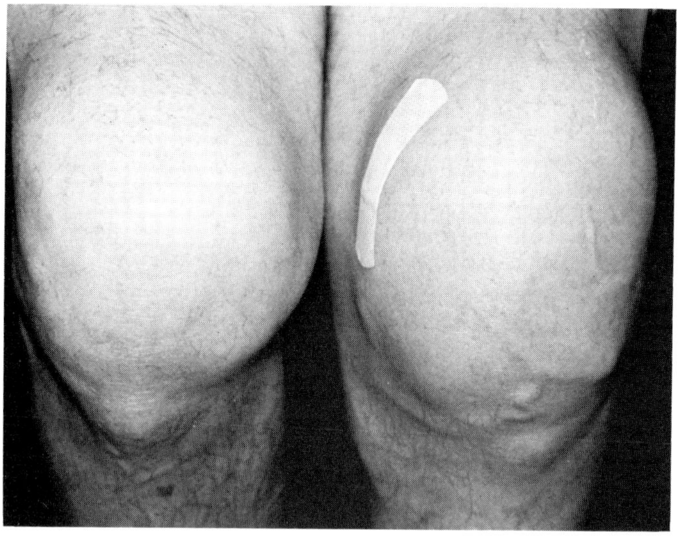

FIGURE 15–12
Ochronosis. The skin is slightly darkened and there are marked deformities of the knees, both reflecting the deposits of homogentisic acid.

skin pigmentation begins in fourth decade of life; less common and less severe than cartilaginous or scleral involvement (see later)

occasional ochronosis of mucosa, nails, cerumen, sebum, apocrine sweat, or eccrine sweat

Non-Skin

alkaptonuria (urine that darkens on exposure to air) present at birth; characteristic "black diapers"

only half of patients with alkaptonuria develop systemic ochronosis

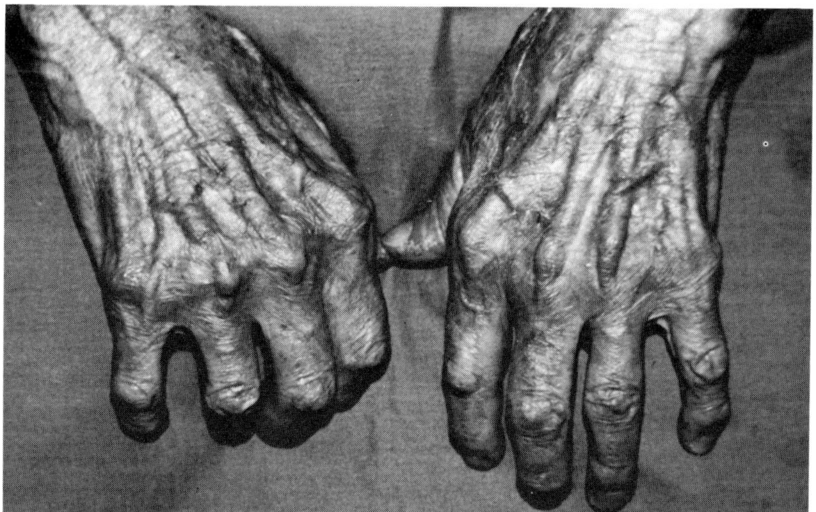

FIGURE 15–13
Ochronosis. The skin on the back of the hands is markedly darkened. The same phenomenon occurs in other light-exposed areas and around joints. (Courtesy of Neil A. Fenske, MD, Tampa, Florida.)

grayish blue discoloration of tendons, cartilage, and sclerae (areas with scant nerve and blood supply) usually occurs by fifth decade of age, but sometimes as early as the third decade; calcification may follow

cartilage pigmentation most easily seen in ears, occasionally in nose

tendon discoloration most easily seen in dorsa of hands and feet and around knees

ocular hyperpigmentation of tarsal plates and the nasal and temporal areas of perilimbal sclerae

joint cartilage ochronosis results in arthritis, especially of spine and large joints (knees, shoulders, and hips); other sequelae include kyphosis and gait abnormalities

occasional deafness (involvement of cartilage of inner ear bones) and hoarseness

occasional involvement of intima of endocardium or large vessels

perspiration may stain clothing brown and cerumen becomes black

Genetics

AR

Pathophysiology

deficiency of homogentisic acid oxidase, a hepatic and renal enzyme

Laboratory Data

freshly voided urine darkens (pigment is due to polymerization of oxidized homogentisic acid) on exposure to air or on addition of 10% NaOH

Fishberg test: alkalinized urine turns photographic paper black

histopathology: thickened, darkened dermal collagen

radiographs: calcified intervertebral disks and ligaments

Prognosis

myocardial infarction may occur

arthropathy may be disabling

Discussion

acquired cutaneous ochronosis may be caused by numerous drugs, including quinacrine, topical phenol, topical resorcin, and topical hydroquinone; urinary and systemic signs are lacking

REFERENCES

McK 203500

Albers SE, Brozena SJ, Glass LF, Fenske NA. Alkaptonuria and ochronosis: case report and review. J Am Acad Dermatol 1992; 27:609–614

Christensen K, Manthorpe R. Alkaptonuria and ochronosis: a survey and 5 cases. Hum Hered 1983;33:140–144

La Du BN. Alcaptonuria. In: Scriver CR, Beaudet AL, Sly WS, Valle D, eds. The Metabolic Basis of Inherited Disease. 6th ed. New York, McGraw-Hill, 1989:775–790

Layman CW. Ochronosis. Arch Dermatol 1953;67:553–560

Lee EB. Metabolic diseases and the skin. Pediatr Clin North Am 1983;30:597–608

O'Brien WM, La Du BN, Bunim JJ. Biochemical, pathologic and clinic aspects of alcaptonuria, ochronosis and ochronotic arthropathy: review of world literature (1584–1962). Am J Med 1963;34:813–838

PHENYLKETONURIA

Synonym

- PKU
- hyperphenylalaninemia
- Folling disease
- phenylpyruvic oligophrenia

Skin

hair, skin and eyes are lighter than expected for the family phenotype; blond hair and blue eyes are typically described

dermatitic eruption, often in a flexural distribution, in 20% to 40% of patients; may improve with time

occasional progressive sclerodermoid induration of skin and subcutaneous tissue with onset in infancy, predominantly affecting buttocks and thighs initially, then spreading to other areas including upper extremities and trunk; hands and feet are spared, unlike in systemic scleroderma

occasional widely spaced incisors

Non-Skin

excessive phenylalanine in blood causes progressive and irreversible mental deterioration; rarely, patients have near-normal intelligence

disease may first manifest with seizures, vomiting, irritability, and a peculiar musty or mousy body odor due to phenylacetic acid in sweat and urine

other neurologic abnormalities include athetoid movements, catatonic posturing, hyperactivity, and gait abnormalities

microcephaly, short stature, syndactyly, pes planus, and epicanthal folds common

Genetics

AR

1 in 10,000 to 15,000

Pathophysiology

a wide range in deficiency of phenylalanine hydroxylase may be seen; the enzyme converts phenylalanine to tyrosine

retained phenylalanine is metabolized and excreted as phenylpyruvic acid in the urine

although tyrosine levels are normal, phenylalanine competitively inhibits tyrosinase from converting tyrosine to melanin

Laboratory Data

blood phenylalanine levels more reliably elevated than urine phenylpyruvic acid levels, hence screening should be performed on blood samples

the Guthrie test is the most commonly used screening test

abnormal electroencephalogram in 80%

Prognosis

diet low in phenylalanine prevents mental retardation and mental delay; must be instituted as soon after birth as possible; phenylalanine is especially damaging to brain during first 6 months of life

diet may help normalize skin and hair pigmentation and improve the dermatitis, the severity of which tends to parallel the biochemical deficiency

diet should be continued until child is of school age

pregnant females with phenylketonuria must resume diet during pregnancy to protect fetus from increased phenylalanine levels, which may cause mental retardation, microcephaly, congenital heart disease, or other abnormalities

mandatory neonatal screening in North America is responsible for increased early detection

Discussion

otherwise asymptomatic heterozygotes have decreased levels of phenylalanine hydroxylase, which can be demonstrated using phenylalanine tolerance tests; these carriers may develop dermatitis during tolerance tests

hyperphenylalaninemia types II through V are due to less severe deficiencies of phenylalanine hydroxylase and deficiencies in its co-enzymes tetrahydrobiopterin reductase and dihydropteridine reductase

REFERENCES

McK 261600
Farishian P, Shittaker J. Phenylalanine lowers melanin synthesis in mammalian melanocytes by reducing tyrosine uptake: implications for pigment reduction in phenylketonuria. J Invest Dermatol 1980;74:85–89
Fisch RO, Tsai MY, Gentry WC Jr. Studies of phenylketonurics with dermatitis. J Am Acad Dermatol 1981;4:284–290
Guillet GY, Dore N, Hehunstre JP, et al. Pseudoscleroderma and phenylketonuria. Int J Dermatol 1983;22:422–426
Lee EB. Metabolic diseases and the skin. Pediatr Clin North Am 1983;30:597–608
Levy HL, Waisbren SE. Effects of untreated maternal phenylketonuria and hyperphenylalaninemia on the fetus. N Engl J Med 1983;309:1269–1274
Nova MP, Kaufman M, Halperin A. Scleroderma-like skin in a child with phenylketonuria: a clinicopathologic correlation and review of the literature. J Am Acad Dermatol 1992;26:329–333
Scriver CR, Kaufman S, Woo SLC. The hyperphenylalaninemias. In: Scriver CR, Beaudet AL, Sly WS, Valle D, eds. The Metabolic Basis of Inherited Disease. 6th ed. New York, McGraw-Hill, 1989:495–546

HISTIDINEMIA

occasional atopic dermatitis–like eruption

tendency for fair hair and blue eyes, similar to patients with phenylketonuria

occasional mental retardation and speech disorders

AR and AD cases

urine ferric chloride test (also used for screening for phenylketonuria) is often positive in children with histidinemia but may be negative in infants

skin histidine alpha-deaminase (histidase) levels and urocanic acid levels are absent or greatly reduced

most persons detected by newborn screening with metabolic histidinemia are found to be asymptomatic

McK 235800
Baden HP, Hori Y, Pathak MA, Levy HL. Epidermis in histidinemia. Arch Dermatol 1969;100:432–435
Levy HL. Disorders of histidine metabolism. In: Scriver CR, Beaudet AL, Sly WS, Valle D, eds. The Metabolic Basis of Inherited Disease. 6th ed. New York, McGraw-Hill, 1989:563–576
Scriver CR, Levy HL. Histidinemia: I. Reconciling retropective and prospective findings. J Inher Metab Dis 1983;6:51–53
Society transactions, Minnesota Dermatological Society meeting of September 10, 1967. Histidinemia and atopic dermatitis. Arch Dermatol 1968;98:317–319

TYROSINEMIA TYPE II

Synonym

- Richner-Hanhart syndrome

Skin

punctate palmoplantar keratoses, especially of fingertips and thenar and hypothenar eminences (Fig. 15–14); sometimes keratoses preceded by painful erosions

onset in infancy or childhood

hyperkeratotic papules and plaques on elbows and knees

leukokeratosis of tongue reported

Non-Skin

occasional corneal erosions, dendritic ulcers, photophobia, lacrimation, and ocular pain in first months of life, often before skin findings; progressive keratitis and scarring may cause blindness

neurologic abnormalities include developmental delay and mental retardation

Genetics

AR

Laboratory Data

hepatic tyrosine aminotransferase deficiency

elevated tyrosine in plasma and urine

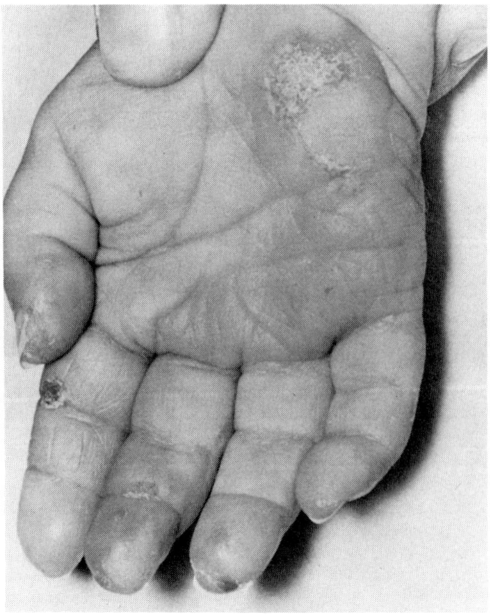

FIGURE 15–14
Tyrosinemia type II. Hyperkeratotic scaling lesions of the palms are typical in this condition. (Courtesy of Lowell Goldsmith, MD, Rochester, New York; reprinted with permission from Goldsmith LA. Tyrosinemia. In Fitzpatrick TB, Aisen AZ, Wolff K, Friedberg JM, Austen KF, eds. Dermatology in General Medicine. New York, McGraw-Hill, 1987, pp 1634–1639.)

Prognosis

low tyrosine and phenylalanine diet may prolong life, improve symptoms, and, if early enough, may prevent mental retardation

most patients, however, die before adulthood

Discussion

tyrosinemia type I (tyrosiluria) has no skin findings

REFERENCES

McK 276600

Goldsmith LA, Laberge C. Tyrosinemia and related disorders. In: Scriver CR, Beaudet AL, Sly WS, Valle D, eds. The Metabolic Basis of Inherited Disease. 6th ed. New York, McGraw-Hill, 1989:547–562

Goldsmith LA. Tyrosinemia II: a large North Carolina kindred. Arch Intern Med 1985; 145:1697–1700

Machino H, Miki Y, Kawatsu T, et al. Successful dietary control of tyrosinemia II. J Am Acad Dermatol 1983;9:533–539

HYPERLYSINEMIA

fine, sparse hair; synophrys

lax ligaments

most patients with hyperlysinemia are normal; mental retardation and other abnormalities reported

AR

lysine-ketoglutarate reductase deficiency results in hyperlysinemia and hyperlysinuria

REFERENCES

McK 238700

McK 238710

McK 238750

Brown JH, Fabre LF Jr, Farrell GL, Adams ED. Hyperlysinuria with hyperammonemia: a new metabolic disorder. Am J Dis Child 1972;124:127–132

Menkes JH. Textbook of Child Neurology. 4th ed. Philadelphia, Lea & Febiger, 1990:55–57

ISOVALERIC ACIDEMIA

bromhidrosis with the general "odor of sweaty feet" in patients either in the acute, frequently fatal neonatal form or in the chronic intermittent form

alopecia of scalp in the intermittent form

AR

isovaleryl-CoA dehydrogenase deficiency

McK 243500

Berry GT, Yudkoff M, Segal S. Isovaleric acidemia: medical and neurodevelopmental effects of long-term therapy. J Pediatr 1988;113:58–64

Budd MA, Tanaka K, Holmes LB, et al. Isovaleric acidemia: clinical features of a new genetic defect of leucine metabolism. N Engl J Med 1967;277:321–327

MAPLE SYRUP URINE DISEASE

sweet-smelling ear cerumen is often the earliest specific sign and may be noted by 2 months of age

periorificial or widespread dermatitis reported in patients with classic form of maple syrup urine disease while undergoing dietary therapy (restriction of protein intake); cutaneous eruption associated with decreased plasma isoleucine and/or leucine levels

exfoliative erythroderma reported with inadequate dietary intake of branched-chain amino acids

urine has a sickly maple syrup–like odor

different defects in the mitochondrial multienzyme complex, branched-chain alpha-ketoacid dehydrogenase (BCKD)

McK 248600

Clow CL, Reade TM, Scriver CR. Outcome of early and long-term management of classical maple syrup urine disease. Pediatrics 1981;68:856–862

Indo Y, Akaboshi I, Nobukuni Y, et al. Maple syrup urine disease: a possible biochemical basis for the clinical heterogeneity. Hum Genet 1988;80:6–10

Koch SE, Packman S, Koch TK, Williams ML. Dermatitis in treated maple syrup urine disease. J Am Acad Dermatol 1993; 28:289–292

Northrup H, Sigman ES, Hebert AA. Exfoliative erythroderma resulting from inadequate intake of branched-chain amino acids in infants with maple syrup urine disease. Arch Dermatol 1993;129:384–385

Spraker MK, Helminski MA, Elsas LJ. Periorificial dermatitis secondary to deficiency of isoleucine in treated infants with maple syrup urine disease. [Abstract]. J Invest Dermatol 1986;86:508

Wendel U, Lombeck I, Bremer HJ, et al. Maple syrup urine disease. N Engl J Med 1983; 308:1100–1101

Mucopolysaccharidoses

The mucopolysaccharidoses (MPS) are inherited deficiencies in lysosomal enzymes that result in metabolic storage defects. The dermatologist usually neither makes the diagnosis nor decides the treatment for these patients. The skin may be biopsied for fibroblast culture for enzyme analysis. Of the many MPS diseases, only Hunter syndrome manifests characteristic dermatologic features, namely, papules on the upper back. Patients with any of the MPS diseases may have coarse hair or thickened skin. Only MPS I H (Hurler disease) and MPS II (Hunter disease) are described below; see Table 15–3 for information on the other MPS and related syndromes.

MUCOPOLYSACCHARIDOSIS I H

Synonyms

- Hurler syndrome
- MPS I H
- Hurler-Pfaundler syndrome
- gargoylism
- lipochondrodystrophy
- dysostosis multiplex

Skin

thick, inelastic, frequently hyperpigmented skin, predominantly in exposed areas; develops in infancy or early childhood

lips are thick and tongue is enlarged and protuberant

hypertrichosis of scalp, neck, eyebrows, trunk, and extremities

dental abnormalities include small and widely spaced teeth and dentigerous cysts; gingival and alveolar bony hypertrophy common

Non-Skin

nonspecific signs in early infancy include hernia, macrocephaly, limited hip abduction, and recurrent respiratory infection

growth failure after infancy

hepatosplenomegaly

skeletal changes called "dysostosis multiplex" causing bizarre skeletal deformities in almost all patients

other musculoskeletal abnormalities include short stocky stature, thoracic and lumbar kyphosis with hip and knee flexion (patients appear semi-crouched), and pectus excavatum and carinatum that develop during first year of life, skull and sella turcica distortion, genu valgum, coxa valga, pes planus, and talipes equinovarus

TABLE 15–3
MUCOPOLYSACCHARIDOSES AND RELATED DISORDERS

MPS Type (Eponym)	Inheritance	Defective Enzyme	Excessive Urinary AMPS	Comments
MPS I H (Hurler)	AR	Alpha-L-iduronidase	DS HS	Hyperpigmentation and thickening of skin; hypertrichosis
MPS I H/S (Hurler-Scheie)	AR	Alpha-L-iduronidase	DS HS	Similar to MPS I H
MPS I S (Scheie)	AR	Alpha-L-iduronidase	DS HS	Similar to MPS I H
MPS II A (severe) (Hunter severe)	XLR	Iduronate sulfate-sulfatase	DS HS	Occasional white papules and nodules on back, arms, and thighs; classically, "pebbling" of skin on, below, or between scapular areas or on the deltoid areas; connective tissue nevus gives a similar clinical appearance; skin and hair similar to MPS I H
MPS II B (mild) (Hunter mild)	XLR	Iduronate sulfate-sulfatase	DS HS	Mild variant; cutaneous lesions as with MPS II A
MPS III A (Sanfilippo A)	AR	Heparin-N-sulfatase	HS	Hair may be coarse
MPS III B (Sanfilippo B)	AR	Alpha-N-acetyl-glucosaminidase	HS	
MPS III C (Sanfilippo C)	AR	Acetyl CoA:alpha-glucosaminidase-N-acetyltransferase	HS	
MPS III D (Sanfilippo D)	AR	Alpha-n-acetylglucosaminide-6-sulfatase	HS	Skin thickened and inelastic but "loose"
MPS IV A (Morquio A)	AR	Galactosamine-6-sulfate-sulfatase	KS	
MPS IV B (Morquio B)	AR	Beta-galactosidase	KS	
MPS V—no longer used				
MPS VI A (Maroteaux-Lamy A)	AR	Arylsulfatase B	DS	Macroglossia
MPS VI B (Maroteaux-Lamy B)	AR	Arylsulfatase B	DS	
MPS VII (Sly)	AR	Beta-glucuronidase	DS HS	Occasional skin laxity
MPS VIII—no longer used				
GM1 Gangliosidosis	AR	Beta-galactosidase		Similar phenotype to MPS I H; angiokeratomas, telangiectasia and atypical mongolian spots (Color Fig. 15–6)

AR, Autosomal recessive; XLR, X-linked recessive; DS, dermatan sulfate; HS, heparan sulfate; KS, keratin sulfate.

Modified from Neufeld EF, Muenzer J. The mucopolysaccharidoses. In: Scriver CR, Beaudet AL, Sly WS, Valle D, eds. The Metabolic Basis of Inherited Disease. 6th ed. New York, McGraw-Hill, 1989:1565–1587.

craniofacial abnormalities include large head, prominent forehead, depressed bridge of nose, broad nasal tip with wide nostrils, and ocular hypertelorism

flexion contractures involve shoulders, elbows, and fingers (characteristic claw hand)

ocular findings include bilateral diffuse corneal clouding (70% to 80%), which presents by age 3 years (rarely present at birth), and retinal degeneration; blindness may occur

genitalia appear normal but do not mature

frequent cardiomegaly

mental retardation develops after first year of life

Genetic

AR

Laboratory Data

alpha-L-iduronidase deficiency, which can be assayed in leukocytes or cultured skin fibroblasts; prenatal diagnosis using amniocytes or chorionic villous tissue possible

urinary mucopolysaccharides: dermatan sulfate (chondroitin sulfate B) and heparan sulfate (heparitin)

occasional metachromatic-staining granules in leukocytes

Prognosis

most die in first decade of life; chief causes are congestive heart failure or pulmonary infection

REFERENCES

McK 252800
Gardner DG. The oral manifestations of Hurler's syndrome. Oral Surg 1971;32:46–57
Hambrick GW Jr, Scheie HG. Studies of the skin in Hurler's syndrome. Arch Dermatol 1962;85:455–471
Neufeld EF, Muenzer J. The mucopolysaccharidoses. In: Scriver CR, Beaudet AL, Sly WS, Valle D, eds. The Metabolic Basis of Inherited Disease. 6th ed. New York, McGraw-Hill, 1989:1565–1587

MUCOPOLYSACCHARIDOSIS II

Synonyms

- Hunter syndrome
- MPS II

Skin

skin and hair findings similar to Hurler syndrome

in addition, "pebbling" of skin on, below, or between scapular areas or on the deltoid areas (Fig. 15–15); occasional whitish papules and nodules on back, arms, and thighs

occasional café-au-lait macules

Non-Skin

normal at birth

signs and symptoms are similar to Hurler syndrome (abnormal craniofacies, hepatosplenomegaly, cardiac anomalies, and musculoskeletal abnormalities) but are milder and appear later

no corneal clouding

no kyphosis

mental deficiency occurs later than in Hurler syndrome

Genetics

XLR

Laboratory Data

enzyme deficiency: iduronic sulfatase

urinary mucopolysaccharides: dermatan sulfate (chondroitin sulfate B) and heparan sulfate (heparitin)

metachromatic-staining granules (Alder-Reilly granules) in leukocytes

radiographs: skull and sella turcica distortion, "dysostosis multiplex"

prenatal diagnosis is possible

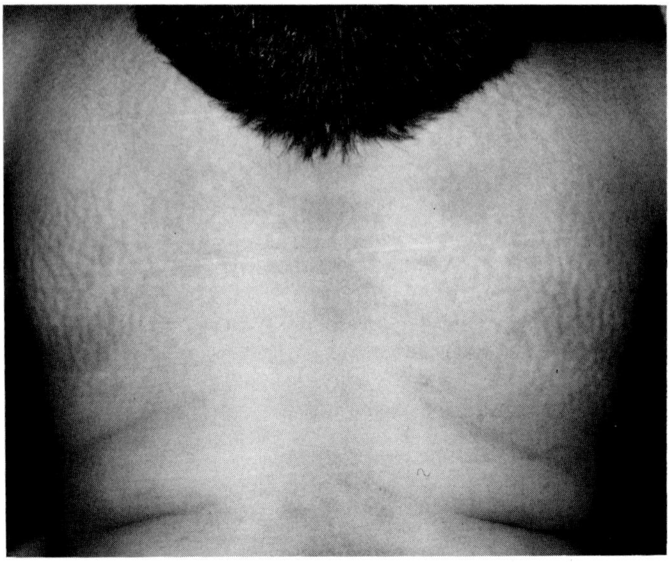

FIGURE 15–15
Mucopolysaccharidosis II (Hunter syndrome). Bilateral plaques composed of multiple skin-colored papules on the upper back.

Prognosis

death usually before age 15 years due to cardiac, pulmonary, or neurologic sequelae

Discussion

female carriers have metachromatic granules in some skin fibroblasts; enzyme assay may allow carrier detection

mild variant exists in which mental function is normal; patients survive into fourth to seventh decades; cutaneous papules and plaques are more frequent; XLR

a variant with AR inheritance and variable clinical features may exist

REFERENCES

McK 309900

Finlayson LA. Hunter syndrome (mucopolysaccharidosis II). Pediatr Dermatol 1990; 7:150–152

Gerich JE. Hunter's syndrome: beta-galactosidase deficiency in skin. N Engl J Med 1969;280:799–802

Gorlin RJ, Cohen MM Jr, Levin LS. Syndromes of the Head and Neck. 3rd ed. New York, Oxford University Press, 1990:99–117

Neufeld EF, Muenzer J. The mucopolysaccharidoses. In: Scriver CR, Beaudet AL, Sly WS, Valle D, eds. The Metabolic Basis of Inherited Disease. 6th ed. New York, McGraw-Hill, 1989:1565–1587

SKELETAL DYSPLASIA WITH TELANGIECTASES AND MESODERMAL DYSGENESIS OF THE IRIS

possible AR

McK 270240

Greaves MW, Inman PM: Cutaneous changes in the Morquio syndrome. Br J Dermatol 1969;81:29–36

Spellacy E, Gibbs DA, Watts RWE: A newly recognized syndrome of connective tissue dysplasia in siblings (previously described as a variant of Morquio disease). Q J Med 1981;200:377–415

NIEMANN-PICK DISEASE

Synonyms

- Niemann-Pick disease, type I
- sphingomyelin-cholesterol lipidosis

Skin

xanthomas with predilection for face, extremities, hands, and shoulders occur in about one fourth of patients

skin is yellowish brown, waxy, and indurated

black macules on mucosa common

Non-Skin

jaundice is the most common initial symptom and is usually present at birth; resolves in 3 to 4 months

patients develop apathy, progressive abdominal enlargement due to hepatosplenomegaly, growth retardation, and muscle weakness in first months of life

cherry-red spots in macular area of optic fundi in one fourth to one half of patients cause partial or complete blindness

ataxia and supranuclear gaze paresis

deafness

Genetics

AR

over half of cases are seen in Jewish families

Pathophysiology

a sphingolipidosis

sphingomyelinase deficiency results in sphingomyelin accumulation in lysosomes

"Niemann-Pick cells" are cells of the mononuclear phagocytic system having a mulberry or foamy appearance due to intracytoplasmic sphingomyelin-containing vacuoles

Laboratory Data

cytoplasmic vacuoles are seen in circulating monocytes and lymphocytes

leukocytosis, moderate anemia, and thrombocytosis (a late finding)

prenatal diagnosis is reliable (cultured fibroblasts)

histopathology: increased melanin in basal layer of epidermis

Prognosis

death usually occurs before the third year of life due to pulmonary infection

Discussion

there are two broad types of Niemann-Pick disease, each of which has three subtypes:

1. Niemann-Pick disease, type I: these patients have sphingomyelinase deficiency, resulting in principal accumulation of sphingomyelin and cholesterol in tissue
   a. Acute form (type IA): chief features are hepatosplenomegaly and neurologic symptoms in early infancy; disease progresses rapidly and death before age 6 years is usual
   b. Subacute form (type IS): chief features are hepatosplenomegaly in infancy or childhood; progresses less rapidly and has less neurologic disease than type IA
   c. Chronic form (type IC): chief features are hepatosplenomegaly first discovered in adulthood; some patients have central nervous system involvement
2. Niemann-Pick disease, type II: these patients are not sphingomyelinase deficient; sphingomyelin accumulation, when present, is less severe than in type I
   a. Acute form (type IIA): chief features are jaundice, hepatosplenomegaly, and neurologic symptoms in early infancy, but severity and progression are to a lesser degree than type IA
   b. Subacute form (type IIS): chief features are variable psychomotor retardation, hepatosplenomegaly, seizures, and vertical supranuclear ophthalmoplegia in the first decade of life; progressive central nervous system disease causes death in the second decade
   c. Chronic form (type IIC): chief features are dementia, extrapyramidal signs, and variable organomegaly in adulthood

■ *familial sea-blue histiocytosis*

occasional irregular brown gray patches on face and trunk; facial nodules

infiltrates of histiocytes in multiple viscera including spleen and bone marrow; usually begins in early adulthood

mild thrombocytopenia

AR

death from pulmonary or hepatic failure

histopathology: histiocytes with lipid granules that stain blue or blue-green with Giemsa or Wright stains; however, blue staining of histiocytes is not a specific finding for this or any other disease

some cases may represent a form of Niemann-Pick disease

McK 269600

REFERENCES

McK 257200
McK 257220
McK 257250
Brady RO, Filling KMR, Barton NW, Pentchev PG. Niemann-Pick disease types C and D. Neurol Clin 1989;7:75–88
Crocker AC, Farber S. Niemann-Pick disease: a review of 18 patients. Medicine 1958; 37:1–95
Levade T, Salvayre R, Douste-Blazy L. Sphingomyelinases and Niemann-Pick disease. J Clin Chem Biochem 1986;24:205–220
Mardini MK, Gergen P, Akhtar M, Ghandour M. Niemann-Pick disease: report of a case with skin involvement. Am J Dis Child 1982;136:650–651
Sawitsky A, Rosner F, Chodsky S. The sea-blue histiocyte syndrome, a review: genetic and biochemical studies. Semin Hematol 1972; 9:285–297
Silverstein MN, Ellefson RD. The syndrome of the sea-blue histiocyte. Semin Hematol 1972;9:299–307
Spence MW, Callahan JW. Sphingomyelin-cholesterol lipidoses: the Niemann-Pick group of diseases. In: Scriver CR, Beaudet AL, Sly WS, Valle D, eds. The Metabolic Basis of Inherited Disease. 6th ed. New York, McGraw-Hill, 1989:1655–1676
Zina AM, Budino S. Familial sea-blue histiocytosis with cutaneous involvement: a case report with ultrastructural findings. Br J Dermatol 1983;108:335–361

GAUCHER DISEASE, TYPE I

Synonyms

- adult Gaucher disease
- nonneuropathic Gaucher disease
- cerebroside lipidosis

Skin

generalized yellow-brown pigmentation in about half of patients

scattered hyperpigmented macules (café-au-lait macules) and easy tanning reported

occasional purpura due to hematologic abnormalities, most commonly pretibial

hyperhidrosis, even in cool weather

Non-Skin

typical signs include weakness, mild bone pain, and bleeding diathesis; these are usually apparent in early adulthood but may occur at any age

splenomegaly is the earliest and most common presenting sign; frequent hepatomegaly and generalized lymphadenopathy

infiltration of bone marrow by Gaucher cells results in both acute fever and diffuse pain, as well as generalized osteoporosis and pathologic fractures

bilateral pingueculae-like wedge-shaped thickenings of nasal and temporal conjunctivae (Fig. 15–16)

osteoporosis

neurologic symptoms usually absent

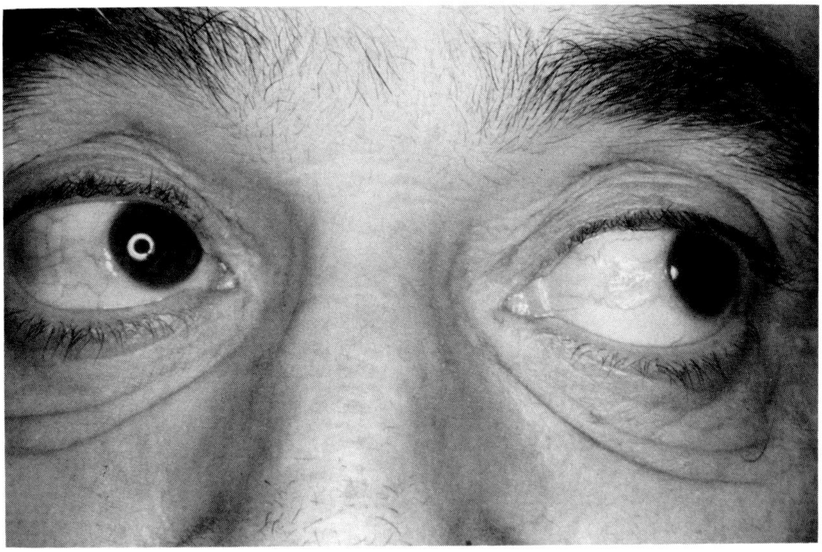

FIGURE 15–16
Gaucher disease. Wedge-shaped thickening of the nasal and temporal conjunctiva (pingueculae).

Genetics

AR

Pathophysiology

a sphingolipidosis

glucocerebrosidase (beta-glucosidase) deficiency results in accumulation of glucocerebroside in lysosomes of cells of the mononuclear phagocytic system

heterozygote carriers have intermediate glucocerebrosidase activity, which is measured in white blood cells or fibroblasts

Laboratory Data

osteoporosis demonstrated radiographically

thrombocytopenia, leukopenia, and anemia (usually hypochromic and microcytic, rarely macrocytic) due to hypersplenism

increased serum acid phosphatase

asymptomatic heterozygotes may have Gaucher cells (lipid-infiltrated macrophages) present in bone marrow

prenatal diagnosis is possible using either amniocytes or chorionic villi

Prognosis

life span may be normal; patients with a later onset have a better prognosis

intravenous enzyme replacement therapy beneficial

bone marrow transplantation has been used with partial restoration of deficient levels of enzyme in the monocyte

Discussion

Gaucher disease is the most prevalent lysosomal storage disorder, and type I accounts for most cases

the distinctive hyperpigmentation from knees to below ankles reported in the early literature was not seen in a recent large case series

although the classification of Gaucher disease into the various types is often clinically useful, great genetic and phenotypic variability is seen; thus, patients with type I Gaucher disease range from disabled children to asymptomatic octagenarians

Gaucher types II and III are described with earlier onset, neurologic symptoms, more severe course, and absence of skin manifestations

REFERENCES

McK 230800

Barranger JA, Ginns EL. Glycosylceramide lipidoses: Gaucher disease. In: Scriver CR, Beaudet AL, Sly WS, Valle D, eds. The Metabolic Basis of Inherited Disease. 6th ed. New York, McGraw-Hill, 1989:1677–1698

Barton NW, Brady RO, Dambrosia JM, et al. Replacement therapy for inherited enzyme deficiency: macrophage-targeted glucocerebrosidase for Gaucher's disease. N Engl J Med 1991;324:1464–1470

Beutler E. Gaucher's disease. N Engl J Med 1991;325:1354–1360

Goldblatt J, Beighton P. Cutaneous manifestations of Gaucher disease. Br J Dermatol 1984;111:331–334

FABRY DISEASE

Synonyms

- Fabry-Anderson disease
- angiokeratoma corporis diffusum

Skin

numerous angiokeratomas, which begin as red macules that develop into papules as they increase from pinpoint to several millimeters in size

angiokeratomas, often grouped, usually appear on lower trunk, umbilicus, groin, and genitalia (Color Fig. 15–7 and Fig. 15–17); other sites may be involved

angiokeratomas usually present before puberty, occasionally as early as the first years of life; lesions increase in number with time, but eventually stabilize

occasional flushing of skin on extremities and leg edema unrelated to cardiac, renal, hepatic, or protein abnormalities

Non-Skin

burning dysesthesias and paresthesias, often excruciatingly severe, are constant early features in childhood and usually predate the skin eruption

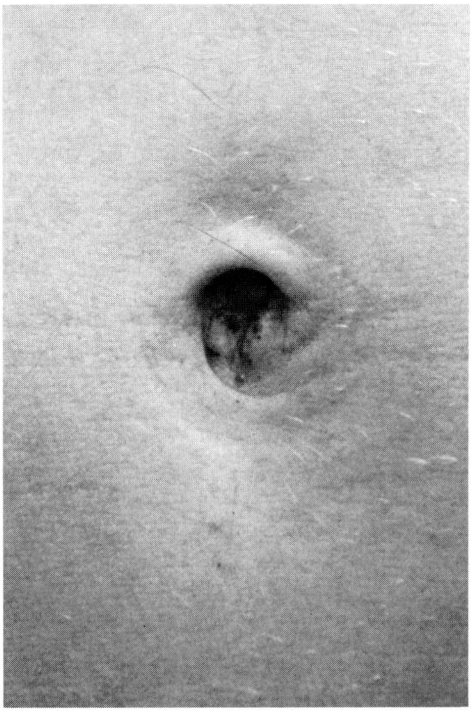

FIGURE 15–17
Small angiomatous papules in the umbilicus, a characteristic site for the angiokeratomas of Fabry disease.

pain occurs in episodic Fabry crises associated with fever and may last minutes to several days; crises typically occur in the later afternoon and involve the hands and feet

other neurologic signs and symptoms include headaches and cerebrovascular accidents

whorled corneal opacities (cornea verticillata) seen on slit-lamp examination are the most characteristic eye findings; other findings include posterior capsule cataracts (including characteristic spoke-like granular material termed *Fabry cataracts*), vascular lesions of lids, periorbital and retinal edema, and conjunctival or retinal vessel tortuosity

renal and urinary findings include proteinuria, cellular casts, and birefringent lipid globules with a characteristic “Maltese cross” pattern (found free in urine or within “mulberry cells”); insidious development of hypertension and uremia

cardiac findings include angina, myocardial infarction, hypertensive heart disease, cardiomyopathy, and heart failure

pulmonary disease, which may be fatal, includes chronic bronchitis and emphysema

gastrointestinal phenomena include intermittent abdominal pain, diarrhea, and bleeding (which may be the cause of chronic anemia) that may last days to months; signs and symptoms may mimic an acute abdomen or ulcerative colitis

recurrent attacks of painful arthritis of the terminal phalanges associated with fever and an elevated erythrocyte sedimentation rate

myositis-like signs and symptoms with severe atrophy of forearm muscles

occasional decreased libido and/or fertility in males

Genetics

XLR

fullest expression in males

mostly occurs in western Europe and the Mediterranean area

Pathophysiology

a sphingolipidosis

a deficiency in alpha-galactoside A (ceramide trihexosidase) results in abnormal lipid deposits of galactose-galactose-glucose-ceramide molecules in affected tissues

electron-dense intracytoplasmic lamellar lipid granules detectable by electron microscopy are diagnostic of Fabry disease

Laboratory Data

sphingolipid levels in the urine are elevated

alpha-galactosidase activity in serum and hair roots can be assayed

prenatal diagnosis possible

Prognosis

in males, death in fourth or fifth decades is most common, usually due to uremia or stroke, coronary artery or other cardiac disease, or pulmonary disease

affected females have a normal life span

Discussion

rarely, skin lesions are absent

cornea verticillata lesions may also be seen in patients on long-term chloroquine or amiodarone therapy

other rare metabolic disorders associated with angiokeratomas include beta-galactosidase deficiency, sialidosis with combined deficiency of beta-galactosidase and neuraminidase, aspartyl glycosaminuria, mannosidosis, partial combined deficiency of fucosidase and alpha-galactosidase, and alpha-N-galactosaminidase deficiency; several well-studied patients with angiokeratoma corporis diffusum with and without systemic abnormalities but without enzyme defects have also been reported

- *Fabry disease in female heterozygotes:*

  milder disease, (e.g., a few angiokeratomas on the trunk)

  detection of corneal opacities in 80% to 90% (most reliable means of carrier identification)

  elevated sphingolipid levels in the urine

REFERENCES

McK 301500
Chesser RS, Gentry RH, Fitzpatrick JE, Harrington AC. Perioral telangiectases: a new cutaneous finding in Fabry's disease. Arch Dermatol 1990;126:1655–1656
Desnick RJ, Bishop DF. Fabry disease: alpha-galactosidase deficiency. In: Scriver CR, Beaudet AL, Sly WS, Valle D, eds. The Metabolic Basis of Inherited Disease. 6th ed. New York, McGraw-Hill, 1989:1751–1780
Gasparini G, Sarchi G, Caviochini S, Bertagnolio B. Angiokeratoma corporis diffusum in a patient with normal enzyme activities and Turner's syndrome. Clin Exp Dermatol 1992;17:56–59
Kang WH, Chun SI, Lee S. Generalized anhidrosis associated with Fabry's disease. J Am Acad Dermatol 1987;17:883–887
Kanzaki T, Wang AM, Desnick RJ. Lysosomal α-N-acetylgalactosaminidase deficiency, the enzymatic defect in angiokeratoma corporis diffusum with glycopeptiduria. J Clin Invest 1991;88:707–711
Wallace HJ. Anderson-Fabry disease. Br J Dermatol 1973;88:1–23

FUCOSIDOSIS TYPE III

angiokeratomas (similar morphologically to those in Fabry disease) first appear on scrotum and in perineal area; subsequently, become more widespread, including palms and mucosae

onset in infancy to early childhood

skin thickened

thick lips and tongue

hypohidrosis or hyperhidrosis in some

purple bands across distal aspects of nails; nailbeds have pale appearance

coarse facial features

progressive psychomotor retardation, spasticity, growth retardation, dysostosis multiplex, short stature, recurrent respiratory tract infections, and tortuosity of conjunctival and retinal vessels

AR

absent or decreased alpha-L-fucosidase

histopathology: dilated blood vessels in dermal papillae and swollen, vacuolated cells in secretory coils of sweat glands

carriers detected by decreased enzyme activity in cells and serum

prenatal diagnosis possible through enzyme detection in amniotic fluid cells

fucosidosis types I and II has no skin findings; death by age 5

McK 230000
Dvoretzky I, Fisher BK. Fucosidosis. Int J Dermatol 1979;18:213–216
Kornfeld M, Snyder RD, Wenger DA: Fucosidosis with angiokeratoma: electron microscopic changes in the skin. Arch Pathol Lab Med 1977;101:478–485
Willems PJ, Gatti R, Darby JK, et al. Fucosidosis revisited; a review of 77 patients. Am J Med Genet 1991;38:111–131

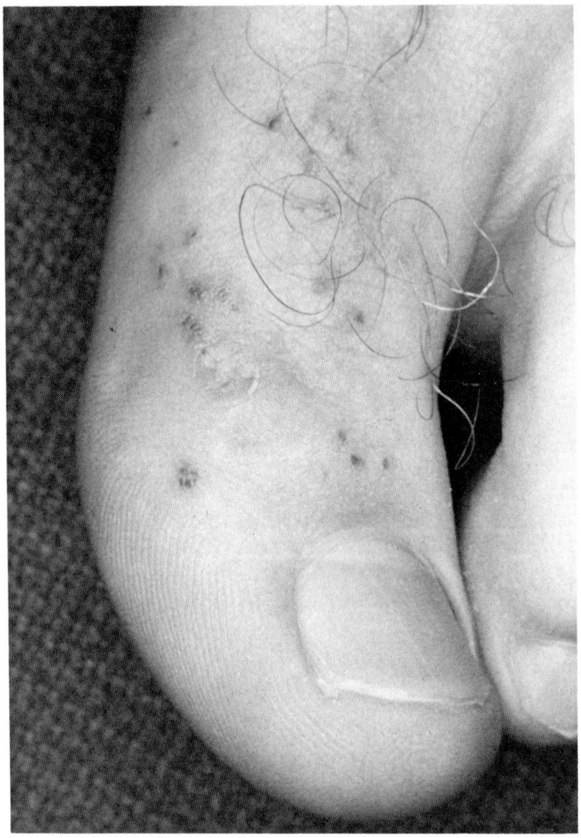

FIGURE 15–18
Angiokeratoma of Mibelli. Multiple dark-red hyperkeratotic papules scattered over the great toe. (Courtesy of Benjamin K. Fisher, MD, Toronto, Ontario.)

ANGIOKERATOMA OF MIBELLI

Skin

bright red macules and warty darker red papules up to 5 mm on fingers, toes, dorsa of hands, and feet (Fig. 15–18); occasionally on elbows and knees, calves, and buttocks

onset at age 10 to 15 years

antecedent cold injury common

Genetics

mostly sporadic, but AD cases reported

male to female ratio: <1

REFERENCES

Dave VK, Main RA. Angiokeratoma of Mibelli with necrosis of fingertips. Arch Dermatol 1972;106:726–728

Smith RB, Prioir IA, Park RG. Angiokeratoma of Mibelli: a family with nodular lesions of the legs. Australas J Dermatol 1968;9: 329–334

FARBER DISEASE

Skin

erythematous papules and subcutaneous nodules near joints, over tendons, and at pressure points, especially of the hands and feet

onset in infancy

Non-Skin

hoarseness, progressive and painful joint deformities result from deposition of sphingolipid material; liver, lung, brain, spleen, and heart are also affected

failure to thrive and breathing difficulties

Genetics

AR

Pathophysiology

a sphingolipidosis

lysosomal acid ceramidase deficiency results in accumulation of sphingolipid material

Prognosis

death in infancy or childhood usually results

Discussion

wide variety in phenotypic expression

REFERENCES

McK 228000

Amirhakimi GH, Haghighi P, Ghalambor MA, Honari S. Familial lipogranulomatosis (Farber's disease). Clin Genet 1976;9:625–630

Jameson RA, Holt PJ, Keen JH. Farber's disease (lysosomal acid ceramidase deficiency). Ann Rheum Dis 1987;46:559–561

Moser HW, Moser AB, Chen WW, Schram AW. Ceramidase deficiency: Farber lipogranulomatosis. In: Scriver CR, Beaudet AL, Sly WS, Valle D, eds. The Metabolic Basis of Inherited Disease. 6th ed. New York, McGraw-Hill, 1989:1645–1654

Metabolic Disorders—Abbreviated Entries

INFANTILE FREE SIALIC ACID STORAGE DISEASE

lysosomal storage disorder with increased free sialic acid in tissues and excreted in urine; manifestations noted at birth or in early infancy

generalized pigment dilution of skin and hair

systemic findings include axial hypotonia and hypertonia of extremities, severe psychomotor retardation, recurrent pulmonary infections, skeletal abnormalities, hepatosplenomegaly, and ascites

AR

death in early infancy in some; those who survive are severely impaired

REFERENCES

McK 269920

Stevenson RE, Lubinsky M, Taylor HA, et al. Sialic acid storage disease with sialuria: clinical and biochemical features in the severe infantile type. Pediatrics 1983; 72:441–449

Paschke E, Trinkl G, Erwa W, et al. Infantile type of sialic acid storage disease with sialuria. Clin Genet 1986;29:417–424

Tondeur M, Libert J, Vamos E, et al. Infantile form of sialic acid storage disorder: clinical, ultrastructural, and biochemical studies in two siblings. Eur J Pediatr 1982;139:142–147

CHAPTER

16

Chromosome Disorders

The cutaneous manifestations of syndromes caused by chromosomal abnormalities are rarely distinctive enough to permit definitive diagnosis. Rather, clinical diagnosis is usually based on a combination of dysmorphic features and multisystemic abnormalities. For this reason, we have presented only a few of the more common syndromes in full format and have briefly listed the cutaneous features and associated chromosomal abnormalities of less common syndromes in Table 16–1. Nail abnormalities in chromosomal syndromes are listed in Table 10–4. The reader is referred to some excellent sources of information on chromosomal syndromes in the reference sections of individual diseases.

DOWN SYNDROME

Synonyms

- trisomy 21
- mongolism
- Langdon Down disease

Skin

doughy skin, cutis marmorata, and ruddy cheeks common in newborn

skin thickens and roughens (especially palms and soles) in childhood

increased incidence of atopic dermatitis (lichenified plaques on posterior neck, arms, dorsal thighs, and volar wrists and ankles) and keratosis pilaris (Fig. 16–4)

actinic damage (e.g., ephelides and atrophy) is manifest early

TABLE 16–1
SELECTED CHROMOSOMAL SYNDROMES WITH MUCOCUTANEOUS FINDINGS*

Syndrome	Mucocutaneous Findings
Cat eye syndrome	Preauricular tags and fistulae
Chromosome 4 short arm deletion syndrome (4p- syndrome)	Aplasia cutis congenita of scalp; facial port wine stain; preauricular tags and sinuses; sparse and high-arched eyebrows
Chromosome 5 short arm deletion syndrome (cri-du-chat syndrome; cat's cry syndrome; 5p- syndrome)	Preauricular tags; premature canities
Ring chromosome 7 syndrome	Multiple congenital melanocytic nevi and/or café-au-lait spots
Trisomy 8 syndrome (Fig. 16–1)	Deep plantar (occasionally palmar) furrows; short nails
Trisomy 9 syndrome	Deep palmar and/or plantar creases; occasional preauricular tags
Trisomy 13 syndrome (Patau syndrome) (Figs. 16–2 and 16–3)	Nevus flammeus, especially of forehead; low posterior hairline; skin of neck redundant; scrotal-type skin extending to tip of penis; hypoplastic toenails, fingernails narrow and hyperconvex; scalp defects in the parietal and occipital areas; distal palmar axial triradii
Ring chromosome 13 syndrome	Alopecia and occasional scalp defect; symmetrical arciform hypopigmentation
Prader-Willi syndrome	Interstitial deletion in the proximal long arm of chromosome 15; cutaneous and ocular hypopigmentation; skin-picking behavior
Trisomy 18 (Edward syndrome)	Nevus flammeus; skin of neck redundant; hypoplasia of fingernails and toenails, especially fifth digits; increased hair on back and forehead; eyebrows and eyelashes may be thicker or thinner than normal; fingerprints show low-arch dermal ridge pattern

*See main text for main chromosomal syndromes with mucocutaneous findings.

References: Borgoankar DR. Chromosomal Variation in Man: A Catalogue of Chromosomal Variants and Anomalies. 4th ed. New York, Alan R. Liss, 1984; Butler LJ, Snodgrass GJAI, Sinclair NE, et al. (16-18) Trisomy syndrome: analysis of 13 cases. Arch Dis Child 1965;40:660–671; Butler MG. Hypopigmentation: a common feature of Prader-Labhart-Willi syndrome. Am J Hum Genet 1989;45:140–146; Clarke Fraser F. Gross chromosomal aberrations. In: Avery ME, Taeusch HW, eds. Diseases of the Newborn. 5th ed. Philadelphia, WB Saunders, 1984; DeLozier-Blanchet CD, Masouye I, Vollenweider S. Ring chromosome 7, hyperpigmented skin lesions and malignant melanoma. Am J Med Genet 1992;43:1039–1040; Hodes ME, Cole J, Palmer CC, et al. Clinical experience with trisomies 13 and 18. J Med Genet 1978;15:48–60; Lubs HA, Ulman Koenig E, Brandti K. Trisomy 13-15: a clinical syndrome. Lancet 1961;2:1001–1002; Warnock JK, Kestenbaum T. Pharmacologic treatment of severe skin-picking behaviors in Prader-Willi syndrome. Arch Dermatol 1992;128:1623–1625.

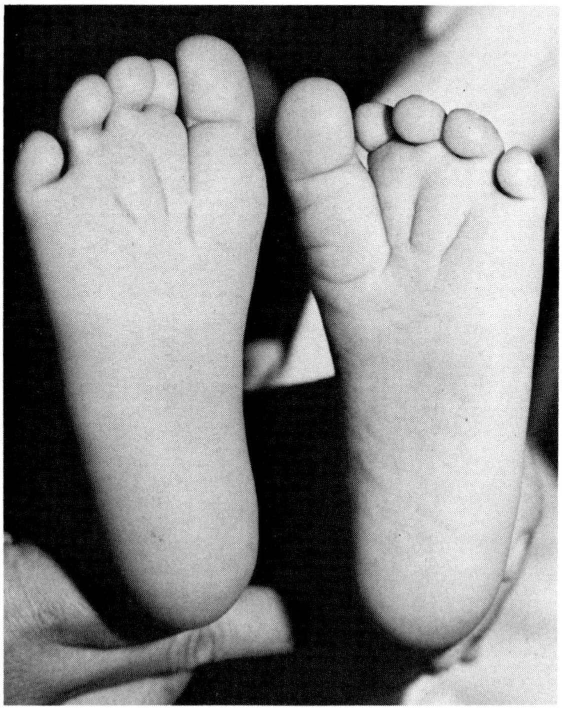

FIGURE 16–1
Trisomy 8. The characteristic deep vertical creases are seen on the plantar surface of both feet.

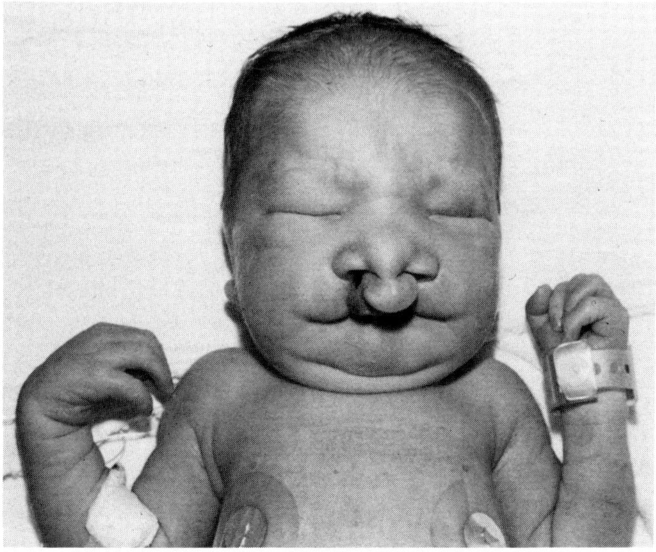

FIGURE 16–2
This infant with trisomy 13 has the characteristic facies and positioning of the hands.

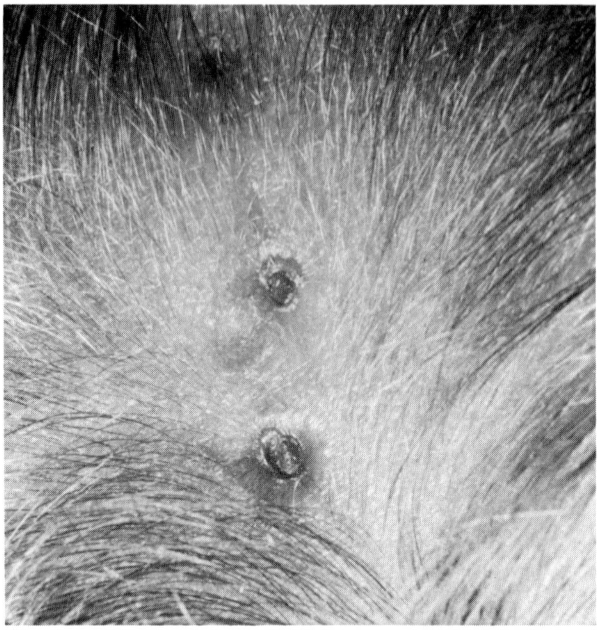

FIGURE 16–3
Partially healed localized scalp defects in a newborn with trisomy 13 syndrome (same infant as in Figure 16–1).

increased frequency of elastosis perforans serpiginosa; more widespread and of longer duration than in idiopathic form

increased incidence of syringomas (more often in females), seborrheic dermatitis, superficial fungal infections, vitiligo, and Norwegian scabies

connective tissue nevi (skin-colored nodules in cobblestone-like pattern) on neck, trunk, buttocks, and proximal extremities reported (Fig. 16–5)

dermatoglyphic abnormalities including simian crease on one or both palms, hallucal small distal loop, and distal axial triradius of palm

enlarged lips with increased tendency to fissure; multiple labial frenula

open mouth and protruding, widened scrotal tongue with prominent filiform and fungiform papillae

white thickening of mucous membranes and angular cheilitis

scalp hair is straight and fine; beard may be absent; eyelashes sparse; hair of axillae, pubes, trunk, and extremities is sparse (rarely, hirsutism is present); synophrys and low occipital hairline is common; increased incidence of alopecia areata

dental abnormalities include delayed dentition, small teeth with abnormal alignment, periodontal disease, and reduced caries

Non-Skin

hypotonia and hyperextensibility of joints

gross and fine motor developmental delay

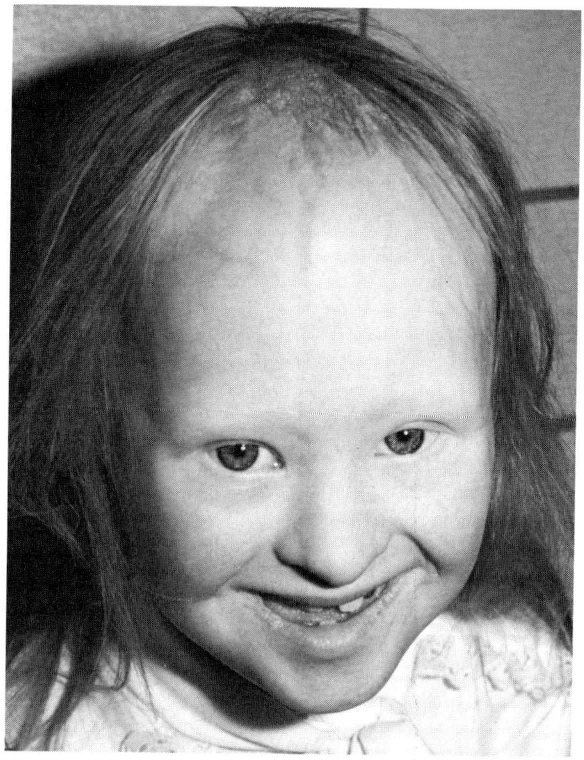

FIGURE 16–4
Alopecia areata affecting the frontoparietal scalp in a patient with Down syndrome.

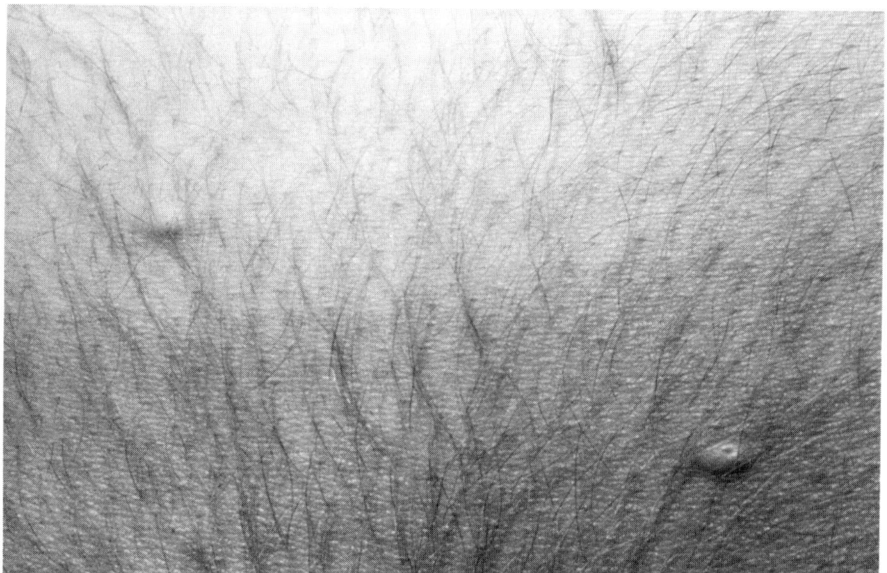

FIGURE 16–5
Multiple nodules representing connective tissue nevi are present on the torso of an adolescent woman with Down syndrome.

increased incidence of epilepsy

abnormal craniofacies including small skull, short broad neck, flattened face and occiput, short nose with depressed bridge, and short ears with overhanging helices, overt cleft palate increased and occult (submucous) cleft palate common

short neck with excess loose skin on posterior aspect

mild to moderate mental retardation; presenile dementia common

eye abnormalities include ocular hypertelorism, small palpebral fissures with "mongoloid" slant, epicanthal fold (which often disappears by end of first decade), cataracts, Brushfield spots on iris close to pupillary margin in 85%, and fine lens opacities

pectus carinatum and excavatum; dysplastic pelvis

shortening of extremities, most marked in hands and feet, which are short, broad, thick, and flabby

fingers shortened, fifth digits incurved (clinodactyly; single flexion on fifth finger due to rudimentary middle phalanx)

wide space between first and second toes

spina bifida common

cardiovascular abnormalities include ventriculoseptal defects and tetralogy of Fallot

protuberant abdomen, umbilical herniae, obesity, and poorly developed genitalia; males sterile

duodenal atresia

lymphatic hypoplasia

increased prevalence of hypothyroidism and less commonly hyperthyroidism; antithyroid antibodies common

Genetics

"regular" trisomy 21 in approximately 95%, translocation trisomy 21 in 4% to 5%; mosaic trisomy 21 in 1% to 3%; different etiologies not separable clinically

1 in every 600 to 800 births

most common autosomal chromosomal abnormality

incidence of Down syndrome rises with increasing maternal age; however, translocation trisomy is not age dependent

Pathophysiology

immunologic abnormalities include impaired cell-mediated immunity and increased occurrence of autoantibodies

Laboratory Data

in first year of life, radiograph of the pelvis is often pathognomonic, showing pelvic dysplasia and diminished acetabular and iliac lines

Prognosis

increased incidence of lymphatic and myelogenous leukemia

life expectancy decreased; when death occurs in infancy and childhood it is most often related to congenital heart disease, respiratory disease, and leukemia

physical and mental stigmata are stable

REFERENCES

Carey AB, Park HK, Burke WA. Multiple eruptive syringomas associated with Down's syndrome. [Letter]. J Am Acad Dermatol 1988;19:759–760

Carter DM, Jegosothy BV. Alopecia areata and Down's syndrome. Arch Dermatol 1976; 112:1397–1399

Down JLH. Observations on an ethnic classification of idiots. Clin Lect Rep Lond Hosp 1866;3:259–262

Kopec AV, Levine N. Generalized connective tissue nevi and ichthyosis in Down's syndrome. Arch Dermatol 1979;115:623–624

Rasmussen JE. Disseminated elastosis perforans serpiginosa in four mongoloids: recognition of residual changes. Br J Dermatol 1972;86:9–13

Scherbenski JM, Benson PM, Ritchford JP, James WD. Cutaneous and ocular manifestations of Down syndrome. J Am Acad Dermatol 1990;22:933–938

Smith DW, Wilson AA. The Child with Down's Syndrome. Philadelphia, WB Saunders, 1973

Urban CD, Cannon JR. Eruptive syringomas in Down's syndrome. Arch Dermatol 1981; 117:374–375

KLINEFELTER SYNDROME

Synonym

- XXY syndrome

Skin

scalp hair is abundant with low occipital and frontal hair lines; however, beard and body hair is sparse and female pubic escutcheon is present

increased frequency of leg ulcers reported

abnormal dermatoglyphics including low ridge count

Non-Skin

boys appear normal at birth, but small testes may be noted on careful examination

tall stature (mostly increased in lower body segment), eunuchoid appearance, and increased weight due to prepubertal hypogonadism; unilateral or bilateral gynecomastia in half

infertility, impotence, lack of libido, high-pitched voice, small testes and prostate (normal sized penis), and osteoporosis due to testicular dysgenesis

clinodactyly and cubitus valgus common

intelligence is usually normal, but personality and psychiatric disorders common and may manifest in childhood

Genetics

47 XXY, so-called classic Klinefelter syndrome comprises 80% of chromatin-positive males (see Discussion for "variants")

1 in 400 to 500 live-born males

Laboratory Data

karyotypes should be done to detect mosaicism or extra X or Y chromosomes

increased urinary gonadotropins and low 17-ketosteroids

plasma testosterone below normal

Discussion

the most common single cause of hypogonadism and infertility

- *46XY/47XXY, 48XXXY, 48XXYY, 49XXXXY, 49XXXYY syndromes*

  account for approximately 20% of chromatin-positive males, so-called variants of Klinefelter syndromes

  increasing X-aneuploidy associated with decrease in stature, increased mental retardation, leg ulcers, and varicosities

REFERENCES

Becker KL, Hoffman DL, Underdahl LO, Mason HL. Klinefelter's syndrome: clinical and laboratory findings in 50 patients. Arch Intern Med 1966;118:314–321

Caldwell PD, Smith DW. The XXY (Klinefelter's) syndrome in childhood: detection and treatment. J Pediatr 1972;80:250–258

Campbell WA, Price WH. Venous thromboembolic disease in Klinefelter's syndrome. Clin Genet 1981;19:275–280

Donlan MA, Dolan CR, Metcalf MJ, et al. Trisomy Xq in a male; the isochromosome X Klinefelter syndrome. Am J Med Genet 1987;27:189–194

Klinefelter HF, Reifenstein EC Jr, Albright F. Syndrome characterized by gynaecomastia, aspermatogenesis with A-Leydigism and increased excretion of follicle-stimulating hormone. J Clin Endocrinol 1942; 2:615–627

Osawa T, Furuse-M, Kikuchi Y, et al. Roentgenographic manifestations of Klinefelter's syndrome. AJR 1971;112:178–184

Robinson A, Lubs HA, Nielsen J, Sorensen K. Summary of clinical findings: profiles of children with 47,XXY, 47,XXX and 47,XYY karyotypes. Birth Defects 1979;15(1):261–266

Topper E, Dickerman Z, Prager-Lewin R, et al. Puberty in 24 patients with Klinefelter syndrome. Eur J Pediatr 1982;139:8–12

TURNER SYNDROME

Synonyms

- Ullrich-Turner syndrome
- Bonnevie-Ullrich syndrome
- XO syndrome
- ovarian agenesis

Skin

see Figure 16–6 and Color Figure 16–1

webbing of neck (pterygium colli), usually bilateral

multiple pigmented nevi

low posterior nuchal hairline; pubic and axillary hair often scant

congenital lymphedema of dorsal hands and feet; resolves during first 2 to 3 years of life

redundant skin on neck

thinning and wrinkling of palmar skin; thenar, hypothenar, and interdigital pads remain normal

transient pedal hemangiomas reported

nails narrow, hyperconvex, or deep set

premature eruption of teeth

dermatoglyphic abnormalities including distal axial triradius and high ridge counts

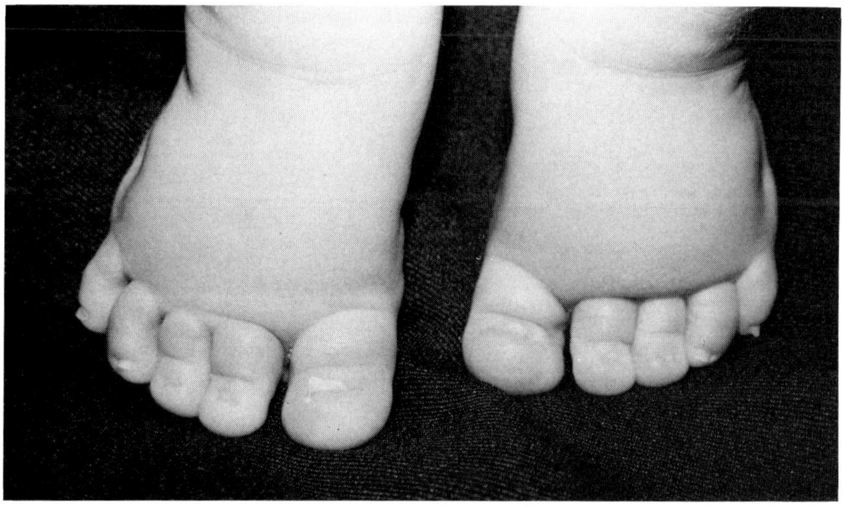

FIGURE 16–6
Lymphedema and nail hypoplasia in an infant with Turner syndrome.

Non-Skin

short stature

gonadal dysgenesis (streak ovaries); ovaries vary from virtual absence to normal size

retarded sexual development, including amenorrhea and underdeveloped breasts, vagina, and uterus

abnormal craniofacies including ptosis of eyelids, broad nasal bridge, prominent and low-set ears, high-arched and occasionally cleft palate, and micrognathia

ocular abnormalities include hypertelorism, epicanthal folds, blue sclerae, and corneal opacities

broad, shield-shaped chest and widely spaced nipples; cubitus valgus (wide carrying angle)

other skeletal abnormalities include kyphoscoliosis, maxillary and mandibular hypoplasia, and skull and facial bone asymmetry

cardiovascular abnormalities include coarctation of the aorta and patent ductus arteriosus

renal abnormalities include horseshoe kidneys

frequent nerve deafness

mental retardation, if present, is mild

Genetics

45,XO (chromatin negative) in 60% to 80%; many are mosaics (e.g., XX/XO and XXX/XO) or have 46 chromosomes with partial deletion of one of the X chromosomes and are chromatin positive

incidence of about 1 in 2500 female births

95% of 45,XO fetuses are spontaneously aborted

Laboratory Data

low estrogen levels and increased pituitary gonadotropins

histopathology of ovaries after infancy: absence of follicles and only long streaks of white connective tissue present

Prognosis

lymphedema may recur during estrogen therapy

prognosis good unless renal or cardiac defects supervene; 1% to 2% die in childhood

Discussion

about one third of cases are diagnosed during the infancy, childhood, and teenage years, respectively

REFERENCES

Carr RF, Ochs RH, Ritter DA, et al. Fetal cystic hygroma and Turner's syndrome. Am J Dis Child 1986;140:580–583

Grumbach MM, Conte FA. Disorders of sex differentiation. In: Williams RH, ed. Textbook of Endocrinology. Philadelphia, WB Saunders, 1981

Hall JG, Gilchrist DM. Turner syndrome and its variants. Pediatr Clin North Am 1990; 37:1421–1440

Lemli L, Smith DW. The XO syndrome: a study of the differentiated phenotype in 25 patients. J Pediatr 1963;63:577–588

Nora JJ, Nora AH, Sinha AK, et al. The Ullrich-Noonan syndrome (Turner phenotype). Am J Dis Child 1974;127:48–55

Paller AD, Esterly NB, Charrow J, Cahan F. Pedal hemangiomas in Turner syndrome. J Pediatr 1983;103:87–88

Turner HH. A syndrome of infantilism, congenital webbed neck and cubitus valgus. Endocrinology 1938;23:566–574

NOONAN SYNDROME

Skin

see Figures 16–7 and 16–8

coarse, curly fair scalp hair and low occipital hairline; in males, scant pubic, axillary, and beard hair and female escutcheon

transient lymphedema of dorsa of hands and feet in infancy; stationary or progressive lymphedema into adulthood

soft elastic skin

increased tendency to keloid formation

occasional ulerythema ophryogenes

numerous pigmented nevi occasionally

short and wide nails

dermatoglyphics include distal axial triradius

Non-Skin

short stature

broad short neck; occasionally webbed

abnormal craniofacies including hypertelorism, downward slanting palpebral fissures, blepharoptosis, malformed ears, high-arched palate, and micrognathia

musculoskeletal abnormalities include pectus carinatum (superiorly) and pectus excavatum (inferiorly) and clinodactyly

cardiac abnormalities include pulmonary stenosis

mild mental retardation more common in males

genital abnormalities include cryptorchidism

Genetics

AD; many sporadic cases representing new mutations

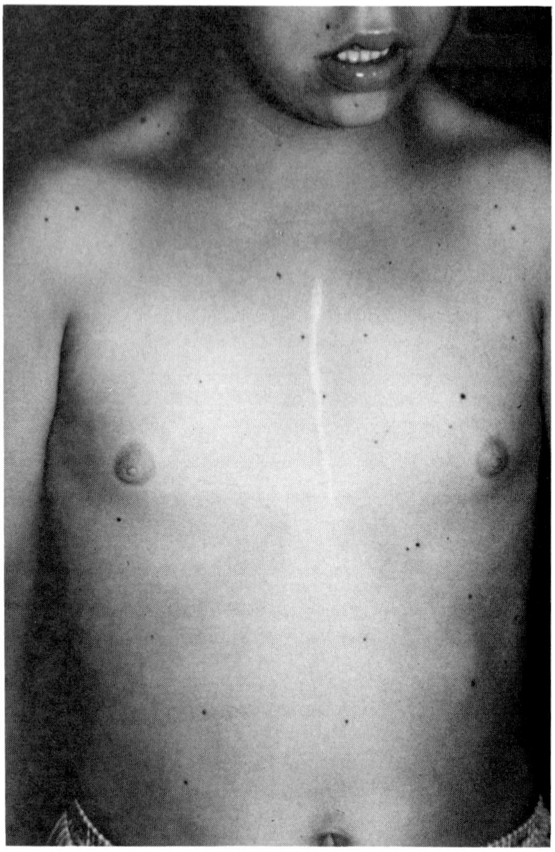

FIGURE 16–7
Noonan syndrome. Note the pectus excavatum and midline scar secondary to repair of a congenital heart defect. Numerous melanocytic nevi are scattered over the anterior torso.

FIGURE 16–8
The facies in Noonan syndrome, as in this young man, are characterized by ptosis, hypertelorism, low-set auricles, and anterior dental malocclusion.

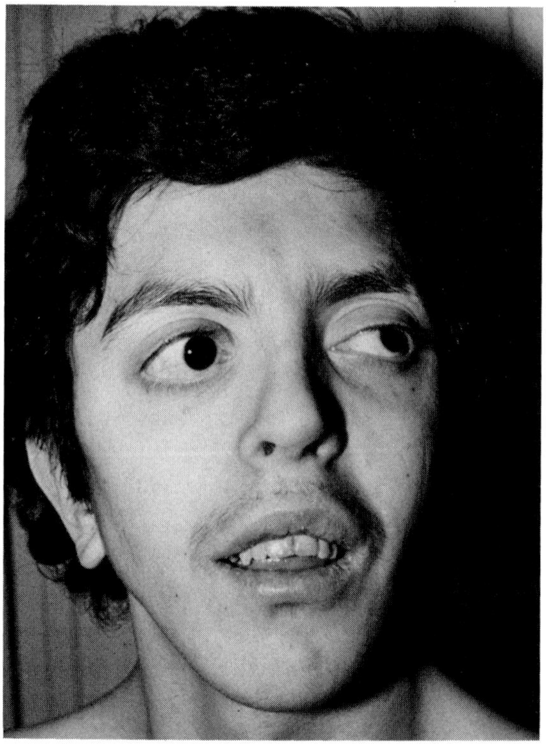

Discussion

phenotypically resembles Turner syndrome but karyotype normal; differences from Turner syndrome include occurrence in both sexes, presence of pectus excavatum or carinatum, downward slant of palpebral fissures, valvular pulmonary stenosis (cf. coarctation of aorta), and possibly higher incidence of mental retardation

- *cardiofaciocutaneous syndrome (Noonan-like short stature syndrome)*

sparse, short, curly, slow-growing scalp hair; sparse eyebrows and eyelashes

patchy to widespread ichthyosiform eruption

congenital lymphedema of hands and feet; after lymphedema resorbs, skin on dorsa of hands and feet may be redundant

generalized hypotonia

short stature

widely spaced hypoplastic nipples

abnormal craniofacies similar to that in Noonan syndrome, including high forehead, round face with macrocephaly, hypertelorism, posteriorly angulated ears, and depressed nasal bridge

cardiac defects include pulmonic stenosis, atrioseptal defect, and cardiomyopathy

AD

McK 115150

REFERENCES

McK 163950

Allanson JE, Hall JG, Hughes HE, et al. Noonan syndrome: the changing phenotype. Am J Med Genet 1985;21:507–514

Borradori L, Blanchet-Bardon C. Skin manifestations of cardio-facio-cutaneous syndrome. J Am Acad Dermatol 1993;28:815–819

Matthews CA, George P, Hood AF. Cardiofaciocutaneous syndrome. Arch Dermatol 1993;129:46–47

Mendez HMM, Opitz JM, Noonan syndrome: a review. Am J Med Genet 1985;21:493–506

Pierard GE, Soyeur-Broux M, Estrada JA, et al. Cutaneous presentation of the cardio-facio-cutaneous syndrome. J Am Acad Dermatol 1990;22:920–922

Pierini DO, Pierini AM. Keratosis pilaris atrophicans faciei (ulerythema ophryogenes): a cutaneous marker in the Noonan syndrome. Br J Dermatol 1979;100:409–416

Reynolds JF, Neri G, Herrmann JP, et al. New multiple congenital anomalies / mental retardation syndrome with cardio-facio-cutaneous involvement: the CFC syndrome. Am J Med Genet 1986;25:413–427

Sharland M, Morgan M, Smith G, et al. Genetic counselling in Noonan syndrome. Am J Med Genet 1993;45:437–440

Somer M, Peippo M, Aalto-Korte K, et al. Cardio-facio-cutaneous syndrome: three additional cases and review of the literature. Am J Med Genet 1993;44:691–695

Witt DR, Hoyme E, Zonana J, et al. Lymphedema in Noonan syndrome: clues to pathogenesis and prenatal diagnosis and review of the literature. Am J Med Genet 1987; 27:841–856

Wyre HW Jr. Cutaneous manifestations of Noonan's syndrome. Arch Dermatol 1978; 114:929–930

APPENDIX 1

Organizations for Information and Assistance Regarding Inherited and Congenital Disorders

General Organizations

NATIONAL CENTER FOR EDUCATION IN MATERNAL AND CHILD HEALTH (NCEMCH)
2000 15th N, Suite 701
Arlington, VA 22201-2617
(703) 524-7802

ALLIANCE OF GENETIC SUPPORT GROUPS
35 Wisconsin Circle, Suite 440
Chevy Chase, MD 20815
(301) 652-5553
(800) 336-GENE

NATIONAL ORGANIZATION FOR RARE DISORDERS (NORD)
P.O. Box 8923
New Fairfield, CT 06812
(203) 746-6518
(800) 999-6673

Disease-Specific Organizations

ALBINISM

NATIONAL ORGANIZATION FOR ALBINISM AND HYPOPIGMENTATION (NOAH)

1500 Locust Street, Suite 1816
Philadelphia, PA 19102-4329
(215) 545-2322
(800) 473-2310

ATAXIA-TELANGIECTASIA

NATIONAL ATAXIA FOUNDATION

600 Twelve Oaks Center
15500 Wayzata Blvd.
Wayzata, MN 55391
(612) 473-7666

COCKAYNE SYNDROME

SHARE AND CARE (family support group)

1294 S Street
North Valley Stream, NY 11580
(516) 825-2284

Thaddeus Kelly, MD (patient referrals)
(804) 924-2665

DYSAUTONOMIA

DYSAUTONOMIA FOUNDATION, INC.

20 E. 46th Street, Room 302
New York, NY 10017
(212) 949-6644

ECTODERMAL DYSPLASIAS

NATIONAL FOUNDATION FOR ECTODERMAL DYSPLASIAS

219 Main Street
Box 114
Mascoutah, IL 62258
(618) 566-2020

EHLERS-DANLOS SYNDROME

EHLERS-DANLOS NATIONAL FOUNDATION
P.O. Box 1212
Venture Center, Suite 125A
15100 N. Line Rd.
Southgate, MI 48195
(313) 282-0180

EPIDERMOLYSIS BULLOSA

DYSTROPHIC EPIDERMOLYSIS BULLOSA RESEARCH ASSOCIATION OF AMERICA (D.E.B.R.A.)
141 Fifth Ave, Suite 7-S
New York, NY 10010
(212) 995-2220

HEREDITARY HEMORRHAGIC TELANGIECTASIA

HEREDITARY HEMORRHAGIC TELANGIECTASIA FOUNDATION, INTERNATIONAL (patient support group)
P.O. Box 8087
New Haven, CT 06530

Patient Referrals
(203) 785-6938

ICHTHYOSIS

FOUNDATION FOR ICHTHYOSIS AND RELATED SKIN TYPES (FIRST)
P.O. Box 20921
Raleigh, NC 27619-0921
(919) 782-5728
(800) 545-3286

KLIPPEL-TRENAUNAY SYNDROME

KLIPPEL-TRENAUNAY SYNDROME SUPPORT GROUP (family support group)
4610 Wooddale Avenue
Edina, MN 55424
(612) 925-2596

LYMPHEDEMA

NATIONAL LYMPHATIC AND VENOUS FOUNDATION, INC. (NLVF)

P.O. Box 80
Cambridge, MA 02140

MARFAN SYNDROME

NATIONAL MARFAN FOUNDATION

382 Main Street
Port Washington, NY 11050
(516) 883-8712
(800) 862-7326

NEUROFIBROMATOSIS

NATIONAL NEUROFIBROMATOSIS FOUNDATION, INC.

141 Fifth Avenue, Suite 7-S
New York, NY 10010-7105
(800) 323-7938 (outside New York)
(212) 460-8980
fax: (212) 529-6094

NEUROFIBROMATOSIS INC. (patient and family support oriented)

8855 Annapolis Road, Suite 110
Lanham, MD 20706-2924
(301) 577-8984

PORPHYRIA

AMERICAN PORPHYRIA FOUNDATION

P.O. Box 22712
Houston, TX 77227
(713) 266-9617

PROGERIA

PROGERIA INTERNATIONAL REGISTRY

New York State Institute for Basic Research
Department of Human Genetics
1050 Forest Hill Road
Staten Island, NY 10314
(718) 494-5363
Dr. Ted Brown; patient referrals only

STURGE-WEBER SYNDROME

STURGE-WEBER FOUNDATION

P.O. Box 460931
Aurora, CO 80015
(303) 693-2986
(800) 627-5482

TUBEROUS SCLEROSIS

NATIONAL TUBEROUS SCLEROSIS ASSOCIATION

8000 Corporate Drive, Suite 120
Landover, MD 20785
(800) CALNTSA
(301) 459-9885

XERODERMA PIGMENTOSUM

XERODERMA PIGMENTOSUM REGISTRY

UMDNJ, New Jersey Medical School
Department of Pathology, Room C-520
Medical Science Building
185 S. Orange Avenue
Newark, NJ 07103-2714
(201) 982-4405

APPENDIX

2

Dermatologic Disorders, Commonly Sporadic but Occasionally Familial (and Rare Familial Disorders Not Included Elsewhere)

■ acne conglobata, hidradenitis suppurativa, pili torti, and cataracts

Gold SC, Delaney TJ. Familial acne conglobata, hidradenitis suppurativa, pili torti and cataracts. Br J Dermatol 1974;91 (Suppl 10):54–57

Quintal D, Jackson R. Aggressive squamous cell carcinoma arising in familial acne conglobata. J Am Acad Dermatol 1986;14:207–204

■ ainhum

McK 103400

Simon KMB. Ainhum, a family disease. JAMA 1921;76:560

■ alopecia areata

McK 104000

Valsecchi R, Vicari O, Frigeni A, et al. Familial alopecia areata—genetic susceptibility or coincidence? Acta Dermatol Venereol 1985;65:175–177

Zlotogorski A, Weinrauch L, Brautbar C. Familial alopecia areata: no linkage with HLA. Tissue Antigens 1990;35:40–41

■ androgenetic alopecia

McK 109200

Snyder LH, Yingling HC. The application of the gene-frequency method of analysis to sex-influenced factors, with special reference to baldness. Hum Biol 1935;7:608–615

■ familial anetoderma

Friedman SJ, Venencie PY, Bradley RR, Winkelmann RK. Familial anetoderma. J Am Acad Dermatol 1987;16:341–345

■ familial Becker melanosis

Fretzin DF, Whitney D. Familial Becker's nevus. [Letter]. J Am Acad Dermatol 1985;12:589–590

Schnyder UW, Panizzon R. Familial Becker's nevus. Dermatologica 1988;176:275–276

■ carotenemia

McK 115300

Frenk PE. Etat keratodermique avec taux serique abaissé de la vitamine A et hypercarotinemie. Dermatologica 1966;132:96–98

■ cicatricial pemphigoid

McK 164185

Ahmed AR, Foster S, Zaltas M, et al. Association of DQw7 (DQB1*0301) with ocular cicatricial pemphigoid. Proc Natl Acad Sci USA 1991;88:11579–11582

■ colloid milium

Bosellini PL. Sur deux-cas de pseudo-milium colloide familial. Ann Dermatol Syph 1906;7:751

Handfield-Jones SE, Atherton DJ, Black MM, Hashimoto K, McKee PH. Juvenile colloid milium: clinical, histological and ultrastructural features. J Cutan Pathol 1992;19:434–438

Percival BH, Duthie DA. Notes on a case of colloid pseudomilium. Br J Dermatol 1948;60:399

■ dermatitis herpetiformis

Meyer LJ, Zone JJ. Familial incidence of dermatitis herpetiformis. J Am Dermatol 1987;17:643–647

■ elastofibroma dorsi

Nagamine N, Nohara Y, Ito E. Elastofibroma in Okinawa: a clincopathologic study of 170 cases. Cancer 1982;50:1794–1805

■ erythema nodosum

McK 132990

Elkayam O, Caspi D, Segal R, et al. Familial erythema nodosum. Arthritis Rheum 1991;34:1177–1179

■ hereditary multiple granular cell tumors

Rifkin RH, Blocker SH, Palmer JO, et al. Multiple granular cell tumors: a familial occurrence in children. Arch Surg 1986;121:945–947

■ granuloma annulare

Friedman SJ, Winkelmann RK. Familial granuloma annulare: report of two cases and review of the literature. J Am Acad Dermatol 1987;16:600–605

■ hemangiopericytoma

McK 234820

Plukker JT, Koops HS, Molenaar I, et al. Malignant hemangiopericytoma in three kindred members of one family. Cancer 1988;61:841–844

■ hidradenitis suppurativa

McK 142690

Fitzsimmons JS, Guilbert PR, Fitzsimmons EM. Evidence of genetic factors in hidradenitis suppurativa. Br J Dermatol 1985;113:1–8

■ hyperhidrosis palmaris et plantaris

McK 144110

■ keratoses of actinic distribution, internal malignancy, and cellular hypersensitivity to UVA

McK 148390

Atherton DJ, Botcherby PK, Francis AJ, et al. Familial keratoses of actinic distribution associated with internal malignancy and cellular hypersensitivity to UVA. Br J Dermatol 1989;120:671–681

■ keratosis spinulosa

Boyd AS. Lichen spinulosus: case report and overview. Cutis 1989;43:557–560

Meyer D, Stolp A, Knapp A. Ueber eine Familie mit Keratosis follicularis spinulosa bei vermuetlich dominantem Erbgang.

■ lichen planus

McK 151620

Mahood JM. Familial lichen planus: a report of nine cases from four families with a brief review of the literature. Arch Dermatol 1983;119:292–294

Valsecchi R, Bontempelli M, di Landro A, et al. Familial lichen planus. [Letter]. Acta Derm Venereol 1990;70:272–273

■ lichen sclerosus et atrophicus

McK 151590

Shirer JA Jr, Ray MC. Familial occurrence of lichen sclerosus et atrophicus: case reports of a mother and daughter. Arch Dermatol 1987;123:485–488

■ discoid lupus erythematosus

Durmichev A, Pramatarov K, Mateev G. Familial lupus erythematosus chronicus discoides. Hautkrankheit 1986;61:128–132; abstracted in J Am Acad Dermatol 1986;15:264

■ melanonychia striata

Colver GB, Beveridge GW. Familial acquired pigmented streaks in the nail. Clin Exp Dermatol 1991;16:158–159

■ morphea

Wuthrich RC, Roenigk HH Jr, Steck WD. Localized scleroderma. Arch Dermatol 1975;111:98–100

■ nail clubbing

McK 119900

Curth HO, Firschein IL, Alpert M. Familial clubbed fingers. Arch Dermatol 1961;83: 828–836

■ idiopathic atrophy of nails

Suarez SM, Scher RK. Idiopathic atrophy of the nails: a possible hereditary association. Pediatr Dermatol 1990;7:39–41

■ subungual pterygium of nails

Christophers E. Familiäre subunguale pterygien. Hautarzt 1975;26:543–544

Dugois P, Amblard P, Martel C, et al. Pterygium inversum unguis familial. Bull Soc Fr Dermatol Syph 1975;82:283–284

Odom RB, Stein KM, Maibach H. Congenital, painful, aberrant hyponychium. Arch Dermatol 1974;110:89–90

■ giant pigmented hairy nevus

McK 137550

Goodman RM, Caren J, Ziprkowski M, et al. Genetic considerations in giant pigmented hairy naevus. Br J Dermatol 1971;85:150–157

■ pemphigus vulgaris

McK 169610

Ahmed AR, Wagner R, Khatri K, et al. Major histocompatibility complex haplotypes and class II genes in non-Jewish patients with pemphigus vulgaris. Proc Natl Acad Sci USA 1991;88:5056–5060

Ahmed AR, Yunis EJ, Khatri K, et al. Major histocompatibility complex haplotype studies in Ashkenazi Jewish patients with pemphigus vulgaris. Proc Natl Acad Sci USA 1990;87:7658–7662

Brenner S. Familial pemphigus vulgaris. [Letter]. J Am Acad Dermatol 1987;16:1270

Laskaris G, Sklavounou A, Stavrou A, Stavropoulou K. Familial pemphigus vulgaris with oral manifestations affecting two Greek families. Oral Pathol 1989;18:1–53

■ perifolliculitis capitis abscedens et suffodiens

Bjellerup M, Wallengren J. Familial perifolliculitis capitis abscedens et suffodiens in two brothers successfully treated with isotretinoin. J Am Acad Dermatol 1990;23:752–753

■ pustulosis palmoplantaris with arthrosteitis

Isoda M. Familial cases of pustulosis palmoplantaris with arthrosteitis. Arch Dermatol 1992;128:699–700

■ pigmented purpuric eruption

McK 172900

Gould WM, Farber EM. A familial pigmented purpuric eruption. Dermatologica 1966; 132:400–408

■ pityriasis rubra pilaris

Gelmetti C, Schiuma AA, Cerri D, Gianotti F. Pityriasis rubra pilaris in childhood: a long-term study of 29 cases. Pediatr Dermatol 1986;3:446–451

■ psoriasis

McK 177900

Abele DC, Dobson RL, Graham JB. Heredity and psoriasis: study of a large family. Arch Dermatol 1963;88:38–47

Suarez-Almazor ME, Russell AS. The genetics of psoriasis: haplotype sharing in siblings with the disease. Arch Dermatol 1990; 126:1040–1042

■ pyoderma gangrenosum

Shands JW Jr, Flowers FP, Hill HM, Smith JO. Pyoderma gangrenosum in a kindred: precipitation by surgery or mild physical trauma. J Am Acad Dermatol 1987;16: 931–934

■ scleroderma

McK 181750

Greger RE. Familial progressive systemic scleroderma. Arch Dermatol 1975;111:81–85
Sheldon WB, Lurie DP, Maricq HR, et al. Three siblings with scleroderma (systemic sclerosis) and two with Raynaud's phenomenon from a single kindred. Arthritis Rheum 1981;24:668–676
Valenta LJ, Elias AN. Familial scleroderma in a kindred with high incidence of autoimmune disease: correlation with HLA-A1/B8 haplotype. Arch Dermatol 1987;123:1438–1440

■ striae distensae

McK 185200

McKusick VA. Transverse striae distensae in the lumbar area in father and two sons. Birth Defects 1971;7(8):260–261

■ emotional eccrine sweating

James WD, Schoomaker EB, Rodman OG. Emotional eccrine sweating: a heritable disorder. Arch Dermatol 1987;123:925–929

■ geographic tongue

McK 137400

Dawson TAJ, Pielou WD. Geographical tongue in three generations. Br J Dermatol 1967;79:678–681

■ pigmented tongue

McK 275250

Koplon BS, Hurley HJ. Prominent pigmented papillae of the tongue. Arch Dermatol 1967;95:394–396
Rao DC. Tongue pigmentation in man. Hum Hered 1970;20:8–12

■ scrotal tongue

McK 137400

Tobias N. Scrotal tongue and its inheritance. Arch Dermatol Syph 1945;52:266

■ aquagenic urticaria

McK 191850

Bonnetblanc JM, Andrieu-Pfahl F, Meraud JP, Roux J. Familial aquagenic urticaria. Dermatologica 1979;158:468–470

Index

Page numbers in *italics* refer to illustrations; numbers followed by t indicate tables.

ISBN 0-7216-3803-1

90038

9 780721 638034